Pharmaceutics for Pharmacy Students

Pharmaceutics for Pharmacy Students

Indiran Pather, DPharm
Chair and Professor
Department of Pharmaceutical Sciences
College of Pharmacy
Howard University
Washington, DC

Pharmaceutics for Pharmacy Students

1 2 3 4 5 6 7 8 9   LWI   29 28 27 26 25 24

ISBN 978-0-07-181832-2
MHID 0-07-181832-4

This book was set in Minion Pro by MPS Limited.
The editors were Michael Weitz and Peter J. Boyle.
The production supervisor was Catherine Saggese.
Project management was provided by Karan Rana, MPS Limited.

Library of Congress Cataloging-in-Publication Data

Names: Pather, Indiran, author.
Title: Pharmaceutics for the pharmacy students / Indiran Pather.
Description: New York : McGraw Hill, [2024] | Includes bibliographical
    references and index.
Identifiers: LCCN 2023048505 (print) | LCCN 2023048506 (ebook) |
    ISBN 9780071818322 (paperback) | ISBN 9780071818360 (ebook)
Subjects: MESH: Dosage Forms | Drug Delivery Systems | Drug Administration
    Routes
Classification: LCC RS403 (print) | LCC RS403 (ebook) | NLM QV 786 |
    DDC 615.1/9—dc23/eng/20231129
LC record available at https://lccn.loc.gov/2023048505
LC ebook record available at https://lccn.loc.gov/2023048506

McGraw Hill books are available at special quantity discounts to use as premiums and sales promotions, or for use in corporate training programs. To contact a representative, please visit the Contact Us pages at www.mhprofessional.com.

This book is dedicated to the memory of my late colleague, Dr. Chandra Sekhar Kolli. Chandra joined our new college of pharmacy in California in 2008 as an assistant professor. He soon impressed everyone, faculty and students alike, with his wit and charm. He was an excellent teacher and dedicated researcher. He rose through the ranks and was a full professor by the time he returned to India to be with his family after many years of illness.

He and I enjoyed many good conversations and debates, mainly about pharmaceutics, and long hours working in a new lab that we had set up and initiated. Despite the big difference in our ages, we were truly good friends. From the time he joined our college and through his long years of medical treatments, until our last few video calls to India, he was always a friend.

Chandra displayed great inner strength and fortitude through his many years of illness. This book is dedicated to his memory and his resilience in the face of adversity.

Contents

Preface

As a pharmaceutics professor of many years standing, I have assigned reading material to my students more times than I can easily count. I have often thought, when doing so, about how I would have written a chapter about one topic or the other to fit the needs of the students more closely. These casual musings have culminated, eventually, in this book.

First, a little about myself. I worked in hospital pharmacy briefly, in community pharmacy for a few years, and have taught for nearly 30 years. The teaching experience was broken by a spell of approximately 10 years in the pharmaceutical industry where I focused mainly on the development of buccal and sublingual dosage forms, leading the pharmaceutical development of two products that were marketed. During this period, I rose to the level of Director of Pharmaceutical Sciences. During much of my academic life, I served as a consultant to, or undertook university-based laboratory work for, pharmaceutical companies; and during my industry life, I served as either an industrial advisory board member or an adjunct faculty member. Thus, with respect to pharmaceutics, teaching at a university and working in the pharmaceutical industry are intertwined in my consciousness and outlook. I currently serve as Chair and Professor of Pharmaceutical Sciences at Howard University, College of Pharmacy in Washington, DC.

One aspect of the safe and appropriate utilization of medicines deals with human physiology, pathology, and pharmacology, as the theoretical basis. To me, the other important aspect is a fundamental understanding of what goes into the production of medicines and the patient-centric issues that arise from this process. Pharmacists should understand both aspects to be suitably equipped to advise their patients. In addition, drug delivery concepts should not only be of research importance, since they already affect medicines consumed daily. The pharmacist is handling these products or must offer consultation about them to patients and medical staff, and they are becoming increasingly important. Hence, a fundamental understanding of this topic is also needed. This book is written to encompass these concepts. Innovation is a cornerstone of pharmaceutical development, largely responsible for vastly improved patient care in recent years. Many research developments are worthy of mention, even in a student textbook, because they are likely to lead to products that the aspiring pharmacist will handle in the future. Mentioning them also serves the important function of giving the reader an indication of the dynamic and vibrant nature of the subject area and the forward thinking of its practitioners. In this regard, I should mention that I have 20 US patents to my credit.

In the United States, pharmacy curricula are guided by the Center for the Advancement of Pharmacy Education (CAPE) outcomes. These outcomes are amended from time to time and schools and colleges must cover them in their teaching. Obviously, educational institutions may go beyond these outcomes to some extent. In the pharmaceutics area, there is room to offer some additional material over and above what is conventionally taught. It is suggested that some basic concepts in drug delivery and pharmaceutical production may provide pharmacists with tools to be better at their job function, without detracting from the clinical focus of the degree. This book will be found useful in this regard, offering the instructor more-detailed material that they can incorporate into their teaching. In addition, graduate students may find these pages a useful starting point in their exploration of different dosage forms or routes of drug delivery.

My thanks go to my family for supporting me in this effort. I also thank my student, Amari Manigault, for helping to find some of the illustrations. My administrative assistant and laboratory technician, Mr. Otis Hooper, took some of the photographs in this book and, as always, was ever-eager to assist. Michael Weitz and Peter Boyle at McGraw-Hill Education were patient and always had constructive ideas and I thank them for this. Karan Rana, Project Manager, and his team at MPS Limited in India were super-efficient and I thank them for their work.

Indiran Pather
Washington, DC
September 2023

Introduction

1

PREVIEW

- Why another pharmaceutics textbook?
- Overview of drug development
- Unique attributes of this book
- What are mind maps and why are they useful?

The reader may well ask: why another pharmaceutics textbook? This is a valid question but before it can be answered, the development of pharmacy and the pharmaceutical sciences must be briefly discussed to provide the background for the answer to this fundamental question.

Modern pharmacy grew out of the art of the apothecary who cultivated medicinal plants and harvested the leaves, roots, seeds, or other parts as needed. These materials may have been dried, ground and incorporated into relatively simple final dosage forms. Alternatively, they may have been extracted with appropriate solvents to form tinctures and other types of extracts which were subsequently incorporated into the final liquid dosage forms. The apothecary was extremely adept at identifying medicinal plants and distinguishing them from either closely related plants that did not have medicinal properties, or from those with a similar appearance that were toxic and unsuitable for human use. The apothecary was also skilled at formulating these extracts or crushed plant tissues into pastes, poultices, and other dosage forms that are no longer used in the practice of pharmacy. In some instances, animal tissues, or extracts from such tissues, were incorporated into pharmaceutical formulations.

Some aspects of modern pharmacy began with a study of these extracts and concoctions to determine which had scientific merit, and which, did not. While, in many instances, products were found to have no effect (and some could even be harmful), others were found to be beneficial. Upon further characterization and scientific investigation of such products, a specific chemical could be identified as being responsible for the beneficial pharmacological action. In other cases, a specific chemical could not be identified, yet it could be scientifically demonstrated that the material (such as the crushed, dried root of a plant) as a whole had a beneficial effect. In other instances, a crude extract (containing a large number of chemicals from the original source) could similarly be demonstrated to be beneficial. Demonstration of a beneficial action, such as the lowering of elevated blood pressure, does not necessarily mean that the mechanism of action (ie, an exact physiological, or biochemical, series of events) is known. It may be surprising to note that this may, not infrequently, be true even with modern medicines. In addition, the extent of side effects could be demonstrated in well-developed scientific experiments. Typical side effects include the increase in blood pressure, heart rate, or other measurable parameters. The mechanisms by which such actions occur may also have been elucidated in similar experiments.

Where a specific chemical could be identified as the active ingredient eliciting the pharmacological effect, attempts were made to isolate this ingredient and to purify it. The pure active chemical compound is more potent than the crude plant extract which contains a multitude of other chemical substances. The pure chemical could also be more easily compounded into a patient-acceptable final formulation. As chemistry evolved, it became easier to determine the structure of the active chemical. This led to a consideration of structure-activity relationships. In other words, which aspects of a complex chemical structure were important for the observed pharmacological action? Which aspects detracted from this action, or led to decreased potency, or to side effects? Questions along these lines led to considerations of what would happen if the molecule were modified in specific ways. Would the addition of a specific chemical group to the molecule, for example, lead to greater potency? Modifications of the chemical structure of active molecules followed this line of reasoning, as did the synthesis of chemical analogues of the active substance. These developments were aided by the development of pharmacology as a modern science, utilizing rigorous scientific principles and well-developed test methods. The impact of a modification of a molecule could be assessed. The refinement of the concept of a receptor, and that of the interaction between a molecule and its receptor to elicit a specific pharmacological action, led to a deeper understanding of the actions of drug substances. Chemical manipulations of molecules were then seen as a way to create more potent activity at the receptor (a stronger agonist), or conversely, of blocking the receptor in a more potent manner (a stronger antagonist).

Modern molecular biologists elucidate pathways for physiological effects and also determine aberrations or defects that are present in specific disease conditions. They may also suggest points along this pathway where drugs having specific characteristics may act to bring about desirable responses. Synthetic medicinal chemists will, thereafter, attempt to create molecules with these desirable properties. Numerous variants of the basic chemical structure may be produced so that pharmacologists could perform tests to determine the effects of these different, but related, chemicals. Such tests may be performed using a cell culture model, that is, on cells grown in a laboratory, or on whole organs that are excised from animals. Those chemicals that are shown to be effective at this level may be tested on live animals. Molecules that continue to show efficacy in multiple studies (without demonstrating significant side effects) may, eventually, be the subject human clinical trials.

The pharmaceutics specialist's role is to incorporate these chemicals, or drugs, into suitable dosage forms for patients. There are many aspects to this work including pre-formulation studies during which the potential for interaction between the drug and a range of excipients is tested, prior to the actual formulation studies. Next is the actual formulation work. When a suitable formulation has been developed, it will be tested for its bioavailability attributes: what is the rate and extent of absorption of the drug from the developed dosage form? For how long will a significant amount of drug be present in the body to elicit a measurable drug response?

The concept of what constitutes an acceptable formulation has also evolved over time. Patient acceptability has been regarded as an important criterion for dosage forms for a long time. A product that is not patient acceptable will not be regularly taken, as prescribed, and this inconsistency usually affects the therapeutic outcome. One aspect of patient acceptability is the pharmaceutical elegance of the dosage form. This concept relates to the dosage form's color, shape, size, taste, mouthfeel, etc. Historically, a great deal of emphasis was placed on the elegance of the dosage form and on the fact that it should contain the correct amount of the drug. However, it soon became apparent that many elegant dosage forms that contained the correct amount of the drug, did not release the drug appropriately for adequate absorption to occur. Despite some advances, emphasis was still largely placed on the drug and its effects, up to a few decades ago. The dosage form was considered merely the vehicle to carry the drug. Notwithstanding their increasing sophistication, dosage forms continued to be of secondary importance during this time.

The modern formulator must prepare the dosage form in such a manner that the drug is released at the desired rates, in the appropriate place, for adequate absorption. This requirement is in addition to considering pharmaceutical elegance and other quality control measures. For a particular product, drug release in the small intestine may be better than in the stomach, whereas for another product, rapid initial release with a slower subsequent release may be the best profile.

Modern dosage forms do much more than provide the drug in a unit that is (a) suitable for consumption, (b) consistently produced, and (c) subject to the highest quality standards. While the release of the drug at the right location in the body and at the correct rate for optimal absorption are important, many modern dosage forms are formulated to do much more than even this. For example, many of the newer drugs do not inherently have the appropriate physico-chemical properties for good absorption, that is, their molecular structure does not confer such properties. Modern formulations, therefore, frequently contain ingredients that promote drug absorption. These include pH-adjusting substances that alter the micro-environment close to the dosage form and the absorbing membrane, or absorption enhancers that may temporarily change the nature of the biological membrane that is the barrier to drug absorption. One mechanism, by which the latter is achieved, is to make the phospholipids constituting the lipid cell membrane more "fluid," permitting drug molecules to more easily permeate the membrane. Another common mechanism is to open the tight junctions between cells, so that molecules may more easily pass through the "barrier" membrane.

Drug release from the dosage form has to occur at a predetermined rate (not too fast and not too slow) in order that absorption may occur at a desirable rate. In many instances, the fastest absorption is not necessarily the best rate. Absorption, sometimes, must also occur in a predetermined portion of the gastrointestinal tract (GIT). The chosen portion of the GIT may be one in which acidity or enzymes do not destroy the drug. After absorption, the blood (laden with the drug) flows directly to the liver. This is disadvantageous since drugs are broken down in the liver, which is considered the primary metabolizing organ (see "avoiding the first-pass effect" in the next section). Sophisticated coatings may be included to ensure that the drug is not released prematurely from the dosage form, that is, drug release should only occur when the dosage form, such as a capsule, reaches a particular portion of the GIT. In addition, many dosage forms have been developed for delivery of the drug by novel routes. Such routes of administration involve absorption of the drug through the skin, through the lining of the mouth, or that of the nasal passages, as examples. The latter is referred to as drug delivery technology.

It is suggested that in the most recent times, the dosage form has advanced so much that the drug and dosage form must be considered together as an integral unit. In some instances, the nature of the observed therapeutic effect is due to both the drug and the dosage form, and this phenomenon requires a paradigm shift. The following sections illustrate a few cases where the dosage form acts as more than a simple carrier for the drug.

TARGETING, AND MODIFICATION OF INTENSITY OR DURATION

A few examples of modification of drug action by the dosage form are given below with the clinical application.

Treatment of Periodontal Disease

The periodontal sulcus is the socket in which the tooth resides. This socket and the surrounding gum tissue may become inflamed and infected. Oral antibiotics are ineffective for treatment of this disease since a very small proportion of an administered dose actually reaches the fluid in the periodontal sulcus. The antimicrobial effect of such a drug is directly related to the drug's concentration in the periodontal fluid. While the blood concentration of a drug is frequently used as a measure of the magnitude of the drug's action, it is of no relevance in this situation. This is because the drug concentration in the periodontal sulcus is very low at the usually used oral drug doses, in spite of blood levels being reasonable. The oral route (swallowed drug) is, therefore, not an effective route of drug administration for the treatment of periodontal disease. Another way to think about this is to consider that an abnormally high dose of an antibiotic drug, such as tetracycline, has to be administered orally in order to obtain a sufficiently high concentration of the drug in the periodontal fluid. This is impractical in the sense that the required dose would produce very serious side-effects.

Drug solution directly instilled into the periodontal sulcus would rapidly flow out into the oral cavity. Even frequent re-instillation would not result in significant drug levels for long periods of time. For this reason, such a method cannot be used to treat this condition. The development of small inserts (small pieces of thin film) which are drug loaded is a useful approach. After scraping to remove plaque, the dentist inserts a thin film into the periodontal sulcus. The thin film is left in place in the sulcus where it slowly releases the contained drug. The thin film will usually be removed at the next dental visit. One example of such a product is the Periochip° which contains chlorhexidine, released over approximately 10 days. Drug concentration in the periodontal fluid reaches a high value in this period. Since, a very small amount of this drug is absorbed into the general circulation, blood levels remain low. Therefore, this form of treatment for periodontal disease does not produce systemic

side effects, even though chlorhexidine is toxic when absorbed. Repeat visits, usually at 3-month intervals, are required for the insertion of additional chips for long-term treatment.

Drug-eluting Stents

Arterial stenosis is a condition in which the lumen of the artery becomes smaller (the narrowing of a cavity is referred to as "stenosis"). This usually occurs due to the buildup of cholesterol-containing plaques, the result of high blood cholesterol levels. Blood flow through the affected artery is restricted. The formation of fibrous tissues, in conjunction with the plaques, blocks a portion of the artery (not its entire length). One approach to correcting this problem is the insertion of a stent into the artery. The stent is a mechanical metal device having the basic form of a short tube, with a mesh structure. It is placed within the artery, expands, and becomes embedded in the arterial tissue, helping to keep the artery open. This effect is extremely important in the case of the coronary artery, which supplies blood to the muscle of the heart. If this artery is blocked, the muscle tissues are deprived of essential nutrients and oxygen.

Drug-eluting stents are an improvement upon the basic stent in that the metal mesh is coated with a polymer containing a drug which is capable of reducing cell proliferation, thus preventing the growth of excess fibrous tissue. The problem of restenosis (blockage of the artery after placement of a stent) is less frequent with drug-eluting stents. After surgical insertion into the coronary artery, the stent releases the drug into the arterial tissue over a prolonged time, typically a few years. In this way, the artery is kept open and constantly supplies blood to the heart muscle for improved oxygen delivery. This enables the heart to continue functioning effectively, decreasing chest pain and reducing adverse cardiac events, such as myocardial infarction and death.

The drug that is slowly released has a local effect for a long time, as indicated, but the drug concentration in other parts of the body does not reach significant levels. Again, appropriate formulation allows the desirable effect to occur locally, without affecting other tissues of the body significantly, with the net result that a useful device (the drug and stent combination) has been created. The utility lies in the combination: the drug in a simple formulation, such as a tablet, has no utility for this indication and the stent alone is less effective. Many other drug-device combinations are currently in the research phase for various conditions.

Avoiding the First-Pass Effect

Orally administered drugs are absorbed, usually, in the small intestine. They then pass directly to the liver which is the major metabolizing organ of the body. From nature's perspective, this is an ideal situation since any chemical that is not recognized as a nutrient, and is therefore considered foreign and potentially toxic, is rapidly detoxified. From the drug delivery scientist's perspective this is not ideal: the amount of drug that enters the liver, after absorption from the gastrointestinal tract, is often far greater than the amount of drug that leaves the liver. This reduced amount of drug, eventually, goes into the general circulation and carries out its pharmacological action.

Upon passage through the cells of the gastrointestinal tract during the absorption process, drugs also become metabolized by enzymes contained within the cells. "Pre-systemic metabolism" is a term that is used to consider all metabolism that occurs prior to the drug reaching the systemic circulation. This includes metabolism by cells within the gastrointestinal tract and liver metabolism. Pre-systemic metabolism is also referred to as the first-pass effect.

In many instances, this first-pass effect can reduce the amount of drug reaching the general circulation by 50% and, in some instances, by 90% or even more. It should be borne in mind that this occurs before the drug reaches the systemic circulation and, therefore, has not had the opportunity to begin its intended action. Obviously, this is a serious limitation to the science of drug delivery. To overcome this limitation, drug delivery scientists have developed alternate routes of administration. Examples include delivery of the drug across the lining (or the mucosa) of the mouth, or that of the nose, or through the skin. The drug delivered via these routes does not go directly to the liver, and hence, a significantly larger portion of the absorbed drug reaches the systemic circulation. Once in the systemic circulation the drug will be diluted in a large volume of blood. It should be noted that some of the blood from the systemic circulation will flow to the liver and its drug content will be subject to metabolism. However, only a small portion of the blood flows through the liver at any given moment and its drug concentration is low. The drug contained in this small volume of blood will be subjected to liver metabolism. Hence, these alternate delivery routes avoid gut and liver first-pass metabolism and are more effective in getting a large amount of drug into the systemic circulation.

In most instances, the drug to be delivered via an alternate route does not naturally permeate the tissues encountered. Therefore, absorption via these routes would be very limited after administration of a simple formulation, such as a solution. Special methods need to be developed in order to obtain effective penetration of the drug through these tissues, and to do so in a manner that is safe to the patient. The development of one pharmaceutical product, for absorption by one of the alternative routes, may take a team of scientists several years to develop. The FDA has regulatory oversight and will not approve a product unless demonstrated to be safe and efficacious.

Circadian Rhythm and Timing of Drug Action

Many body functions, such as the production of hormones, or of enzymes, vary with the time of day. This is a natural rhythm of the body which has been built into our genetic system over millennia. Many attributes of the body, such as blood pressure, also vary with the time of day. This variation in body function with the time of day is referred to as the circadian rhythm. Analogously, malfunctions of the body may also follow this rhythm or cycle, corresponding approximately with the natural cycle of secretion of hormones, enzymes, and other physiological chemicals. Naturally, it may be desirable to control drug release, from a device or dosage form, to follow this rhythm so that the drug is available in larger quantities when most needed. Conversely, very small amounts are released when less is needed. Dosage

forms to accommodate the circadian rhythm are special formulations which are discussed in the section "Chronotherapeutics" in Chapter 11, Modified-Release Oral Dosage Forms.

Recap Questions

1. Do you think chlorhexidine mouthwash, used daily, will work as well as a chlorhexidine chip inserted into the periodontal sulcus?
2. Do you think a drug-eluting stent will be more effective at counteracting coronary artery disease than the same drug administered intravenously into the patient's arm daily?
3. What is the major function of the liver and what advantage is gained by delivering a drug in such a way that its absorption bypasses the liver?
4. In which way is the circadian rhythm a protective physiological function?

CHANGING DRUG EFFECT OR FUNCTION

The knowledge of the formulation scientist has been used for some time to improve the intensity of a specific, known drug action; to prolong that action; or to direct the action to a specific organ or part of the body. The examples in the previous section illustrate these effects. What is relatively new, and exciting, is the fact that formulation science may be used to obtain a different end result, or therapeutic effect, from the same drug. The type of formulation, the rate at which it releases the drug, the extent to which the formulation aids drug absorption, and the targeting of the drug (to a particular organ) may all be manipulated. The summation of the effects of these changes could be directed to obtaining a different therapeutic response. This is illustrated in the following examples.

Fentanyl

Fentanyl was developed as an anesthetic in the 1960s. Given by intravenous injection, it rapidly and smoothly induces anesthesia. For surgical procedures of short duration, it may be used as the only anesthetic. When anesthesia is required for a longer duration, another anesthetic may be administered after induction by fentanyl. For these indications, fentanyl has been well established for many years. In the 1990s, the Duragesic patch was developed to provide fentanyl for relief of pain which is severe, and of prolonged duration. It is not intended for pain that is likely to be of short duration, for example, postoperative pain. Pain experienced by cancer patients may be treated with this patch. One patch gives relief for 72 hours.

A cancer patient whose pain is well controlled by long-acting medication such as the Duragesic patch may, nevertheless, experience excruciating pain of short duration, for example,

15 to 30 minutes. This may occur several times a day. This pain is sometimes associated with events such as moving the patient (for medical procedures, for example) and sometimes pain occurs for reasons that are not clear. It is undesirable to increase the dose of the long-acting pain medication since the patient would be under the influence of this higher dose throughout the day, whereas the extreme pain only occurs for a short duration (several times a day). What is needed, for this situation, is a fast-acting, and potent, pain medication that can provide relief of the pain rapidly. When the pain subsides, ideally, the effect of the medication should taper off. This medication would be administered at the time the pain is experienced and would be given in addition to the long-acting pain medication which is routinely administered to the patient. Actiq, and later Fentora, were developed to provide relief of breakthrough cancer pain. They are administered in low doses through the lining (mucosa) of the mouth.

The fentanyl contained in Atiq and Fentora provides the required rapid relief of symptoms in a dosage form that is short-acting so that the patient does not experience the side effects of the drug for a prolonged time. It should be borne in mind that a potent drug is needed for the intense pain and that, as a consequence, the side effects may also be severe. The fentanyl from Actiq and Fentora are supplemental to that from the Duragesic patch, or to other long-acting medication. The success of Actiq and Fentora has spurred the development of other low-dose, quick-acting fentanyl medications for breakthrough cancer pain and these are discussed in more detail in Chapter 20, Buccal and Sublingual Drug Delivery.

From the above description, it can be seen that the drug, fentanyl, may be used as an anesthetic when delivered by intravenous injection, as a long-acting analgesic (72 hours) when delivered by a transdermal patch and as a rapidly-acting pain reliever of short duration (approximately 15–30 minutes) when delivered by an oral mucosal delivery system. The intravenous injection provides a rapid anesthetic effect by providing the drug directly into the venous system; the transdermal formulation provides slow absorption since the drug must first be released by the patch and then slowly absorbed through the skin. On the other hand, the oral mucosal delivery system provides delivery that is rapid but slower than the intravenous injection. The injection is low dose, the oral mucosal delivery system has an intermediate dose and the patch is relatively high dose. Thus, fentanyl can have very different effects depending on the dose and the delivery system that is used.

Naloxone

Opioids are potent drugs used in very small doses, frequently for the relief of pain. They fall into the category of drugs referred to as narcotic analgesics. Apart from their analgesic effect, they have sedative effects as well as being euphoric. The latter is the main reason for the development of dependence and addiction. The major problem with these drugs, especially in high doses, is respiratory depression. The drug blocks the respiratory center in the brain and, if not treated, the patient will die. In mild cases of respiratory depression, the subject can be reminded to take deep breaths. The real danger is in severely overdosed patients who are not conscious: respiration can cease, resulting in death. Opioids also cause severe constipation.

Naloxone is a drug that blocks opioid receptors and is used to reduce the respiratory depression associated with opioid use. For example, when fentanyl is used to induce anesthesia, naloxone is administered toward the end of the surgery to reverse the effects of fentanyl and to reduce respiratory depression. For this purpose, naloxone must cross the blood brain barrier to reach the respiratory center. Injectable naloxone can do so rapidly and, thereby, very quickly reverses respiratory depression. Similarly, naloxone can be used to reduce respiratory depression in non-surgical patients who have overdosed on an opioid. In this context, a naloxone injection or inhalation may be life-saving.

Obviously, if a patient was experiencing pain (for which purpose the opioid was prescribed in the first place), the administration of naloxone would also tend to block the pain relieving effect of the drug. In addicts, the decrease in pain relief is less important; the reversal of respiratory depression is of the greatest importance and, as mentioned, it could save the patient's life. If the addiction arose from a legitimate use of the opioid to relieve pain, the patient may no longer be experiencing pain but is now addicted to the drug. In many instances, however, the addiction arises from the use of street drugs rather than prescription pain relievers.

With the above brief introduction to the use of naloxone, let us consider a specialized formulation of this drug. The constipating side effect of naloxone has already been mentioned. For patients who experience severe pain for a prolonged time and who obtain relief by using an opioid, continued administration of the drug is required for a significant length of time. A cancer patient may fall into the category that requires chronic opioid drug administration for control of their pain. (This is in contrast to surgical patients, eg, who may need potent drugs for pain relief for only a few days, before they can be changed to less potent, non-narcotics for relief of lower intensity pain.) While long-term administration of opioids offers relief of chronic pain, the prolonged constipation that the patient experiences will be very uncomfortable. Naloxone will relieve constipation but conventional formulations of this drug will also inhibit pain relief, negating the reason that the drug was used in the first place.

A new formulation of naloxone, Movantik® (Astra Zeneca LP), is administered in a special formulation for local action in the colon only. It is a reaction product of polyethylene glycol (PEG) and naloxone, called noloxegol, while the reaction is referred to as "PEGylation." Colonic delivery requires the incorporation of special formulation ingredients so that the dosage form does not release the drug in the stomach or small intestine. When released in the colon, it blocks the mu opioid receptors in this organ and reduces the constipating effect of the opioid. Since drug absorption into the general circulation is minimal, the amount that crosses the blood brain barrier is negligible and, therefore, naloxone from this formulation does not block the pain relieving effect of the opioid. From the above, it can be seen that by PEGylating the drug, naloxone may be used to treat the constipating effects of opioids with practically no central effect. The desirable properties of the opioid, pain relief, may continue to be experienced without the undesirable side effect.

Recap Questions

1. Do you think fentanyl is slowly or rapidly absorbed from the buccal area after administration of a Fentora tablet?

2. Do you think fentanyl is slowly or rapidly absorbed through the skin after application of a Duragesic patch?

3. Why does the naloxone in Movantik not reduce the pain-relieving effect of the opioid?

SOPHISTICATION AND QUALITY CONTROL

The above hints at the increasing sophistication of pharmaceutical dosage forms; the complexity of pharmaceutical manufacturing science has increased enormously over the last few decades and is continuing to develop. To match this increasing sophistication and complexity, there has, of necessity, been an improvement in the finesse of quality control departments. What impacts does this have on the pharmacist?

In the first instance, instructions for the correct utilization of medication have become far more complex than they were even 10 years ago. The pharmacist has an increasing role to ensure that patients follow these instructions carefully and use their medication appropriately. A transdermal formulation, for example, usually involves removal of the backing strip and the correct placement of the formulation onto the correct part of the body. More complex formulations of this type may involve some degree of assembly of the components, for example, placement of the medication pad onto a backing pad after removal of the protective liner. It is imperative that the components be correctly assembled before application to the skin to ensure appropriate delivery of the medication.

Drugs for delivery through the lining of the mouth may also carry special instructions. One such formulation requires that the tablet be placed above the premolar tooth, between the gum and cheek. The patient should be instructed not to eat or drink while the dosage form is in place. Another oral mucosal dosage form, Actiq, has the appearance of a lollipop. The candy portion has to be rubbed against the lining of the cheek, then twirled and rubbed against the lining of the other cheek. The dosage form, which dissolves as it is rubbed against the cheek, must be completely consumed within 15 minutes. Thus, the patient or caregiver must adjust the rate of application to comply with this time requirement. Longer, or shorter, administration times may not provide the correct blood levels. Not only should the pharmacist herself understand these instructions in order to be able to correctly convey them, but there is a need to understand why these

requirements are expected. In the case of Actiq, the rate of administration is linked with the rate at which the drug can be absorbed through the mucosa. If the application rate is too fast, the drug released from the dosage form is swallowed with the saliva. This results in a loss of drug from the intended primary absorption site.

It is also important for the pharmacist to understand that Fentora, while it resembles a conventional tablet, is not rapidly disintegrating; that the lack of significant disintegration action comes about through omission of the disintegrant that conventional tablets contain. Further, that the hardness of the tablet was selected to give the optimal time in the mouth before the tablet slowly disintegrates, allowing the drug to dissolve. Information, such as this, may be useful to answer questions that patients might have.

In many instances, it is important for the pharmacist to have some knowledge of pharmaceutical formulation and manufacturing methods. For example, when can a transdermal patch be safely cut? In general, it may not be advisable to cut transdermal patches. However, patches are made in a limited number of strengths. As a practical matter, therefore, it becomes necessary to cut a patch to obtain the correct dose for a particular patient. Some types of patches, because of the way they are manufactured, should not be cut. These so-called reservoir patches would have the sustained-release mechanism destroyed if cut and would not be safe to use. Matrix patches, on the other hand, may be cut.

In other instances, some knowledge of pharmaceutical manufacturing operations and quality control may allow the pharmacist to answer patient questions in a very informed manner. For example, a person with mathematical knowledge once asked how one would know whether every tablet of a low dose formulation (eg, 0.1 mg) contained its drug load. Is it not probable that some tablets contained no drug while others contained 0.2 mg? The questioner had knowledge of probability theory and to provide an informed answer, one had to have some knowledge of tablet manufacture and quality control procedures.

GENERIC DRUGS

The advent of generic drugs and their increasing popularity requires that, first, the pharmacist be able to answer questions regarding the comparability of generics, as a group, to brand-name products; and, second, about the comparison of two generic products. These are complex questions and the simplistic answer that both were approved by the FDA is not sufficient at the present time. To be in a position to answer these questions adequately, one must have some understanding of manufacturing processes and quality control. This question is discussed in detail in Chapter 17, Introduction to Bioavailability.

The pharmacist may also find himself on the formulary committee at a large hospital. One task of the committee could, conceivably, be to select a generic formulation from three or four competitive brands, with the intention that the hospital would carry one generic only. By so doing, the hospital may obtain an economic advantage by purchasing a high volume from one manufacturer. A good decision in this regard would not be to simply select the brand that offers the lowest pricing. An ability to evaluate the quality of the product from company data would be useful. What is the probability that the initial high quality of the generic from this manufacturer would be maintained consistently over several batches? To answer this question well requires knowledge of pharmaceutical formulation and manufacturing and an ability to evaluate the quality over several batches.

COMPOUNDING

Traditionally, compounding involved the extemporaneous preparation of medication for one patient. This medication was supplied to that patient, or the caregiver, at the compounding pharmacy. In recent years, the compounding pharmacy has, frequently, not supplied the product directly to the patient but, instead, provided several units, for example, 100-g containers of compounded medicinal cream to a doctor's office which, in turn, supplied the product to the patient. Compounding pharmacies are also able to provide clinical supplies for phase one clinical trials. This may involve many units of medication, or a few hundred tablets or capsules.

The above describes the supply of larger quantities of product than was the case in traditional compounding pharmacies. Regulations were relaxed to allow the preparation of a relatively small number of units, as described above. The regulatory environment was not intended for the pharmacist to manufacture hundreds of thousands of units and thus usurp the role of the pharmaceutical manufacturer. However, it has come to the notice of the FDA that significantly larger quantities, than intended by FDA regulation, were being produced by some compounding pharmacies. In addition, in recent times, there were several incidents of substandard products being prepared with consequently negative effects on the patient. Some of these involved sterile products, which were subsequently found not to be sterile. Due to these circumstances, the FDA has developed new guidance documents for pharmacy. The controls and oversights that are now required are far more rigorous than in the past. In this situation, compounding records and other control measures begin to resemble the batch manufacturing records and quality control of manufacturers. A basic understanding and some knowledge of pharmaceutical manufacturing processes and quality control would place the pharmacist in a good position to understand the rigorous preparation methods and control measures that are required for compounding.

NOW TO ANSWER THE QUESTION ...

In the light of recent developments in pharmaceutics, the observed therapeutic effect in many complex, modern dosage forms is brought about by the interplay of the drug and its dosage form. The effect of the dosage form may be to target drug action to a specific organ or tissue (including delivery to a tissue in which drug levels would be insignificant with conventional dosage forms); modification of the intensity and duration of drug effects; or changing the nature of the therapeutic effect compared to that obtained with a conventional dosage form.

Because the drug effect is so intimately related to the dosage form, it becomes imperative that the pharmacist understand the principles underlying dosage form formulation and manufacturing and, to some extent, the way in which their quality is tested. This approach will provide an appreciation of the impact of scientific principles, and formulation and manufacturing conditions, on the dosage form and its effects on the human body.

Modern dosage forms are extremely sophisticated as are the quality control systems utilized to ensure consistent products. The pharmacist who works with these products, and who explains their use to patients and medical staff, should have a basic understanding of formulation development, manufacturing processes, and aspects of pharmaceutical quality control to be able to do this well. In addition, the widespread use of generics makes it necessary that the pharmacist be able to compare generics, in general, with the innovator (original) products. Additionally, the pharmacist should be able to compare two generic products of the same drug. The latter, for example, may be important when a large institution prefers to stock one generic formulation of a particular drug.

The increasing control of compounding activities by the FDA and other bodies necessitates a more controlled functioning of a compounding pharmacy, with more rigid control systems and documentation in place. This book intends to present a more thorough discussion of manufacturing systems for pharmaceuticals, than is presently the case. While this is important for the reasons mentioned above, it would also be useful for understanding the efficient conduct of a compounding pharmacy, since the underlying principles are similar.

Drug delivery science has developed enormously in the last few decades. This science involves the following aspects: controlling drug release in terms of rate and, in many instances, the part of the body (organ) where drug release occurs; absorption rate(s) which may differ at different time points; and maintaining a blood drug concentration-time profile that is specific to the needs of patients for the drug in question when it is used to treat a specific disease. Whereas this was a research area, there are now several marketed products embodying this science and, hence, there is a need for pharmacists to have some knowledge and awareness of this area of pharmaceutical endeavor and development. The presentation of drug delivery science in Pharmaceutics textbooks has not been consistent. This book aims to provide a brief encapsulation of the science which will give the pharmacist a basic understanding of the drug delivery products she will encounter, and in respect of which, she may be asked questions.

The author hopes to express these ideas in relatively straightforward language that is readable to the student. The intention is to provide a textbook that is not unduly long, and which is user-friendly. Readability and user-friendliness are important characteristics for the modern student who depends, to a greater extent, on active learning in the classroom than did the student of a decade ago. There are many active learning techniques that have been described in the scholarship of teaching and learning. These techniques often result in a deeper understanding of the taught materials but consume time in the limited lecture period. Hence, with liberal use of active learning strategies, the instructor may not be able to discuss every aspect of a topic in the classroom session. This necessitates giving students the opportunity to engage in self-study of some aspects of a topic. Alternately, the instructor may provide the broad strokes and permit the student to read the details.

As an experienced teacher of Pharmaceutics, the author has used active learning techniques and has faced the dilemma of what to cover in class and which aspects of a topic can be assigned as self-study. The problem he faced was that students said the prescribed textbooks were not easy to read. This book attempts to overcome that problem while, at the same time, providing a modern perspective on Pharmaceutics.

WHAT THIS BOOK IS NOT ABOUT

The book is not intended to make the reader fully capable of researching and manufacturing pharmaceutical products. For this, most often, a doctoral degree in the pharmaceutical sciences is required. Instead, the book attempts to provide relevant information so that the pharmacist is able to discuss modern dosage forms and to answer questions from patients. Examples of such questions are sprinkled liberally throughout the text. Where issues that relate to the dosage form are encountered in pharmaceutical practice, it may become necessary to discuss these with the manufacturing company or its representative. The pharmacist should have sufficient knowledge and understanding of the subject matter (including aspects of manufacturing science and technology) to present such questions in a clear fashion.

MIND MAPS

Mind maps are a useful tool to present complex, and possibly confusing, ideas in an easy-to-understand diagram (Mind Map 1-1). Each concept is represented by a few words enclosed in a box of a particular shape. This makes for a representation that is more readily grasped by the mind. Ideas are depicted stemming from a central idea, and with layers of ideas stemming from their predecessors. It is said that the representation of ideas in lines of text is not the easiest way to assimilate concepts. This book makes liberal use of mind maps, and the student is encouraged to draw his or her own mind maps which creates an opportunity for them to handle and work with the information. This helps the student to make the knowledge their own. More information on mind maps can be obtained from numerous websites.

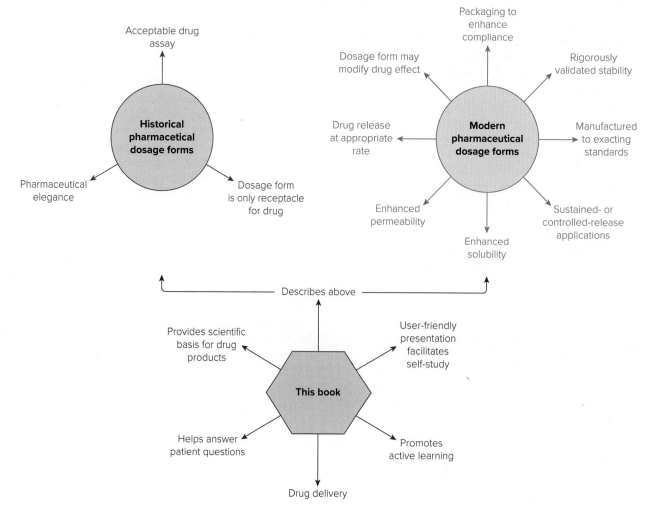

MIND MAP 1-1 Summary of Book Objectives (Revised)

Recap Questions

1. The increasing complexity of dosage forms is something that the research scientist in the pharmaceutical industry must contend with, it is not important to a community pharmacist. Do you agree or disagree with this statement? Support your answer with appropriate information.

2. The time taken to consume an Actiq unit relates to .... (fill in the blank).

3. A mind map is a pictorial representation of many facts and is likely to help with understanding and recollection. Is this statement true or false?

What do you think?

1. Developments in pharmaceutics necessitate a paradigm shift. Do you agree or disagree with this statement? Give reasons for your answer.

2. Name two developments in pharmaceutics, mentioned in this chapter, that you think will have the most far-reaching consequences. Motivate your answer.

3. Are mind maps worth the time it takes to draw them? Explain your answer.

SUMMARY POINTS

- The book intends to introduce the reader to the complexities of modern pharmaceutical products.
- A basic understanding of pharmaceutical processes will foster a better understanding of the functioning of the dosage form.
- The book provides a basis for answering patient questions and provides a good pharmaceutical background.
- The knowledge provided may facilitate some aspects of compounding pharmacy but does not supplant the training needed to operate such a facility.

Dosage Forms and Routes of Drug Administration

2

PREVIEW

- Why are dosage forms needed?
- Extended functions of dosage forms
- What is a "route of drug administration"?
- Why are different routes of drug administration needed?
- What is the ideal in drug delivery and why is this ideal not easy to achieve?
- Overview of common routes of drug administration

INTRODUCTION

Chapter 1 deals with the approach that this book takes to the study of pharmaceutics. It makes the point that the drug and its dosage form must be considered together. The dosage form may significantly alter the impact of the drug and, in certain instances, actually change the nature of the observed pharmacological response. Several examples were given to explain the expanded role of the dosage form, illustrating the modified effects obtained as a consequence of the drug being placed within specialized dosage forms. This chapter starts off with a discussion of dosage forms to illustrate why we need them from a practical point of view, even when they do not materially affect the pharmacological response. It then briefly describes the different routes of drug administration. These two topics serve as the prelude to a book that deals largely with dosage forms and routes of drug administration (Mind Map 2-1).

With respect to dosage forms, the following aspects are important:

1. What they are
2. Why we need them
3. What goes into them (ingredients)
4. How they are made
5. How they are tested
6. What effect they have on the body (biological system)
7. How the body affects them
8. Their stability
9. The advantages and disadvantages of each type
10. How to choose from the different types of dosage forms, of the same drug, for a particular patient

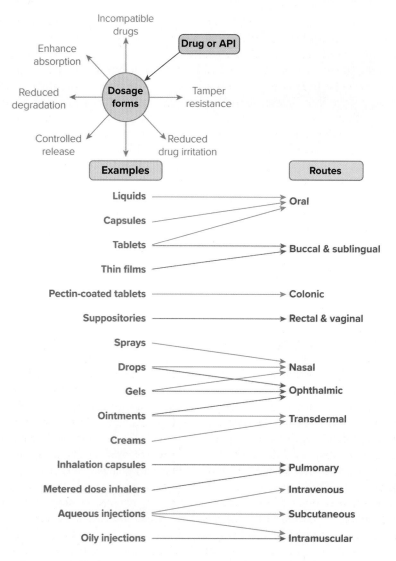

MIND MAP 2-1 Some Dosage Forms and Their Most Important Routes of Administration

In addition, the mechanisms of drug release from the dosage form are important, as are the mechanisms and physiological factors that affect its absorption. A general approach adopted in this book is to outline the principles and give a few examples for illustrative purposes. Given that the book takes this approach, it is useful to start with a very basic concept: *what are dosage forms and why do we need them?*

NEED FOR DOSAGE FORMS

Dosage forms are the physical unit or form in which drugs, or active pharmaceutical ingredients (API), are supplied to the patient. Tablets, capsules, suppositories, injections, and lozenges are dosage forms in common use at the present time. Besides the active ingredient, the dosage form also contains inactive ingredients, or excipients, which help to create the dosage form, or confer specialized attributes to the dosage form. Over time, older dosage forms cease to be popular and are discontinued. They may be superseded by more effective dosage forms. The pill was a dosage form made from licorice which was rolled out as a thin long cylinder, then cut into shorter pieces and finally formed into the round or ovoid pill shape. This dosage form is no longer in use. What is commonly called a "pill" or a "sugar-coated pill" in the lay press is actually a tablet and a coated tablet, respectively.

Conversely, new or novel dosage forms are the subject of research and development and, from time to time, one reaches the marketplace. New dosage forms are often created to follow a therapeutic need. For example, orally disintegrating tablets (ODT) are pleasant tasting, and disintegrate in the mouth. The residue can then be swallowed without the need for water to aid consumption. This fills a therapeutic need for patients who have difficulty swallowing. In addition, it is very practical for busy people who can take the medication at any time or place without stopping activities. For example, someone in a meeting or driving a car can take an ODT with minimal interference to their activity.

The thin film is a relatively new dosage form consisting of a very thin polymer layer which contains a drug. Typically, this is placed under the tongue or adjacent to the inner cheek for absorption of the drug through the mucosa (lining membrane) of the oral cavity. Alternately, the thin film can be placed on the tongue for rapid disintegration, followed by swallowing of the saliva and the components of the thin film. In the latter case, the drug is absorbed through the GIT in the conventional way and the dosage form is used for patient convenience only. This is an example of an evolving dosage form. Thin films are described in Chapter 20, Buccal and Sublingual Drug Delivery. New research is also indicating the utility of the thin film for vaginal drug delivery and this is mentioned in Chapter 24, Rectal and Vaginal Drug Delivery.

The number of different dosage forms available to the consumer is limited only by the ingenuity of the formulation scientist and new dosage forms appear periodically. Some dosage forms may also be created for novelty or to distinguish the company in the marketplace. From the above, it is clear that a comprehensive list of dosage forms, assuming it is possible to produce one, may be soon outdated. A list of the more important dosage forms is given in Table 2-1.

To understand the need for dosage forms, consider how the patient would be forced to take the drug in the absence of dosage forms. For example, how would a powdered drug be taken? In many instances, taking the drug powder alone would be very difficult, or practically impossible. For example, if the dose of the drug is very small, such as 1 mg or less, it would be very difficult to measure, and to administer, an accurate dose. Larger amounts of powder may be easier to measure but the taste and palatability of the powder would deter regular consumption of the medication. In the case of the very small dose, it would also be very difficult to handle the extremely small volume of powder. Similarly, it would be very difficult for the patient to measure, and to handle, very small volumes of liquid drugs (microliter quantities). The simplest method to overcome the size limitations of small doses is to incorporate the drug in a diluent, which could take the form of a powdered material or a liquid. In a blend of a powdered drug with lactose (as an example), the lactose serves the function of the diluent, whereas water may serve as the diluent in a suspension or solution dosage form. Water may also serve as the diluent for a liquid drug. The diluent, as the name implies, dilutes the potent drug by incorporating it in an inert powder or liquid, with mixing to distribute evenly. In this instance, the diluent may be considered as the vehicle in which to present the drug.

Starting with an initially well-dispersed drug mixture, it is important that the drug does not separate from its diluent. Suppose a mixture of a potent powdered drug with other powders can be verified, by chemical analysis, to contain an accurate concentration of the drug. At some point in time, this well-mixed powder may not contain an even distribution of the drug. This phenomenon may be due to separation, or segregation, of the drug particles, a problem which is described more fully in Chapter 5, Pharmaceutical Powders. Contrary to this situation, the constituents of a tablet or capsule formulation, for example, are contained within the dosing unit with practically no possibility for altering the drug concentration in the tablet or capsule by physical separation. The notable exceptions are volatile drugs that may vaporize out of tablets.

Manufacturing is also done using rigorously developed written methods for the consistent production, and also the testing,

of dosage forms. This ensures that each unit from a production batch contains an accurate amount of the drug. Low-dose tablets (eg, those containing 1 mg of drug in a tablet weighing 150 mg) generally contain close to 1 mg of drug in every tablet of a batch, even when the batch contains as many as 1 million tablets, or even more. Wide variations in drug content, such as 0.5 mg to 1.5 mg, in the above example, are not expected in modern dosage forms. On the other hand, suppose the patient had been provided with a container of a potent drug blended with a diluent, and was instructed to take one teaspoonful of this mixture each day. Wide swings in the amount of drug consumed could be anticipated, even when the patient manages the dose as accurately as is possible with a teaspoon. Such variation may be due to segregation of the drug particles within the container upon handling and transport.

The above description is not intended to imply that a slow decrease in drug content, due to degradation, does not occur in manufactured products over an extended period. However, over the shelf life of a drug product, typically two years, the drug content of each tablet or capsule remains within acceptable, predetermined limits in spite of slow degradation. Many drug powders if dispensed in a container for the patient to measure out the required dose, as needed, will reveal significant degradation over time, making the product unacceptable to use. Hence, the dosage form, in many instances, contributes to the stability of the contained drug. Some pharmaceutical products, which embody the described desirable characteristics are given below, by way of example. The dosage form contributes to the stability of the drug in these instances.

Fentora® (fentanyl citrate) is a potent opioid that is available in accurately controlled doses of 100 μg (0.1 mg) or 200 μg (0.2 mg) per tablet. These are very small doses and the manufacturer performs rigorous testing to show that the actual amount of drug in the tablets is close to the *theoretical* dose stated on the label. This testing is done before the product is released for sale. (Some of the tests that are typically conducted on tablets are discussed in Chapter 9, Tablets.)

Lanoxin® tablets are another example of a very low-dose tablet formulation. The tablets contain as little as 0.125-mg digoxin per tablet. Taking this tablet provides a far more accurate dose of the drug compared to the patient taking digitalis leaf (the plant material from which the active ingredient is obtained). The difference in accuracy of the dose is due, firstly, to the fact that plant materials may vary in their drug content, depending on soil conditions, the geographical region where the plant was grown, the condition of the soil, and the amount of rain experienced that season, etc. In addition, in most situations, it would be difficult for the patient to accurately measure the required amount of plant material. Similarly, a reserpine tablet has a far more accurate dose than would be the case if the patient attempted to measure a small quantity of reserpine powder for consumption.

Nitroglycerin is a highly volatile chemical used in low doses. However, stabilized nitroglycerin tablets (eg, 0.4 mg) have a fair shelf life when stored under the proper conditions. Similarly, Isordil® tablets contain a stable dose (eg, 5 mg) of isosorbide dinitrate, if the tablets are properly stored. This includes storage at room temperature, away from light and moisture. Thus,

TABLE 2-1	Routes of Drug Administration with the Corresponding Dosage Forms*		
ROUTE	**DOSAGE FORMS**	**ROUTE**	**DOSAGE FORMS**
Oral	Syrups Elixirs Emulsions Tablets Orally disintegrating tablet Floating tablets Rapidly disintegrating films Sustained-release tablets Enteric-coated tablets Capsules Enteric-coated capsules Sustained-release capsules Softgels	Nasal	Creams Ointments Gels Drops Sprays Metered-dose sprays Nasal metered-dose aerosols (mostly discontinued)
Oral Mucosal	Tablets Solutions Thin films Discs Wafers Gels Creams Ointments Pastes	Pulmonary	Metered-dose inhalers Dry powder inhalers Capsules for dry powder inhalation Nebulized solutions
Colonic	Specially coated (eg, pectin) tablets Capsules containing specially coated beads Rectal foams	Ocular	Drops Suspensions Gels Topical devices Inserts Intraocular injections
Rectal	Creams Ointments Gels Suppositories Liquid suppositories Aerosol foams Enemas	Intravenous	Aqueous solutions
Vaginal	Creams Ointments Gels Suppositories Softgels (ovules) Vaginal tablets Liquids	Intra muscular	Aqueous solutions Oily solutions Suspensions (oily and aqueous)
Topical	Creams Ointments Gels Transdermal patches Lotions	Sub cutaneous	Aqueous solutions Aqueous suspensions Implants
Otic	Aqueous drops Oily drops	Intradermal	Aqueous solutions

*This is not a comprehensive list.

in these cases, the formulation of nitroglycerin powder into a pharmaceutical product provides a great deal of stability to a drug that is inherently unstable.

While the dosage form provides an enhanced stability to the drug in many instances, it is important that the dosage form, itself, is stable. Examples of instability of the dosage form include a capsule shell that degrades, or a tablet that softens to an extent that makes it difficult to handle. Softening of the tablet could, also, change the delivery rate of the drug. Modern dosage form research and development incorporates rigorous testing to detect such changes and develops mechanisms to overcome them.

From the above, it can be seen that one goal of the preparation of dosage forms is *to provide an accurate amount, or dose, of the drug in a physical entity or unit that is convenient to administer, that provides stability to the drug, and in which the entity, itself, is stable.* While the above characteristics are vitally important, modern dosage forms provide several additional benefits as the following examples indicate:

Separate Incompatible Drugs

The dosage form may contain two incompatible drugs that are separated in such a way as not to interact with each other. For example, the drugs may be present in separate layers of a tablet. In some instances, this degree of separation is sufficient to prevent reaction between the two drug components. In other instances, a third layer containing no drug (a placebo layer) is needed in order to maintain complete separation and non-reactivity of the two drugs. In other cases, each drug may be incorporated into different individual units (such as granules), where numerous such granules comprise the dosage form. The granules of one, or both, drugs are coated to maintain separation of the reactive components. Such coated granules may be contained within a capsule (where each granule remains a separate entity) or compressed into a tablet, where the individual granule is no longer a separate entity. Nevertheless, the coating material still separates the different active components. These are some of the methods by which the dosage form prevents incompatible drugs from reacting with one another. Obviously, there are many instances where two drugs, by their chemical nature, do not react with each other and such components may simply be compressed together, or otherwise combined, into one dosage form with no interventions to prevent their reaction.

In a novel invention,[1] two incompatible drugs, tramadol and diclofenac were combined into one dosage form. Tramadol is a potent pain reliever and diclofenac is a non-steroidal anti-inflammatory drug (NSAID). The World Health Organization (WHO) claims that the combination of opioid analgesic and NSAID is a potent pain reliever and that the dose of opioid may be reduced if the combination is used. However, tramadol and diclofenac react chemically to form a poorly soluble complex. Thus, in a conventional dosage form, such as a tablet, the drugs would react. Upon consumption, absorption of the drugs would be reduced due to the slow dissolution of the drugs from this complex. Most drugs must be in solution in order to be absorbed. By incorporating these drugs in separate layers of a tablet, with at least one placebo layer in between the drug layers, an effective combination product is produced.

Many dietary supplements claim the separation of incompatible ingredients in multiple-layered tablets. Since the layers are often colored differently, the tablet looks attractive. It is often not clear if these supplements and herbal products were produced as layered tablets mainly for aesthetic reasons. Herbal products may also be presented as bi-layered tablets where one layer is for rapid release of the drug, while the other is a sustained-release layer. Again, they may be colored differently, possibly for marketing appeal. Prescription drug products may also consist of bi-layered tablets where each layer has a different release rate. Thus, this type of product is formulated for various purposes, not only the prevention of instability.

Provide a Mechanism to Enhance the Absorption of Poorly Absorbed Drugs

Cyclosporine has been used for many years to counteract rejection in transplant patients. The old formulation, Sandimmune®, was replaced several years ago by a microemulsion formulation, Neoral®, which shows much-improved absorption and better control of rejection. The nature of the microemulsion allows the drug to be absorbed to a much greater extent. When Griseofulvin tablets were reformulated many years ago, micronized drug particles were utilized, and this increased absorption so greatly that the dose had to be reduced to 500 mg, the present dose for adults. Although Griseofulvin is not used much at the present time, due to the advent of newer drugs, this example is still interesting because it shows that grinding of the drug to a micrometer particle size allowed the use of a lower dose. Hence, the type of formulation is important. In some instances, big differences in the amount of drug absorbed, or of side effects, can be seen with different formulations of the same drug.

While the above, "historical" examples are well known, there are also newer instances where the reduction in dose has been possible as a result of better drug delivery systems. When Actiq (the fentanyl "lollipop") was developed, it was seen as an innovation in the treatment of breakthrough cancer pain. The dosing units were produced in a range of different strengths ranging from 200 μg to 1600 μg. Fentora is a newer buccal/sublingual tablet formulation which utilizes half the dose, that is, 100-μg Fentora is equivalent to 200-μg Actiq.

Reduce Degradation in Biological Fluids

A dosage form may be constructed so as to reduce a specific drug's natural tendency to be degraded in a biological fluid. All enteric-coated tablets and capsules protect sensitive drugs from the highly acidic conditions of the stomach. In the less acidic conditions of the small intestine, the coating dissolves to release the drug for absorption. Nexium® (esomeprazole), also known as "the purple pill," is such an example. Enteric coating is discussed in Chapter 9, Tablets.

The above examples illustrate how it may be possible to allow the passage of a dosage form through a part of the body that degrades the drug, without significant degradation occurring. An alternate approach would be to introduce the drug into the body by another route in which the harsh, drug-degrading conditions are not present. For example, a drug that is degraded in the stomach may be delivered through the buccal membrane of the mouth. The oral cavity does not have the strongly acidic conditions of the stomach and, hence, the drug is not degraded. Some drug-containing saliva may be swallowed unintentionally and a portion of this drug is degraded in the stomach. This inadvertent loss is relatively small. It is important to bear in mind that all acid-sensitive drugs cannot simply be administered via the buccal mucosa to avoid drug degradation. The drug may not, naturally, permeate the biological membrane of the oral cavity and a buccal tablet will not necessarily deliver the drug adequately via this route. In general, special formulation approaches are utilized to enhance drug absorption and these methods may have varying degrees of success. Alternately, routes other than the buccal may be selected to deliver the drug. Again, special mechanisms may be needed to promote absorption through the membrane of the alternate route. For example, peptides (used as drugs) are very susceptible to the action of gastric acid and are rapidly degraded in the stomach. They are not degraded during transdermal delivery but enhancement mechanisms must be used to make this alternate route practical. Since the drug does not penetrate the skin easily, it cannot simply be applied in the form of a transdermal patch. A special formulation must be used to promote the passage of the drug through the skin.

Controlled Release

The dosage form may contain mechanisms to control the drug release rate for a steady, slower rate of absorption of the released drug. This produces the desired effect, relief of pain for example, without the intense side effects that may be caused by high drug levels in the body. Conversely, the drug effect does not decline rapidly as would occur in the absence of the sustained-release mechanism which ensures continued absorption for a longer period. The product may be an oral (swallowed) dosage form (such as Sudafed 12-hour extended-release tablets or Ambien CR). The pharmaceutical product may, alternately, utilize permeation of the drug through another part of the body, for example, the fentanyl patch, or the Scopolamine patch, which both utilize permeation through the skin.

Fentanyl patches are available for administration once in 3 days which is much more convenient than taking injections every 6 hours (the alternative since this drug is not well absorbed through the GIT and is rapidly cleared from the body). The patch also provides more or less constant blood levels of the drug for better control of pain. The Scopolamine patch provides sustained release of this drug to eliminate or reduce motion sickness over a period of 72 hours, without causing drowsiness. The latter side effect would occur with rapid absorption, and high blood levels, from a conventional dosage form. Other transdermal patches provide convenience of administration and offer several days' wearing of one extended-release patch. These patches release the drug steadily to achieve nearly constant blood levels over an extended period of a few days, to 1 week in the case of hormonal formulations. Patches will be discussed in more detail in Chapter 22, Dermal and Transdermal Drug Delivery.

Reduce Drug Irritation

Many drugs are irritant to the tissues with which they come into contact. A dosage form could be developed to decrease such drug irritation. Aspirin is a drug that has irritant properties. The irritation can be due to the physical characteristics of aspirin, that is, crystals with sharp edges, or the drug may cause irritation through a chemical reaction. Microfined aspirin has smaller aspirin particles to reduce the physical irritation caused by the crystals which abrade the stomach surface as they rub against it. Buffered aspirin, on the other hand, reduces the acidity caused by aspirin in the local area of the drug particles. The first example utilizes a physical mechanism, whereas the second utilizes chemistry to reduce drug irritation. In the absence of such mechanisms, gastric irritation would prevent the continued use of aspirin.

Provide Tamper Resistance

Gel tabs are capsule-shaped tablets with a thin coating of gelatin. These tablets offer ease of swallowing, comparable to capsules, but they have a far greater tamper resistance than capsules. The products were developed by the McNeil Company after incidents of willful tampering of the company's acetaminophen capsules. This product represents a convenience to the patient while greatly improving safety. Tamper-evident packaging is discussed in Chapter 14, Packaging.

Recap Questions

1. If you were talking to a friend, how would you describe the following in lay terms?
   a. The size or volume of 1 mg of a powdered drug
   b. The volume of 1 mg of a liquid drug
2. In the absence of pharmaceutical dosage forms, how would you administer to a patient the quantities of drugs considered in question 1?
3. Mention three functions of dosage forms, other than being a vehicle to convey the drug.
4. Why is it important to achieve blood levels that do not fluctuate greatly, that is, go high, and then low, only to go high again some hours later?
5. Two pairs of incompatible drugs are each prepared in a tablet dosage form, using only the ingredients that are essential. In case A, the drugs are simply contained in separate layers of the tablet whereas, in case B, a placebo layer is incorporated between the drug layers. Both tablet products are considered successful. Which pair of drugs, A or B, contains more highly incompatible drugs?
6. How can a dosage form be instrumental in reducing drug irritation? Mention three different ways.

DRUG DELIVERY SYSTEMS

The more complex dosage forms are referred to as "drug delivery systems." In recent times, their complexity has increased with each passing year. Such complex dosage forms are usually patented. The patent allows the pharmaceutical company protection from competition for a limited period, usually 20 years, but also forces the company to disclose the nature of the invention in a publicly accessible document, the patent. The patent may contain several examples of the disclosed art. These must include the best example, known to the company, at the time of filing. The mere reading of a patent may stimulate another scientist to develop other, novel drug delivery systems. Of course, these should not infringe the original patent. Once the patent period has expired, other companies may produce the same formulation as described in the invention. Thus, the patenting system ultimately makes new inventions accessible to everyone. It will be readily understood that patents are valuable documents and are therefore frequently the subject of litigation. Company A may claim that Company B infringed its patent by producing a similar product. It would then be Company B's responsibility to show that their product is different from that of company A's and that they do not infringe the patent.

If the need for a dosage form, as a suitable unit in which to present the drug for delivery into the body is appreciated and accepted, then it becomes obvious that many different types of dosage forms, or units of presentation, are possible. Furthermore, these units may be presented to the body via different apertures, or other modes of entry into the body. These modes of entry are referred to as "routes of drug administration" or "drug delivery routes." While the oral route has historically been the most important route of drug delivery, it was not the only route that was known to man, even from the earliest times. Ointments, creams, and other topical formulations have been in use for a very long time (albeit with variable effectiveness); there is also historical evidence of the use of nose, and ear, drops and even inhalation therapy. In recent times, other routes of drug delivery, such as the oral transmucosal, rectal and vaginal, have become increasingly important.

In addition to providing an introduction to the concept of dosage forms (as described above), this chapter also provides an introduction to the different routes of drug administration (as described in the remainder of the chapter). This is done so that the pharmacist will have an understanding and an appreciation of the advantages, and limitations of the different routes currently utilized for drug administration.

Other chapters in this book will discuss selected, individual routes in more detail providing, in addition, a description of the most common dosage forms used for that route, and of the formulation factors that influence the quality of the products. This will provide the pharmacist with a knowledge of the products he handles and recommends and will enable him to be able to talk to both industrial formulation scientists and clinicians with an understanding of the issues. Consideration will also be given, in these chapters, to the biological barriers that must be overcome for absorption to occur, and to the rate of drug absorption. In addition, the influence of the route of administration on the effect of the drug will be described, where appropriate. Some routes, for example, give a faster rate of absorption while others provide a slower but more sustained rate. Each of these effects may be desirable for certain pathological states but inappropriate for others. The drug may cause irritation when administered via certain routes, but not by others. However, the routes may also influence the dosage form. For example, the drug may degrade faster when administered via certain routes. This approach to understanding the influence of the body on the dosage form (including the drug) and the influence of the dosage form on the body, falls into the subject area of Biopharmaceutics. This subject also includes the biological mechanisms of drug absorption and pharmaceutical methods utilized to enhance absorption.

ROUTES OF DRUG ADMINISTRATION

The ideal therapy would be to administer to a patient a single drug which has only one effect. This effect would be the one that is desired to treat the disease and there would be no unwanted or side effects. In this ideal situation, the drug would pass directly to the site of action, which is normally, but not always, a drug receptor in an organ, or part of an organ, where the effect is required. In this way, the desired response, such as the relief of pain, it is brought about in that part of the body only, without affecting other organs. Such an ideal drug does not exist. In the first place, all drugs have multiple effects, and the pain-relieving drug may also cause euphoria and drowsiness, or reduce coordination. Alternately, a pain medication may irritate the stomach and increase bleeding time.

In reality, medicinal chemistry has not progressed to the point where we have drugs with a single effect, or "pin-point" pharmacology as depicted idealistically above. Hence, pharmaceutical scientists, clinicians, and the patient population have to contend with drugs with multiple effects, including many undesirable effects. The drug's beneficial effects and its side effects are a "package deal": it is not possible to have one without the other at the present time. Generally, the drug is administered at some convenient site for absorption into the body. The "route of drug administration" means the passage or path by which the drug is introduced into the body which, historically, has been through the mouth. The dosage form is swallowed, passes into the stomach and releases its drug content. The drug then, generally, passes into the small intestine, which is the major absorptive region of the gastrointestinal tract (GIT). Upon absorption, the drug passes into the bloodstream. The blood carries the drug to the liver where a portion of it is metabolized to an inactive form, or one that is excreted more readily (the liver sees the drug as a foreign substance that must be eliminated). The remaining, intact, drug passes into the general circulation and is carried to the site of action (as well as to other parts of the body).

The vascular system has been described as the body's highway system. Just as an actual highway system can be used to deliver packages throughout the country, the circulatory system is able to deliver drugs to all parts of the body. After passage into the circulatory system, the drug becomes diluted in the blood and this central compartment serves as the source of the drug that is supplied, over a period of time, to the entire body.

If it is accepted that, at the present time, drugs with multiple effects are the reality, the next question that must be asked is the following: *Is it possible to administer the drug only to a localized area, that is, the afflicted part of the body; or the specific organ where the drug's effect is needed; or, in the best case scenario, only to specific receptors in a particular organ?* In other words, if multiple effects cannot be avoided, is it possible to limit drug effects, beneficial and unwanted, to specific areas of the body?

If this goal could be achieved, the rest of the body would not experience the drug's effects, both desirable as well as unwanted. Specialized drug delivery systems achieve this goal partially in that the target area receives a higher concentration of the drug than the rest of the body. With most medications, however, there is a lack of drug targeting. Pharmaceutical scientists are continually making strides toward obtaining higher drug concentrations at target sites (with correspondingly lower concentrations elsewhere in the body). To innovatively develop drug delivery systems with improved drug targeting, a thorough knowledge is needed of drug and excipient properties, drug delivery systems, and physicochemical principles such as diffusion. This knowledge must be coupled with an intimate understanding of the human body and the disease condition being treated.

Consider catheterization for drug delivery, that is, administration of the drug through a tube inserted into a particular organ with the intention of treating only that organ. Theoretically, a drug may be delivered this way and the process may be more effective in a hollow organ that has thick walls. Under these conditions, the technique may produce a high drug level in the organ concerned, with practically no drug to the general blood circulation. This spares the rest of the body exposure to the drug which is in contrast to what occurs with most other modes of administration. Since a significantly lower dose can be given as a consequence of the drug not being distributed throughout the body, it also reduces drug costs. Generally, however, catheterization is not a practical means of drug delivery since it may be difficult to perform, requiring a clinic visit in some instances. Because of such practical difficulties, the technique is only used in special cases. However, it does provide a theoretical model of how the drug may be delivered to a single organ.

It should be noted that the drug leaks out of the organ, to some extent, even with this mode of administration. Some of the leaked drug may enter into the blood circulation. Hence, the drug effect is not totally located in one organ. The leakage may not be significant where the wall of the organ is thick, due to its resistance to diffusion. In the case of the bladder, this technique may be used effectively since the bladder wall is thick.

Another example is the delivery of a drug to the tooth socket. Each tooth is located in an individual socket or periodontal sulcus which can become infected and inflamed in periodontal disease. A problem with treating this disease conventionally is the fact that very high amounts of antibiotics, or other anti-infective agents, would have to be administered via the oral route to attain a significant concentration of the drug in the periodontal fluid. Frequently, such doses would be toxic to the patient and, therefore, this mode of administration is unacceptable. It is also not a simple matter of applying a gel to the gums with a finger or other applicator since the drug will not penetrate the periodontal sulcus in sufficient quantity with this mode of application. Specialized slow-release anti-infective drug treatments are placed within the tooth socket and are effective in treating the disease. While the drug placed into the sulcus in this form displays some perfusion into local tissues, very little perfusion into blood vessels occurs, virtually eliminating systemic drug distribution.

Periodontal films are thin strips, or films, of biocompatible material that are impregnated with the drug. The Periochip® is an example of a thin film. It contains chlorhexidine gluconate for the adjunctive treatment of periodontal disease. After scaling and root planing, a dentist or oral hygienist inserts the chip into the periodontal sulcus where it releases the chlorhexidine over a period of approximately 10 days (Figure 2-1). Each chip contains 2.5 mg of chlorhexidine gluconate. Repeat visits, at 3-month intervals, are required for the insertion of additional chips for long-term treatment. By the use of this device, high concentrations of the antiseptic, chlorhexidine, can be reached in the periodontal sulcus. Bacteria are effectively killed without causing systemic toxicity. This selective effectiveness

(A)

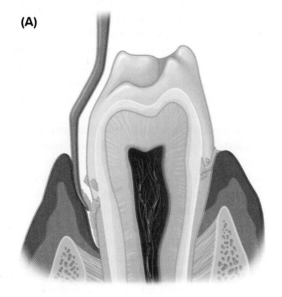

(B)

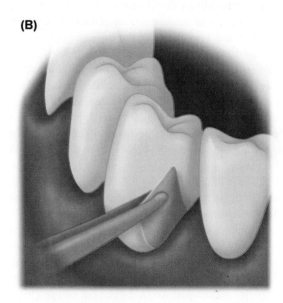

FIGURE 2-1 The Periochip. A. Scaling removes plaque and tartar from around and below the gum line in preparation for B. **B.** Insertion of the Periochip for local delivery of chlorhexidine.

is achieved in spite of the fact that chlorhexidine is toxic if absorbed in large amounts.

Another formulation, of this type, that is popular in the US is Arestin® (Figure 2-2). It contains 1 mg of the antibiotic, minocycline, within microspheres which are embedded in a viscous gel. After scaling and root planing, the oral hygienist delivers the viscous gel into the dental sulcus from a prefilled syringe. The drug slowly diffuses out of the microspheres and through the gel base and has a prolonged effect killing microorganisms within the sulcus. The extent of permeation into the bloodstream is low resulting in low blood drug concentration in the vicinity of the treated sulcus. This concentration becomes diluted by distribution throughout the blood volume. Hence, systemic levels of minomycin are low and side effects are negligible.

A stent is a device placed into the coronary artery to help keep it open when disease conditions, mainly artherosclerosis, have caused a narrowing of the artery. (Stents have also been used off-label to keep other arteries open but their main use is in the coronary artery.) The stent reverses the restriction of blood flow, and oxygen supply, to the heart muscles. The stent may also contain drugs that prevent the artery from becoming blocked once more, a process known as restenosis (Figure 2-3). Such stents are referred to as drug-eluting stents, and the drugs they contain prevent cell proliferation, due to inflammation, as well as the formation of scar tissue. The latter tends to form as a result of injury during the surgical procedure. The drugs used in the first drug-eluting stents were paclitaxel or sirolimus, while analogues of these drugs are used in the newer stents.

The stent may be equated to a hollow tube with a mesh wall. The latter allows for expansion and contraction of the stent as the vascular wall changes diameter. The drug is coated over the surface of the stent. Usually, several polymer coatings are also applied over the stents for different purposes. One or more of these coats may be used to decrease the rate of drug release from the stent and, hence, also the absorption rate into the vascular tissue. With the stent touching the vascular wall, the drug is effectively placed at the site of action. While there may be slow lateral drug diffusion within a small portion of the arterial wall, the extent of diffusion into the systemic circulation is very little.

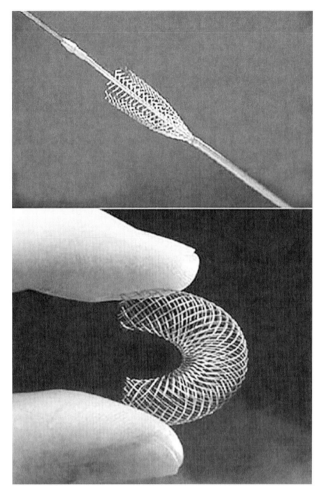

FIGURE 2-3 A drug-eluting stent. (Reproduced, with permission, from Brunicardi FC, Andersen DK, Billiar TR, et al. *Schwartz's Principles of Surgery.* 11th ed. New York, NY: McGraw Hill; 2019.)

This small amount is rapidly diluted by the large volume of blood and, therefore, its concentration is insignificant. Hence, this form of drug administration targets the site of action very well.

The above examples illustrate that it is possible for a system to deliver practically all of its drug load to one predetermined location in the body. However, these examples are extreme cases which are invasive, to varying degrees. Their development was primarily motivated by the difficulty in delivering drugs to the organ in question, using conventional delivery systems. These are not delivery systems that may be applied, generally, to commonly-used drugs. At the present time, it is usually not possible, or not practical, to administer a drug to the site of action, or even to one area of the body, without significant penetration of other organs. In terms of localizing drug delivery, the examples described in this chapter may be considered "ideal," for the present state of the technology. It is an aspirational goal to achieve similar drug profiles, without invasive procedures, for a wide range of drugs used in general therapy.

Traditionally, drugs were administered by swallowing, resulting in them being absorbed, with varying efficiency, and circulated throughout the general circulation. This process transferred a portion of an ingested drug to the part(s) of the body where it

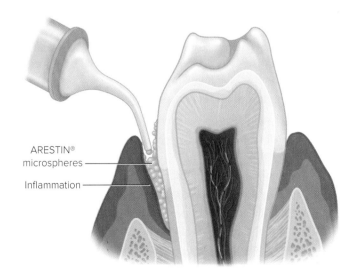

ARESTIN® microspheres
Inflammation

FIGURE 2-2 Application of Arestin.

was needed. In most instances, the portion of the dose actually eliciting the desired pharmacological effect, at the desired sites, is small. The majority of the absorbed drug circulates through body structures where it is not needed. For example, if a patient has a headache and takes acetaminophen, only a small amount of the drug is needed to relieve the pain at the site of action in the head. In contrast, most of the absorbed drug is either metabolized by the liver or carried through the circulation to other parts of the body. Some of the circulating drug reaches the kidneys where it has undesirable effects. On the other hand, it is not possible to supply sufficient oral (swallowed) drug, in the case of periodontal disease, to treat this local condition, without causing serious toxicity to the rest of the body. Some of the limitations of oral drug delivery may be summarized as follows:

1. A large dose must be administered in order to supply a relatively small amount of the drug to the part(s) of the body where it is needed.

2. The circulating drug causes systemic side effects.

3. Conversely, the dose may be reduced out of concern for side effects in a critical organ system which results, in some instances, in the administration of doses of questionable efficacy.

At the present time, pharmaceutical science is, with few exceptions, far from the ideal situation regarding drug delivery at a controlled rate to one location only. Nevertheless, pharmaceutical scientists are constantly trying to enhance, and even alter, the therapeutic effect of administered drugs by means of novel dosage forms. This is done by controlling how fast the drug is released from a dosage form, the rate at which it is absorbed by the body and, most importantly, the route of drug administration. The choice of routes affects the tissues through which the drug is absorbed. Examples of the latter are delivery through the skin (transdermal delivery), through the lining of the mouth (oral transmucosal delivery), and the lining of the nose (nasal delivery). The development of dosage forms for delivery through these routes is usually not easy. To create a dosage form from which the drug is absorbed *advantageously* at these alternate sites requires scientific knowledge, skill, and, most importantly, inventiveness.

To have a drug delivered from an oral dosage form at a controlled rate, and not be destroyed by prevailing conditions in the GIT, also requires significant research and development. The natural tendency with respect to swallowed drugs is for the dosage form to pass through the GIT, along with food contents. The time available for drug release from the dosage form, and also for absorption, is related to the rate of passage of the dosage form through the GIT. A tablet dosage form intended for multi-day treatment, for example, would pass from the stomach to the small intestine and then leave the small intestine in a matter of several hours, carrying a significant portion of its drug load. This would defeat the objective of multi-day treatment since the dosage form would have gone beyond the major organ for absorption, the intestine.

A subject of intense scientific study and invention has, therefore, been the idea of altering the rate at which a dosage form moves through the GIT. Can this time be prolonged to allow an extended period for slow, sustained drug release within the sections of the GIT that absorb effectively? Such questions have led to the development of devices that float on the stomach contents, thereby remaining longer in the stomach before eventual passage of the dosage form to the small intestine. While the released drug usually passes rapidly from the stomach into the intestine for absorption, this innovation allows a longer duration during which the dosage form may remain in the stomach and steadily release its drug load. Other experimental approaches have led to the development of dosage forms that adhere to the mucosa of the GIT. The drug load is released from this position over an extended period. Such dosage forms are described and illustrated in Chapter 11, Modified-Release Oral Dosage Forms.

The oral route is also known as the *enteral* route. The term "enteral" refers to the "enteron" or GIT. Generally, a drug that is absorbed through the GIT has entered the body via the enteral route. All other routes are *parenteral*. Note that the injection route is one example of a parenteral route. In common usage, though, the term parenteral is sometimes taken to mean an injection route only. Types of injections include intravenous (IV) or into a vein, intramuscular (IM) or into a muscle, subcutaneous (SC) or under the skin, and intrathecal or into the spinal cord.

The recent increase in popularity of drugs delivered through the lining of the mouth has caused some confusion in terminology. Since the drug is delivered through the mouth, it has sometimes been referred to as "oral" delivery. This is not technically correct since "oral delivery" has been used for a long time to signify drugs that are swallowed for absorption in some part of the GIT. A different term is needed to distinguish the more recent utilization of the lining of the mouth, or oral mucosa, as the tissue through which drugs are delivered. Some authors have used the term, *oral mucosal delivery* and this term is preferred. It is used throughout this book as the descriptive term for drugs delivered through the lining of the mouth. It should be noted that this is a collective term encompassing absorption through any part of the oral cavity. Oral mucosal delivery may be divided, for example, into the major areas of buccal delivery (through the inside lining of the cheek) and sublingual delivery (under the tongue).

Often there is a choice of the route of drug administration to utilize. The choice will depend on factors such as the nature of the drug, the therapeutic need (eg, rapid delivery or slow, sustained delivery), the stability of the drug in biological fluids, the permeability of different tissues to the drug in question, and the condition of the patient. Some questions that a pharmaceutical formulator may wish to ask, before choosing a route and developing a product, are the following:

1. What are the properties of the drug under consideration?
   a. Water soluble or oil soluble
   b. A small molecule or a large molecule of biological origin, for example, a peptide

2. Is a systemic effect, or a localized effect, desired?

3. What is the metabolic profile of the drug and in which locations is it metabolized?

4. What is the stability profile of the drug, for example, is it affected by the highly acidic conditions of the stomach?

5. Is the drug irritant to sensitive tissues?

6. Is the typical patient ambulatory or hospitalized?

The physico-chemical properties of the drug may provide sufficient information to deduce the likely routes of absorption. However, pre-formulation studies can be performed to determine the relative permeability of the biological barriers at the routes under consideration using surrogates for human tissues. From these early results, an indication of the expected rate of absorption can be obtained for such routes. The estimates of absorption and bioavailability of the drug facilitate a decision regarding the route of administration to be used in drug product development. Sophisticated software is also available to predict bioavailability, distribution to specific tissues, and other parameters. These predictions are based on early, limited data. Consider a drug that is not well absorbed through the skin, but which is absorbed adequately through the mucosa of the oral cavity, the nasal cavity, and the rectum. The formulator must consider which of the latter three routes is most suitable for the condition being treated, considering all aspects of the proposed treatment, including patient convenience. If the patient is nauseous, for example, oral mucosal delivery may not be acceptable.

The overview of the different routes, in the remainder of this chapter, will help the reader to understand the complexities involved in making such a choice. It also serves as an introduction to the individual routes of drug delivery, which are each dealt with in a separate chapter in this book. Such knowledge will also guide the pharmacist in making a choice of route and dosage form when this information is requested by a physician.

Recap Questions

1. Can you see any inefficiency or problem associated with the use of the circulatory system for the distribution of a drug to a specific site of action?
2. Why is it usually not feasible to simply administer a drug through the most convenient route (eg, transdermal)?
3. In which way is the stability of the drug related to the choice of route of drug administration?
4. When considering which route of administration to use, why is it important to consider both the chemical factors, related to the drug, and the biological factors, related to the route of administration?

ORAL OR ENTERAL ROUTE

The oral route has been used from the earliest times for the ingestion of drugs. Historically, it was the most obvious route for administration of substances considered beneficial to the health of man. Today, it is still considered a very safe route and an easy route for self-administration. The dosage forms used via the oral route are relatively cheap to manufacture compared to novel dosage forms administered by other routes. For example, tablets are much cheaper to produce than transdermal patches. However, this route is not without its problems, as the following examples demonstrate:

1. Patients with difficulty in swallowing: Children and geriatric patients may have difficulty swallowing, especially with larger doses. As a separate matter, apart from an actual physical problem, the process of swallowing also requires a specific physical effort on the part of the patient. Hence, oral drug administration is difficult to achieve if the patient is uncooperative. Drug administration via this route can prove to be extremely difficult with such a patient, as the parents of many young children will attest! This may also be the case with a mentally-impaired patient who is uncooperative. (Orally disintegrating tablets are a potential solution to this problem and are described in Chapter 9, Tablets.)

2. The taste of the drug may dissuade patients from taking the medication: This problem is more acute with liquid dosage forms but may be partially overcome with flavors, taste-masking agents, and viscosity enhancers, as described more fully in Chapter 4, Solutions. The taste may be experienced even in a tablet that is swallowed whole but may be completely overcome by coating the tablet. However, the formulation scientist has to ensure that the coating does not significantly delay absorption of the drug which occurs in the intestine. In the case of orally disintegrating tablets, the drug-containing particles may be coated, again taking the precaution that the release of the drug is not impeded to an unacceptable level. The coating of tablets and drug particles is described in Chapter 9, Tablets.

3. The drug may cause nausea or irritation: Most bad-tasting drugs are bitter but the taste of some drugs may be nauseating. This is a difficult problem to overcome. Some drugs are irritating to the tissues into which they come into contact. Ibuprofen is irritating to the mouth and throat, even after the short contact time involved with swallowing the medication. In this case, the irritation potential is overcome by coating the tablet, or by the use of a viscous suspension, in which the high viscosity reduces the contact of the drug with the mucosal membranes.

4. The highly-acidic environment in the stomach may promote drug degradation: Enteric coating of dosage forms or drug-containing particles results in the drug only being released in the small intestine, which is considerably less acidic, thus reducing drug degradation due to contact with stomach contents.

5. Enzymes in the GIT may degrade the drug: Pepsin's function in the stomach is to help digest proteins. It may break down peptide drugs that are administered, resulting in less drug being available for absorption. Gastric lipase is responsible for lipid hydrolysis of food materials and can affect lipid drugs. Pancreatic lipase is secreted in the small intestine and needs a higher pH to similarly hydrolyze lipid drugs. Various peptidases in the small intestine convert peptides originating from food into amino acids and can, similarly, affect peptide drugs.

6. Absorption may be limited, especially with respect to poorly soluble drugs: A drug, in practically all instances, must be in aqueous solution for absorption to occur. Thus, absorption of poorly soluble drugs is limited. It should be noted that many new drugs are poorly soluble.

7. Variable absorption: Variability may be observed from patient to patient, and even within the same patient from one day to the next. Absorption may be influenced, for example, by whether food is taken with the drug and also by the nature of the meal. A fatty meal with a few glasses of wine may change absorption significantly compared to absorption after a light salad.

8. Short absorption window: In some cases, only a small part of the GIT is capable of absorbing the drug. The drug, mixed with intestinal contents, may pass this window too rapidly for significant absorption to occur.

BUCCAL AND SUBLINGUAL DELIVERY

Buccal delivery refers to delivery of drugs through the inside lining of the cheek, whereas sublingual delivery refers to delivery through the mucosa on the floor of the mouth, and/or through the lining on the under-surface of the tongue. While there are some differences between these routes of drug delivery (which will be dealt with in Chapter 20, Buccal and Sublingual Drug Delivery), they also share some similarities. For the purpose of this introduction, we can consider these routes to be essentially the same, and discuss them together as "oral mucosal drug delivery." The mucosa lining both areas shares many similarities. Since it is the mucosa that serves as the barrier to drug permeation, the similarities allow one to consider the two routes together. Below the mucosa lies a rich supply of blood vessels which lead directly into the systemic circulation. Thus, absorbed substances directly enter into the systemic circulation, avoiding the liver during the first pass. A drug that is absorbed from the small intestine (the most effective, and common, part of the GIT for drug absorption) passes initially to the liver where a portion of the drug is metabolized. This so-called, "first-pass" metabolism will not occur for drugs absorbed through the oral mucosa. As a consequence, more of the drug will reach the systemic circulation when administered via the latter route. One of the roles of the liver is to metabolize toxins, including drugs, that are ingested, converting them to substances that are less toxic. With such a change in chemical structure, the substance may no longer function as a drug. Alternatively, metabolic changes may make the drug more water-soluble and thus more easily excreted.

The disadvantages of oral mucosal delivery include the taste of the drug. It is not pleasant to hold a bitter drug under the tongue for several minutes while it is slowly absorbed. The drug-containing tablets cannot be coated, as in other instances, to mask the taste. The reason for this limitation is the fact that the drug must dissolve in saliva, in order to be absorbed, and the coating retards dissolution. The major advantage of this type of drug delivery is the fact that it is possible to get rapid absorption; often the absorption is much faster than occurs via the oral route. Since absorption is more efficient, a lower dose can usually be administered. Special delivery systems may be needed to enable the drug to be transferred across the barrier (oral mucosa). This will be discussed in more detail in Chapter 20, Buccal and Sublingual Drug Delivery.

COLONIC DELIVERY

Some drugs are destroyed by the harsh conditions of the stomach or the small intestines but are effectively absorbed in the colon. The problem, therefore, may be approached as the oral delivery of drugs to the colon, while enabling them to escape destruction or metabolism in other parts of the GIT. The stomach contents are highly acidic and many drugs will be destroyed by these conditions. In addition, it contains pepsin for the digestion of proteins into smaller units called peptides. The small intestine contains enzymes (eg, peptidases) that further break down peptides into smaller peptides. Thus, peptide drugs will be enzymatically broken down and, therefore, this route of administration cannot be utilized for such drugs without incorporating protective mechanisms. Examples of peptide drugs are insulin for diabetes and calcitonin for osteoporosis. (Insulin is currently administered by subcutaneous injection and calcitonin by nasal spray, although there is intense research interest in developing oral dosage forms of these drugs.)

The colon contains few enzymes but bacteria are present. The latter help break down residual matter from food. Hence, a material resistant to acid as well as to enzymes, but which succumbs to bacterial breakdown, could be used to coat the drug particles, or the drug product. Using such a coating, it would be possible to administer oral medication for drug delivery to the colon, without degradation of the drug in either the stomach or the small intestine.

Typically, a drug product, such as a drug-containing tablet, is coated with the resistant material. When the tablet is swallowed and reaches the stomach, it is not affected by the acid due to the coating material. Since the coating does not allow the permeation of water, the tablet passes intact through the stomach, without breaking up or disintegrating. Subsequently, it continues down the small intestine, unaffected by the enzymes present. When the tablet reaches the colon, the coating degrades due to the action of bacterial enzymes. This exposes the tablet to the aqueous medium and ingress of water disintegrates the tablet to release the drug for colonic absorption. The disintegration process is facilitated by the presence, within the tablet, of chemicals which imbibe water and/or swell. Such chemicals are referred to as disintegrants.

RECTAL DELIVERY

The rectum is well supplied with blood vessels and drugs applied to the rectum may be absorbed readily and rapidly. Aminophylline suppositories for the treatment of asthmatic attacks were popular. Generally, suppositories are not popular in the US but they remain popular in Europe and South America. They are still used in the US for certain conditions such as nausea and vomiting, for example, Stemetil® suppositories and Cyclizine suppositories. The pharmacist may be called upon to compound suppositories for a particular patient. This may occur when a specific formulation, which is not available commercially, is required for the patient, or in instances where the dose may have to be adjusted in comparison to commercially available products. The formulation of suppositories is described in Chapter 24, Rectal and Vaginal Drug Delivery.

NASAL DELIVERY

The nasal mucosa is relatively permeable to small molecular weight compounds. If the drug is able to pass the mucosa, it is rapidly taken up into the general circulation. Although the surface area of the nasal mucosa is small, it is large enough for adequate absorption of many drugs. Cocaine is rapidly and extensively absorbed. The rapid absorption which leads to rapid onset of the euphoric effect is responsible for its popularity as a street drug. Small peptides can be sufficiently well absorbed, especially with the aid of absorption enhancers, for this route to be useful. On the other hand, larger peptides may not cross the barrier well. Miacalcin® is a preparation of salmon calcitonin that is administered intranasally to treat osteoporosis and Paget's disease, both conditions involving loss of calcium from bones with the resultant weakening of bones.

TRANSDERMAL DELIVERY

The skin has a very large surface area and, for successful drug administration, only a relatively small part of the skin need be utilized. In addition, transdermal dosage forms can be applied to different areas of the body, at each dosing interval. This allows the skin to recover from possible ill effects of drug administration. Such effects may be as simple as a slight irritation due to the adhesive contained in a transdermal patch. A potentially more serious effect may be caused by chemicals incorporated into the patch to improve the penetration of the drug (penetration enhancers). In contrast to these advantages, it should be noted that the epidermis of the skin contains densely packed cells which contain keratin (a wax-like substance) and the epidermal layer is a barrier to drug absorption. Lipophilic drugs pass through the skin but the transit time may be long. This may be advantageous in certain chronic conditions in order to provide slow drug permeation resulting in consistent drug levels for extended periods.

Nitroglycerin, fentanyl, scopolamine, nicotine, and progesterone are some of the drugs that have been studied for transdermal delivery. Hydrophilic drugs, generally, will not permeate the skin unless special techniques are used. If a drug does cross the barrier, this route is an effective means to deliver the drug since it avoids the GIT and the problems associated with it in the context of drug administration. These include irritation of the stomach, degradation of the drug in the acidic contents of the stomach, or metabolism of the drug by pancreatic enzymes, for example. Since the drug passes directly to the circulatory system after transdermal administration, it avoids first-pass metabolism by the liver. This route can provide a long duration of action from a single dosage form, for example, 72 hours for fentanyl patches. Transdermal drug delivery is more fully described in Chapter 22, Dermal and Transdermal Drug Delivery.

PULMONARY DELIVERY

Presently, pulmonary delivery is used mostly for local delivery of drugs, that is, bronchodilators and anti-inflammatory steroids for asthma and chronic obstructive pulmonary disease. However, there is interest in using this organ to deliver drugs to the general circulation and this is an important research area with many compounds in development. The following attributes of the lungs make this route of delivery advantageous:

1. The surface area is large.
2. It is well supplied with blood vessels.
3. The drug passes directly into the bloodstream and the effect is, therefore, very rapid.
4. The route avoids hepatic first-pass.

The size of particles administered by means of inhalation influences the part of the lung which they reach and, therefore, the usefulness of the therapy. Large particles, for example, do not go down far enough into the lung where the drug is needed. Drug delivery to the lung is described in more detail in Chapter 19, Pulmonary Drug Delivery.

INTRAVENOUS ADMINISTRATION

When a drug is injected intravenously, it enters directly into the bloodstream, that is, there is no absorption phase. After reaching the blood, it is pumped very rapidly throughout the body, including to the site of action. Because of direct entry into the circulatory system, without an absorption phase, IV injections have the fastest onset of action. However, one must not assume that the drug passes directly to the site of action.

The venous blood returns to the heart and is then pumped to the lungs where some drugs may be partially metabolized. If the drug has a high vapor pressure, a fraction of the drug reaching the lungs is excreted in the exhaled air. The blood with the drug that was not metabolized or excreted flows from the lungs back to the heart for circulation to the entire body, including the organ where the drug is needed. While the route from injection site to site of action is not direct, it does not delay drug action appreciably. This is because blood flow is fast, and the sequence of passages to the different organs occurs rapidly. From this brief picture we can see the following:

1. The drug is diluted tremendously before it reaches the site of action.
2. The rest of the body will also experience the effect of the drug, as well as its side effects.

3. Other organs may participate in the elimination (excretion and metabolism) of the drug.

SUBCUTANEOUS INJECTION

When a drug solution is injected into the subcutaneous space (space under the skin), the drug diffuses to, and is absorbed into, the subcutaneous blood vessels. Thus, the drug does not enter directly into the blood vessels, as in the case of an IV injection. There is an uptake or absorption phase. Therefore, a slower pharmacological response can be expected at the site of action than is the case for an IV injection. After the drug passes into the veins, it is carried to the heart, the lungs, back to the heart, and then distributed throughout the body, as described above for an IV injection.

The subcutaneous (SC) route is good for peptides (which are degraded to a large extent in the GIT). For example, insulin is administered in this way. The slower absorption is not a negative attribute, in this case, since a sudden drop in blood sugar would be undesirable. Conversely, delayed absorption means that excessively high blood glucose levels cannot be rapidly counteracted by this method. After a meal, blood glucose levels rise rapidly in diabetics. However, an insulin injection, administered after a meal, will not reduce the blood glucose level quickly. The injection has to be well-timed, and given shortly before the meal, and/or other drugs have to be administered to achieve effective control of blood glucose levels after a meal. The type of insulin (some are long-acting) and the schedule of administration are topics that are discussed in therapeutics courses.

INTRAMUSCULAR INJECTION

Drugs administered into the muscle tissue diffuse through the tissue, reach blood vessels in the muscle, and are absorbed into these vessels. This is similar to the absorption phase for SC injections but diffusion through muscle tissue will be slower than the diffusion of the same drug through the subcutaneous space. The slower absorption rate is due to the dense muscle tissue in comparison to the subcutaneous region, resulting in a slower initial response. However, the response is sustained over a longer period. When the intramuscular injection consists of a slowly dissolving salt, the duration of action may be even longer. In some instances, for example, some chemical forms of penicillin, the duration of action may be several days.

One factor that may affect the absorption rate, is the blood flow rate which, in turn, is affected by the muscle into which the drug is injected. The deltoid muscle has a much faster blood flow rate, and therefore faster absorption, than the gluteus muscle.

OPHTHALMIC DELIVERY

One of the most difficult drug delivery situations is encountered with delivery of drugs to the interior of the eye. Effective drug concentrations in the gel-like interior are difficult to achieve due to the natural protective mechanisms of the eye. These mechanisms are designed to keep foreign molecules out of the eye. Several invasive techniques are in use to deliver drugs to the interior of the eye. However, the sensitivity of the eye and the care which must be taken with invasive drug delivery techniques are further factors limiting delivery of drugs to the eye.

Intraocular injections, intra-vitreal inserts, and other devices, which are surgically placed into the eye, may be utilized to deliver a drug needed to treat a condition in the interior of the eye. These highly invasive methods are warranted because of the serious diseases being treated and the fact that blindness frequently results if the conditions are left untreated. These methods are described in Chapter 24, Ophthalmic Drug Delivery, which also contains illustrations of some devices.

Recap Questions

1. Considering the fact that the oral route of drug administration is convenient to the patient, why should efforts be made to find alternatives routes of drug administration?

2. Name two advantages of the buccal route of drug administration.

3. Why is the slow absorption of fentanyl through a transdermal patch (administered for relief of pain) advantageous to the patient?

4. Name a drug with a higher vapor pressure than water, which is excreted through the lungs. Hint: drugs that are excreted through the lungs can be smelled on a person's breath.

5. In your own words, explain why an intravenous injection can be expected to give a faster response than a subcutaneous injection.

SUMMARY POINTS

- Dosage forms are necessary for several primary reasons including: to provide accurate dosing, convenience of administration, and protect the drug.
- Dosage forms may also control the rate of drug release, mask the taste of the drug, separate incompatible ingredients, etc.
- The oral route of drug administration is well known but several alternative routes are used to confer specific advantage, or used when specific drugs cannot be administered via the oral route.
- Innovative, novel drug delivery systems can supply drugs to an organ that is difficult to reach by conventional routes, without causing systemic toxicity.

What do you think?

1. Should cost be taken into account when developing novel drug delivery systems?

2. Do patents simply hinder competition and prevent the widespread availability of needed drugs?

3. Why is so-called "pin-point pharmacology" important in drug delivery to humans?

4. Distinguish colonic delivery from oral delivery. Under what circumstances is the former method needed?

REFERENCE

1. Bartholomaeus J, Ziegler I. Multilayer tablet for administering a fixed combination of tramadol and diclofenac. United States Patent 6,558,701. Issued May 6, 2003.

Oral Route of Drug Delivery

3

PREVIEW

- Understand the basic mechanisms by which drugs may be absorbed
- Understand the factors that affect drug absorption through the oral route
- Assess whether pathology or co-administered drugs will affect drug absorption via the oral route
- Logically predict whether, and to what extent, a patient's lifestyle choices will impact the effect of drugs administered by the oral route

INTRODUCTION

After the administration of most systemically-acting drugs, there is an absorption phase. The notable exception is an intravenous injection which requires no absorption since the drug is delivered directly into the blood compartment.

Since orally administered dosage forms are by far the most common, we will discuss drug absorption as it occurs from the oral route in some detail. From this, a basic understanding of absorption from other routes may be gleaned. Any special effects or processes, pertinent to alternate routes, will be discussed further in the topics covering the specialized dosage forms/routes of drug delivery, such as transdermal delivery. The oral route is so common (most likely due to ease of administration) that there is a tendency to take this route for granted and to think that any orally-administered drug will be absorbed. However, drug absorption from the oral route (ie, via the gastrointestinal tract [GIT]) is complex as these pages attempt to illustrate. The absorption of all of the administered drug, or even a fixed fraction (eg, 50%) *consistently*, from a standardized dosage form cannot be taken for granted. Drug absorption can be extremely variable for a multitude of factors. The reader is expected to have a basic understanding of GIT anatomy and physiology. If this is not the case, basic texts covering these areas should be consulted.

A very brief overview of a few aspects of gastrointestinal anatomy and physiology will be covered as a lead into the main topic of discussion, namely, how drugs are absorbed and what factors affect their absorption. For immediate-release products (ie, products in which the rate of release of the drug is not controlled or sustained), one would like rapid and complete absorption into the bloodstream for the following reasons:

1. For most drugs, the higher the concentration in the blood, the greater the pharmacological effect.

2. The quicker significant blood concentrations are reached, the sooner the pharmacological effect will begin.

3. The greater the extent of absorption, the less the variability in the amount absorbed by a patient on different days, or between different patients.

4. The more rapidly the drug is absorbed the less the extent of pre-absorption degradation or of interactions between the drug and other substances present in the gastrointestinal lumen.

5. Rapid and complete absorption is associated with more reproducible pharmacological responses (drug effects). Erratic absorption is associated with erratic responses.

Peptides and proteins are large-molecular-weight, potent compounds that have, increasingly, been used as drugs in recent years. They have special challenges for delivery via the GIT and, most often, cannot be delivered via this route. Complex delivery systems are often needed to deliver these drugs via other routes. Most of the discussion in this chapter, therefore, focuses on the absorption of small organic molecules which are by far the most common type of drug.

All nutrients needed by the body for normal functioning must be ingested orally, digested, absorbed into the bloodstream, and then distributed to the whole body. Therefore, the GIT of a complex organism, such as man, is an efficient organ to carry out this function. Drug delivery can make use of this well-tuned absorption system to achieve the absorption of certain drugs. In some instances, drugs are actually actively absorbed by physiological mechanisms that are designed to transport nutrients. An example is the case of drugs that resemble amino acids. The GI system, on the other hand, is system is also designed to recognize and eliminate foreign substances, especially toxins, from the body. This system recognizes several drugs as foreign and toxic, and eliminates them. Mechanisms to rid the system of ingested toxins include:

1. Vomiting

2. Diarrhea

3. An efflux mechanism to actively pump, out of intestinal cells, foreign molecules that have just been absorbed

4. Metabolism of the drug by intestinal cells as it is being absorbed

5. Transfer of absorbed materials, via the bloodstream, to the liver prior to distribution to the rest of the body. The liver metabolizes the toxin or drug with the result that the blood that flows from the liver has reduced quantities of the drug. The liver is like a "first stop clearing house" in the journey of absorbed substances.

The last item is an important mechanism to eliminate toxins or drugs. Nutrients, on the other hand, are recognized as beneficial and pass out of the liver, to the general circulation, in approximately the same quantities as those that reach the liver.

Recap Questions

1. Why is a drug degraded to a lesser extent in the lumen of the intestine, if it is absorbed faster?

2. Why is vomiting, as a mechanism to reduce toxic effects of ingested substances, only effective soon after ingestion?

3. Why does the body attempt to eliminate drugs which are intended to alleviate an unhealthy condition?

ANATOMICAL AND PHYSIOLOGICAL OVERVIEW

Stomach

The main functions of the stomach are storing of consumed food, mixing and reducing all components to a slurry with the aid of gastric secretions, and emptying these contents at a controlled rate into the upper small intestine. The stomach is made up of three basic parts: the fundus, body, and antrum. This is shown in Figure 3-1. Note that the "pyloric part" is also known as the antrum. We will use the latter term.

Food enters the stomach and is stored in the fundus and body. The walls of these parts of the stomach have little muscular activity and the stomach can therefore swell. The epithelial cell surface of the stomach is covered by a layer of mucus (1-1.5 mm thick) consisting of mucopolysaccharides. This mucus layer protects the stomach and keeps the stomach surface lubricated. The latter is important when food material rubs against the surface as the food is mixed.

Food is layered in the fundus and body region in the order in which it arrives (the latest material on the top; oldest closest to the stomach wall). Gastric glands secrete about 2 L of gastric

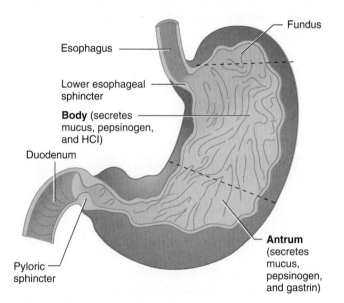

FIGURE 3-1 Regions of the stomach. (Reproduced, with permission, from Widmaier EP, Raff H, Strang KT. *Vander's Human Physiology: The Mechanisms of Body Function*. 11th ed. New York, NY: McGraw Hill; 2008, Fig. 25-2.)

fluid per day. This fluid is acidic due to a high content of HCl. The antrum is the major site of mixing motions since it is more muscular and is capable of strong contractions. It also acts as a pump to accomplish gastric emptying. The pyloric valve is situated between the stomach and the small intestine. It controls the movement of the contents of the stomach between these organs, that is, an open pyloric valve, coupled with strong contractile motion of the antrum, propels the stomach contents into the small intestine. When the pyloric valve is closed in the absence of antral contractions, the stomach contents remain in the stomach.

The contractions of the antrum have an additional, important function. When the pyloric valve is closed and there are simultaneous strong contractions of the antrum, the stomach contents are propelled toward the pyloric valve. Because the pyloric valve is closed, the slurry is ejected backwards toward the body of the stomach. Repeated motions of this type, result in the food material, together with stomach secretions, being well churned or mixed.

Small Intestine

The small intestine has the shape of a convoluted tube and it makes up the major portion of the length of the GIT. The small intestine consists of the following parts (from the stomach onwards):

Duodenum

Jejunum

Ileum

At the junction of the stomach and the duodenum is the pyloric valve, as mentioned. In addition to its functions with respect to the movement of material during stomach (antral) contractions, it also has functions related to the contractions of the *duodenum*, which are discussed below. The valve closes during the strong contractions of the duodenum which propels food material along the small intestine toward the large intestine. The closed valve prevents regurgitation of material back into the stomach. The small intestine's unique structure is the result of modifications to make it ideal for absorption. These structural adaptations greatly increase its internal, or luminal, surface area without increasing its volume. In other words, within a limited space, the intestine has a tremendous internal surface area (luminal surface area) so that it can efficiently absorb materials presented to it. The increase in surface area is achieved in the following ways (Figure 3-3):

1. There are folds of mucosa within the lumen (space) known as the folds of Kerckering.
2. Lining the internal surface, including on the folds of Kerckering, are finger-like projections known as villi.
3. Projecting from the villi are fine structures, the microvilli. The microvilli are actually projections of the individual epithelial cells which make up the wall of the villus. Consequently, they are very fine. For this reason, these cells are described as having a brush border, a term which refers to the microvilli.

While the length of the small intestine is approximately 22 ft only, all of these adaptations taken together give the small intestine an internal surface area equivalent to approximately two-thirds of a tennis court. Considering a cross-section of the small intestine, it can be divided into four distinct layers from the outside of the "tube" to the inside (Figure 3-2):

1. First is the serosa or lining of the small intestine.
2. Second is the muscularis mucosa: two thin sheets of smooth muscle.
3. Third is the lamina propria: the connective tissue which contains blood vessels, lymph vessels, and nerve fibers.
4. Last is the innermost layer, the mucosa or surface epithelium. The epithelial cells form a continuous sheet that lines the entire length of the small intestine. The epithelial cells, or enterocytes, are columnar in shape. The mucosa lies on a submucosa.

The lamina propria and epithelium form the villi. The part of the epithelial cell that faces into the lumen is called the luminal surface. The microvilli are located on the luminal cell membrane. The microvilli are coated with mucus consisting of mucopolysaccharides. This viscous layer probably keeps bacteria and other foreign particles away from the microvilli. On the opposite side of the cell (away from the lumen) is the basal plasma membrane. This can be seen in Figure 3-2(e). The basal plasma membrane rests on a basement membrane which separates it from the lamina propria.

The Large Intestine

The large intestine, also referred to as the colon, consists of three parts:

1. The ascending colon on the right of the human body (seen on the left in the illustration)
2. The horizontal colon, also known as the transverse colon
3. The descending colon on the left of a human body (seen on the right in the illustration)

The small intestine joins the large intestine at the ileocecal junction. The wall of the ileum at this point is very muscular and forms the ileocecal sphincter, the main function of which is to prevent backflow of fecal material from the colon into the small intestine. The structure of the large intestine is similar to the small intestine but it lacks villi.

The large intestine has two primary functions:

1. The absorption of water and electrolytes which occur in the ascending colon and the initial part of the transverse colon
2. Storing and mass movement of fecal matter which occur in a part of the transverse colon, the descending colon, and the rectum

Recap Questions

1. List the ways in which the stomach is different from the small intestine.
2. List the ways in which the small intestine is different from the large intestine.
3. Both the stomach and the large intestine have storing functions. In which way are these storing functions different?
4. Why is the blood from the intestines (rich in nutrients) sent to the liver before circulation throughout the body for distribution of the absorbed nutrients?

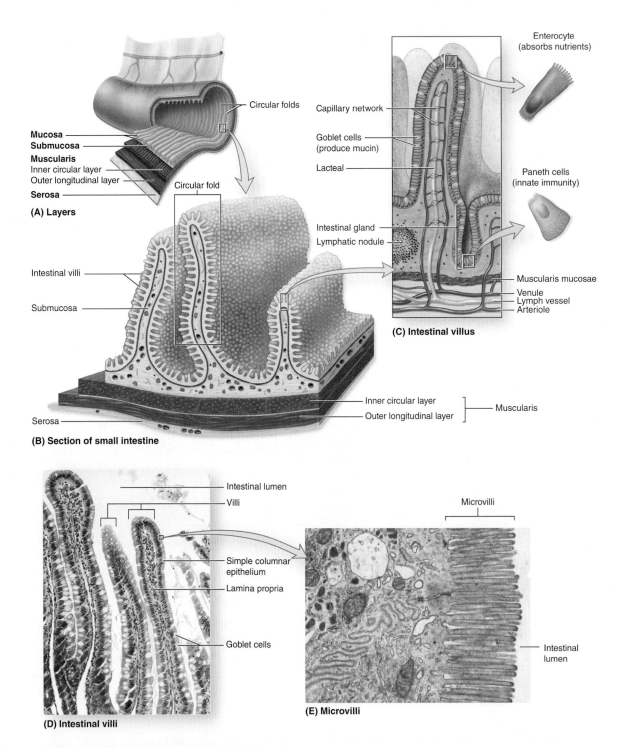

FIGURE 3-2 Villi of the small intestine. (Reproduced, with permission, from Mescher AL. *Junqueira's Basic Histology: Text & Atlas*. 16th ed. New York, NY: McGraw Hill; 2021, Fig. 15-22.)

DRUG ABSORPTION PATHWAYS

Once a drug is in solution, it has the potential to be absorbed. Whether it will be absorbed depends on its permeability, that is, whether its chemical characteristics allow it to permeate biological tissues. The biological environment of the drug also affects permeability to some extent. Does the environment change the drug to a form which cannot be absorbed, or which is absorbed very slowly? One of the most important aspects of the biological environment is its pH which has the potential to change certain drugs to a form which is poorly absorbed.

To enable absorption to occur, the drug must diffuse from the lumen of the gut through the intestinal fluids to the luminal surface of the GIT. If the drug can penetrate the intestinal membrane (actually several membranes) and appear unchanged (unmetabolized) in the blood vessels of the GIT, absorption is

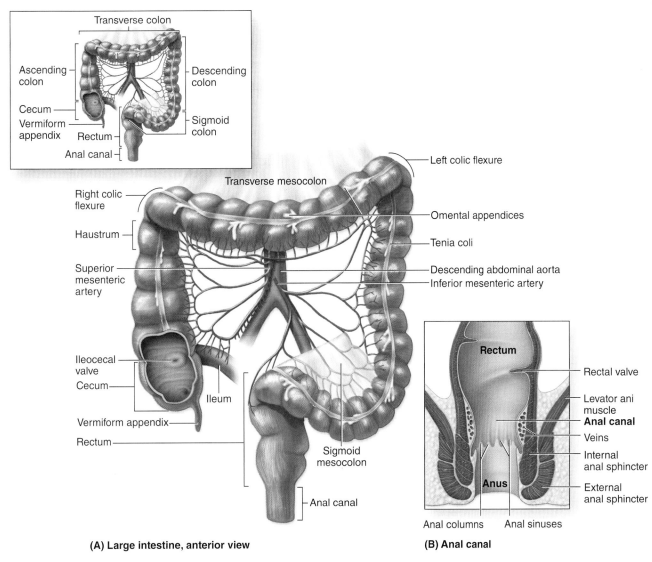

FIGURE 3-3 The large intestine. (Reproduced, with permission, from Mescher AL. *Junqueira's Basic Histology: Text & Atlas*. 16th ed. New York, NY: McGraw Hill; 2021, Fig. 15-31.)

said to have occurred. Consider a drug molecule which is in solution in the GIT. What transport steps must take place for this molecule to be transferred from the luminal fluid environment of the GIT to the interior of the blood vessels, that is, to be absorbed? It is actually a long and harrowing journey for the drug molecule, as denoted by the following steps in its transition:

I. Diffuse through the intestinal fluids.

II. Penetration of the mucus layer.

III. Permeation of the brush border of the enterocyte.

IV. Diffuse through the cytoplasm of the enterocyte.

V. Passage through the basal membrane of the enterocyte.

VI. Passage through the basement membrane.

VII. Passage through the connective tissue region of the lamina propria.

VIII. Passage through the external cell membrane of the capillary endothelial cell.

IX. Passage through the cytoplasm of the capillary cell.

X. Passage through the internal cell membrane of the capillary endothelial cell.

From the above, it is clear that the term "intestinal membrane," that is commonly used to describe the barrier to absorption, is a misnomer. What is meant is the above list of barriers. The term is so well accepted that its usage will be continued in this book, implying all of the above barriers.

Once a drug molecule has passed the lamina propria step (VII), there are two possibilities for absorption: the drug may pass into the blood capillary as noted above (the more general case) or it may pass into the central lacteal and reach the lymph. Most small molecule and lipid-soluble drugs can penetrate both lymph ducts and capillaries. However, drug absorption will, generally, proceed primarily through the blood circulation because blood flow to the GIT is approximately 500 to 1000 times greater than lymph flow. However, the capillary membrane is a barrier to very large molecules or molecular complexes. These substances may pass more easily into the central lacteal because of pores in some cells of the central lacteal wall. These pores or fenestrations allow the passage of large molecules or complexes. While capillaries also have fenestrations, they are significantly smaller. The lymphatic route is important for fats (such as tri-glycerides) and oils that are emulsified with bile salts to form large units known as chylomicrons. The latter may be as large as 0.5 μm which is gigantic by molecular standards.

Returning to the more common absorption mechanism through the blood vessels, the following fact regarding ter-minology should be noted. The drug that has passed into the blood vessels in the small intestine is the absorbed drug; it is not the bioavailable drug, that is, the drug available to the body for pharmacological action. This drug must first be transported to the liver, which is the main metabolizing organ of the body. It is only after passage through the liver, that the blood from the intestines is transferred to the general circulation and, via this system, to all parts of the body. The arrangement whereby blood from the GIT, carrying absorbed substances, passes first to the liver, is so designed to prevent toxic substances from entering the systemic circulation in large quantities. The liver has an early opportunity to rid the body of the toxic substance (includ-ing drugs which the body sees as foreign substances). This results in a portion of the drug being metabolized very soon after absorption and only a fraction of the absorbed drug reach-ing the systemic circulation. This fraction varies widely with the nature of the drug.

There are many factors that may affect drug absorption. These factors may be divided into the following categories: physicochemical factors, physiological factors, and dosage form factors (Mind Map 3-1). Attention is focused on the first two categories in this chapter. Dosage form factors will be dealt with in greater detail as each dosage form is discussed, in later chap-ters, while some outstanding factors will be briefly mentioned in this chapter.

PHYSICOCHEMICAL FACTORS

Oil/Water Partition Coefficient and Chemical Structure

Consider a drug in solution adjacent to a biological membrane. The biological membrane is a lipid bilayer and the cell surface is, therefore, lipid in nature. A drug in aqueous solution expe-riences attractive forces from the water molecules (to keep it in solution) and also from the adjacent lipid molecules of the cell membrane. The **balance** between the lipid attraction and the hydrophilic attraction of the water (hydrogen bonding) will determine the extent to which the drug leaves the water phase to dissolve in the lipid cell membrane. From the cell membrane, the drug could pass into the cytoplasm of the cell if it has the appro-priate hydrophilic-lipophilic balance. The relative balance of the two attractive forces is given by the partition coefficient ($K_{o/w}$).

For non-electrolytes that are not very small, lack of perme-ability depends to a large extent on the number of hydrogen bonds. The larger the number of hydrogen bonds, the greater the tendency to be attracted to water than to the lipid. The impor-tance of hydrogen bonding is strengthened by the following example. In a homologous series, it has been estimated that the members with a longer carbon chain length are more permeable not primarily due to an increase in lipid solubility but by the fact that the hydrocarbon chain is "pushed out" of the water due to a lack of hydrogen bonding. The impact of very small molecular size is given in the section on molecular weight and shape below.

pH and pKa

The non-ionic (unionized) form of a drug is more lipid soluble than the ionized form. The relative amounts of unionized and ion-ized drug will depend on the drug's pKa and the solution pH. This is referred to as the pH-partition hypothesis and is described by the Henderson-Hasselback equation. This theory is well recognized

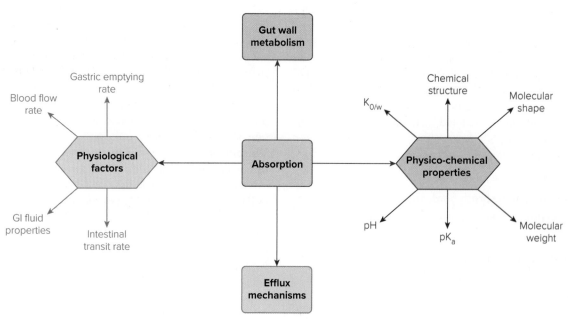

MIND MAP 3-1 Factors Affecting Drug Absorption

and is used daily around the globe. However, the pH partition hypothesis, although important, is only one factor in considering drug absorption and other factors may have a greater impact. For example, although the stomach may have a more favorable pH for the absorption of a particular drug (more of the drug will be in the unionized form), most drugs will be predominantly absorbed in the small intestine. This is because the small intestine is very well-designed for drug absorption due to its large surface area, relatively thin membrane, and high blood flow. In other words, the small intestine's structure is so well-designed for absorption that the structural advantage more than compensates for the smaller percentage of drug in the unionized form in the small intestine, relative to that in the stomach. The stomach also has a thick wall through which drugs, generally, permeate with difficulty.

Molecular Weight and Shape

The above discussion regarding partition coefficient and relative lipid solubility does not apply to very small, highly polar molecules or ions which are able to pass through the biological membrane. Small ions, such as Na^+ and K^+, easily permeate biological membranes, and many biochemical functions are dependent on the relatively rapid transfer of ions through a biological membrane. Since these molecules and ions are not lipid soluble, this behavior appears to contradict the general principle that a molecule is required to be somewhat hydrophobic for permeation of lipid membranes. This can be explained as follows.

Extremely small molecules that are very water soluble, including those in the charged form, pass through pores in the membrane. Urea is an example of a very water-soluble molecule (low $K_{o/w}$ value) that can easily pass through biological membranes. The substance is polar and extensively hydrogen-bonded and does not fit the description of permeable substances given above in "oil/water partition coefficient and chemical structure." However, it may, because of its small size, pass through the pores of membranes. The existence of actual physical pores, or holes in the membrane, has been debated as the charged species may simply be passing through much more polar regions of the membrane.

Another exception to the general rule given in "oil/water partition coefficient and chemical structure" is related to highly branched lipids. Some of these compounds do not permeate biological membranes in spite of a high $K_{o/w}$ value. This can be explained by the fact that the cell membrane is a highly organized structure with parallel orientation of the long chains of fatty acids of which it is made. The branched lipids would have to disrupt this structure in order to penetrate through the membrane. Straight-chain lipid materials, on the other hand, "slip through" the parallel hydrocarbon chains more easily.

PHYSIOLOGICAL FACTORS AFFECTING DRUG ABSORPTION

Components and Properties of Gastrointestinal Fluids

Since the gastrointestinal (GI) fluids are the medium in which a dosage form is presented to the GIT, the properties of these fluids are very important with regard to the fate of the dosage form

and the drug. Ultimately, the nature and properties of these fluids also have an impact on drug absorption. An example of a dosage form effect is the influence of the GI fluids on the disintegration and dissolution of a tablet. Since these processes are preliminary steps to drug absorption, the nature and properties of the GI fluids could affect the rate and extent of absorption. An effect of the GI fluids on the drug is demonstrated by the potentially negative effect of these fluids on the stability of the dissolved drug. Extensive degradation, obviously, limits the amount of drug available for absorption. Thus, a lower amount of absorbed drug may largely be due to the extent of degradation of the drug in the GI fluids. This is a commonly encountered problem.

An important property of GI fluids is their pH which varies considerably along the length of the GIT. The gastric fluids are highly acidic, ranging in pH from 1 to 3.5, when measured in subjects with an empty stomach, and when the test is conducted under normal circumstances. There may be considerable variation in these values, depending on the general health of the subject, her age, and the presence of GI diseases. The gastric fluid appears to be more acidic at night and fluctuates throughout the day, primarily in response to food ingestion. The pH increases after eating and then slowly decreases during the next several hours. The pH range, during the day, is approximately 1 to 5, largely due to the absence, or the presence, of food.

There is an abrupt change in pH in the duodenum. Pancreatic secretions of 200 to 800 mL/day, which have a high concentration of bicarbonate, which is basic, rapidly neutralize the gastric fluid entering the duodenum. This neutralization is important for the following reasons:

1. Protection of the intestinal epithelium since it does not have the stomach's thick mucus coating to protect the underlying cells from damage by acid.

2. To prevent inactivation of the pancreatic enzymes

3. To prevent precipitation of bile acids which are poorly soluble in acidic media

The pH of the intestinal contents gradually increases with distance from the stomach. The pH is approximately 5.7 at the pyloric valve whereas it is approximately 7.7 at the proximal jejunum. The fluid in the large intestine has a pH between 7 and 8.

Since the rate of dissolution is affected by pH (as mentioned), the part of the GIT where a dosage form is located, as it releases the drug, affects the rate at which the drug dissolves, and at which it is subsequently absorbed. Acidic drugs will dissolve more readily in the less acidic/slightly basic contents of the small intestine. In the solution state in this part of the GIT, the drug will be present in both ionized and unionized forms, with an equilibrium between the two species. The relative proportion of each are dependent on the pKa of the drug and the pH of the medium. The unionized form of the drug is generally absorbed faster. Therefore, for fastest absorption, the ideal pH of the biological medium is the one that provides the highest proportion of the unionized form.

Basic drugs will dissolve in the acidic contents of the stomach more rapidly. Again, the drug in solution will be present in the unionized and ionized forms with the unionized portion being more absorbable. Due to the thickness of the stomach wall, however, only a small portion of the unionized form will be absorbed in the stomach. The major portion of the drug in solution will usually pass into the small intestine for absorption. In the small intestine, a portion of the drug will be converted to the free base (unionized), since the pH is higher than that in the stomach. The extent of conversion, again, is dependent on the pH of the medium and the pKa of the drug, as reflected by the Henderson-Hasselback equation. The unionized drug will be efficiently absorbed.

It is worth noting that a basic drug, presented to the small intestines for dissolution, will have a slower dissolution rate than it would in the stomach. (A basic drug will dissolve faster in an acidic medium.) Such a situation will arise if the basic drug is formulated as an enteric-coated tablet. The reason for coating such a drug may be the fact that the drug is irritating to the stomach, or that it is degraded more rapidly in an acidic medium. In addition to dissolution, the disintegration rate may be affected by the pH of the solution. Some disintegrants work better in an acidic environment.

If drug release from a dosage form is a necessary step for absorption, does it follow that the faster the drug is released the better the absorption? This is not always true since fast dissolution may lead to fast degradation of a drug that is not stable in the fluid into which it is released (eg, gastric fluid at low pH). In such a case, slower dissolution may lead to less degradation and, therefore, more drug absorbed. In the case of erythromycin, fast dissolution in the stomach leads to fast degradation. The esters of erythromycin that are usually used (eg, erythromycin estolate and stearate) do not dissolve appreciably in the stomach and, therefore, degradation is limited. When the undissolved erythromycin ester passes into the small intestine, the drug dissolves in the less acidic fluid and is absorbed there more efficiently.

Physiological components of the GIT may increase or decrease drug absorption, in addition to their normal function. The bile emulsifies fats and oils, present in the food, and helps digestion. Increased absorption of a drug after a fatty meal is often the result of bile being secreted in response to the meal. The bile salts, present in the bile, are highly surface active agents. They increase the dissolution rate of many poorly soluble compounds. This leads to faster absorption of such compounds, including the drug taken by the patient. In addition, enzymes which are present in the small intestine to help to digest food may also have a beneficial effect on drug delivery. For example, pancreatic enzymes hydrolyze chloramphenicol palmitate, enabling the free chloramphenicol to be absorbed.

On the other hand, bile salts may form insoluble complexes with certain drugs, for example, neomycin and kanamycin, and thus retard absorption. In addition, mucin may bind with certain quaternary ammonium compounds to reduce, or prevent, absorption. The mucin, as a viscous layer coating the stomach, also presents a barrier to drug diffusion through the membrane.

Cocaine is administered to humans in small doses for medicinal, or recreational, purposes. It is well known that it is not absorbed through the GIT and is not administered by this route. The lack of absorption is due to esterase activity. The latter are enzymes that hydrolyze ester bonds. In the case of cocaine,

the esterase action in the gut renders the drug inactive. For this reason, cocaine is administered by other routes such as intravenous injection or nasal administration However, if a very large dose is taken, the esterase enzymes are overwhelmed and do not hydrolyze a large part of the dose, with disastrous results for the subject. This may occur when a bag of cocaine, swallowed for concealment, bursts and releases a large dose of the drug into the GIT, often with fatal consequences for the drug courier.

Gastric Emptying

As mentioned above, the small intestine is the major organ for absorption of drugs. Even when the drug's pKa implies that a drug should be preferentially absorbed in the stomach, it will, frequently, be mostly absorbed in the small intestine. This is due to the latter's functional adaptation for absorption. It stands to reason, therefore, that a delay in the drug reaching the small intestine, for any reason, will manifest itself as a delay in drug absorption. Since the drug must pass from the stomach to the small intestine, a delay in stomach emptying (with a few exceptions) represents a delay in the arrival of the drug at its major absorptive site and, hence, a delay in absorption. The contents of the stomach are, largely, separated from the small intestine by a closed pyloric valve. Except for small amounts of liquid that may pass through the valve, the major portion of the transfer of the contents of the stomach into the small intestine, happens as a result of a deliberate process referred to as gastric, or stomach, emptying.

What factors delay stomach emptying? Since this question is fundamental to an understanding of drug absorption, the process of stomach emptying is briefly reviewed before going on to describe the factors affecting gastric emptying, and their consequences on drug absorption in different situations.

Emptying of the Full Stomach

Emptying is different in the full stomach compared to the empty stomach. After a meal, the ingested food is mixed with gastric secretions by means of contractions originating in the antrum. Non-viscous fluid flows into the antrum for this purpose, passing around any solid mass. This mixing action has the effect of liquifying the gastric contents, since larger particles are broken down to smaller ones and mixed with the liquid contents to form a slurry. Once a considerable portion of the gastric contents has become sufficiently liquid, to pass through the pylorus, gastric emptying begins. A specific set of events occurs to cause gastric emptying. Peristaltic waves begin in the fundus, travel down the stomach, and become more intense near the pylorus. The antrum contracts, propelling material forward, while the pyloric sphincter is relaxed. Then, the pyloric sphincter contracts and the proximal duodenum relaxes. This sequence of events causes fluid to move into the duodenum. A moment later, the antrum relaxes and the duodenum regains its tone. When this happens, the pyloric sphincter remains contracted to prevent regurgitation, while the contents of the duodenum are propelled forward.

Several factors can affect the rate of stomach emptying: a large meal hastens stomach emptying due to the fact that the stomach is distended. Distension is a trigger causing faster stomach emptying. Fat in the meal is a potent factor to delay stomach emptying; the delay can be as long as 3 to 6 hours. The presence of certain nutrients (such as sugar), high osmotic pressure, and acids delay stomach emptying. In addition, viscous stomach contents and depression delay stomach emptying as does the simple act of lying on the left side of the body. Conversely, anxiety and stress increase the emptying rate. On the other hand, certain drugs delay, while others speed up, stomach emptying. These drugs thus have an effect on the bioavailability of other drugs that may be consumed at about the same time. Anticholinergics and narcotic analgesics reduce emptying rate, while metoclopramide increases this rate.

Emptying of the Empty Stomach

When the stomach is empty, except for a small amount of residual food material, the situation is quite different. The stomach and small intestines experience a sequence of events referred to as the inter-digestive migrating motor complex (MMC). This is a series of contractions (propulsive movements) starting at the top of the stomach and ending at the distal portion of the ileum. These events can be divided into four stages:

Stage 1: There is minimal muscular (contractile) activity during this phase which lasts about 1 hour.

Stage 2: This stage lasts 20 to 45 minutes and is characterized by irregular contractions that gradually increase in strength. These uncoordinated contractions do not lead to effective propulsion of residual stomach contents.

Stage 3: This stage only lasts 5 to 15 minutes but there are intense peristaltic waves (starting at the top of the stomach and progressing downwards), resulting in the emptying of the remaining gastric contents into the small intestine. This phase is referred to as the "housekeeper" wave.

Stage 4: The fourth phase consists of decreasing peristaltic activity, leading to the first phase once again.

As long as the stomach is empty, it and the small intestine will experience this series of repetitive wave actions at regular intervals, for example, every 2 hours. This means that if a subject does not eat for a prolonged period and the stomach is empty for 10 hours, the above sequence of events will be repeated five times in that period.

Non-viscous liquids leave the stomach freely without consideration of the stomach emptying rate. Therefore, such liquids and low viscosity liquid drugs, such as aqueous solutions, will pass freely into the small intestine and not be held up by a delay in stomach emptying. Particles 2 mm in diameter or smaller, in general, will also leave the stomach unhindered. While very large particles, such as 10-mm-diameter non-disintegrating tablets, will not be able to leave the stomach until the housekeeper wave sweeps them away, particles of intermediate size may leave at a slower rate. The size of particles that may leave during this phase (albeit at a slower rate) is determined in each individual by the size of the pylorus (diameter) and the strength of the propulsive force.

For these reasons, many newer dosage forms are developed as multiparticulates, for example, beads in a capsule. As long as the beads are less than 2 mm in diameter they will empty from the stomach freely (like liquids). Their passage to the small intestine, the release of the drug in that part of the GIT, and subsequent absorption will not be compromised by a delay in stomach emptying. Such beads are frequently enteric coated, that is, they are coated with a material that does not dissolve in the acidic contents of the stomach but will dissolve in the less acidic to basic contents of the small intestine. This application is used if the drug is irritating to the stomach, or if it will be destroyed by the acidity of the stomach contents. Due to the insoluble coating material, the drug is not released from the beads in the short time that they are in the stomach. Obviously, this factor is of more significance, the larger the size of the beads or if a small tablet is considered. If the latter is not enteric coated, the drug will be released in the stomach, especially if stomach emptying is delayed. If the drug is soluble in the acidic medium, a drug solution will form in the stomach. This solution will flow through the pyloric sphincter into the small intestine. If drug degradation or stomach irritation is possible in the acidic stomach contents, these processes will occur until the solution passes into the small intestine.

If the drug is poorly soluble in the acidic medium, very little would be released in the stomach from a non-coated, non-disintegrating dosage form. If the poorly soluble drug is in a disintegrating dosage form, such as a disintegrating tablet, the drug powder or small granules, resulting from disintegration, will pass through the pyloric sphincter.

The efficient absorption of the drug from larger enteric-coated tablets might be a problem as these tablets will remain whole (undisintegrated) in the stomach. They will not pass into the intestines until the stomach is empty and the housekeeper wave passes over the stomach. Frequently, there will be variation in the patient's food intake and the regularity of meal times. Therefore, the time taken after consumption of the medication for the housekeeper wave to transport the enteric-coated tablet into the small intestine will not be the same each day.

Intestinal Transit

The main function of the small intestine is the absorption of nutrients. It does this through its well-developed absorptive capacity and pharmaceutical scientists have taken advantage of this capacity for the delivery of drugs. Absorption occurs as the food material passes through the small intestine. The material passes along due to propulsive movements of the small intestine, known as peristalsis. Peristalsis increases after a meal as a result of the gastroenteric reflex initiated by the distension of the stomach. The average transit time reported in the literature for tablets and pellets moving through the small intestine is about 3 hours with a range of about 1 to 6 hours. The physical nature of the material in the small intestine (liquid or solid; large or small particles) does not affect the rate of passage of the material through the small intestine. In general, the transit times through the small intestine do not vary greatly, and stomach emptying rate remains the major variable. Nevertheless, variation in transit time is possible for various reasons, including the administration of drugs that either increase or decrease transit time. The effects of variation in the transit time will now be discussed.

Since the small intestine is the primary site for drug absorption, the longer the drug remains in this area, the more complete the drug absorption, provided the drug is stable in the intestinal environment and does not complex with any other material present. A longer transit time is particularly desirable for drugs that dissolve slowly (if they are not already dissolved when they reach the small intestine) and for sustained-release products. If the tablet reaches the small intestine whole and must first disintegrate before dissolution and absorption can occur, a longer time is desirable, generally, to allow for these additional steps. Metoclopramide increases the stomach emptying rate as well as the intestinal transit time which will have opposite effects on drug delivery: speeding up stomach emptying rate enhances drug absorption since the drug reaches the primary absorption site sooner. Faster movement through the small intestine, on the other hand, reduces the time available for absorption in the preferred absorption area and may retard overall absorption. If the drug is very rapidly absorbed, the shorter transit time may not have any impact on the extent of absorption.

Intestinal transit time is also very important for drugs that can only be absorbed from a small segment of the small intestine. The segment from which absorption is possible is referred to as the absorption window. If the transit time is too fast the drug may pass the absorption window. Riboflavin is absorbed from an absorption window in the proximal duodenum only. If the drug passes this part of the small intestine, it will not be absorbed at all. For, this reason, it is best to administer substances like riboflavin in several small doses, to increase the probability of a significant portion of the total dose being absorbed.

There are also mixing movements in the small intestine. Segments contract while others remain relaxed, the net appearance being similar to a chain of sausages. The mixing movements mix intestinal contents with secretions several times a minute. The mixing movements are also important for absorption since the absorbing membrane is exposed to fresh contents repeatedly. In addition, the contracting muscle layers produce folds which increase the surface area. The villi also contract during this process, resulting in milking of the central lacteal. Mixing motions may also be influential in bringing about disintegration and dissolution of a dosage form.

This poses a problem for the administration of sustained-release medication, especially dosage forms to be administered every 24 hours. If the transit through the small intestine is so rapid, the administered medication would reach the colon long before the 24-hour period ends, and the colon is not well adapted for drug absorption. To achieve once-a-day dosing for a sustained-release medication, pharmaceutical scientists have proposed engineering the formulation for a longer residence time in the stomach (assuming the drug is not destroyed by the acid). A second option is to modify the formulation to achieve absorption in the colon.

Blood Flow

Drug molecules that are absorbed, that is, reach the bloodstream, will be quickly carried away by the flow of blood. If this were not the case, their presence would impede the continued absorption of drug molecules, keeping in mind the fact that molecules diffuse from a region of high concentration to one of lower concentration. When a large concentration difference exists between the donor region and the receiver region,

"sink" conditions are said to be maintained. This occurs when the concentration of the diffusing molecules is zero, or very low, in the receiver compartment or vessel, with a high concentration in the donor compartment or vessel. Blood flow to the GIT is extensive and so fast that the absorbed drug is cleared from the absorption site immediately. Thus, perfect sink conditions are usually maintained. Hence, blood flow is ordinarily not a rate-limiting factor for drug absorption. One exception is in cases of cardiac failure where there is pooling of blood in certain parts of the body. Under these circumstances, it is possible that blood flow to the GIT becomes sufficiently slow that it decreases absorption.

Recap Questions

1. Will a basic drug with a pKa of 8 be unionized to a greater extent in a fluid of pH 7 or a fluid of pH 2? (If you cannot easily answer this question, please review the application of the Henderson-Hasselbach equation in a chemistry textbook or online.)
2. Why are bile acids poorly soluble at an acidic pH?
3. Pharmaceutical scientists place much emphasis on stomach emptying rate. Why is this factor given more consideration, in general, than intestinal transit time or the rate of blood flow to the GIT?
4. Explain why beads do not cause a delay in drug absorption, in the small intestine, even if stomach emptying is delayed.

MECHANISMS OF DRUG ABSORPTION

A drug that is in solution in the lumen of the GIT must pass through the GI membranes, typically the wall of the small intestine, to reach the blood vessels for absorption (as mentioned in the drug absorption pathways section of this chapter). There are two major mechanisms of drug absorption through the GI membranes. These are as follows:

1. Passive absorption in which absorption occurs by diffusion in observance of physical laws and without the active participation of the cell membrane or expenditure of energy.
2. Active absorption is an absorption process where the membrane participates in the process and there is the expenditure of energy.

Most drugs are absorbed by passive absorption. The driving force for this type of absorption is the concentration gradient, or the activity gradient, and is described by Fick's first law. In terms of this law, the rate of absorption is proportional to the concentration of the drug in the donor compartment, or donor area, minus the concentration in the receiver compartment, or receiver area. In most practical GI absorption situations, the rate of absorption is proportional to the concentration in the GI fluids only. This is because the concentration of the drug in the blood, at the site of absorption, is very low (in comparison to the concentration in the GI fluids). Hence, the former can is considered essentially zero and need not be taken into account.

There are two major routes by which the drug may enter the tissue: the transcellular route (through the cells) and the paracellular route (between the cells). Most drugs use the transcellular route (drugs with a $K_{o/w}$ value between 1 and 5). Small polar molecules ($K_{o/w}$ < 1) may pass through pores or gap junctions. The latter is the space, or channel, between cells through which small molecules may pass. The cells form a tight junction near the luminal surface (the surface facing the lumen). For the paracellular route, in which drugs pass around the cells, the molecular weight should not be greater than about 500 Da.

For essential nutrients (monosaccharides, amino acids, and vitamins), there are special absorption processes involving the cell membrane. In the absence of these processes such molecules would be poorly absorbed. Some drugs may share these mechanisms, for example, L-dopa uses the route for amino acids. For this reason, L-dopa absorption after a protein-rich meal may be depressed. The absorption of amoxicillin and cefixime, both amino acid derivatives of antibiotics, is linked to cellular amino acid or peptide transporters.

EFFLUX MECHANISMS

In contrast to transporters (such as amino acid transporters) which help some drugs to be absorbed, there are also efflux transport systems that take absorbed molecules out of the cell. They function to reduce absorption. This mechanism exists in numerous epithelial cells including in the GIT. P-glycoprotein (P-gp) is a cell surface glycoprotein which is partially within the cell. It is responsible for this action. It attaches to the drug molecule and escorts it out of the cell into the lumen of the GIT (much like a "bouncer" at a nightclub). This action reduces the amount of drug absorbed into cells and the mechanism affects many drugs and drug classes. Furthermore, P-gp may be induced by another drug that is co-administered. Induction involves increased production of P-gp and hence the drug of interest will be escorted out of the cell to a greater extent. Inducers include rifampicin and St. John's wort. Suppose a patient was taking a drug and the physician had titrated the dose until the patient's symptoms were controlled with little side effects. The patient then decided to take St. John's wort as a supplement to treat mild depression. After some time, the induction of P-gp by the supplement may be sufficient to increase efflux of the prescribed drug to an extent that symptoms of the treated condition became apparent, that is, the amount of the absorbed prescription drug is too little to treat the condition adequately.

Conversely, P-gp can be inhibited by other substances co-administered. In this case, the lower production of P-gp results in less of the drug of interest being removed from the cell. This results in an apparently greater bioavailability of the drug. The commonly used antibiotics, clarithromycin and erythromycin, can inhibit P-gp. The HIV drug, ritonavir, and the antihypertensive, verapamil, are also inhibitors. Consider a patient who was stabilized on a drug which is subject to the action of P-gp. In spite of P-gp causing less of the drug to be absorbed, the patient's dosage was such that it accounted for this loss and, thus, the patient was receiving an appropriate dose of the drug. If the physician then added erythromycin for a respiratory tract infection, the latter would inhibit P-gp and more of the first drug would be absorbed, potentially leading to side effects.

The inhibition or induction of P-gp is the mechanism for many drug interactions. Different from inhibition or induction is the situation where P-gp is able to act on two drugs that are co-administered. The efflux mechanism may become saturated by the larger number of drug molecules present. This results in P-gp escorting a smaller amount of each drug out of the cell. When this happens, more drug is absorbed, and the level of each drug in the blood may be higher than if either drug were administered alone. In such a situation, side effects may be more pronounced.

METABOLISM

Intestinal cells contain many metabolizing enzymes, especially those responsible for Phase I oxidative metabolic reactions (the Cytochrome P450 family; CYP450). These enzymes are also present in the liver where they very effectively metabolize drugs. Here, the gut wall metabolism is emphasized in this description of absorption through the GIT. The most important of these enzymes is CYP3A4 which is less selective of the substrate and can metabolize many drugs. Again, if one considers induction or inhibition of this enzyme by other drugs, this mechanism is responsible for many drug interactions. In addition, administration of more than one drug that is metabolized by the same enzyme can also lead to reduced drug metabolism, and higher blood levels of the drug, since the enzyme would now have multiple substrates.

CYP3A4 and P-gp are found at the same locations, even within the same cells, and they often (not always) work on the same substrates. They appear to work in concert: the efflux caused by P-gp results in the drug molecules potentially entering the cells multiple times, with repeat opportunities for metabolism by CYP enzymes. Hence, it is usually difficult to say which of these two mechanisms, efflux or intestinal metabolism, has the greater effect on decreasing drug absorption.

Recap Questions

1. How does active transport differ from passive transport?
2. What is meant by "efflux"?
3. How do metabolic enzymes lead to drug interactions?

SUMMARY POINTS

- The GIT is designed for digestion of food and the effective absorption of nutrients but this system can be utilized for drug absorption as well.

- The following factors affect the absorption and stability of ingested drugs:
  - The fluid environment in different parts of the GIT
  - The way in which food material is transported through different sections of the GIT
- Mechanisms to eliminate foreign chemicals co-ingested with food, which are protective in nature, may reduce drug absorption significantly. These consist of gut wall metabolism, gut efflux mechanisms, and hepatic circulation and metabolism.
- The physicochemical properties of the drug influence its stability and potential for effective absorption in the GIT; there is also an interplay between these factors and the environment in different parts of the GIT.

What do you think?

1. Draw the structures of glyceryl tristearate and oleic acid. Below these structures, draw the basic structure of a lipid bilayer (biological membrane). From your observations, which of these molecules would pass through the membrane more easily? Give reasons for your answer.

2. Drug A and Drug B are each administered as 12-mm diameter, non-disintegrating tablets and they are equivalent pharmacologically. Both drugs dissolve rapidly, and are stable, in intestinal fluid. Drug A takes 6 hours to dissolve in gastric fluid in which it is stable. Drug B dissolves in 30 minutes in gastric fluid and degrades in this medium at the rate of 5% in 24 hours. Both drugs are rapidly absorbed in the small intestine and rapid onset of the pharmacological action is desired.

   If gastric emptying is delayed, which treatment is the better option?

3. Metoclopramide hastens stomach emptying and increases the rate of intestinal transit. What is the effect of co-administration of metoclopramide on the absorption of the following?

   a. Riboflavin which has a very small absorption window in the proximal duodenum

   b. Drug X which is administered as a 10-mm enteric-coated tablet, if X is rapidly and completely absorbed in the small intestine

Pharmaceutical Solutions, Dissolution, and Diffusion

4

PREVIEW

- Know the principal strategies used to formulate a pharmaceutical solution
- Know the major excipient types incorporated into solutions
- Develop a basic knowledge of the compounding of solutions
- Develop a basic understanding of the concepts of dissolution and diffusion
- Distinguish between rate of solution and solubility
- Distinguish disintegration from dissolution
- Understand the relationship between dissolution and bioavailability
- Understand the physical events involved in converting two components, a drug and a solvent, into a solution

INTRODUCTION

As a practical matter, a drug substance as a single entity cannot be directly consumed by the patient in most instances. A dosage form, in which the drug is combined with other ingredients, has to be prepared. For example, tablets and capsules are solid dosage forms, and solutions, suspensions, and emulsions are liquid-dosage forms. In these dosage forms, the drug is combined with several other ingredients to provide a unit that is easier to consume, has the correct amount of the drug, and, frequently, contains other components, or excipients, which confer additional desirable attributes to the dosage form. The pharmaceutical solution is one of the simplest dosage forms in pharmaceutical practice. All the components are already in solution. This has a tremendous advantage since the drug is in a form that is absorbable. For practically all drugs, the drug has to be in aqueous solution before it can be absorbed, that is, the solid drug in a tablet or a capsule must first dissolve to enable absorption. Dissolution is more complex than it appears at first sight and involves several steps which will be discussed in more detail later in this chapter. When a solution dosage form is administered, there is the elimination of the steps involved with transmuting a drug from the solid state into the solution state, for absorption. Considering the above, it may be appropriate to start our discussions on pharmaceutical dosage forms with this chapter on solutions.

The process of a drug going into solution has already been alluded to. It is an important physical event that affects most dosage forms once taken, in that the drugs they contain must go into solution before the drug can be absorbed and any pharmacological action can take place. To gain an appreciation of drug action, especially its rate, it is important to understand the process of a drug going into solution. What actually occurs when something "goes into solution"? From such an understanding, the factors that affect this process can be discerned. This would help to answer the question: what is the rate of solution and how can it be increased? In addition, a pharmacist may have to produce solutions in the course of compounding. It is important that the pharmacist understand this common process that she may utilize daily.

The United States Pharmacopoeia (USP) defines solutions as "liquid preparations that contain one or more chemical substances dissolved in a suitable solvent or mixture of mutually miscible solvents." This definition implies that a single drug dissolved in the single solvent may constitute a pharmaceutical solution, and such solutions do exist. In practice, however, most solutions contain other ingredients and a pharmaceutical solution, used as a dosage form, differs from a solution used in chemistry. If a weighed amount of a chemical substance is stirred with a fixed amount of water, this may produce a chemical solution. If the substance is a drug, the solution may have to be sweetened, thickened, flavored, and preserved before it can be used in the context of a pharmaceutical dosage form. In other instances, it may have to be made sterile and pyrogen free.

Generally, the stability of the pharmaceutical solution must be good. This includes the requirements of adequate drug potency, no microbial growth, and no unacceptable physical changes for an extended time, usually 2 years or more for oral solutions. Examples of physical changes that may occur in solutions include color changes, development of an off-odor, and changes in viscosity. For these reasons, a pharmaceutical solution dosage form differs from a simple chemical solution. When pharmaceutical solution dosage forms are discussed in this chapter, the emphasis will be on oral solutions. Solutions for delivery via alternative routes of drug administration will be mentioned in the chapters dealing with these routes.

There are some special terms used to describe pharmaceutical solutions:

1. Syrups are aqueous solutions that contain a high amount of sugar, usually sufficient to increase the viscosity of the solution.
2. An elixir is a solution of a drug in water and alcohol (ie, a hydroalcoholic mixture) that is sweetened.
3. A tincture is a hydroalcoholic extract from natural materials, such as plant leaves, containing a high alcohol concentration (about 50%, or even more). A tincture may also refer to a solution of a pure chemical in a hydroalcoholic mixture, for example, tincture of iodine.
4. A fluid extract is similar to a tincture but the concentration of *extracted materials* is much higher.

Recap Questions

1. What are the practical difficulties involved with a patient consuming 2 mg of drug on a dosage regimen of three times a day for 30 days if the drug is not constituted as a pharmaceutical dosage form?
2. Name three types of pharmaceutical dosage forms that are solutions. (Hint: capsules and tablets are two types of solid dosage forms.)
3. Name the factors that are important when considering the stability of solutions.

COMPONENTS OF A PHARMACEUTICAL SOLUTION

The components of a solution, or the ingredients, are the drug and the excipients. The latter two terms need to be explained, and their difference clarified, as they are frequently confused. Ingredients are all components that go into a formulation, and this includes the drug. Excipients are the additional ingredients, apart from the drug, that are incorporated into a formulation to make a suitable pharmaceutical dosage form, in this case a solution. It is important to remember that every non-drug ingredient in a formulation is included in the descriptive term, "excipient." For example, the water in a solution is considered an excipient (in the sub-category, "solvent").

The Drug

Drug solubility and stability are the fundamental properties of importance to the process of formulating a good, pharmaceutically elegant solution. Indeed, if the drug is insoluble or unstable in aqueous solution, an oral solution may not be able to be formulated. In such a case, an alternative preparation needs to be formulated. In the case of poor solubility, a suspension or solid dosage form is likely to be considered. In the case of instability in an aqueous medium, it is likely that a solid dosage form, such as a capsule or tablet, will be formulated.

The formulator, having ascertained that insolubility or instability will not be a limiting factor, still has to obtain solubility information to assess whether the drug in the formulation will dissolve in the intended volume of solvent (usually water for oral solutions). Qualitative descriptions of solubility with their quantitative ranges as described in the USP are given in Table 4-1. The pharmacist is often required to convert from one system of expression to another. For example, a concentration of 1:50 may also be expressed as 2%. Such interconversions are covered in calculations textbooks and courses and will not be dealt with further here.

The Solvent

Water is a good solvent for many drugs, it is cheap and easily available. However, it displays poor solubility for many other

TABLE 4-1	USP Descriptions of Solubility
DESCRIPTIVE TERM	PARTS OF THE SOLVENT REQUIRED PER PART OF SOLUTE
Very soluble	Less than 1
Freely soluble	From 1 to 10
Soluble	From 10 to 30
Sparingly soluble	From 30 to 100
Slightly soluble	From 100 to 1000
Very slightly soluble	From 1000 to 10,000
Practically insoluble	10,000 and over

drugs, especially if they are somewhat hydrophobic. For oral solutions, water is the solvent of choice due to the toxicity of many organic solvents.

Major considerations in relation to an aqueous solvent are the following:

1. Will the amount of drug in the formulation be completely dissolved in the intended volume of solvent?

2. Will the volume of the solvent, and consequentially also the volume of an individual dose, need to be increased to accommodate the drug quantity?

3. Alternatively, should a cosolvent be added?

4. Can it reasonably be expected that the drug will stay dissolved throughout the shelf life of the product?

A cosolvent can be considered a secondary solvent incorporated to improve the solubility of the solvent mixture. Frequently, a solvent and cosolvent have a synergistic effect so that the solubility is more than the combined solubilities of each solvent. If a solution contains close to the maximum amount of drug that the solvent is able to accommodate, then physical changes that may occur during storage of the product, for the duration of its shelf life, may cause the drug to precipitate out of solution. This may result in the patients consuming less than the prescribed dose of the drug.

The shelf life is the period, after manufacture, that the product can be stored, during which there is a reasonable assurance of stability of the product. In the US, the FDA assigns the shelf life, based on stability data that the company collects (see Chapter 15, Dosage Form Stability). Suppose that the solubility of a drug is 100 mg per 5 mL of solution (for a particular solvent) and a compounding pharmacy prepares a solution with 1.9 g of drug per 100 mL. This quantity of drug is close to the solubility limit for the volume of solvent. If mixing of the solution, during preparation, was not sufficiently long, it is possible that some trace of drug remains undissolved. This is not an ideal situation since, during storage, the presence of even a few crystals may act as seeds for drug precipitation. Since the precipitated drug would not be included in the dose poured out of the bottle, the patient would receive a lower dose. Also, most stated solubility values are relevant for a specific temperature. If conditions during storage change, and the product experiences

a cold environment for sufficiently long, some of the drug may precipitate with the consequences mentioned above. A key factor in formulating solutions is, therefore, not to work close to the solubility limit.

If the solubility of the drug needs to be improved, to avoid drug precipitation during storage, then additional, water-miscible solvents are added in small quantities. If the drug does not dissolve completely in a convenient volume of water, for example, 5 mL, some of the water may be replaced by a suitable organic solvent to avoid having to increase the dose volume to 7 mL, for example, if only water was used. Frequently, such aqueous systems offer sufficient solubility without side effects to the patient. When formulating solutions for external use, a greater range, and percentage, of organic solvents may be used due to the reduced toxicity. Solvents for external use include isopropanol or ethanol, typically used as solvent systems with water. In other cases, an oily solution may be used externally.

For oral solutions, which is the main focus of the formulation approaches described in this chapter, an organic solvent may partially replace water in the solution. However, care should be taken when selecting organic solvents due to the fact that they may be toxic. If they can be used, they are used in very small quantities, typically. An additional factor to take into consideration is that the solvent usually affects other properties of the formulation, such as taste, viscosity, and clarity. Consideration of these formulation properties may, additionally, limit the quantity that can be used. For example, glycerin has a warm, cloying taste. A positive consideration is the fact that this solvent may improve resistance to microbial growth. Alcohol and glycerin are two solvents having this effect. Therefore, such solvents may be considered part of the preservative system, in addition to helping to dissolve certain components.

The choice of solvents in a mixed solvent system is critical to the quality of the solution. Commonly used organic solvents in pharmaceuticals are ethanol, glycerin, polyethylene glycol, and propylene glycol. These solvents are miscible with water. It is obvious, from the foregoing, that the solvents must dissolve the drug completely, but frequently the solubility of other ingredients, such as flavor oils and preservatives, must also be considered. Flavor oils are used in very small quantities but they are not water soluble. If formulated without taking their solubility into consideration, the oil will simply float on the top of the solution as a thin layer. Thus, initial doses may have a very high-flavor oil content and a correspondingly potent taste. In addition, certain ingredients, such as the preservative, may migrate to the oil, since the preservative's solubility is higher in the oil. Therefore, such ingredients would also be removed from the bulk solution to the surface of the solution. A result could be the consequent microbial deterioration of the dosage form.

Since the quality of all ingredients in a pharmaceutical product must be carefully controlled, the quality of the water used to make a solution must also be controlled. In a pharmaceutical company, there are several tests performed on the water to be used in pharmaceutical formulations. Only if these tests are passed, can the water be used in such formulations. In a dispensing pharmacy, it is impractical to perform these tests on water. Instead, Purified Water, USP is suitable for making solutions. The term "USP" stated after the name of an ingredient or product denotes that it conforms to the standards mentioned in the United States Pharmacopoeia. This informs one that the ingredient or product is of a high quality. The tests listed in the USP monograph for the product have been performed by the manufacturer to confirm quality and purity.

The above discussion focuses on adding other solvents to water (for oral medications) to create an improved solvent system for the drug. Another useful approach—when the drug is an acidic, or a basic, salt—is to alter the pH of the system. As one can deduce from the Henderson-Hasselbach equation, basic salts will be ionized to a greater extent in an acidic medium. Analogously, acidic salts will be more ionized in a basic medium. Since the ionic species of a compound is more soluble, one can improve the solubility of these compounds by making the solution acidic, or basic, respectively, for basic salts and acidic salts of drugs. This helps to prevent precipitation in the container during storage. For example, alkaloids (which are basic) are prepared as solutions in a weakly acidic medium.

Buffers are solutions that have a specific pH and also contain other component(s) that result in the solution being able to resist change in pH. Buffers usually contain two compounds, known as the buffer pair. For example, citric acid and sodium citrate are a buffer pair that, in solution, resist change in pH upon the addition of small quantities of acid or base. Buffers are commonly used in the preparation of eye drops and injections. The USP contains several formulations for buffers, each having a specific pH range of utility. Examples of USP buffers are given in Table 4-2 with their range of pH values. It is not intended that one buffer covers this range. For each buffer type, the USP gives a table of formulas to obtain several buffers within this range. For example, the hydrochloric acid buffer has formulas for a buffer of pH 1.2, and by varying the quantities of the components one may obtain a buffer of pH 1.4, or 1.6, up to pH 2.2. Hence, one may choose a buffer system according to the pH requirement of the preparation to be made. The pharmacist may prepare such a buffer in his compounding pharmacy, as needed. He may also purchase a range of buffers to have on hand for

TABLE 4-2	USP Standard Buffers
BUFFER	**pH RANGE**
Hydrochloric acid buffer	1.2 – 2.2
Acid phthalate buffer	2.2 – 4.0
Acetate buffer	4.1 – 5.5
Neutralized phthalate buffer	4.2 – 5.8
Phosphate buffer	5.8 – 8.0
Alkaline borate buffer	8.0 – 10.0

quicker compounding of formulations that require buffers. The latter may be more suitable for a busy compounding pharmacy. The constituents of pharmaceutical solutions, the types of solutions encountered in practice, and their quality parameters are summarized in Mind Map 4-1.

It should be noted that a full description of the action of buffers, or of the Henderson-Hasselbach equation, is not within the scope of this book. The interested reader should consult a physical pharmacy textbook for more details.

Other Applications of Solvents

Solvents are also used for extracting drugs from plant materials such as crushed roots or leaves. The solubility of the drug of interest (which is contained within the plant material) is taken into account when choosing a solvent for the extraction. If the plant is known to contain a drug that is alcohol soluble, for example, a water/alcohol mixture will likely be selected. Pure alcohol may not be chosen as the solvent. Since alcohol is expensive, a water/alcohol mixture is more cost-effective. However, the reason for this choice is not simply to reduce costs but has to do, also, with the quality of the extract that is produced.

A plant material may contain many compounds. While pure alcohol may achieve a more efficient extraction of the material of interest, it may, additionally, extract a lot of unwanted materials that are also alcohol soluble. The medicinal chemist working

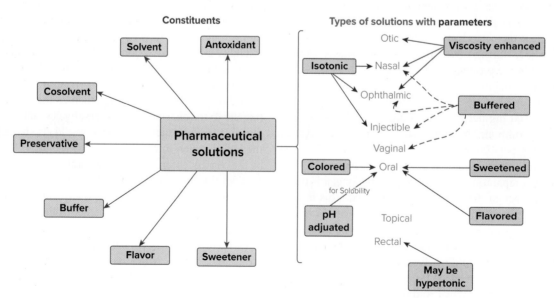

MIND MAP 4-1 Pharmaceutical Solutions

with the extraction will choose the best alcohol/water mixture on the basis that it will extract a reasonable amount of the compound of interest, with the least amount of unwanted materials. Such tinctures were commonly used in pharmacy more than 50 years ago and pharmacies, typically, had rows of bottles of tinctures in the dispensary. The Pharmacist could use these to prepare elixirs or syrups for a particular patient (eg, a tincture of morphine is used to prepare morphine syrup). Tinctures are still used today, but far less commonly. They may be a component of a solution that a pharmacist is compounding.

Other Excipients

Other types of excipients include sweeteners, flavors, colorants, preservatives, and viscosity enhancers. Generally, excipients are needed to make the pharmaceutical formulation elegant and acceptable, from several perspectives. If the excipients confer a pleasant taste, a pleasing color, and no unacceptable odor, they are said to provide patient acceptability. Excipients may also be used to improve pharmaceutical quality and to increase stability. Sometimes, certain excipients may be added for marketing reasons. Dyes and flavors may distinguish the product from its competition.

If the dosage form is acceptable to the patient, he is more likely to take the preparation as prescribed, for example, 1 teaspoon four times a day. If he takes the medication regularly and as prescribed, we say he is complying with the dosage regimen. The issue of compliance is a major concern in pharmacy and will be addressed several times in the pharmacy curriculum. Excipients included in solutions mainly for the purpose of patient acceptability include sweeteners, flavors, and color.

Preservatives

Preservatives are used to inhibit microbial growth. Since solutions usually contain a large amount of sugar, they are a natural microbial growth medium. Commonly used preservatives are the group of compounds known as the parabens, and benzoic acid and derivatives (eg, sodium benzoate). Chemically, the parabens are esters of para-hydroxybenzoic acid. The most common examples are methyl para-hydroxybenzoic acid (methylparaben) and propyl para-hydroxybenzoic acid (propylparaben). The butyl derivative is also fairly commonly used. Each paraben has a slightly different antimicrobial spectrum and two parabens are commonly combined for greater antimicrobial efficiency.

Sweeteners

Sugar may be used as a sweetener, unless the patient is diabetic. There are also several polyols, such as sorbitol, erythritol, and maltitol which are low-calorie sweeteners. In addition, there are a few artificial sweeteners, such as saccharin, acesulfame potassium, and sucralose, that are commercially available. The polyols and artificial sweeteners may be preferable to some nondiabetic patients who may be very conscious of caloric intake. Syrup, which has a high sugar content, may be considered a sweetener. Because of the high sugar content and the need to heat to dissolve the sugar within a reasonable time, some pharmacies may consider it worthwhile to purchase premade syrup.

Colors

Colors are usually used as so-called "lakes." These are pigments adsorbed onto a solid support particle, usually aluminum. Lakes are very fine, insoluble particles. They disperse well in water to give an even color. The particles of the color substance, on their own, do not disperse well but tend to form clumps. This occurs because the dye partially dissolves in the water and the dissolved dye forms a sticky solution which surrounds undissolved dye particles, resulting in the clumps. Because the clumps are very difficult to disperse, the solution has an unappealing appearance. Lakes are used because the very fine particles, consisting of dye substance adsorbed onto a solid support, do not clump easily when mixed with water. This is due to the fact that the lakes are not soluble and do not react, as described above for the pure dye. The insoluble lake particles disperse evenly in water, providing a uniform coloration. Particle size is so fine that they do not have the appearance of separate particles visually.

The lakes are used in very small quantities, frequently a few milligrams for a prescription. Nevertheless, the lake is an excipient and its quality must be controlled, in spite of the low quantity. Indeed, only a limited range of dyes and lakes are approved for use in human medication.

Flavors

There are many synthetic flavors that are used today, and sometimes naturally occurring volatile oils, such as cinnamon, orange, or lemon oil, are used in pharmaceutical formulations. Vanillin and synthetic vanilla flavor are also commonly used. Cherry flavor is a common, older flavor. Many newer flavors such as watermelon, bubblegum, and chocolate have become popular in recent years. The small amount of volatile oil that is used in a solution may not disperse well in water. Therefore, other ingredients are used to aid dispersion. Certain surfactants (solubilizing agents) or potent solvents that are water miscible may be included to dissolve the oil. The oil, dissolved in the small amount of secondary solvent or surfactant, disperses well in the larger volume of water. An example of a surfactant used for this purpose is Tween 20, while an example of a solvent that may be used in this way is ethanol.

Color and flavor are usually matched for aesthetic reasons, for example, a banana-flavored solution is more appealing in a light yellow color than in bright pink. Some flavor/color combinations are used to set the product apart from competitors' products. For example, when Wyeth Pharmaceuticals first marketed Dimetapp as a deep purple syrup with a grape flavor, it distinguished their product over the cough and cold solutions on the market at that time. Previous formulations had the more traditional flavors and colors, such as a cherry flavor in a red syrup.

Viscosity Enhancers

Viscosity enhancers (thickeners) may increase palatability but may also add to the overall effectiveness of a preparation. For example, a viscous cough syrup may be soothing as it slowly goes down the throat upon swallowing. This is purely the effect of the thick syrup base and is in addition to the effect of the drug, which is to relieve the cough. The thickener may also decrease the potential for crystal growth, during storage, in more concentrated drug solutions. In this way, the thickener also enhances pharmaceutical quality.

Recap Questions

1. Distinguish an excipient from an ingredient.
2. Name three types of excipients used in the preparation of pharmaceutical solutions.
3. What effect, if any, would it have on the patient, if the drug did not stay in solution within the bottle?
4. Why is it not a good idea to prepare a solution at a concentration that is close to the solubility of the drug?
5. If you are required to prepare 200 mL of a 5% solution of sodium bicarbonate, how many grams of sodium bicarbonate will you weigh?
6. If water is non-toxic, why do we not use water (only) for all pharmaceutical solutions?

THE PREPARATION OF SOLUTIONS IN A PHARMACY

When preparing solutions, whether in industry or during compounding in a pharmacy, there are several factors to take into account, the most important of which are the solubility of the drug, the nature and properties of the solvent, the other excipients that are needed to make a pharmaceutically acceptable solution, the potential interactions between any of the ingredients, and the chemical and physical stability of the formulation.

Although there are many solution dosage forms marketed by pharmaceutical companies, there are occasions when a pharmacist has to prepare a solution for a patient. This situation may arise for many reasons. For example, a pharmaceutical company may market a tablet or a capsule dosage form for adults, but not a liquid-dosage form suitable for children. Alternately, an adult may have a serious swallowing problem and may, therefore, require a liquid formulation of a drug that is only available in a solid dosage form. Such a solution may be made from the drug powder, if the powder is available commercially. On the other hand, the solution may be prepared from crushed tablets, or the contents of capsules, if the drug is available in these forms. The material, thus obtained, may be utilized in the formulation of the solution. In either case, care must be taken to accurately weigh the powder that will be incorporated into the solution. Similarly, care must be exercised in all other steps required to prepare and dispense the solution.

The typical solvents that one may consider include water, syrup, ethanol, glycerin, and propylene glycol. Syrup may be prepared in the pharmacy or purchased from a commercial manufacturer. Paddock Labs in Minneapolis manufactures a range of syrups with different flavors. It is convenient to purchase syrups, since their small-scale manufacturing can be tedious and involves the use of heat. The use of a heating system, such as a hotplate, carries with it some risk. In addition, the heated solution has an expanded volume. Before making the solution up to its final volume, the solution has to be cooled to room temperature. This may not appear to be difficult but it is tedious when there are multiple activities occurring simultaneously in a busy pharmacy. If it is decided that the syrup will be made in-house, a bulk quantity should be produced and suitably labeled and stored for use in the preparation of individual prescriptions. Sorbitol solution or methylcellulose dispersion can be used, in place of syrup, if the patient is diabetic.

When preparing the solution from drug powder, the weighed powder may be added to a measure containing three-quarters of the volume of the solvent, stirred to dissolve, other ingredients added and made up to volume. This could work well if the drug, as well as other ingredients, dissolves rapidly in the solvent. If the drug does not dissolve easily, the solution may have to be heated, in a beaker. Before transferring to the measure, the solution should be cooled to room temperature. Next, it is made up to three-quarters of the final volume with solvent, and the other soluble ingredients added, before making up to final volume. In general, one wishes to avoid the use of heat because some drugs are thermolabile, and because the solution must be cooled again to room temperature because of volume changes, as alluded to above. The loss of water due to evaporation when heating is not a major problem since the preparation has still to be made up to volume. However, one should avoid heating volatile solvents, even at low temperature at which the possibility of ignition is low, due to solvent evaporative losses which are costly. If such a solvent has to be warmed, this should be done, on a water bath, in a fume hood to avoid atmospheric contamination. The water bath is used at a low setting (with checks on the water temperature) for better control of the solvent temperature.

A prerequisite step, in the preparation of drug solutions, is to check the solubility of the drug in various solvents. A suitable solvent can then be chosen. Often, one chooses a mixture of solvents (a cosolvent system), based on the drug's solubility in various solvents. One should take into account the solubility of all the ingredients of the formulation in that solvent and their compatibility with the solvent(s) chosen. In addition, one has to be concerned with the pH effects of the solvent. Where a combination of solvents is used, with one solvent having a much greater solubility for one (or more) of the ingredients, it makes sense to dissolve these ingredients in that solvent first. Examples of such solvents are propylene glycol and ethanol which may display a much higher solubility for either the drug or other ingredients such as the preservative.

Methylparaben and, especially propylparaben, are cases in point. These preservatives are highly soluble in both propylene glycol and ethanol, while they may be close to maximum solubility in the volume of water present in the solution to be made. Instead of dissolving these preservatives in water, with extended stirring and possibly the use of heat, it would be far better to dissolve these substances in the cosolvent. This solution is then added to the solution of the remaining ingredients in three-quarters of the volume of water. To ensure that the preservative does not precipitate out of the water (in which it is significantly less soluble), the addition of the organic solvent-solution of the preservative should be done slowly with constant stirring. The dissolution of the drug may be handled in a similar way if it is far more soluble in the organic solvent than in water.

If the drug powder is unavailable commercially, the pharmacist may prepare a prescribed solution from tablets or capsules, if available commercially. One reason that the drug substance may not be available commercially relates to patents which the company holds. Such a patent may prohibit any other company from synthesizing the drug, while the patent holder prepares the drug substance for its own use only. In such cases, it is permissible to compound the solution from crushed tablets or the contents of capsules. The liquid product of such an exercise can, strictly, only be referred to as a solution if all the ingredients, including the drug, are soluble in the medium. If the drug is soluble but some of the components are not, then it is a solution of the drug but a suspension of the other ingredients. If neither the drug nor the excipients is soluble, it is a suspension. The preparation of a solution, or of a suspension, from tablets or capsules is similar. The preparation of the suspension requires that a suspending agent be incorporated additionally. The general steps for the preparation of a solution are given below.

1. Crush the tablets using a mortar and pestle.
2. Slowly add syrup into the mortar, with mixing, up to about three-fourths of the final volume.
3. Add additional ingredients (if any).
4. Pour into a bottle and use more syrup to rinse out the mortar (mixing vessel).
5. Add the rinsing liquid to the bottle and make up to volume.

Recap Questions

1. Why is it important to use more solvent than the minimum needed to dissolve the quantity of drug present? (Hint: what happens after the medication leaves the pharmacy and is stored by the patient or caregiver?)
2. Why are mixed solvents used in pharmaceutical formulations? Consider the case of a drug that dissolves better in ethanol than in water, why should we not use ethanol only?
3. What is meant by the term "thermolabile drug"?
4. If sorbitol is a sweetener, why is it acceptable for use by diabetics?

COMMERCIAL SOLUTIONS

Some examples of commercial oral pharmaceutical solutions in the US market are given in Table 4-3 which includes a listing of either the solvents, or of all excipients, in the solution. A review of this information illustrates many of the theoretical considerations mentioned above. For example, the solvent systems,

buffers, and preservatives used in different formulations can be compared. The constituents of one commercial formulation will now be described as an example. The information in Table 4-4, pertaining to this product (Abilify Solution), can be obtained from the package insert of the referenced product, or from the FDA's Orange book.

Abilify solution is used as an adjunct medication for the treatment of depression. As we can see from the table, the active ingredient is Aripiprazole 1 mg/mL. The solvents are distilled water, propylene glycol, and glycerin. The latter has some preservative properties as well. Fructose and sucrose are sweeteners while methylparaben and propylparaben are preservatives. Tetrasodium EDTA is a chelating agent, which traps ions and helps to keep the solution clear. Lactic acid and sodium hydroxide are pH-adjusting agents, used to either decrease or increase the pH, respectively, as needed.

INTRODUCTION TO DISSOLUTION AND DIFFUSION

It is important for the pharmacist to understand the process by which a solid drug goes into solution. This process is termed "dissolution." The conceptual framework for this process is important for two major reasons: first, the pharmacist may be making solutions for patients and he should understand the process involved. An understanding of the process implies knowledge of the factors that affect this process, which affords one, for example, the ability to increase the rate at which dissolution occurs. Second, since most drugs must be in solution in order to be absorbed, an understanding of this process promotes a better appreciation of the speed and onset of drug action. The dissolution of the drug is a necessary first step for eventual drug action. It should be noted that very fine, undissolved particles can be absorbed by the body in a very few instances. This occurs through the process of pinocytosis, in which the particles of drug are engulfed and taken into the cytoplasm of the cell. Since this is not the absorption mechanism for most drugs, the rate of solution of the drug is an important factor to take into account when considering the rate and extent to which a drug is absorbed. The latter, in turn, affects the extent of drug action in the body.

In addition to the concept of dissolution, a second concept, "diffusion", is important for the pharmacist to understand and is described below. Consider a drug that has dissolved in one part of a body of liquid, such as the bottom of a beaker of water (or in a part of the stomach). The dissolved substance then distributes throughout the body of liquid. The distribution process is referred to as "diffusion" and it is important for drug action since the molecules of drug must move through the body of liquid to reach the absorbing membrane.

An understanding of dissolution and diffusion is important for an understanding of how dosage forms function, and how drugs work. Dissolution of the drug contained within a dosage form may not be a simple process. Frequently it is controlled by formulation factors. For example, in a sustained-release tablet formulation, the dissolution and the release of the drug

TABLE 4-3	Some Examples of Commercial Pharmaceutical Solutions	
NAME OF PRODUCT/ COMPANY	**DRUG NAME**	**INDICATION AND NOTES**
CLEOCIN T/Pfizer	CLINDAMYCIN PHOsphate	Antibiotic to treat acne vulgaris. The solvent consists of 50% v/v isopropyl alcohol, propylene glycol, and water. A very small portion of the dose is absorbed systemically from this formulation (oral solutions are also available for other applications).
Neoral Oral Solution/ Novartis	Cyclosporine	Antibiotic. Solvent: 11.9% v/v, corn oil mono-di-triglycerides, polyoxyl 40 hydrogenated castor oil NF, DL-α-tocopherol USP, glycerol, propylene glycol USP.
Baraclude/Bristol Myers Squibb	Entecavir	Antiviral for chronic hepatitis B viral infection. It is an aqueous solution with the following inactive ingredients: maltitol, sodium citrate, citric acid, methylparaben, propylparaben, and orange flavor
Neurontin/Upjohn	Gabapentin	Antiepileptic. Inactive ingredients: glycerin, xylitol, purified water, and artificial cool strawberry anise flavor.
Sporonox/Janssen	Itraconazole	Antifungal solubilized by hydroxypropyl-β-cyclodextrin. It has a target pH of 2 and the ingredients are hydrochloric acid, propylene glycol, purified water, sodium hydroxide, sodium saccharin, sorbitol, and flavors.
Corlanor/Amgen	Ivabradine	Pediatric stable heart failure. Supplied as sterile, preservative-free, colorless solution in LDPE ampoules, for oral administration. The inactive ingredients are maltitol and water.
Xyzal/Sanofi-Aventis	Levocetirizine dihydrochhloride	Antihistamine for allergic rhinitis. Inactive ingredients are sodium acetate trihydrate, glacial acetic acid, maltitol solution, glycerin, methylparaben, propylparaben, saccharin, flavors, and purified water.
Kaltra/Abbvie	Lopinavir/ritonovir	Anti-retroviral for pediatric patients. Inactive ingredients: acesulfame potassium, alcohol, citric acid, glycerin, high fructose corn syrup, flavors, polyoxyl 40 hydrogenated castor oil, povidone, propylene glycol, saccharin sodium, sodium chloride, sodium citrate, and water.
ZOFRAN/ NOVARTIS	ONDANSETRON HYDROCHLORIDE	Prevention of nausea and vomiting associated with chemotherapy and radiation therapy. Inactive ingredients: citric acid anhydrous, purified water, sodium benzoate, sodium citrate, sorbitol, and strawberry flavor.
LYRICA/ PFIZER	PREGABALIN	Neuropathic pain, fibromyalgia, seizures. Inactive ingredients: methylparaben, propylparaben, monobasic sodium phosphate anhydrous, dibasic sodium phosphate anhydrous, sucralose, artificial strawberry #11545, and purified water

TABLE 4-4	Constituents of Abilify Solution
ABILIFY 1 mg/mL SOLUTION	
NDC: 59148-0013-15 Box, 1 bottles, 150 mL Aripiprazole 1 mg/1 ml, Oral Solution and 1 each Oral Dose Cup, calibrated	
Active Ingredients:	Aripiprazole 1 mg/1 mL
Drug Description:	Clear, orange
Inactive Ingredients:	Distilled Water Fructose Glycerin Lactic Acid Methylparaben Propylene Glycol Propylparaben Sodium Hydroxide Sucrose Tetrasodium EDTA

is determined by the chemicals which make up the matrix of the tablet. Similarly, in some dosage forms, water may penetrate the dosage form and dissolve the drug relatively easily, but the diffusion of the drug, from within the dosage form to the outside, may be controlled by the base in which the drug is formulated. For example, an ointment or a suppository may contain an undissolved drug within a base which is the major constituent of these dosage forms. The dissolution and diffusion of the drug in such a system is influenced by the nature of these bases.

The diffusion of water vapor also comes into play in the drying of solids such as granules. Granulation is a preliminary step in the manufacture of tablets and the wet granules must be dried before further processing. Likewise, the diffusion of water vapor from the atmosphere into tablet containers may affect the stability of the tablets. The discussion of diffusion will occur first since some of the described concepts are needed for a consideration of the dissolution rate.

DIFFUSION

Diffusion is defined as the movement of mass in response to a spatial gradient in chemical potential which is brought about by random molecular motion (Brownian movement). "Chemical potential" in this definition is most often represented by the concentration of a substance. Hence, "differences in chemical potential" can be thought of as differences in concentration. Differences in chemical potential are also more easily measured in terms of concentration differences. In the following discussion, therefore, "concentration" will be used instead of "chemical potential." We may think of "spatial gradient" as a gradient in concentration within a certain volume (of liquid in a beaker, for example). Diffusion occurs from a region of high drug concentration to one of low concentration. From the above description, it should be clear that diffusion is a mass transfer process, in contrast to heat, or energy, transfer.

Fick's First Law of Diffusion

While one could study the rate at which a drug diffuses through a thin segment of a body of liquid, or a "slice of water," it is more convenient to look at diffusion through a membrane. Consider a drug passing through such a membrane, which acts as a partial barrier. This process could arise in several situations that we come across in pharmaceutical sciences. Let us consider two such situations:

1. Suppose a patient swallows 10 mL of a solution of a drug. The drug solution, in due course, passes into his small intestines. In order that the drug can exert its effect and be useful, absorption must occur. For absorption, the drug has to pass through a biological membrane to enter a body compartment.

2. Suppose the patient swallows a tablet that is coated with a membrane that does not dissolve. Water diffuses through the intact coating membrane, dissolves the drug within the tablet, and then the drug solution has to pass through, or diffuse out of, the membrane in order to leave the dosage form.

Now that it has been established where these situations might arise, the rate at which the drug passes through this membrane will be considered. Usually, there is a lag time (when practically no diffusion occurs), then the diffusion rate increases up to a constant rate, and finally the rate falls off again as the source of the drug becomes depleted. Consider the steady state, that is, when the amount of matter passing through unit surface area of the membrane, in unit time, is constant.

First, the concept of "flux" must be understood. Definition: The flux (J) is the amount of matter passing through unit surface area of membrane in unit time, for example, 2 mg of drug pass through 1 cm^2 of membrane in 1 hour. Equation (4-1) describes flux.

$$J = \frac{dM}{dt.S} \qquad (4\text{-}1)$$

where M is the mass of the drug passing through the membrane in time, t, and S is the surface area of the membrane.

To further explain these concepts, the following experimental setup is considered. Two bodies of liquid are separated by a membrane. The drug is added to one body of liquid, the donor side, and has to pass through a membrane to reach the other side, the receiver side (Figure 4-1). According to Fick's First Law, the flux is proportional to the concentration gradient across the membrane.

$$J \propto \frac{dC}{dx}$$

Where C is concentration and x is distance (dC/dx refers to the change in concentration with distance from the source).

This proportionality can be written as an equation as follows:

$$J = -D\frac{dC}{dx} \qquad (4\text{-}2)$$

where D = diffusity;

and the negative sign indicates that the flow is from a high concentration to a low concentration, that is, it merely indicates direction.

The coefficient, diffusity, is a function of the molecular structure of the diffusant (the substance that is diffusing), the properties of the barrier material (the membrane), and the temperature. It is constant only for a narrow set of defined conditions. The properties of the diffusant that are important include molecular size (large molecules diffuse more slowly than small molecules) and molecular structure (branched molecules diffuse more slowly than a similar straight-chain molecule).

Referring to the model depicted in the diagram, Eq. (4-2) can be written as follows:

$$J = -D\frac{C_{DM} - C_{RM}}{h} \qquad (4\text{-}3)$$

Where C_{DM} = membrane conc on the donor side
C_{RM} = membrane conc on the receiver side
h = thickness of the membrane
D = diffusity

Substituting for J according to Eq. (4-1):

$$\frac{dM}{dt.S} = -D\frac{C_{DM} - C_{RM}}{h} \qquad (4\text{-}4)$$

One can observe that Eq. (4-4) requires the concentration of the drug on the donor side of the membrane, and the concentration of the drug on the receiver side of the membrane. Since it would be highly impractical to determine the concentration in

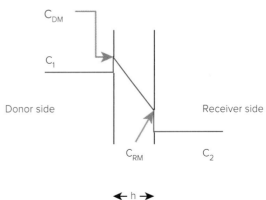
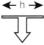

FIGURE 4-1 Diffusion through a membrane.

the membrane, we could attempt to use the concentrations in the donor and receiver liquids as substitutes for the concentration of the drug on the respective sides of the membrane. It is far easier to measure drug concentration in liquids. How can this substitution be scientifically justified? Consider the partition coefficient which is defined as follows:

$$K = \frac{C_{DM}}{C_1} = \frac{C_{RM}}{C_2} \qquad (4\text{-}5)$$

This equation states that the concentration of the drug on the donor side of the membrane divided by the concentration in the donor-compartment liquid is equal to a constant, K; and that the concentration of the drug on the receiver side of the membrane divided by the concentration in the receiver-compartment liquid is also equal to the constant, K. This constant describes the propensity of the drug to distribute between the liquid and the membrane, and its value is the same on either side of the compartment.

Therefore, we can substitute KC_1 for C_{DM} and KC_2 for C_{RM} in Eq. (4-4):

$$\frac{dM}{dt.S} = -D\frac{KC_1 - KC_2}{h} \qquad (4\text{-}6)$$

If the concentration in the receiver side is very low, we can omit C_2. (Typically, the receiver is filled with aqueous buffer at the start of the experiment, ie, the drug concentration equals zero; and experimental conditions are selected such that the drug concentration stays low throughout the experiment.) Taking this into account, rearranging terms, and dropping the negative sign (which indicates the direction of the reaction only), the usual form of this equation is:

$$\frac{dM}{dt} = \frac{DSKC}{h} \qquad (4\text{-}7)$$

For a constant set of experimental conditions, the factors D, K, and h are constant. Hence, we may define a new constant, permeability, taking these factors into account as follows:

$$P = \frac{DK}{h} \qquad (4\text{-}8)$$

Hence,

$$\frac{dM}{dt} = PSC_1 \qquad (4\text{-}9)$$

The permeability of a drug is an important concept in pharmacy. It takes into account the following:

- Molecular properties of the drug (such as size), membrane resistance, and temperature (D)
- Relative solubility in the membrane versus water (K)
- The thickness of the membrane (h)

EXPERIMENTAL STUDIES

A drug developer may want to know how fast a newly-synthesized drug will permeate a biological membrane. This will give the scientists in the company an idea of how fast the drug will be absorbed compared to other drugs in the same

category. To deteremine this, they could set up a donor cell and a receiver cell separated by a membrane. A drug solution is added to the donor cell and the receiver cell is sampled at fixed time intervals, that is, a small quantity of liquid is taken out of the receiver cell and analyzed for drug content. In this way, the rate at which the permeant (the chemical that is permeating) passes through the membrane can be determined. The Franz cell (Figure 4-2) is one kind of experimental cell that is commonly used in these studies which are designed to provide information useful for drug development. However, results have to be carefully interpreted so that one does not make erroneous conclusions.

Some of the ways in which the above type of experiment can be usefully employed in drug development are the following:

1. Is a new chemical entity (NCE) absorbed through biological membranes such as the gastrointestinal (GI) membrane?

2. Will a drug, which has previously been successfully administered orally, permeate the skin or the buccal mucosa?

3. If the drug does not permeate these tissues sufficiently for it to be useful as a drug product, which absorption enhancers can be used to increase its permeation?

4. Is the permeation-enhancing mechanism damaging to the membrane? One can look for overt damage, such as pinholes, by using a microscope. Also, biochemical tests can be done to determine changes in the tissues.

5. Some types of sustained-release medication have a coating that retards the release of the drug from the dosage form. One may test the effectiveness of the coating by inserting the membrane into the Franz cell and conducting a permeation experiment. The membrane is prepared by spreading the liquid coating material on a glass slab (or other support), drying and removing the membrane which is then cut into suitably-sized pieces.

For studies of the general type described above, one can use the following:

a. Pig skin as a surrogate for human skin

b. Pig buccal mucosa as a surrogate for human mucosa

c. Cadaver skin

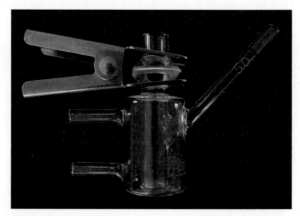

FIGURE 4-2 Frantz Diffusion Cell. (Used with permission from Permegear.)

d. Human vaginal tissue (from hysterectomies) as a surrogate for human buccal tissue

e. Cultured membranes

f. Synthetic membranes

Recap Questions

1. If a researcher wants to know if a drug is absorbed, why can't he simply administer the drug to a human and measure blood levels?

2. Why is diffusity a function of molecular structure? Is it not simply a function of the resistance of the membrane?

3. What do you understand from the term, "flux"?

4. Why is pig skin and oral mucosa used in a Frantz diffusion cell?

DISSOLUTION

Consider a single drug crystal placed into water which is then stirred mechanically. The stirring helps to dissolve the drug faster. Let us look at this process in more detail and try to understand the factors that affect the dissolving of the drug.

Dissolution occurs from the surface of the solid, that is, molecules leave its surface to enter the liquid phase and do so as discrete, individual molecules (Figure 4-3). Close to the surface of the solid, there is a stagnant liquid layer or film of liquid. In spite of the stirring of the body of water, this layer remains unstirred. The thickness of the film is affected by the stirring rate, that is, a faster stirring rate results in a thinner film. The concentration of drug in the unstirred layer (film) decreases regularly across the film, that is, there is a gradient of concentration across the film. The level of the drug in the bulk solution, generally, is low.

The Noyes-Whitney equation {Eq. (4-10)}was derived from the above theoretical model and describes the rate of drug dissolution (ie, the rate at which drug molecules leave the solid crystal to enter the bulk liquid). The mass of the crystal decreases with time, while the mass of drug in solution increases. The change in the mass of the dissolved drug is affected by:

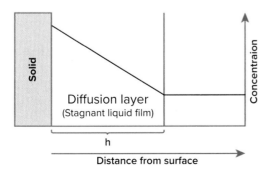

FIGURE 4-3 Theoretical model for dissolution of a solid.

• The difference between the solubility of the drug and the amount of drug in the bulk solution—it is directly proportional. If the concentration in the bulk solution becomes high, the rate of dissolution goes down; ideally, one must maintain sink conditions when conducting such an experiment, that is, C (concentration of drug in solution) is less than, or equal to, 20% C_s (the solubility of the drug). This may also be expressed as the amount of drug in solution should not exceed 20% of the solubility of the drug.

• Surface area of the solid—directly proportional. If one wants to dissolve the drug rapidly, the drug must be finely ground. The faster dissolution occurs because of the larger surface area of all the drug particles in total, for a fixed mass of the drug. This occurs because dissolution occurs from the surface of drug particles, and the greater surface area results in faster dissolution.

• The thickness of the unstirred layer—inversely proportional. If stirring occurs more rapidly, faster dissolution results because of the thinner unstirred layer.

The diffusion coefficient for most small molecule drugs in water at room temperature is very similar.

Noyes-Whitney Equation

$$\frac{dM}{dt} = \frac{DS}{h}(C_s - C) \qquad (4-10)$$

Where, M = mass dissolved

$\frac{dM}{dt}$ = dissolution rate

D = diffusion coefficient

S = surface area of solid

C_s = solubility of solid

C = concentration of solid in bulk solution

h = thickness of diffusion layer

If we divide both sides of the equation by volume (V), we get the following equation:

$$\frac{dC}{dt} = \frac{DS}{Vh}(C_s - C) \qquad (4-11)$$

(Note that M/t divided by V is $M/V/t = C/t$)

This equation is easier to work with as we get concentration values directly from experiments. The left-hand side of the equation is the dissolution rate, that is, the change in concentration with time. When $C << C_s$, we can eliminate C. For example, if the solubility of a drug is 100 mg per 100 mL and the concentration of the bulk solution, at time t during an experiment, is 1 mg per 100 mL, then by this simplification, $100 - 1 \approx 100$. Therefore, Eq. (4-10) can be written as:

$$\frac{dM}{dt} = \frac{DS}{h}C_s \qquad (4-12)$$

For fixed conditions, D and h are constant. (Since D is affected by temperature and h by stirring speed, these factors must be kept constant.) Hence, we may define a new constant, $k = D/h$, such that:

$$\frac{dM}{dt} = kSC_s \qquad (4\text{-}13)$$

and

$$\frac{dC}{dt} = \frac{kSC_s}{V} \qquad (4\text{-}14)$$

where k is the dissolution rate constant.

Example:

To prepare a particular solution, 10 g of the drug is added to 100 mL water and stirred to dissolve. The solubility of the drug is 10 mg/mL and the total surface area of the drug particles is 0.25 m². After 10 minutes, 1 g of the drug has dissolved. Assuming sink conditions, find the dissolution rate constant in cm/s.

$$\frac{dM}{dt} = kSC_s$$

1 g/10 min = k (0.25 m²) × 10 mg/mL
100 mg/min = k × 2500 cm² × 10 mg/cm³

$$k = \frac{100}{2500 \times 10} cm/min$$
$$= 0.004 \text{ cm/min}$$
$$= 0.0000667 \text{ cm/s}$$
$$= \mathbf{6.667 \times 10^{-5} \text{ cm/s}}$$

Recap Questions

1. In the above calculation example, what would be the impact of
   a. Changing the volume of the water to 200 mL?
   b. Changing the volume of the water to 40 mL?
   c. Changing the total surface area of the solid to 0.5 m²?
2. Why does dissolution occur faster when the particles of the test substance are ground to a finer size?

DISSOLUTION AND BIOAVAILABILITY

Dissolution, as we have discussed, is the process whereby molecules of a substance leave the surface of the solid phase and go into solution. For the above theoretical model and calculations, a single, pure substance was considered. We can also consider a drug going into solution not as a pure chemical but as a component of a dosage form. This is a more complex process and there are several steps involved. This process is also referred to as dissolution, or drug release, and there are standardized procedures to test the rate of drug release from dosage forms. Thus, the term "dissolution" has two connotations in pharmaceutics (dissolution of pure drug; and dissolution and release of the drug from a complex dosage form). Drug dissolution from solid oral dosage forms has several steps which are considered in more detail in Chapter 9, Tablets.

It is very important that the drug be released from a solid dosage form at a suitable rate, for absorption to occur at an acceptable rate. Since drug release is a prior step to absorption, it follows that the rate at which a drug is released from the dosage form is important. Note that a "suitable" dissolution rate is not necessarily the fastest rate.

Bioavailability

One cannot assume that all of the drug in a dosage form is released and absorbed after consumption. In fact, for most available products, only some fraction of the dose actually reaches the systemic blood circulation. With reference to swallowed dosage forms, some portion of the drug is unabsorbed and excreted with the feces, and some portion is destroyed during the absorption process by enzymes in the gut wall. The drug that enters the blood vessels in the gut is carried to the liver where a fraction is metabolized by the liver enzymes. Hence, only a smaller fraction of the administered dose reaches the systemic circulation and is available for drug action and this is referred to as the bioavailable drug. Factors that delay dissolution make the drug unavailable for absorption during the delay. Hence, these factors may affect the rate of absorption and the bioavailability of the drug, and should be avoided where possible. The exception is the situation where the medication is intentionally formulated to provide a slower drug release. This occurs with modified-release medication, the subject of Chapter 11, Modified-Release Oral Dosage Forms, whereas bioavailability is discussed in more detail in Chapter 17, Introduction to Bioavailability.

BIOPHARMACEUTICAL CLASSIFICATION SYSTEM

The following question has been asked for long: Does the dissolution rate give an indication of bioavailability? As may be discerned from the information that follows, this question may be more usefully stated as: When does dissolution give an indication of bioavailability?

In recognition of the fact that certain drugs have properties that allow them to be more easily absorbed, and that others have properties that make absorption by the body difficult, the FDA has relatively recently accepted the biopharmaceutical classification system. This system places drugs in classes 1 to 4 (Table 4-5), the lower the number the more easily will the referenced drug be absorbed by a biological system. Since class 1

TABLE 4-5	Biopharmaceutical Classification System	
	HIGH SOLUBILITY	**LOW SOLUBILITY**
High Permeability	1	2
Low Permeability	3	4

drugs will be readily absorbed, the FDA will place more reliance on dissolution testing of products containing these drugs as a measure of bioavailability. For class 4, the FDA will not accept dissolution testing results alone and human studies must be performed to show that the drug is bioavailable. The two drug factors that are used to determine placement into these categories are solubility and permeability. From the table, it can be seen that a high reliance can be placed on dissolution testing if solubility and permeability are both high for a specific drug. On the other hand, we cannot place any reliance on dissolution testing **to indicate biological availability** if the solubility of the drug and its permeability are low (Class 4). For classes 2 and 3, the reliance is intermediate and must be viewed on a case-by-case basis. However, the test can still be relied upon to indicate batch-to-batch difference and will be used by manufacturers to control their products.

NON-ORAL SOLUTIONS

Apart from oral medications, there are other routes of administration of solutions in pharmacy practice. Injections, eye drops, nose drops, eardrops, vaginal and rectal solutions, and topical solutions are other applications of solution dosage forms. These dosage forms are formulated along the lines of the general principles mentioned in this chapter. A few differences will be highlighted here. Whenever a non-aqueous solvent is used, the formulator must ensure that the solvent is non-toxic and is acceptable to use by the contemplated route of administration.

Most injections are solutions, while some may be suspensions. Water is the most common solvent used in injections. For this purpose, the water should be sterile, particle-free, and also pyrogen-free. Pyrogens are products of microbial metabolism that, when injected, cause the temperature of the patient to rise. Some injections, particularly controlled-release injections, may be oily solutions or suspensions and are injected into a muscle where the injected material remains as a depot. The drug slowly dissolves, from the depot, into aqueous interstitial fluids for subsequent absorption into blood vessels and distribution throughout the body.

Eye drops must be sterile, buffered, and isotonic with tears to limit irritation to the sensitive tissues of the eye. In addition, many eye drops contain a viscosity-enhancing agent (thickener) to delay the leakage of the eye drops over the lower eyelid, and also drainage into the naso-lacrimal system. Nose drops must also be isotonic so that they do not irritate the sensitive nasal mucosa. An increase in the viscosity of nasal solutions helps to retard the leakage of drops out of the nose onto the upper lip, and also into the pharynx. Enhanced viscosity keeps the nose drops where they are required. Eardrops are especially viscous for the same reason, limiting the leakage of the drops out of the ear. Glycerin and propylene glycol are frequently used as solvents in eardrops due to their viscosity-enhancing effect in addition to their solvent properties. Propylene glycol is a much better solvent than glycerin. Vaginal and rectal solutions have

applications as douches and enemas, respectively, besides other applications.

Isopropyl alcohol is frequently used as a solvent for solutions to be applied to the skin since it is non-toxic and a good solvent for several drugs. Isopropyl rubbing alcohol is an aqueous dilution of this alcohol with water (usually 70% concentration). Rubbing alcohol contains 70% ethanol and is used for rubbing the body to reduce pain and swelling, which are similar to the indications for isopropyl rubbing alcohol.

Examples and some details of non-oral solution dosage forms are provided in the respective chapter dealing with the route of administration in which a particular solution dosage form is used. For example, information on eye drops can be found in Chapter 23, Ophthalmic Drug Delivery; and specific information on injections are mentioned in Chapter 12, Injections.

Recap Questions

1. Is there a difference between solubility and dissolution rate?
2. Why is a dissolution test not always a reliable indicator of bioavailability?
3. Assume that the dissolution test has been shown to be an unreliable indicator of bioavailability for a test drug. Should the manufacturer bother to use the test at all? Provide reasons for your answer.
4. When evaluating non-aqueous solvents, is there a difference between topical dosage forms and oral? Why is there such a difference?

SUMMARY POINTS

- A solution dosage form is different from a conventional solution in several critical ways.
- One solvent may be insufficient to fully dissolve a drug in the concentration required; cosolvents may be needed.
- A solution should not be formulated close to its solubility limit and a solution should be stable for its intended shelf life.
- Taste, color, and appearance are important considerations because such aesthetic properties affect the willingness of the patient to take the medication as prescribed.
- Understanding the theoretical principles of dissolution helps the pharmacist to develop efficient ways to make solutions.
- Dissolution theory provides an understanding of a process that is critical to drug action.
- Diffusion is encountered in many formulation steps and is also basic to the understanding of drug action.
- The basic concepts of non-oral solutions are provided.

What do you think?

1. Examine the following pairs of compounds. What is the chemical difference between the members of the pair? What difference would it make to the patient if you used one member of the pair instead of the other? (Answers are not in this chapter.)

   a. Methanol and ethanol

   b. propylene glycol and ethylene glycol

   c. ethylene glycol and polyethylene glycol

2. Describe the function of each of the ingredients in Prozac solution which contains fluoxetine hydrochloride, alcohol, benzoic acid, distilled water, glycerin, and sucralose.

3. Draw a lipid bilayer, as found in biological membranes. Now add to this drawing, just above the membrane representation, the chemical structure of any small molecule (molecular weight less than 50) and the chemical structure of a large molecule (molecular weight above 500). Which molecule would permeate the membrane more easily? Why?

Pharmaceutical Powders

5

PREVIEW

- Types of medicated powders used in pharmacy
- How powders are mixed and how mixed powders should be handled
- Why particle size is important in pharmacy and therapeutics
- How the size of particles is reduced and how particle size is measured
- Methods to represent, and perform calculations on, particle size data

The term, pharmaceutical powders, has two connotations. First, the term may refer to a type of dosage form and, second, it may be used to describe the material used to manufacture other dosage forms. Powdered dosage forms are provided to patients either as bulk powders in a bottle or other container (to be measured out and dissolved or dispersed in water before consumption) or as individually packaged doses. While the wrapped powder is not very common any longer, we do have the more modern dosage forms, such as inhalations, which contain, and deliver, the medication in the form of a powder. (It should be noted that there are other types of inhalations that contain solutions.)

Many dosage forms contain powders (either as the drug or as some other excipient) and the particle size of the powder is usually important for ease of pharmaceutical processing, or the utility of the dosage form, or for both. For instance, the rate of solution is affected by the size of the particles to be dissolved. If the drug is not very soluble, the time required to form the solution becomes a significant parameter that is dependent on the size of the solute. Particle size has a much smaller effect on the dissolution rate of a very soluble drug. For suspensions, the particle size of the suspended particles affects the rate of settling of the particles with larger particles settling faster. Hence, particle size has an impact on the ability to remove a consistent dose from the bottle of suspension. Ultimately, particle size also has an impact on the stability of the product. If the particle size of one powder is large and that of another powder is small, they will not be able to be mixed effectively. Consequently, the mixed powder will not have an even distribution of the drug. The dosage forms made from such a powder may have varying amounts of drug in the individual dosing units (eg, tablets or capsules). A coarse drug particle size could also result in grittiness in ointments. These examples illustrate that the nature of powders may affect the ease of production, utility, quality, and therapeutic effect of the dosage form comprising the powders (Mind Map 5-1).

Recap Question

1. Can you name the equation that predicts that larger particles take longer to dissolve? It has been mentioned in a previous chapter.

TYPES OF MEDICATED POWDERS

Medicated powders fall into two basic categories: those that are taken internally (swallowed), and those that are applied externally. Swallowed powders may be presented to the consumer in two forms. First, as bulk powders provided in a bottle, or other container, from which the patient measures a dose, for example, sodium bicarbonate, which is used to alleviate hyperacidity. Using a calibrated scoop or teaspoon, the patient measures out the required dose and dissolves it in water before drinking the solution. Metamucil (psyllium husk powder), provided in a bulk container, is another example. Second, the powders may be provided as individual doses wrapped in paper. A special method of folding the paper limits the loss of the powder during handling. The patient unfolds the paper and dissolves the powder in water, or places the powder on the back of the tongue and swallows it with the aid of water. Such powders, individually wrapped in paper, with a few doses packaged in a box were more common previously, for example, headache powders. Individual powders have largely been replaced by other dosage forms, including the recent addition of orally disintegrating tablets (ODT) for patients who cannot swallow. Briefly, ODT are tablets which, when placed in the mouth, disintegrate rapidly and the resulting powder, mixed with saliva, is swallowed without the need for water. ODT will be covered in more detail in Chapter 9, Tablets. Metamucil is also provided in individually packaged doses. The amount of the laxative, psyllium seeds, is too much to be placed into a tablet or conveniently wrapped in paper. Hence, it is packaged into a sachet to be emptied into water in a glass. The sachet protects the powder from the ingress of water. Fine powders, in

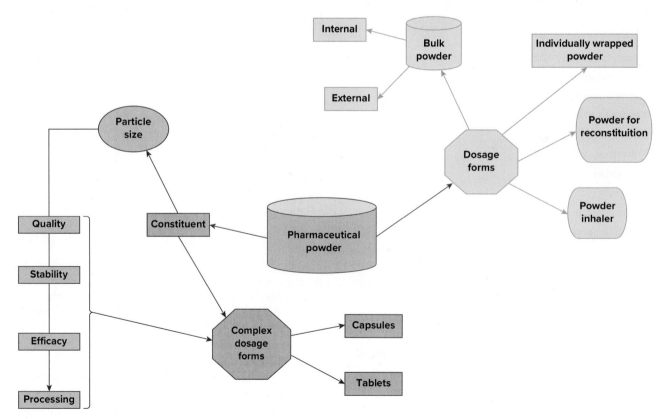

MIND MAP 5-1 Overview and Types of Pharmaceutical Powders

general, can adsorb water and form lumps. The damp powder may also not flow well.

External powders are commonly represented by dusting powders. These are very fine powders provided in a bulk container with a sifter top. Medicated powders for external use resemble dusting powders but they contain a drug, for example, tolnaftate for treatment of athlete's foot. The powders are very fine to ensure a non-gritty feel when applied to the skin and to allow a small mass to be spread over a large area. Finer powders tend to adsorb more moisture and this is a functional advantage when the powder is intended to adsorb perspiration and allow the area of application to have a "dry" feel. When the fine powder in the container takes up moisture to form clumps, it is a negative attribute. The sifter top is intended to break up small aggregates, if they form in the container. It also controls the rate at which powder is dispensed from the container and makes it easier to disperse a small amount over a wide area, that is, it enables the provision of a "light" powder.

Powders, or granules, could also be provided for reconstitution by the pharmacist, doctor, or nurse, before being supplied to the patient. Antibiotics, such as penicillin for example, are commonly dispensed this way because the antibiotic powder is stable, whereas the solution or suspension in water has limited stability. Commonly dispensed antibiotics of this type are Amoxil (amoxicillin trihydrate), Augmentin (amoxicillin trihydrate and clavulanate potassium), and Keflex (cephalexin monohydrate). Injections may be supplied as a powder in a prefilled syringe. The doctor draws up the required amount of Water for Injections to dissolve the drug.

Recently, there has also been the advent of dry powders for inhalation. These are chiefly for asthma or chronic obstructive pulmonary disease (COPD). Examples of such products are Spiriva (tiotropium bromide) and Advair Diskus (fluticasone propionate and salmeterol). The powders are used with an inhalation device which delivers one dose each time the patient actuates the dispenser. In this way, the patient inhales an accurate dose. In many instances, this form of inhalant device has replaced the propellant-containing aerosol. A much higher dose can be supplied using this method. A very specific particle size range is required to deliver the drug to the correct part of the lungs. The provision of particles of the required size is much more complex than it might seem and this topic is discussed in greater detail in Chapter 19, Pulmonary Drug Delivery.

Recap Questions

1. Why do you think Metamucil is provided in both a bulk container and sachets?
2. If a powder for external use is provided as a very fine powder in a bulk container, why is a sifter top needed?

MIXING

Often, we are required to blend a small amount of drug powder with other ingredients. The drug content of a tablet, for example,

may sometimes be as little as one or 2 mg, or even a fraction of a milligram. This amount may, literally, fit on the head of a pin. To incorporate this small amount of drug into a reasonably sized tablet that can be manufactured and handled conveniently, a diluent (in the form of a powder) is added. If we assume 1 mg drug in a 150 mg tablet, the amount of drug for 1000 tablets is 1 g in 149 g of diluent (and other excipients). How does the manufacturer incorporate this small amount of powder evenly with the rest of the materials used to make the tablet? The compounding pharmacist may also face this situation when a prescription calls for a small amount of a potent drug to be mixed with a much larger amount of other ingredients.

In each case, industry or compounding pharmacy, the powders would have to be well blended. The small-scale blending of powders will be discussed before a brief overview of industrial blending is provided. The small-scale blending of powders can be done by one of four techniques: trituration, tumbling and rolling, spatulation, or sifting.

Trituration

"Trituration" for mixing is performed using a glass mortar and pestle. The mortar has a smooth inner surface. A light pressure is applied with the pestle which is also smooth. The circular motion of the pestle provides an adequate mixing action. Under these conditions, there is little, if any, size reduction between the smooth surfaces of the mortar and the pestle.

Tumbling and Rolling

Tumbling and rolling can be done in a glass jar. The powders to be mixed are placed in a jar, which is closed with a lid, and then the jar is rolled between the hands. It is important to note that with rolling, only the surface of the powder is mixed. For a better mixing action, the whole jar needs to be tumbled. This brings large amounts of powder to the surface and takes the previous surface powder to other parts of the jar. Continued rolling then mixes the material brought to the surface. The process of rolling with intermittent, repeated tumbling provides a good mix of the powders. Obviously, the pharmacist must take great care not to drop the jar and it would be wise to work above a solid surface, such as a tabletop.

Spatulation

Spatulation is performed on a glass slab using a spatula. The two powders are placed in adjacent heaps on a glass slab and the edge of the spatula is used to mix them together in a chopping action, moving through the bed of powders from end to end. This action breaks up lumps as well as mixes the powders.

Sifting

Sifting is another way of mixing powders. The drug powder and the diluent powder are added together onto a sieve. Then, by shaking, the powders go through the sieve together. They end up on the receptacle in a light form of the powder that is a blend of the two components.

As the reader may well imagine, sifting is not a very efficient way of mixing and neither is spatulation. Therefore, to mix a more potent drug, on a small scale, trituration or tumbling and

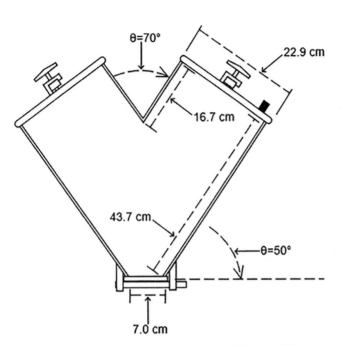

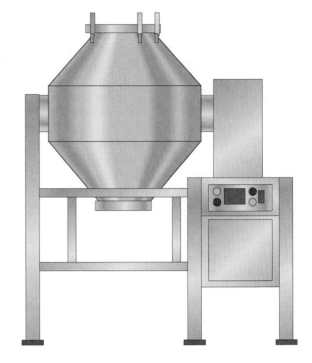

FIGURE 5-1 V-Blender (A) and double-cone blender (B).

rolling should be chosen instead. With both techniques, geometric dilution may be applied as described below.

If a very small amount of powder has to be mixed with a much larger amount of diluent, geometric dilution is used to improve the distribution of the small amount of powder throughout the bulk of the diluent. The procedure is as follows: the small amount of drug powder is placed on the bottom of the mortar. Then, the weighed, large amount of diluent, on a clean sheet of paper, is placed next to the mortar. An amount of diluent, equal in apparent volume to the amount of powder contained within the mortar, is removed from the paper and added to the mortar. The powders in the mortar are mixed well. Note that mixing equal amounts of two powders gives the best chance for an even mix, that is, the distribution of powder A throughout powder B and *vice versa*. Then, the volume of mixed powders within the glass mortar is observed and an amount of diluent approximately equal to the amount of powder in the mortar is added and mixed again. This process is repeated until all the diluent has been added to the mortar. This ensures a good chance of even mixing of the powders, that is, the mixed powder is expected to have a consistent amount of drug in every portion of the powder.

It should be noted that visual observation of the amount of powder in the mortar is an estimation of the *volume* of powder. Hence, with this method, an attempt is made to mix one powder (the one in the mortar) with an equal volume of another powder (the diluent). The volume of powder in the mortar doubles at each step.

In the pharmaceutical industry, the blending of powders is performed, for example, for the production of hundreds of thousands, or a few million, tablets in one batch. The pharmaceutical scientist has to ensure that the powder blend is uniform so that all tablets contain an equal amount of the drug.

If the powder from which the tablets are made is not uniform, some tablets would be super-potent while others would be sub-potent. A uniform drug content is assured by appropriate blending and then ensuring that the powder remains well blended throughout the production process, for example, until tablets are compressed or capsules are filled. Powders are blended at an industrial scale using various types of mechanical blenders which either rotate the whole vessel, or the large vessel has blades which rotate inside of it. Common industrial blenders of the first type are the V-blender and the double-cone blender (Figure 5-1). Examples of the second type are the planetary mixer (Figure 8-2 in Chapter 8) and high-shear mixer/granulator (Figure 8-5 in Chapter 8). The planetary mixer has an impeller that rotates on an axis as well as revolves around the inside of the container, its action resembling that of the planets rotating and revolving around the sun. A high-shear mixer has an additional blade that is used to break up lumps of powder with a chopping action during wet mixing (Mind Map 5-2).

IMPORTANCE OF PARTICLE SIZE IN PHARMACY AND THERAPEUTICS

The size of powder particles has an influence on many pharmaceutical manufacturing processes and also on several biological effects. Some of these may be obvious to the reader while others may be encountered for the first time.

Dissolution Rate of Solids

As the particle size is decreased, the specific surface area (the surface area per unit mass of the substance) is increased. This leads to faster dissolution since dissolution is a surface phenomenon, as

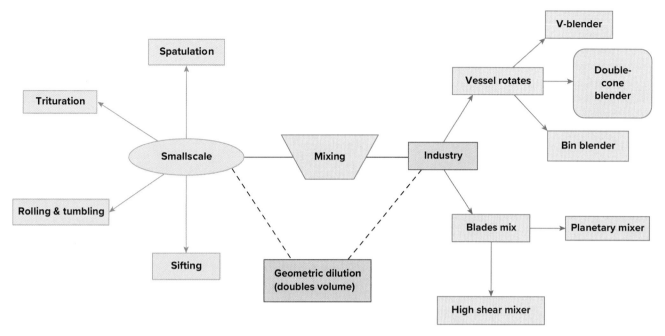

MIND MAP 5-2 Mixing of Powders

discussed in Chapter 4, Pharmaceutical Solutions, Dissolution, and Diffusion. This phenomenon may have important consequences, depending on the drug in question:

1. A shorter preparation time for solutions, especially on an industrial scale, is an obvious advantage. If the drug is slowly soluble, then grinding it to obtain a faster solution rate is valuable; whereas, if it is rapidly soluble, not much advantage is to be gained by reducing the particle size.

2. The bioavailability of solid dosage forms such as tablets and suppositories may increase since the drug goes into solution rapidly and may be absorbed rapidly. This does not apply to all drugs since the absorption rate, and not the dissolution rate, may be the rate-limiting step. Reduction of particle size to micron dimensions, also known as micronization, may have a major impact on the bioavailability of the drug. In the case of griseofulvin, the micronized drug provides better absorption and bioavailability and, hence, it was possible to decrease the dose of this antifungal drug. This example illustrates the utility of fine milling, even though this drug is not used very much in recent times. In recent years, reduction of particle size down to the nanometer range has greatly enhanced bioavailability in some cases (see Chapter 13, Nanotechnology).

3. Smaller particles produce less gastrointestinal (GI) disturbance. As smaller particles dissolve, the rough particles are rapidly replaced by a solution within the gastrointestinal tract (GIT). Hence, less GI irritation occurs. An example of a commercial product that utilizes this approach is "microfined" aspirin. Note: the chemical nature of some drugs, and not their surface roughness, causes GI irritation. In such cases, reducing particle size has little effect on GI irritation.

Suspension Settling Rate

Finer particles in a suspension settle more slowly (in the bottle) and the fine particles also dissolve more rapidly when the suspension is diluted in GI fluids. However, fine particles are also subject to greater caking (the formation of a hard sediment) at the bottom of the bottle after standing for a long time. Some injections are formulated as suspensions and the size of the suspended powder particles affects the properties of the injection. For example, the particle size affects the viscosity of the injection which, in turn, influences the ease with which the injection flows from the syringe. Similarly, the ease of pouring oral suspensions, and the ease of spreading topical suspensions, are affected by particle size. Suspensions with finer particles are more viscous for the same powder load.

Location of Inhaled Particles

The respiratory system consists of a branching network of progressively smaller tubes. Drugs may be administered directly to the respiratory system via inhalation systems which may contain a solution or a dry powder. When a dry powder device is used, the particle size of the powder affects how deep the medication penetrates into the branched respiratory system, with finer particles penetrating deeper. How deep should the particles penetrate?

While very large particles are not suitable because they may deposit in the mouth and throat, it may be surprising to learn that the finest particles are also not ideal. Particles with a slightly larger size (6 μm) are trapped in the bronchioles where their effect is needed and do not reach the deeper parts of the lungs. While one generally thinks of particle size reduction, if the particle size of the synthesized drug is too small, it must be increased for this application. Fisons Pharmaceuticals has a patent on the adsorption of fine particle sodium cromoglycate onto lactose. The complex particle, due to its larger size, reaches the part of the respiratory system where it will cause the greatest anti-allergic effect.

Rate of Solvent Extraction

During solvent extraction of drugs from plant tissues, the smaller the particle size, the faster is the extraction generally.

The solvent has a smaller distance to penetrate the particles and the drug solution has a shorter distance to diffuse out of the particles. However, small particles also result in the extraction of more unwanted material, such as coloring matter, carbohydrates, proteins, and sugars. In small particles of plant tissue, more cells are broken open during size reduction and, consequently, they spill their entire contents into the solvent. An optimum particle size of the plant material will give relatively fast extraction, with little of the unwanted matter, since many cells within the particle remain intact.

Rate of Drying

Since drying is a surface phenomenon, the greater specific surface area of fine particles results in faster drying. With small particles, moisture or solvent has a shorter distance to travel from the interior to the surface of the particle. Finer particles are, also, able to be dried to a lower moisture content value and, hence, moisture-sensitive drugs are more stable, that is, residual moisture is less after sufficient exposure to the drying conditions.

Blending of Powders

Two important effects of particle size on the mixing of powders are readily observed:

1. The blending of multiple ingredients is easier if the particles are approximately the same size. If the sizes are very different, there will be segregation (separation of particles based on size) upon standing and handling, with the finer particles falling through the gaps between the larger particles.

2. Consider two powders, A and B, which have to be mixed. If particles of equivalent size are chosen, in accordance with (1) above, does it make a difference whether relatively large particles (eg, 500 μm) or relatively small particles (eg, 100 μm) are used? The smaller particles will produce a more uniform blend because there will be a greater number of particles per unit mass and, therefore, a greater probability that a particle of "A" will be next to a particle of "B." The effects of the flow and static charge of very small particles on good mixing, as discussed below, should also be taken into account.

Powders in Semi-Solids

Although it is sometimes necessary to include powdered solid substances in semi-solid pharmaceutical formulations, the result may be an unacceptable product unless correctly processed. Creams, pastes, and ointments can have a rough and gritty feel when applied to the skin if the particle size is large. Due to a poor texture, the appearance of these formulations may also not be appealing to the patient. The solution is to subject the final product (semi-solid) to a milling process in a colloid or roller mill.

Organoleptic Properties

The color of dyes is affected by the particle size of the dye powders. The taste of materials may also be perceived to be different depending on the particle size. In the first place, smaller particles dissolve faster and therefore are tasted more readily (chemicals must be in solution for taste to be perceived). In addition, there may also be a qualitative difference between the perceived tastes of smaller, versus larger, particles.

Surface Activity

Powders used for their surface effects are more active when smaller-sized particles are used.

1. Since adsorption is a surface phenomenon, the smaller the particles, the greater the specific surface area and the greater the adsorptive power. Kaolin and charcoal are used as adsorbents in poisoning cases. The finer the particles, the greater the adsorptive power and the more effective is the treatment.

2. Lubricants and glidants are used in tableting. The former lubricates the particles making up the tablet so that they can slip past each other easily under high compression in the die of the tablet press and also allows the compressed tablet to be more readily ejected from the die. Fine particles of magnesium stearate coat the larger particles of drug and tablet excipients to provide the desired lubricant effect.

Huge differences in the effectiveness of magnesium stearate, used as a lubricant, have been noted in the literature when different particle size grades were used. The finer particles are more effective as lubricants. However, magnesium stearate is a very hydrophobic material which, generally, retards wetting and water penetration. Hence, when powders are coated with magnesium stearate, the tablets made from them have a tendency to slower dissolution and disintegration since the rate of water penetration into the tablet is slower. This phenomenon explains the lower bioavailability obtained from tablets containing finer magnesium stearate. The finer particles of magnesium stearate are more effective in coating the powder particles resulting in efficient lubrication but they, simultaneously, are also more effective in adding a hydrophobic layer to the particles. This retards water penetration into the tablet to a greater extent and results in a slower drug release rate.

A glidant allows bulk powders to flow more easily from the storage hopper to the processing area of pharmaceutical machines, such as tablet presses. Glidants are more effective when used as fine particles. For example, silicon dioxide is much more effective as an ultra-fine powder. Cab-O-Sil® M5 and Aerosil® 200, two brands of silicon dioxide are so fine that 1 g has a surface area of 200 m².

Hardness of Tablets

The smaller the particles, the harder the compact formed during tableting since small particles pack closely, with less void spaces between them. However, smaller particles, in general, flow less well and a compromise between flow rate and the ability to form a compact has to be achieved (Mind Map 5-3).

PARTICLE SIZE REDUCTION

Particle size is reduced in industry using mills of various types. Industrial scale particle size reduction is beyond the scope of this course and we will not discuss it further. However, there are

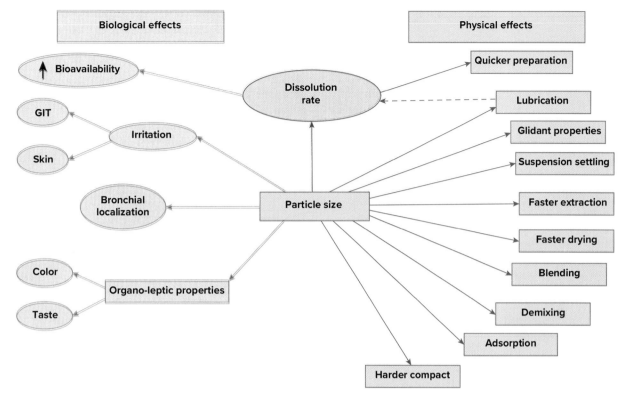

MIND MAP 5-3 Physical and Biological Effects of Particle Size

small-scale methods which a pharmacist could use for particle size reduction related to compounding. There are chiefly two ways to do this: trituration and levigation.

Trituration

Trituration is performed using a porcelain mortar and pestle. This is also commonly referred to as a "Wedgewood" mortar and pestle, which is actually a brand name. The coarse powder is placed into the mortar and, using steady, firm pressure, the pestle is rotated within the mortar. The particles of the powder are reduced in size as they are rubbed between the rough surfaces of the mortar and the pestle. A glass mortar is not good for this purpose as the smooth surfaces do not provide the required friction. As previously noted, a glass mortar is good for mixing by trituration.

Levigation

Levigation is the process of grinding an insoluble substance to a fine powder, while wet. The paste that results can be easily incorporated into semi-solid dosage forms. For this procedure, a glass slab with a spatula, or a mortar and pestle, is used in conjunction with a suitable levigating agent. The levigating agent is, typically, an oil or some other liquid in which the powder is not soluble. Common levigating agents are light mineral oil or glycerin. By incorporation of the levigating agent, and the mechanical action, either between mortar and pestle or, on a glass slab, between the glass and the flat face of the spatula, the particle size of the powder becomes reduced. If the formula contains an ingredient that is suitable to use as a levigating agent, a portion of it can be used in this first part of the preparative method. If it does not, a small amount of liquid paraffin or

glycerin may be added, if it is compatible with the rest of the ingredients. The mixture of levigating agent and powder is then incorporated with the rest of the ingredients. In the latter case, obviously, the material has an extra component, the mineral oil or the glycerin, at the end of the process. Therefore, the formulation in which this powder is being used has to be able to accommodate the selected levigating agent. This is usually acceptable if an ointment is made. Similarly if suppositories (solid dosage forms for insertion into the rectum or vagina) are made, a levigating agent may be useful when powdered drugs have to be incorporated. A hydrophobic levigating agent (such as mineral oil), or a hydrophilic levigating agent (such as glycerin) can be used, depending on the nature of the base, or bulk material, to be used in the preparation of such formulations.

POWDER FLOW

The flow properties of powders may have a tremendous influence on the process of powder mixing and on the homogeneity (or lack thereof) of the mixed powder. Tablets made from a non-homogeneous powder are likely to have some tablets with a higher drug level, while others may contain a lower drug level than required. During processing on an industrial scale, the powder is stored in a large hopper (a part of the machine) and flows, often through curved and narrow channels, to a part of the machine where the powder is processed. The processing may consist of the filling of capsules or the flow of powder into a die of a tablet press for compression into a tablet. Poor flow to the processing area leads to products of poor and variable quality.

Since a pharmacist may be called upon to dispense mixed powders, an understanding of the flow and other properties of powders may be useful. The pharmacist may also be asked to compare two brands of a commonly prescribed tablet. Is the generic product good enough and should the pharmacy stock only this brand at a tremendous saving to the patient? The comparison of the two brands may involve examination of manufacturing methods and ingredients. If the product is a major item for a hospital, this level of review may be justified. An understanding of powder properties and the factors that facilitate mixing, or promote demixing, is important in this regard.

The following factors affect the flow properties of powders:

Particle Shape

Particles that approximate a spherical shape flow well whereas irregular particles do not. If the shape is highly irregular it may severely impede the flow of particles. On the other hand, spherical particles also demix more easily when subjected to shaking and vibration, for example during transport. Highly irregular particles may lock together and prevent demixing (although difficult to mix in the first place).

We often refer to the diameter of a particle, implying that it is a perfect sphere, whereas particles are usually irregular and the spherical approximation is only used for convenience of description, comparison, and calculation.

The shape of the particle depicted in Figure 5-2 is close to spherical and the use of a circle to describe it seems reasonable. A circle is uniquely described by one parameter, its diameter. The use of one dimension to characterize the size of particles becomes more difficult to justify when particles deviate greatly from the spherical shape. In such cases, one has to make more than one measurement on each particle (measure the length, breadth, and, possibly, thickness). Heywood's ratios may be used to characterize the shape of highly irregular particles. Several ratios have been described relating length (L) to breadth (B) to thickness (T). An example is the elongation ratio, $(n) = L/B$. Acicular (needle-shaped) crystals have a high n-value (eg, > 5). Typical cuboidal crystals have L:B:T approximating 3:2:1. Cuboidal crystals are known to compact well (form hard tablets) and to be directly compressible (the powder does not have to be converted to granules first for tableting). Examples of cuboidal crystals are NaCl and KCl.

Moisture Content

When the moisture content of a powder is above the optimal value, it will result in poor flow of the powder. All powders are not equally affected. For example, microcrystalline cellulose can gain a few percent of moisture without severely affecting its flow rate whereas lactose will lose some of its flow properties

for the same moisture gain. However, some moisture is needed for pharmaceutical processing, such as tableting and, therefore, one cannot remove moisture completely in an attempt to aid flow. In any event, if a powder is over dried, it will rapidly regain moisture when taken out of the oven and exposed to the atmosphere. The moisture gain will continue until the powder attains its equilibrium moisture content. This value depends on the moisture content of the atmosphere and the nature of the material, that is, if two different dried powdered materials are exposed to the same relative humidity, one may gain moisture until its equilibrium moisture content is reached, for example, 1% whereas the other may only attain equilibrium at 3%.

Electrostatic Attraction

Powders that have gained static (due to mixing for example) will not flow well. Mixers should be grounded to reduce static charge and so avoid explosion risk.

In many processes, consistent powder flow is extremely important. Capsule filling and tablet production are two processes in which good, consistent flow is essential to avoid the following problems:

1. Mass variation of dosage form
2. Decreased drug load
3. Thin tablets (too little material in the die of the tablet press results in thin tablets after compression)
4. Soft tablets (too little material in the die offers low resistance to the compression force and forms a soft tablet)

In the worst cases, poor flow of powder from the hopper of a production machine results in bridging which is the formation of a dense mass of material across the hopper (Figure 5-3). When this occurs, flow ceases. Rat holing is the formation of a narrow hole in the center of the powder bed with compacted material on the sides. Very poor flow, through the rat hole, occurs in this case which is also illustrated in Figure 5-3.

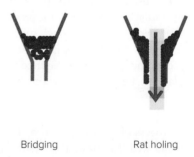

Bridging   Rat holing

FIGURE 5-3 Diagrammatic representation of two common flow problems.

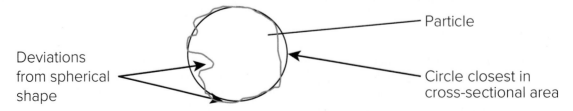

Particle

Deviations from spherical shape

Circle closest in cross-sectional area

FIGURE 5-2 Cross-sectional area of an irregular particle and a comparator circle.

How can poor flow be improved? Particle size reduction may improve flow down to a size of about 100 μm, in general. With further size reduction below this level, flow usually gets slower. This is due to the fact that very small particles have a high specific surface area and friction and cohesive forces, which are related to surface area, become very high. The notable exception to this general rule is material prepared by supercritical fluid technologies which produce very small, spherical particles that flow very well.

Before we can discuss the measurement of powder flow, we have to develop an understanding of powder density since this parameter may be used in the assessment of powder flow (Mind Map 5-4).

Recap Questions

1. If two powders are dried overnight at the same temperature, will they have the same moisture content after taking them out of the oven and leaving the open containers to cool for 6 hours?
2. If two powders have particles of the same size, will the powders flow equally well?

DENSITY OF POWDERS

The density (ρ) of a solid is given by:

$$\text{Density} = \frac{\text{Mass}}{\text{Volume}} \quad (5\text{-}1)$$

From this equation, we can see that we have to determine the mass of the powder and its volume, and divide the former by the latter to find the density of the powder. Mass determination is easy, but how does one determine the volume? There are several, different, volumes that can be described for a powder.

Bulk Volume

When a powder is poured into a container, such as a measuring cylinder, without tamping or compressing the powder, the volume that it occupies is the bulk volume, and

$$\text{Density}_{\text{bulk}} = \frac{\text{Mass}}{\text{Volume}_{\text{bulk}}} \quad (5\text{-}2)$$

Tapped Volume

The tapped volume is the volume occupied by the bulk powder after tamping or compacting to a controlled, predetermined extent. The tapped density is given by:

$$\text{Density}_{\text{tapped}} = \frac{\text{Mass}}{\text{Volume}_{\text{tapped}}} \quad (5\text{-}3)$$

The tapped density is an important parameter in pharmacy and commercial equipment is available for its measurement. Figure 5-4 is an example of such equipment.

Granule Volume and True Volume

The granule volume is the volume of the powder particles omitting the large void spaces between particles, but including the volume of cracks and fissures within the particle. The granule volume is measured by the volume of fluid displaced by the particles, using a fluid that fills the void volume between the particles but cannot flow into the cracks (eg, mercury).

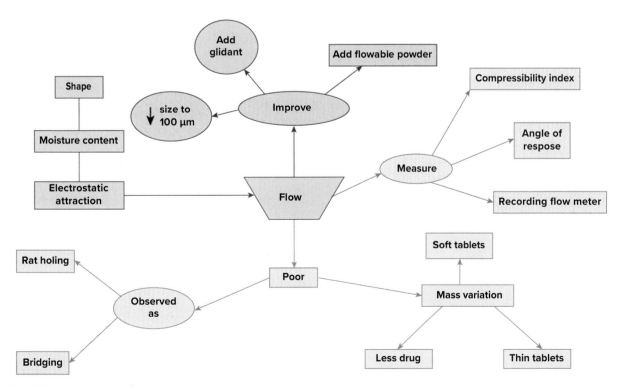

MIND MAP 5-4 Flow Properties of Powders

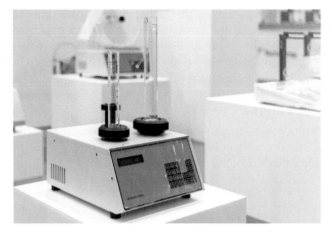

FIGURE 5-4 **Sotax tapped density tester.** (Used with permission from Surasak_Photo/Shutterstock.)

The true volume omits, additionally, the volume occupied by fissures and cracks in the material. It is measured in terms of the displacement of a fluid, such as helium, which flows into cracks and fissures. In Figure 5-5, the distinction between true volume and granule volume can be seen. The space that is omitted in the determination of granule volume (the space between particles in a powder) is shown in Figure 5-5B. The true volume is used in Eq. (5-1) to determine the true density, whereas the granule volume is inserted into Eq. (5-1) to determine the granule density.

MEASUREMENT OF POWDER FLOW

There are several methods to measure the flow of powders. Some use sophisticated (and expensive) equipment, whereas others measure, by means of relatively simple equipment, an attribute of the powder that is related to flow.

Compressibility Index

The compressibility index is used to estimate powder flow and is given by the following equation:

$$\text{Compressibility Index} = \frac{\text{Density}_{tapped} - \text{Density}_{bulk}}{\text{Density}_{tapped}} \times 100 \quad (5\text{-}4)$$

A large difference between tapped and bulk densities (and, therefore, a higher compressibility index value) means that the powder compresses under a force, rather than flowing. Where there is only a small difference between tapped and bulk densities, the powder bed utilizes the applied force to flow rather than to contract or reduce the powder volume. Compressibility index values of 5% to 15% indicate excellent flow, 18% to 21% indicate fair flow, and values above 21% show poor flow.

Angle of Repose

The angle of repose is used as an indirect measure of the ability of a powder to flow. Cohesion and friction retard flow. In a heap of powder, surface particles flow down the heap to form an angle with the support surface. This angle is characteristic of the powder in question and of its ability to flow. Powders with good flowability, form a broad heap with a narrow angle of repose (ϕ) (Figure 5-6). Powders with poor

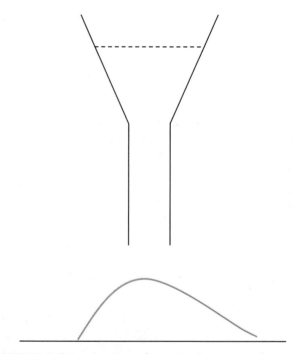

FIGURE 5-6 Setup for dynamic angle of repose testing.

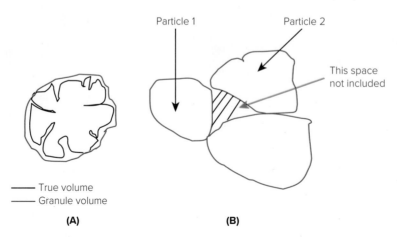

True volume
Granule volume

(A)

(B)

FIGURE 5-5 **True volume and granule volume.**

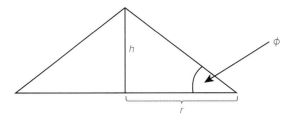

FIGURE 5-7 Determination of the angle of repose.

flowability, on the other hand, form a steep cone with a large angle of repose.

The diagram depicts the setup for one method of conducting the test. Under standardized conditions, powder is filled into a funnel, the stem of which is blocked to prevent the flow of the powder out of the funnel. When the obstruction is removed, the powder flows to form a cone on a piece of paper placed beneath the funnel. The angle φ is determined from the diameter and the height of the powder cone (Figure 5-7).

Tan φ is numerically equal to the coefficient of friction (μ).

$$\mu = \tan\phi \qquad (5\text{-}5)$$

$$\tan\phi = \frac{h}{r} \qquad (5\text{-}6)$$

The angle can be calculated from the experimental setup shown in Figures 5-6 and 5-7 (Box 5-1).

The lower the angle of repose, the better is the flow. The theoretical lower limit is 25°. Above 50°, flow is considered poor. It is probably better to use 45° as the cutoff for good flow. Although the accuracy and utility of the angle of repose as a measure of flowability has been criticized in the literature, this test can provide useful results for a small lab when performed correctly.

Box 5-1	Example of Calculation of Angle of Repose

In an experiment with Starch 1500 powder, the following values were obtained: $h = 19$ mm; $d_1 = 59$ mm; $d_2 = 62$ mm. Calculate the angle of repose for Starch 1500.

$$\tan\phi = \frac{h}{\dfrac{d_1 + d_2}{4}}$$

$$\tan\phi = \frac{19}{\dfrac{59 + 62}{4}}$$

$$\tan\phi = \frac{19}{30.25}$$

$$\phi = \arctan 0.6281$$

$$= 32°$$

Note: Instead of using r (the radius), the sum of the "shortest" and "longest" diameters of the irregular powder heap was divided by 4.

Recording Flow Meter

The recording flow meter is the preferred method of determining the flow rate of powders. It is a direct method of measurement, that is, the actual flow is measured. Particles fall from a funnel onto the pan of a scale. This is connected electronically to a strip chart recorder or a computer. The increase in mass versus time is plotted. The flow rate is given by the slope of the straight-line portion of the curve. The steeper the curve, the better is the flow. One can also detect changes in the flow rate which are denoted by a change in the slope of the curve. A change in flow rate could be due to separation of some components of a mixture, or even to separation of fast-flowing, and slow-flowing, particles of a single compound. This may be observed when the material consists of powders of vastly varying sizes. In Figure 5-8, the powder labeled A is expected to flow better than the one labeled B. Powder C shows evidence of segregation of components. Note that only the straight-line portions of the curves are shown. The curves are generally sigmoidal in shape.

POWDER HANDLING

The properties of powders, as outlined above, dictate how they should be handled.

Adsorption of Moisture and Gases

Because of their large surface area, powders can adsorb moisture and gases readily. Moisture pickup may be an important factor in the degradation of a drug by hydrolysis. Apart from its chemical effects, moisture can also cause agglomeration and, thus, affect the flow properties of powders.

It is important to store powders in well-closed containers and minimize exposure to the atmosphere especially when it is known that the powder is moisture or oxygen sensitive, for example, do not leave the material overnight in an open mixing vessel if the process cannot be completed. Extremely sensitive powders may have to be stored under nitrogen until used. This may also be the case for powders that have to be reconstituted before administration, for example, some powders for injection (for reconstitution with water at the time of injection) may be stored in the vial under nitrogen to prevent oxidation.

The higher moisture content of tablets compressed from exposed powders may have negative effects on the tablets during storage. The moisture present may result in the tablet

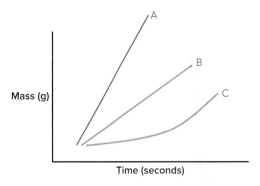

FIGURE 5-8 Recording flowmeter output.

having a soft and crumbly appearance. On the other hand, the moisture may promote a reaction in which the tablet hardens with age.

Effervescent formulations are very moisture sensitive and are usually packaged under special air conditioning. The 40% to 60% relative humidity (RH) usually present in a pharmaceutical factory is not acceptable for effervescent preparations. They may need to be packaged at about 20% to 40% RH to ensure adequate stability on an industrial scale.

In a pharmacy, it is good practice to store all powders in well-closed containers and to minimize contact with the atmosphere by closing containers as soon as possible after they are opened.

Static Charge

Particle size reduction may result in the creation of a great deal of static charge. This is especially true when very small powder particles are created. The static can cause the agglomeration of powder into clumps. When mixing large quantities of fine powder on an industrial scale (eg, 100 kg), the buildup of static charge can be explosive. The mixer has to be adequately grounded to prevent an explosion.

The pharmacist should also be aware of the following effect, due to static, when mixing powders: One component of a mixture may adhere to the wall of the mixing container to a greater extent than the other components. Hence, the dispensed mixture may be deficient in one component (perhaps, the drug). This effect may be decreased by using non-metallic containers and/ or by adding up to 0.5% (usually less) of silicon dioxide ("Cab-O-Sil M5" or "Aerosil 200") to the powders before mixing.

Segregation of Mixed Powders

Mixed powders may segregate due to particle size and density differences. Vibration during transport and handling can cause segregation. The vibration of a tablet press as it compresses tablets, can cause segregation of particles in the material to be compressed which is stored in the hopper, especially on long tablet runs of the order of 12 hours or more. The smaller particles filter through the spaces between the larger particles. If the smaller particles are the drug particles, this leads to variation in the drug content of the tablets. A solution may be to reduce the fill volume of the hopper in which case the powder remains in the hopper for a shorter duration and experiences less segregation. This is not the preferred solution since the hopper would have to be repeatedly filled. In addition, particles that are more dense tend to flow to the bottom of the container, when they are mixed with particles of a less dense material, even if both materials are equally sized. Particles that are more spherical flow well and mix better; but they also demix more easily.

One may appreciate that different drugs have distinct effects and that the chemical structure of the drug is related to its biological effects. It may not be immediately apparent, however, that the particle size of a drug can modulate the body's response to it. The particle size may have a large effect on the dissolution rate of the drug and on its biological availability. An understanding of these effects may help the pharmacist to make appropriate drug therapy choices.

Drugs are usually produced in a solid form (particles) and are then milled to produce powders which are incorporated into dosage forms. While there are coarse, fine, and intermediate mills, the product from each of these mills may include a vast range of particle sizes. It is important to be able to describe the size accurately as the size may affect powder properties.

PARTICLE SIZE MEASUREMENT

The measurement of particle size is difficult due to the fact that powder particles are irregular in shape. Which dimension of an irregular particle should be measured? The fact that powder particles usually cover a vast size range necessitates the use of statistical methods of representation. Is there only one unique way of representing the data? Because of these factors, the stated particle size of a powder is considered an estimate. It is possible that a powder measured by two different techniques and represented using different statistical methods may appear to be fairly different in size. Therefore, when stating the size of a powder, it is usual to give the method of particle size determination that was used.

Sieving

Sieving is the simplest method of size analysis but is employed for larger-sized particles only. Usually, a stack of sieves is used: the sieve with the largest apertures (or mesh size) in the stack is at the top, while the sieve with the smallest apertures, is at the bottom (and the other sieves are of intermediate size and are stacked in decreasing size order, Figure 5-9). A pan and a lid go

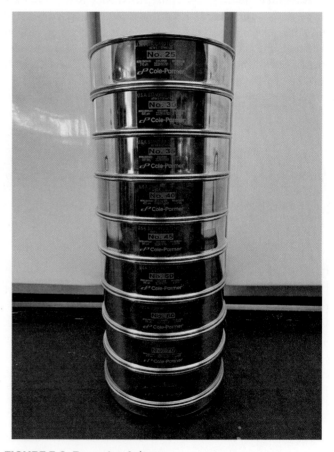

FIGURE 5-9 Example of sieves.

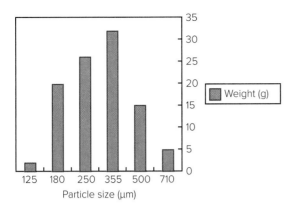

FIGURE 5-10 Mesh size vs weight of powder retained.

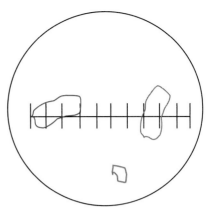

FIGURE 5-11 Diagrammatic representation of particles and eyepiece micrometer.

TABLE 5-1	Weight of Powder Retained on Sieves
MESH SIZE (μm)	**WEIGHT (gm)**
710	5
500	15
355	32
250	26
180	20
125	2

to the bottom, and the top, of the stack, respectively. Changes necessary because the pan and lid are not shown separately in the photo. The weighed sample of powder is placed on the top sieve and the stack is shaken or vibrated mechanically for a fixed length of time, for example, 15 minutes. A sieve shaker is used to create the motion.

Large particles are retained on the largest mesh-size sieve and the rest fall through. Those particles that are smaller than the size of the mesh on the next sieve fall through to the third sieve while the others are retained, and so on. Particles are segregated into size fractions in this way. The weight of powder retained on each sieve is determined. The data is usually represented as follows: the weight (or percentage by weight) of powder retained on each sieve is plotted against the mesh size of the sieve as reflected in Figure 5-10, or weight and mesh size are tabulated as presented in Table 5-1.

Microscopy

Microscopy is a direct method of assessing particle size, that is, a fixed number of particles (eg, 200) are actually observed and measured. This is done by means of an eyepiece micrometer (Figure 5-11). This is a small disc of glass which is placed into the eyepiece of the microscope. Engraved on it is a line with a scale. Each particle is measured using the eyepiece micrometer. In a separate step, the eyepiece micrometer is calibrated by reference to a stage micrometer at the same magnification used for measuring the particles. The problems associated with microscopy include:

1. Clumping of particles can be a problem if the operator mistakes the clump for one large particle.

2. The orientation of the particle can also be an issue: the large particle on the right in Figure 5-11 (blue) is identical to the one on the left (red) but may appear smaller due to a different orientation. A widely accepted rule is to measure each particle in the orientation that it appears on the line. For highly irregular particles, such as needle-shaped crystals (eg, theophylline), it is possible to measure both the length and the width of particles.

3. It is tedious and can cause eye strain.

4. There can be operator bias in that one operator may preferentially choose small particles to measure. A solution is to have only a limited no. of particles in any field of view on the microscope slide and to measure (or "count") every particle in that field.

The Coulter Counter

The Coulter Counter is used to measure the size of smaller particles, generally referred to as sub-sieve–sized particles (smaller than those that can be measured by sieves). In practice, however, there may be an overlap between the largest particles measured with this technique and the smallest measured with sieves.

The Coulter Counter works on the principle that a particle moving between two electrodes immersed in an electrolyte solution will change the conductance of the electrolyte solution. The extent of the change is proportional to the volume of the electrolyte solution displaced by the particle. The volume of electrolyte displaced is, obviously, equal to the volume of the particle.

HIAC Particle Counting Method

"HIAC" is an acronym for HI Accuracy Counter. This particle counting method depends on the extent of light blockage by an individual particle. As particles pass individually between a light source and a photodetector, the particle obstructs some of the light. The obstruction (reduced light reaching the detector) results in a voltage pulse, the extent of which is related to the size of the particle. The particles flow through the space between the light source and the detector and must have a medium in which they are dispersed. This medium can be viscous, non-viscous, aqueous, or non-aqueous liquids as well as gases. The diameter which is given (output) is related to the cross-sectional area of the particle.

The advantage of this system is that it is automated and greatly reduces operator bias. It is also very accurate. A disadvantage is that it relates cross-sectional area to the area of an equivalent sphere. This may not be an issue with particle 1 in Figure 5-12 but may be more of an issue with particle 2.

Laser Particle Size Analysis

Light from a laser is shone into a cloud of particles suspended in a transparent gas, for example, air. The particles scatter the light, smaller particles scattering the light at larger angles than bigger particles. The scattered light can be measured by a series of photodetectors placed at different angles. The way that the light is scattered by a particular powder sample is known as the diffraction pattern of the sample. The diffraction pattern can be used to measure the size of the particles. In the simplest configuration, particle concentration is made so low that the light scattered by a particle, essentially, reaches the detector directly and can be directly measured. It is assumed that light is not re-scattered by other particles before reaching the detector, that is, single scattering occurs. With higher concentrations of particles, the initially scattered light reaches other particles first, to be scattered again, that is, multiple scattering occurs. With laboratory instruments, the user has control over the sample size and a sufficiently dilute sample can be prepared so that multiple scattering does not occur.

Since the instrument measures clouds of particles, rather than individual ones, it is known as an "ensemble" technique. The system measures millions of small particles (eg, 10 micrometers) in the course of one determination. This confers a greater degree of reliability on the results.

This method is commonly used in the industry because of its accuracy. However, the method of sample preparation and handling should be specified to have consistent results by different operators. Laser diffraction is sensitive to the volume of the particle. Again, the particle is assumed to be spherical and

the reported results are the diameters of particles having equivalent volume to the irregular particles that were measured. The report can be customized, that is, one can request the instrument to print out the diameter for which 50% of the particles are larger than the stated size. This gives one an idea of the average size of particles within a sample. Or, one could program for $d_{10\%}$ and $d_{90\%}$ (10% of particles are larger than the stated size and 90% are larger than the stated size, respectively). This would give one an evaluation of the largest, and the smallest, sizes in the sample, respectively.

Recap Questions

1. If small particles dissolve faster, should we always use the smallest particles possible in any dosage form?
2. A pharmaceutical company makes a vast range of products. The lab manager states that he would prefer to only use one particle size measurement method for all samples that he receives. That way, everyone in his lab can be an expert in that method. What's your opinion?

DATA HANDLING AND REPRESENTATION

From the above, one can appreciate that the different methods of particle size analysis can give different results. Sieving provides the proportional weight of particles larger than a particular size, for example, 10% of the particles, by weight, are larger than 200 μm. Microscopy, on the other hand, gives the sizes of individual particles, from direct measurement of their dimensions.

When handling a large amount of data, the individual sizes are placed into size groups for convenience. The result is the *number* of particles within a particular size group. The

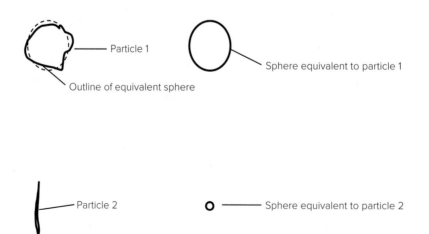

FIGURE 5-12 Depiction of particles and equivalent spheres.

Coulter counter provides the *number* of particles larger than a particular size but this "size" is that of an equivalent sphere having the same volume as the irregular particle. With the HIAC particle size analyzer, it is the number of particles equivalent in cross-sectional area to a perfect sphere of a particular size. For example, the result from a HIAC particle size determination that 20 particles in a sample were larger than 50 μm, means that 20 irregular particles had cross-sectional areas that were each larger than that of a sphere having a diameter of 50 μm.

Example

An example of the handling and presentation of data will now be shown, using results from a microscopy size determination. The individual diameters of 300 particles were determined by optical microscopy. The various sizes obtained were placed into different size groups and the no. of particles in each size group was determined. The data can be presented in a table for review (Table 5-2). Alternately, the number of particles in each size group (n_1, n_2 ..., etc.) can be plotted against the midpoint of the group (d_1, d_2, ..., etc.); or a bar graph can be drawn. Another way to use the data is to calculate the arithmetic mean. Thus, one parameter (the arithmetic mean) may be used to compare several batches of the powder. The arithmetic mean diameter is calculated from the summary data as follows (Box 5-2):

A graph gives a visual picture and shows if the data follows a normal distribution or if it is skewed. Usually, there are more powder particles of small size (skewed to the right). The mode

TABLE 5-2	Summary of Data from Optical Microscopy
SIZE GROUP	NO. IN EACH SIZE GROUP
0 to 10	6
>10 to 20	16
>20 to 30	37
>30 to 40	48
>40 to 50	62
>50 to 60	52
>60 to 70	43
>70 to 80	21
>80 to 90	7
>90 to 100	6
>100 to 110	1
>110 to 120	1

is the maximum in the size-frequency curve. The graph gives a unique description of the data set since many different data sets could, conceivably, give the same mean or mode value (Mind Map 5-5).

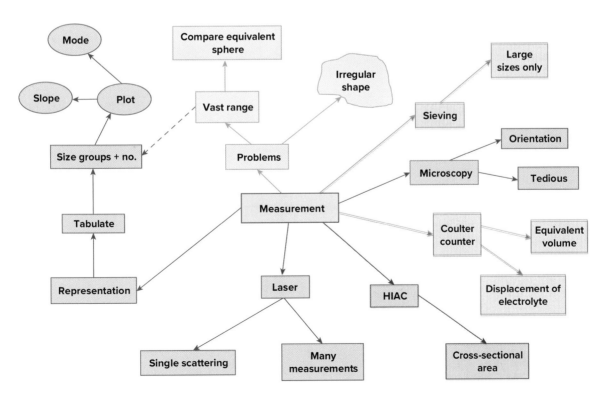

MIND MAP 5-5 Size Measurement and Representation

Box 5-2	Calculation of the Arithmetic Mean Using Data from Table 5-2

$$d_{arith} = \frac{n_1 d_1 + n_2 d_2 + \dots n_n d_n}{n_1 + n_2 + \dots n_n}$$

$$d_{arith} = \frac{\sum (nd)}{\sum n}$$

$$= \frac{6(5) + 16(15) + \dots}{6 + 16 + \dots}$$

$$= \underline{47.98\,\mu m}$$

SUMMARY POINTS

- Particle shape, size, static charge, and moisture content affect the ability of the powder to flow; flow in turn is important for processing. Powder handling, thus, is very important and simple steps such as limiting exposure to atmospheric moisture may be important.
- Particle size is an important attribute that may affect dissolution rate and bioavailability, adsorption and the rate at which a powder will dry. Smaller particle sizes, especially micronized particles, can be used to improve the bioavailability of some drugs.
- In specialized dosage forms, such as inhalations, a specific particle size is required for optimal therapeutic response.
- It is important to mix powders well to ensure uniform doses. On the small scale, trituration, spatulation, tumbling and rolling, and sifting can be used. For low-dose, potent drugs, geometric dilution may be used to ensure an even mix of drug and diluent.
- Size measurement is not as simple as measuring a square or a circle: irregular particles pose additional problems with measurement. Often the measurement relates an attribute of the powder particle (such as its volume or cross-sectional area) to that of a perfect sphere.
- Because of the wide range of particle sizes encountered, the individual sizes are placed into size groups and the number of particles in each size group is determined. Such data may be tabulated or graphical methods may be employed to represent the data.
- It is important for the pharmacist to understand powder properties and the impact that batch differences may have on the therapeutic effect of the dosage form.

What do you think?

1. Considering all the variability that is possible in powdered drugs and powdered excipients, how is it possible to make dosage forms of consistent quality from these powders?
2. Would it be easier to formulate all drugs as solutions and so avoid the problems inherent with solid dosage forms made from powders?

Pharmaceutical Suspensions

6

PREVIEW

- Why are suspensions formulated?
- The two major categories of suspensions: deflocculated and flocculated
- Compounding of suspensions
- Suspension stability
- Popular suspension products

INTRODUCTION

The discussion on suspensions will begin with a brief description of some salient features of solutions. Then, the analogous features of suspensions will be mentioned to illustrate the differences between these two liquid dosage forms. Pharmaceutical solutions are one-phase liquid systems in which the drug is distributed, at a molecular level, in a solvent. Pharmaceutical solutions add an element of complexity in that there may be additional additives above those required to simply form a solution. These include thickeners, sweeteners, flavors and preservatives. Nevertheless, a pharmaceutical solution is still a one phase system. There are no particles of drug (which would be

considered a separate phase) within the liquid. Consequently, the liquid is uniform throughout its volume. We refer to such a system as a one-phase system. There are other liquid formulations in which there are two phases: the drug or other substance is finely distributed in a liquid, but these components can be distinguished from the liquid as a separate phase. The substance distributed is referred to as the dispersed phase (or internal phase), and the liquid in which the distributed substance is dispersed is termed the dispersing phase, or dispersion medium, or external phase. Together, the dispersed phase and the dispersion medium produce a dispersed system. The two main types of dispersed systems are:

1. Suspensions in which the internal phase is a fine powder—discussed in this chapter; and
2. Emulsions in which one liquid is dispersed as fine droplets in another, immiscible liquid—described in Chapter 7, Emulsions.

Types of Suspensions

There are many applications of suspensions in pharmacy and some are administered by alternate routes of administration. The physical forms and applications of pharmaceutical suspensions are summarized in Mind Map 6-1. Examples are otic (ear),

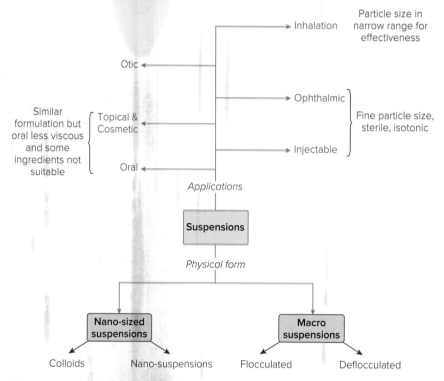

MIND MAP 6-1 Physical Forms and Applications of Pharmaceutical Suspensions

ophthalmic (eye) and injectable suspensions. This chapter will primarily focus on suspensions for oral, or topical, administration, with a brief reference to injectable suspensions. The latter are discussed in more detail in Chapter 12, Injections, while ophthalmic suspensions are described in Chapter 23, Ophthalmic Drug Delivery. Suspensions for inhalation are usually prepared in the propellant and the suspension filled into an aerosol can. Aerosols are described in Chapter 19, Pulmonary Drug Delivery.

While the same principles, generally, apply to the formulation of suspensions administered by any route, some have additional requirements. For example, ophthalmic and injectable suspensions must be made isotonic. Both suspension types must also be sterilized, whereas this is not a requirement for oral and topical suspensions. In addition, the suspended particles, in ophthalmic and injectable suspensions, must be of a very fine particle size. Suspensions for injection have become very important in modern therapy since they provide sustained release (SR) formulations of injectable drugs. The SR properties of suspensions for injection are also discussed in Chapter 12, Injections.

Of the different types of suspensions, topical suspensions are most closely related to oral suspensions and have similar preparation methods. Hence, they are discussed together in this chapter. There are also differences in their respective formulations, for example, topical suspensions can be very viscous whereas oral suspensions are usually not, to allow easy swallowing. In addition, some ingredients that are routinely used for topical applications may not be acceptable for internal consumption. Topical suspensions are sometimes referred to as lotions, for example, calamine lotion. The term "lotion" denotes a liquid dosage form for external use. An emulsion for external use can also be called a lotion.

With respect to the suspensions discussed in this chapter, the particles of the dispersed phase may be relatively large (10-50 μm). A suspension may also contain particles in the size range of 1 to 100 nm. These suspensions are referred to as "nano suspensions" and are of great interest in modern pharmaceutical technology for two reasons. First, they have the ability to promote the absorption of drugs that are poorly absorbed from other formulations. Second, many nano particles display special properties that may be beneficially utilized in drug delivery. For example, some nanoparticles may escape detection by certain body systems that normally trap particles and remove them from circulation. Therefore, the nanoparticles can remain in circulation for a prolonged time, providing a beneficial effect. For this reason, injected nano suspensions have a huge therapeutic advantage, for example, in cancer chemotherapy.

While nano technology is a relatively new idea and requires special processing, there are dispersions consisting of fine particles of natural origin that have been known for a long time. These dispersions have special properties and are therefore of scientific interest. Usually, the particles are in the size range of 500 nm to about 1 nm. The protein found in milk, casein, naturally agglomerates to units of colloidal dimensions, that is, milk can be considered a colloidal dispersion. The special properties of colloidal dispersions include the ability to fluoresce and the advantageous characteristics in biological applications. Colloidal silver and colloidal gold are further examples of colloids.

While nano particles and colloids have been mentioned to provide a perspective on the nature of suspended particles, this chapter will focus on coarse suspensions. Wherever "suspensions" is mentioned in the remainder of this chapter, it is in reference to coarse suspensions. Largely because of their greater size, particles in a coarse dispersion tend to separate from the dispersion medium. Most solids in dispersion tend to settle to the bottom of the container because of their greater density compared to that of the dispersion medium. Complete and uniform redistribution of the dispersed phase is essential to the accurate administration of uniform doses of pharmaceutical suspensions. For a properly prepared dispersion, this should be accomplished by moderate agitation of the container. Nanosuspensions, on the other hand, are much more stable and display no settling.

DESCRIPTION

Suspensions may be defined as two-phase preparations which contain a liquid and finely-divided, poorly-soluble solid drug particles which, after shaking the container, remain distributed more or less uniformly in the liquid for sufficiently long to allow the removal of an accurate dose. The liquid distribution medium in pharmaceutical suspensions is usually water, or a mixture of water with other solvents. Some suspensions are fully prepared at the pharmaceutical factory and are available to pharmacists and patients ready for use. Others are obtained from the pharmaceutical manufacturer as "dry powders for suspension". The dried powder usually contains the required amount of powdered drug to make up a suspension of a predetermined concentration and volume, provided in an oversized bottle. The pharmacist adds the liquid (usually water) and shakes to disperse the powder before supplying it to the patient.

Drugs, such as certain antibiotics, that are unstable in water, if stored for long, are usually supplied as dry powders for suspension. The dry powder is stable for an extended time and contains the correct amount of the drug to make a suspension of the desired concentration. Also included in the powder mixture are suspending agents and other excipients, for example, flavoring agents and coloring agents. This type of preparation is designated in the United States Pharmacopoeia (USP) as "XX (drug name) for Oral Suspension," for example, ampicillin for oral suspension. Suspensions that are fully formed at the pharmaceutical factory (ie, those that do not require constitution by the pharmacist at the time of dispensing) are simply called "oral suspensions" in the USP.

Recap Questions

1. What is the major difference between a solution and a suspension?
2. What is the major difference between a suspension and an emulsion?
3. Name three powders for oral suspension that are mentioned in the USP or other source of drug information.
4. Why are powders for oral suspension provided in *oversized* bottles?

REASONS FOR FORMULATING SUSPENSIONS

There are several reasons for formulating and preparing suspensions, including the following:

1. Many patients prefer liquids because they are easy to swallow.
2. Liquids give greater flexibility for measuring a dose.
3. Certain drugs are unstable in solution but are stable when provided in suspension form. Therefore, the suspension confers stability while providing the advantages of a liquid dosage form, such as ease of swallowing. This is especially important for infants, children, and the elderly, as mentioned above.
4. Suspended particles have little taste while a solution of a soluble salt of the same drug may have a very unpleasant taste.

Alternate salt forms of certain poor-tasting drugs have been developed for the formulation of suspensions. These salts are less soluble than the original salt of the drug (which may have been used in earlier formulations, including experimental formulations). A drug (or any substance, for that matter) has to be in solution to reach the taste buds on the tongue to enable taste perception. Therefore, poorly soluble salts result in less taste perception of the drug. In this way, a palatable liquid dosage form can be prepared even though the drug, in a soluble form, has an unacceptable taste. For example, erythromycin estolate is a less water-soluble ester form of erythromycin. Erythromycin Estolate Oral Suspension, USP is a palatable liquid dosage form. Likewise, when a drug is unstable in solution, converting the drug to an insoluble form promotes chemical stability because the drug has to be in solution for degradation reactions to occur.

It is very difficult to make a poorly-tasting drug acceptable, from a taste perspective, simply by the use of sweeteners and flavors. It is far easier to use an insoluble, or poorly soluble, form of the drug in the formulation. Thus, where the use of an insoluble drug is acceptable in terms of therapeutic efficacy, the formulation of insoluble, or poorly soluble, salts is the approach taken by most formulators. Any added flavor is used to impart a pleasant taste to the product and is not primarily used to mask the bad taste of the drug. The choice of flavor is then based on taste preference of the intended patient population, for example, grape flavor for children. To an extent, flavor preferences are also regional, for example, an acceptable taste in the US may not be acceptable in some Asian countries.

In general, poorly-soluble drugs are also poorly absorbed. Hence, the solution of the taste problem may create another significant problem, namely, poor bioavailability of the drug. Hence, the drug developer who has produced a suspension of acceptable taste has to also ensure that the poorly-soluble drug is absorbed in adequate amounts. One way to achieve this is to ensure that the formulated salt breaks down under biological conditions to the original form of the drug (which is more soluble). For example, erythromycin estolate (an ester) breaks down under the acidic conditions prevalent in the stomach to release erythromycin (a free base). Erythromycin then passes from the stomach to the small intestine where it is absorbed. This effect may also be achieved by additional formulation ingredients, which are added to the product, to enhance the breakdown of the salt once the drug has left the oral cavity.

THE FEATURES OF AN IDEAL PHARMACEUTICAL SUSPENSION

There are many considerations in the development and preparation of a pharmaceutically elegant suspension. A few of the desirable features are specific to pharmaceutical suspensions and are listed below. These are in addition to the usual requirements for all pharmaceutical dosage forms, namely, therapeutic efficacy, chemical and physical stability, and esthetic appeal.

1. Since suspensions settle with the passage of time, the preparation should have an appropriate settling rate and should be easily re-dispersed with shaking.
2. The particle size of the dispersed phase should remain approximately the same throughout the shelf life of the suspension, even with long periods of undisturbed standing, that is, there should not be a significant crystal growth.
3. The suspension should pour readily and evenly from its container to enable the easy removal of a precise dose.

BASIC CATEGORIES OF SUSPENSIONS

In general, there are two categories of suspensions that can be developed, based on the physical behavior of the suspended particles. These two categories can be differentiated by the manner in which the suspended particles settle at the bottom of the container (or come out of suspension). To explain this further, consider what happens when a dose of suspension is to be administered to a patient. Typically, the bottle of suspension is shaken (to evenly disperse the suspended particles) before removing the cap and measuring the volume, for example, 5 mL. What happens to the suspended particles once shaking of the bottle stops? This model provides the basis for a clearer understanding of the two suspension categories.

If the particles settle rapidly, the correct dose may not be provided each time the patient takes the medication for the reason mentioned below. A significant amount of the active ingredient (the suspended particles) would settle out of suspension, and fall towards the bottom of the container, in the time that it takes to unscrew the cap and pour the medication into the spoon or measuring cup. This means that the patient would be taking a lower-than-desired dose. More importantly, if the settling rate is very rapid, the amount of drug that settles may differ with each pouring. The small differences in the time it takes to pour the dose at each dosing interval (once shaking stops) results in different quantities of the particles settling within the container before the suspension can be poured. Therefore, different amounts of the drug are transferred to the measuring spoon each time a dose is poured. Thus, the dose is not only deficient but also variable.

In addition, settled particles can, by the process described below, form a solid cake that is difficult to re-disperse. The settled particles, or sediments, get compressed due to the hydrostatic pressure of the liquid above the sediment. This leads to a progressively more compacted cake as water is squeezed out from between the particles. If this process is allowed to continue, eventually the individual particles are brought so close together that fusion of adjacent particles (crystal growth) may occur. Such a compact cake with crystal growth is very difficult, if not impossible, to re-disperse. How can the particles be prevented from settling very rapidly? Once a sediment has formed, how can the formation of a hard cake be prevented?

There are two divergent solutions to this problem. Each solution leads to a different category of settling behavior. There are two basic categories of suspensions, based on their settling behavior, as previously alluded to. These categories are described below and it is worth remembering that they arise from the solution to the basic problems with suspensions, namely:

1. How can we retard settling sufficiently that the product allows the removal of a uniform dose?
2. How can long term physical stability be assured in suspensions for the product to be of practical utility? For example, it should not form a hard cake that resists dispersion.

Deflocculated Suspensions

One approach to achieve the desired situation is to increase the viscosity of the dispersion medium (usually water) and, thereby, slow down the settling of the particles. The individual particles settle more slowly due to the greater resistance to settling offered by the medium of greater viscosity. This category of suspension, in which particles settle individually, is referred to as a deflocculated suspension. Such suspensions takes long to settle but the sediment, once formed, is generally more difficult to disperse than flocculated systems, which are described next. While the hydrostatic pressure of the liquid above exerts pressure, it is more difficult to squeeze out the viscous medium and to force the particles very close together. Thus, the formation of a hard cake and crystal growth will only occur in extreme cases. This is because the viscosity reduces settling and also because the viscous dispersion medium coats individual particles and retards their ability to fuse and exhibit crystal growth.

Flocculated Suspensions

A second approach to solving the problem of the settling of particles in a suspension is to prepare a flocculated suspension. Flocs are described as loose clumps of particles held together by weak forces, such as van der Waals forces. In a flocculated suspension, the suspended particles are not discrete, individual particles but they group together to form small, loosely-held units of several particles. The units or fluffy clumps, are referred to as *flocs*. A suspension containing flocs is referred to as a flocculated suspension. (On the other hand, a suspension in which the particles are individually dispersed is called a *deflocculated* suspension.)

When settling occurs from a flocculated suspension, each floc settles as a unit; settling does not originate from discrete

particles. In addition, the totality of flocs settles fairly rapidly compared to a deflocculated suspension in which complete settling may take years to occur. The major advantage of a flocculated suspension is the fact that the flocs form a loose sediment that can be redispersed easily.

Considering the rapid settlement of flocs and the fact that all sizes of particles participate in floc formation, the appearance of a flocculated suspension after the suspension is allowed to stand for some time, is very different from that of a deflocculated suspension. In a flocculated suspension, a small volume of clear liquid is formed above the suspended particles, after a few hours of standing. This is the supernatant and it has the appearance of water in an aqueous suspension, because the content of particles in the supernatant is very low. (Water is the most common suspending liquid in pharmaceutical suspensions.) The supernatant may contain dissolved substances, which were added to the suspension to provide desirable attributes, for example, a flavorant. The remaining volume of the suspension, below the supernatant, has a somewhat coarse appearance and is referred to as the volume of the sediment. From this volume, particles, in the form of flocs may continue to settle. The supernatant has no particles and sedimentation cannot occur from the supernatant (Figure 6-1).

The concept of sedimentation volume is used in relation to flocculated suspensions. The sedimentation volume is the ratio (F) of the ultimate volume of the sediment (V_u) to the original volume of the sediment (V_o). Figure 6-2 illustrates the calculation of the sedimentation volume. The sedimentation volume may be calculated at different times, for example, 1 week, 2 weeks, 3 weeks, etc., after allowing the suspension to stand. The

change in sedimentation volume over time gives an indication of the stability of the suspension. Frequently, the sedimentation volume becomes smaller over time, the changes between each successive observation becoming progressively less, until the changes become negligible. However, the sedimentation volume can also become larger than the original volume of the suspension, that is, the suspension expands with floc formation.

Individual particles in a deflocculated suspension, on the other hand, settle at different rates depending on their particle size. Larger particles settle faster than smaller particles. Settling may continue for several years, an indication of how long it takes fine particles to settle. Therefore, no clear supernatant is observed even after standing for some time. While the bottom of the suspension appears more dense with particles, the top of the suspension still has discernible particles, that is, there is no supernatant liquid. In a typical, well-formulated pharmaceutical suspension of the deflocculated category, a clear supernatant may only be observed a few years after the suspension was left to stand undisturbed (Figure 6-1).

The flocs settle *relatively* rapidly, in comparison to deflocculated suspensions, because the flocs are larger clumps of particles. In a properly formulated flocculated suspension, the settling is not so fast as to make the removal of consistent doses questionable. The flocs are easy to redisperse because they are loose aggregates due to the nature of the forces holding the individual flocs together. In addition, there is water (the dispersion medium) between the individual particles making up a floc and there is also water between the different flocs that make up the dispersed phase of the suspension. With this arrangement, individual particles do not get so close together that they form a compact cake, nor do particles get forced together strongly to cause fusion and, ultimately, growth of a large crystal. Even after years of standing, a flocculated suspension is usually easy to redisperse.

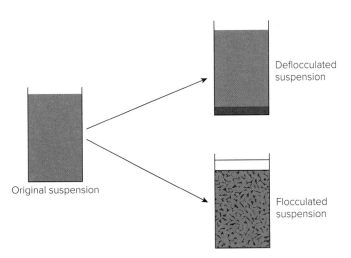

FIGURE 6-1 **Illustration of flocculated and deflocculated suspensions.**

> ## Recap Questions
>
> 1. Why do the individual particles in a deflocculated suspension settle at different rates?
> 2. Why do the flocs, in a flocculated suspension, settle at approximately the same time?

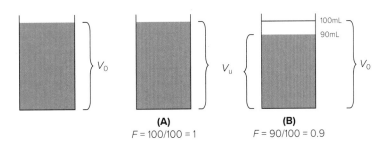

$$F = 100/100 = 1$$

$$F = 90/100 = 0.9$$

FIGURE 6-2 **Illustration of sedimentation volume (sedimentation volume $[F] = V_u/V_o$).**

Mechanism of Floc Formation

Why do flocs form? Flocs form as a result of certain physical interactions within the suspension. Generally, there are two basic types of interactions: electrostatic interactions between suspended particles and interaction of suspended particles and a polymer.

Electrostatic Interactions Between Suspended Particles.

Consider a typical deflocculated suspension, that is, one in which flocculation has not occurred. The dispersed particles of the suspension usually have a charge. There are multiple ways in which suspended particles can acquire the charge but only a few will be mentioned.

1. Ionization of surface groups. In this case, the particle contains ionizable surface groups, such as -COOH groups. When the ionization occurs, the small ion (H^+ in this case) is released into the bulk liquid whereas the remainder of the molecule remains with the particle as a charged group ($-COO^-$ in this case).

2. Selective ion adsorption. When particles are dispersed into a solution of ionic substances, the particle surface may become negatively charged through the following mechanism. The cations of the dissolved ionic substance are more highly solvated than the negatively charged ions. As a result, the positively charged ions have a greater tendency to reside in the bulk liquid, whereas the negatively charged ions reside at the particle surface.

3. Addition of surfactants. These substances have a strong affinity for surfaces, as their expanded name, surface active agents, implies. They can have a strong influence on the charge at a surface. Whether a positive, or negative, charge is applied depends on the chemical nature of the surfactant. They are frequently used to alter the charge on particles to bring about a desired effect in suspension formulation, as described in the next section.

Particles usually have a double layer of charge (Figure 6-3). This charge can be positive or negative and have a fairly high value (positive or negative). The charge can be determined by measuring a factor called the zeta potential of the material. A detailed description of the nature of the double layer is complex and requires a mathematical description for a full understanding. Clearly, such a treatment is beyond the scope of this chapter and what follows below is a very brief and simplified version. This is intended solely to help with an understanding of suspension formulation. There are several methods and commercial equipment available for measuring zeta potential, but the details of these methods are also beyond the scope of this chapter.

This surface charge causes repulsion between particles. In a deflocculated suspension, this repulsion keeps the particles away from each other. The level of the charge (high or low zeta potential) or its nature (positive or negative) can be manipulated as needed for specific formulation attributes. Take the case of dispersed particles having a high positive charge. The formulator may add some negatively charged particles, or ions, to the suspension. The charged particles or ions will be adsorbed onto the positively charged suspension particles. This has the

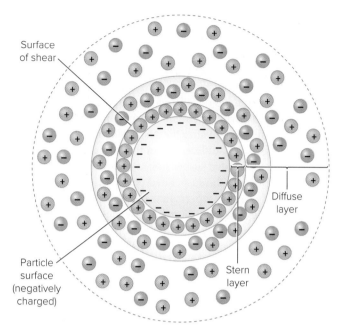

FIGURE 6-3 Electrical double layer around suspended particle.

effect of decreasing the positive charge on the suspended particles. If more negative charge is added to the suspension, the net charge becomes progressively less positive. This can be continued until the net charge on the particles becomes only slightly positive.

When the positive charge is made very low, two randomly moving particles are capable of coming into close proximity with each other. Random movement in a suspension is provided by Brownian motion. With some random movements, the particles may come very close to each other or may touch. When the latter occurs, very short-range attractive forces come into play and these hold the particles together. When this happens repeatedly, a clump of particles, that is, a floc, is formed. Mixing action during suspension formation and the motion of settling particles, among other forces, also bring particles close together.

If the addition of the negative charge is continued a little further than described above, the net charge on the particles becomes slightly negative. The net result, in terms of floc formation, would be essentially the same. The weakly charged negative particles will not repel each other significantly. Such particles are also capable of coming close together and of touching. This, eventually, leads to floc formation as other particles join the agglomeration. Thus, flocs can form from weakly positive, or weakly negative, charged particles.

Polymer Interactions.

A second manner in which flocs may be formed is by the addition of certain polymers to a deflocculated suspension. In solution, the polymer may take the form of a long strand of monomers. Such a strand may be an essentially straight chain, or a chain that coils. A coiled polymer strand is particularly useful for forming flocs. A number of the suspended particles, which are individually dispersed initially, attach to a long, coiled strand of polymer. This aggregation of particles constitutes the floc.

After a relatively short period of standing (days), a flocculated suspension may show a clear supernatant (the liquid above the sediment). This occurs because:

i. The flocs settle rapidly.

ii. **All** the particles (large and small) are involved in floc formation in contrast to a deflocculated suspension, as described below.

Recap Questions

1. Describe two ways to flocculate a suspension.

2. With the information provided up to now, list the differences between a flocculated and a deflocculated suspension.

3. In your *own words* describe the appearance of a flocculated suspension after 10 hours of standing.

4. In your *own words* describe the appearance of a deflocculated suspension after 10 hours of standing.

SEDIMENTATION IN A DEFLOCCULATED SUSPENSION

The description given in this section refers to deflocculated suspensions only. Stokes' law describes the rate of settling of individual particles in a suspension, as found in a deflocculated suspension. It does not apply to agglomerates such as flocs that are present in a flocculated suspension. In addition, Stokes' equation (Eq. [6-1]) was derived for the settling of particles under very specific conditions that are well controlled:

1. The particles are perfectly spherical and of uniform diameter (eg, all particles have a diameter of 20 μm).

2. The suspension is very dilute (1%, or less, solids).

Under these circumstances, the settling particles do not collide with other particles. This is referred to as "unhindered settling." The particles simply fall downward under the influence of gravity. They do not spin as they fall which might happen if they collide with other particles. Therefore, they do not produce turbulence in the liquid medium. There is, also, no chemical or physical attraction or affinity for the dispersion medium.

Practical pharmaceutical suspensions usually contain more than 1% dispersed phase. The concentration of the particles gives an indication that the particles might bump into each other as they settle, potentially producing turbulence. Furthermore, the particles are irregular in shape and the rotation of the irregular particles (as they fall) produces turbulence. In addition, the particles are, generally, also likely to have some affinity for the dispersion medium. For these reasons, which have been briefly stated, Stokes' equation does not apply precisely. In spite of this, we can still consider the equation, and the various factors contained therein, and estimate the effect of formulation changes on the settling rate of particles in a pharmaceutical suspension. The equation is also informative when one has to adjust the formulation of a suspension because it is settling too rapidly. The equation gives the formulator guidance on which formulation

characteristics to adjust in order to make the suspension more physically stable and, therefore, more useful.

$$\frac{dx}{dt} = \frac{d^2(\rho_1 - \rho_2)g}{18\eta} \qquad (6\text{-}1)$$

Where $x =$ the vertical distance that a particle falls in time $= t$;

$dx/dt =$ the rate at which a particle falls;
$d =$ diameter;
$\rho_1 =$ density of the particles;
$\rho_2 =$ density of the dispersion medium;
$g =$ gravity;
$\eta =$ viscosity of the dispersion medium.
From the equation, it is clear that:

1. Larger particles settle at a faster rate than smaller particles (keeping other factors constant). Therefore, if the particle size of the dispersed phase is reduced, the particles settle more slowly. This factor has a major impact since "d" is squared in the equation.

2. The greater the difference in density between the particles and the dispersion medium, the greater will be the rate of settling. If water is the dispersion medium, most particles used in pharmaceuticals will be more dense and will settle to the bottom of the container. It is important to realize that it is the particle density that is applicable, whereas the bulk density may be less than that of water. This is because the bulk density takes into account the powder particles as well as the air spaces between them (see Chapter 5, Pharmaceutical Powders). One may also glean from the above equation that particles with a greater density will settle faster than less dense particles, if other factors are kept constant. If water is the dispersion medium, then the difference in density, as given by the above equation, will be greater for the more dense particles.

3. The rate of sedimentation is inversely related to the viscosity of the dispersion medium. Since this factor is multiplied by 18 in the equation, settling may be appreciably reduced by increasing the viscosity of the dispersion medium. On the other hand, very viscous liquids are difficult to pour. Also, when the suspended particles have settled, it will be difficult to redisperse them, due to the high viscosity of the suspension. For these reasons, it is not practical to use an extremely viscous dispersion medium.

The viscosity characteristics of a suspension may be altered not only by the vehicle and viscosity-enhancing agent (thickener) used, but also by the solids content. As the proportion of solid particles in a suspension increases, so does the viscosity. We measure viscosity by using a viscometer, such as a Brookfield Viscometer. This instrument measures the force required to rotate a uniform spindle or other attachment (analogous to a propeller) in the fluid being tested. The greater the resistance to rotation, the greater is the viscosity. The apparatus uses different attachments for viscous, and for thin, liquids respectively. Each attachment is only capable of measuring viscosity in a specific range.

One cannot adjust the dispersion medium viscosity to a large extent since the suspension becomes too difficult to pour, and may also have a poor appearance, beyond a certain viscosity. Therefore, most often, the physical stability of a pharmaceutical suspension is achieved by an alteration of the dispersed phase, for example, change in the particle size, uniformity of particle size, and maintenance of the separation of the particles. Particle separation ensures that very large agglomerates are not formed due to the cohesion of several particles. The latter, referred to as agglomeration, can form a solid cake upon prolonged standing. The close proximity of the particles in such an agglomerate can lead, ultimately, to crystal growth. This process is different from flocculation in which loose flocs are formed. Such flocs do not promote the formation of a dense cake, neither do they promote crystal growth. Flocs are easily dispersed upon mild agitation of the bottle.

SIZE OF DISPERSED PHASE PARTICLES

An important consideration in a discussion of suspensions is the size of the particles, especially the particles in a deflocculated suspension. In most commonly used pharmaceutical suspensions, the particle diameter is 1 to 50 μm. These are the conventional suspensions, sometimes also called "macro suspensions" to distinguish "nano suspensions" which contain particles in the nanometer (nm) size range. Nano particles and nano-suspensions are of tremendous interest in research for a variety of reasons, including improved bioavailability of the extremely small particles. A detailed consideration of nano-suspensions is beyond the scope of this chapter.

There are several methods, which are commonly used in the industry, to produce particles in the 10 to 50 μm size range. Usually, this is done by milling. Two types of mills that may be used for this purpose are the hammer mill and the ball mill. The fluid energy mill, also known as the jet mill, produces particles under 10 μm. There are no moving parts in the fluid energy mill. Instead, high-velocity compressed airstreams rapidly sweep the particles through narrow, curved tubes. The particles are accelerated to high velocities and collide with one another and with the walls of the mill, resulting in fragmentation. Since particles are in the micron size range, the process is also known as micronization. The process is very effective in that size reduction occurs rapidly, there is no contamination from moving parts (which occurs in other mills), and there is little heat generation. This method may be employed when the particles are intended for parenteral or ophthalmic suspensions because of the very low levels of contamination. One disadvantage is encountered when relatively small amounts of research drug (eg, 1 kg) are to be ground. The percentage of drug retained in the mill, and therefore lost, is relatively high.

Particles of extremely small dimensions may also be produced by spray drying. A spray dryer, essentially, creates very fine drops of drug solution. These drops are sprayed into a large container where they meet a hot air stream. They are rapidly dried before the drop can touch the wall of the container. As the liquid evaporates, the drug precipitates out of solution, and fine drug particles are created. It is not possible for a pharmacist to create such fine particles with a mortar and pestle. However, many micronized drugs are commercially available to the pharmacist for compounding, for example, progesterone.

Recap Questions

1. Why is low heat generation during the milling of drugs important?
2. The fluid energy mill is very effective for micronized drug particles. Name one disadvantage of using this mill.
3. In broad terms, what is the physical difference between a coarse suspension and a nano suspension?

Reducing the size of particles to be incorporated into a suspension improves stability because the rate of settling is slower, as shown by Stokes' equation. Smaller particles settle more slowly and often more uniformly. The latter would occur if the size range of the particles becomes narrower due to size reduction. However, the formulator should avoid reducing the particle size too much since very fine particles have a tendency to form a compact cake when the particles eventually settle. If left in this state (as a settled cake) for a prolonged period, adjacent particles could fuse together to form large crystals, for reasons previously described. Crystal formation is an extreme situation but it does show that very small particles represent a potential problem. (In nano suspensions, a different set of forces are in play and nano-suspensions are, actually, very stable.)

A compact cake will resist breakup upon shaking and this will be the case even when particle growth has not occurred. Particle shape may play a role in the ease with which the compact cake can be redistributed: needle-shaped particles tend to interlock and are difficult to redisperse whereas spherical particles distribute more easily. These are extremes in shape. More generally, irregularly-shaped particles tend to hook onto each other and display some degree of difficulty to redisperse.

In contrast to the above, flocculated suspensions can be considered to be systems in which cake formation is avoided by the intentional formation of loose aggregations of the particles held together by comparatively weak particle-to-particle bonds. The flocculated particles form a lattice, or network, of particles that resists complete settling and cake formation, although flocs settle more rapidly than individual particles. The loose structure, with water between flocs as well as within individual flocs, allows for the easy breakup of the sediment, and facilitates the distribution of the suspended particles when the bottle is shaken.

Probably, the most common way to create a flocculated suspension is to reduce the charge on the particles, as previously mentioned. The charge is added in the form of an electrolyte solution and the electrolyte is said to "reduce the electrical barrier" between the particles. The charge prevented the particles from getting close together and, hence, acted as a barrier. The electrolyte may also, physically, form a bridge so as to link two particles together. A calcium ion (Ca++) may link two negatively charged particles. Sometimes, flocs of the dispersed phase can be produced by simply altering the pH of the suspension towards the value at which the drug has least solubility. At such a pH, there is less ionization of the drug and, consequently, less charge.

The addition of a small amount of polymer may also cause flocculation. Several particles attach to the long polymer strand which is, or becomes, coiled, leading to the formation of a floc. Clays are fine particle material of natural origin. Examples of clays are calamine, bentonite, and hectorite. The clays are used as suspending agents and thickeners in suspensions and lotions. Bentonite and other clays may be purchased as a powder or as a magma which is a very thick dispersion. When using the magma, it should be diluted, by the addition of water, before use.

Bentonite is commonly employed as a flocculating agent in suspensions. It has a negative charge which reduces the positive charge of some drug particles. Clays have a very fine particle size and a tendency for several particles to floc together. This may pull the drug particles together into aggregates. Clays may be too weak as flocculating agents on their own but when used together with polymers, may be effective flocculating agents. Interestingly, clays have been used to flocculate bacteria which are then filtered off.

The degree of flocculation that is created is important both for the appearance and the function of the suspension. A high degree of flocculation may be regarded as unsightly as the suspension has large flocs and appears coarse. Also, the settling rate may be too rapid to accurately remove a dose of the drug from the bottle. Hence, controlled flocculation is desired, that is, the extent to which flocculation occurs, or the degree of flocculation, is controlled. The flocs are small and have a pleasing aesthetic appearance in controlled flocculation. They, also, do not settle too rapidly. Increasing the viscosity of the dispersion medium by, for example, the addition of a polymer may assist in controlling the rate of settling of the flocs. See Dispersion Medium below, for examples of polymers that can be used for this application.

DISPERSION MEDIUM

A suspension may be thickened, that is, its viscosity is enhanced, to decrease its settling rate and to allow the removal of an accurate dose. Viscosity enhancement is particularly important for deflocculated suspensions but may also be used to enhance the functionality of flocculated suspensions.

Examples of viscosity enhancers that are commonly used are carboxymethylcellulose (CMC), methylcellulose, microcrystalline cellulose, polyvinylpyrrolidone, xanthan gum, and bentonite. The cellulose derivatives are of plant origin. Naturally occurring cellulose may be chemically modified to provide a derivative with certain desirable properties. Xanthan gum is also of plant origin. It is important that the thickener not interfere with the bioavailability of the drug. It is interesting to note that in comparison to solutions, a suspension has the following negative attributes with respect to bioavailability:

1. The drug molecule must dissolve from the particle before it can be available for absorption.

2. The drug molecule, once in solution, must diffuse to the body's absorbing membrane through a viscous dispersion medium.

3. The possibility of interaction between the dissolved drug and the suspending agent, or the flocculating agent, may decrease the availability of drug molecules for absorption.

Each of these factors has the potential to decrease the bioavailability of the drug relative to a simple solution in which no thickening agent is used (some solutions may be made viscous, primarily to give a good feel as the drug solution is swallowed). Conceivably, a very viscous dispersion medium may retard diffusion. Since the ability to diffuse is considered in the dissolution equation, slower diffusion may affect both the rate of solution, and the rate at which a solute molecule will diffuse to the absorbing membrane of the body. It must be kept in mind, though, that the suspension will be diluted in physiological fluids after consumption, and the drug particles that were distributed in a viscous suspension will rapidly become distributed in a larger volume of less viscous aqueous medium. Hence, this problem may be less severe than it may initially appear but must, nevertheless, be kept in mind. The dilution effect is dependent on the route of administration, for example, it is much greater in the GIT than in the eye. In vitro dissolution or release tests have to be performed to ensure that the drug is adequately released from a suspension.

OTHER EXCIPIENTS

While the excipients mentioned above are required for the suspension to function as intended, other excipients are required to make the formulation appealing to the consumer. Since most oral suspensions will be administered to children, the suspension should be appealing to this age group in terms of appearance, taste, and smell. To enhance the appearance, a color may be added. In addition to color, the suspension should be visually appealing in terms of texture. A suspension with a high degree of flocculation will appear coarse and may not be considered appealing by the intended consumer. Attention to the degree of flocculation may, therefore, be beneficial in terms of functionality as well as appearance.

The taste of the suspension should also be acceptable to the patient and this concept has been mentioned at the beginning of this chapter in relation to the motivation for selecting poorly soluble salts for the formulation of suspensions that are palatable. Here, some of the flavors that can be added to a suspension will be considered. The added flavor makes the suspension palatable and thus easier to administer to a pediatric patient. Some of the older flavors that are still popular are cherry, mint, peppermint, and vanilla. Some newer flavors are also very popular with children and these include bubblegum, candy floss, toffee, and fizzy flavors. The flavor and color of a preparation should match, that is, a yellow color for a banana flavor. A red-colored, banana-flavored suspension may surprise a child.

Sweeteners are added to enhance the added flavor and to partially mask the taste as well. Syrups are viscous solutions with a high content of sugar. The high viscosity can assist with the suspending of the particles. In cases where a large proportion of syrup is used in the external phase, the viscosity of the syrup may be sufficient to suspend the particles and an additional suspending agent may not be necessary. Of course, this depends on many factors such as the size and density of the suspended particles. For diabetic patients, syrup should not be used and polyol solutions, such as sorbitol solution, may be used. Sorbitol solution is not as viscous as syrup. Various syrups can be purchased from commercial suppliers in bulk. This saves the compounding pharmacist some time since the preparation of a syrup is not quick. Paddock Labs, located in Minneapolis prepares several syrup types, some flavored. Excipients added for other reasons may also improve viscosity and, therefore, assist with the suspending of the particles. For example, glycerin has preservative properties and a somewhat sweet taste. It also increases the viscosity of the external phase to some extent. Thus, this ingredient has multifunctional properties.

Recap Questions

1. Is it likely that the suspended drug particles will dissolve in the saliva as the patient takes the medication?

2. Assuming the drug particles have not dissolved in the saliva, will they dissolve in the stomach or in the small intestine? Explain, providing justification for your answer.

3. Is it possible to make a suspension without a suspending agent? Explain.

RHEOLOGY

The study of the flow characteristics of materials is called "rheology." The flow properties of liquids and semi-solids are important with reference to pharmaceutical products. The liquid components of a suspension, for example, must have a reasonable flow rate to enable the suspension to be adequately shaken for the purpose of mixing the suspended particles with the dispersion medium. Also, liquid formulations must flow well to be easily removed from the container.

A pharmaceutical product, in general, must also not be too "liquid" or "runny" to cause problems in other instances. For example, etching gel may be applied by a dentist to the surface of a tooth and left on for a short time (eg, 1 minute) to etch the surface of the tooth. The etching allows the filling material, that is subsequently applied, to adhere more strongly to the surface of the tooth. The gel must not easily run on to the soft tissues because it contains phosphoric acid and will cause stinging. On the other hand, hair gel should be easily removed from a squeeze bottle and excessive viscosity will impede the removal of the gel.

Since suspended particles will eventually sink to the bottom of a suspension, and a viscosity enhancer (or thickener), retards the rate at which the suspended particles sink, we may think of the viscous medium as "supporting" the suspended particles. This may be compared to a horizontal beam in a building which supports the upper floor and prevents it from dropping onto the lower floor. The extent of the "support" of the suspended particles by the dispersion medium depends on several factors:

1. The density of the suspended material: If the suspended material has a high density, it requires more support, that is, a higher concentration of viscosity-enhancing agent than does a suspended material of lower density. For example, bismuth subnitrate and magnesium hydroxide are actives that are used in antacid formulations. Bismuth subnitrate generally requires a higher level of suspending agent than magnesium hydroxide because the former has a higher density.

2. The solid content of the suspension.

Obviously, a suspension containing 200 mg of drug per 5 mL would require more of the suspending agent than one containing 100 mg per 5 mL of the same active ingredient.

Depending on the dose and the density of the drug, a sufficient amount of suspending agent is chosen to maintain the drug in suspension for long enough to remove an adequate dose. An excessive amount of the suspending agent is not used since it is likely to make the suspension too viscous.

PREPARATION OF SUSPENSIONS

In the preparation of a suspension, the formulator must be concerned with the rate of settling, palatability, and several other factors in order to produce an elegant suspension. It would appear easy to simply add water (the dispersion medium or vehicle) to a drug powder, and shake, to create a simple suspension of an insoluble, or poorly soluble, drug. Assume this simple formulation works in terms of physical stability, that is, the particles do not settle rapidly. In many instances, however, even this simplistic formulation would not be easy to produce. This is because the powder may be hydrophobic and resist wetting by the added water. In this case, the resulting preparation may have the appearance of water and clumps of partially moistened powder; or powder floating on the surface of the water.

What is required, in such a case, is the addition of a wetting agent. A wetting agent is an example of a surface active agent or "surfactant." The wetting agent is able to make contact with the surface of the powder particle, displaces air, and allows the subsequently added water to wet the powder adequately. When making suspensions on a small scale (as done in a compounding pharmacy), this problem may be overcome by simply adding a few milliliters of ethanol to a powder and mixing intimately before the addition of water. It is important that the mixing be intimate. On a small scale, this is done by rubbing the powders with the alcohol using a mortar and pestle. If the mixing is not adequate, some powder particles will not be moistened with ethanol. These (unmoistened) powder particles will not have contact with water, when the final suspension is made, and lumps of powder, within the suspension, may result. The appearance of such a suspension is not elegant and it is not suitable for dispensing. On a large scale, the mixing is done using a high-shear mixer. Other examples of wetting agents, suitable for pharmaceutical suspensions, are propylene glycol and glycerin.

Small Scale Production

There are two basic ways to prepare a suspension on a small scale, depending on the source of the drug. The drug for the suspension may be a drug in powder form that is purchased, for example, from a company that specializes in the supply of materials to compounding pharmacies. Alternatively, the source of the drug may be a tablet, or capsule, or other dosage form.

Preparation Using Drug Powder

The following steps are generally utilized to prepare the suspension:

1. Weigh all solid ingredients and measure all liquids.
2. Add all soluble components, such as colorants, flavors, and preservatives to the dispersion medium and mix thoroughly to dissolve.
3. Add the drug powder and any additional insoluble powder to a clean and dry mortar.
4. If necessary, add a few milliliters of wetting agent and rub into the powder using a pestle.
5. Add the dispersion medium in small amounts to the powder in the mortar and blend thoroughly, using the pestle, before the next addition of the dispersion medium.
6. Continue addition of the medium and mixing until approximately two-thirds of the vehicle has been added.
7. Transfer the contents of the mortar to the final (dispensing) container.
8. Use the remaining dispersion medium to rinse the mortar repeatedly, using a few milliliters each time. Add the rinsing liquid to the bottle and, finally, make up to volume by the addition of dispersion medium.

Preparation Using a Commercial Dosage Form

There are occasions when a pharmacist is called upon to prepare a suspension from a solid dosage form, usually a capsule or a tablet, as the source of the drug. This generally occurs when a suspension is needed for a particular patient, frequently a pediatric patient, but only tablets or other solid oral dosage forms of the drug are available commercially. Note that the pharmaceutical company that owns the product will probably manufacture the suspension if it is routinely needed. Typically, they manufacture a range of product types to cater for marketing needs, for example, tablets for adults and suspensions for children. When the drug is not routinely given to children, but it is required for a specific pediatric patient, the pharmacist is called upon to produce the suspension utilizing the solid dosage form as the source of the drug. The need may also arise when an adult has difficulty swallowing and the physician determines that a suspension would be more convenient for this patient.

When using capsules as the source of the drug, the procedure is approximately the same as described above for compounding with the drug powder. Instead of weighing out a specific weight of drug, the pharmacist would empty the required number of capsules into the mortar, depending on the stated drug content of each capsule. Since each capsule contains the drug as well as other ingredients, a larger amount of powder is incorporated into the suspension than would be the case if the drug powder was used. The additional powder is largely the diluent, in terms of weight. It is used in the capsule to increase the fill weight (the drug content of the capsule is often very small and it is difficult to accurately

fill this weight into the capsules repeatedly). The rest of the procedure for preparing a suspension is the same as that described above. A small volume of the selected vehicle, or solvent mixture, is added and mixed with the powder to create a paste. Then a further small amount of vehicle is added and triturated to evenly dilute the paste. This is repeated several times. As before, the last amounts of the vehicle should be used to rinse the mortar.

When preparing suspensions from tablets, the tablets are crushed in a mortar with a pestle. This may, practically, be more difficult than it appears. The first step would be to break the tablet by gently pounding with the pestle while ensuring that the tablets do not "jump" out of the mortar (cover the mortar!). Once the tablets are broken into large pieces, they must then be evenly ground to a finer size in the mortar. A flat-bottomed Wedgewood mortar of sufficient size is needed. Also, the pestle must be shaped such that it forms a tight fit with the periphery of the mortar, where the sides and bottom of the latter meet the pestle during grinding. If it does not fit snugly, partially ground material locates in this area and is not ground further by the action of the pestle. A glass mortar is suitable for mixing powders, not for grinding them.

As mentioned, more powdered material is added to the suspension when tablets or capsules are used as the source of the drug, compared to using the drug itself. This is because the tablets and capsules contain other ingredients, such as fillers (eg, lactose). If the added material is soluble in the dispersion medium (eg, lactose in water) then the addition of the extra material does not make a big difference to the properties of the suspension. However, if the tablet filler is insoluble (eg, microcrystalline cellulose or dicalcium phosphate dihydrate, which are common insoluble tablet diluents or fillers), then a large amount of inert material, which also has to be suspended, is being added to the suspension. This may require a larger amount of suspending agent.

In addition to syrups that may be purchased commercially as mentioned earlier in this chapter, several manufacturers prepare vehicles that are suitable for the preparation of suspensions. These vehicles, which may contain the suspending agent, a sweetener and a flavor, are available commercially to the compounding pharmacist. This saves the pharmacist several steps in the preparation of a suspension. Examples of commercial products include Ora-Sweet, Ora-Sweet SF or Ora-Plus (manufactured by Paddock Laboratories, Minneapolis).

Up to this point in the chapter, physical instability (which includes settling, ease of redispersion, cake formation, crystal growth etc.) has been emphasized because this is an important aspect of the formulation of suspensions. However, chemical instability, must also be considered. Most often this involves instabilities of the drug, such as degradation, or a change to an inactive form. To minimize chemical instability, the suspension should be dispensed in an airtight, light-resistant container and stored in the refrigerator by the patient. The patient should shake the container well prior to use. While pharmacists fulfill a need each time they compound a suspension for a patient, they should also be aware that drugs in a liquid environment, generally, tend to have lower chemical stability than drugs in a solid form. Other ingredients that may undergo chemical changes include the preservative, polymers (used as suspending agents), and colors (fading).

Stability data on some formulations have appeared in the professional literature and there are journals devoted to providing information for the compounding pharmacist, for example, the *International Journal of Pharmaceutical Compounding*. These journals may contain reports by drug manufacturers on the stability of their compounds and their suitability for inclusion in extemporaneously prepared formulations, including suspensions. Compounding pharmacists may also present the results of their own stability studies, which are usually limited in scope (shorter duration of study and smaller sample size, generally). It is important to keep the stability question in perspective: the patient is expected to keep the compounded drug suspension for a relatively short time (days in the case of antibiotic suspensions). Evidence of instability is far less likely to be observed. This is in contrast to a manufacturer who makes a product and usually gives an assurance of stability for at least 2 years. This period incorporates the time that a suspension might be on the shelf of a pharmacy or drug wholesaler, as well as the time that it may be in the possession of the patient.

While the above serves as general guidelines for compounding suspensions, it must be kept in mind that the pharmacist is preparing a special formulation for an individual patient. Hence, they must use this opportunity to consider the patient's condition as they formulate the suspension or any other formulation. For example, if the patient cannot swallow a tablet due to the presence of throat ulcers, the suspension should not contain a large amount of alcohol that will cause stinging of inflamed tissues.

Likewise, formulations for a neonate should not include alcohol (ethanol) because this solvent can alter liver function, cause gastric irritation, and produce neurologic depression. Benzyl alcohol should be omitted because it can cause a gasping syndrome with a deterioration of multiple organ systems and eventually death. Propylene glycol can cause seizures and stupor in some preterm infants. For the neonate, the formulation should be the simplest that is possible while retaining good formulation characteristics. To reduce the potential for causing undesirable effects, the formulation should have the least excipients. For example, colorings and flavorings should be avoided. This may not be a disadvantage to product quality since the neonate's taste is not well developed. In addition, the suspension may be administered by nasogastric tube in which case taste is not an issue. Preservatives should not be used; the pharmacist may have to prepare a suspension for one, or a few, day's use. In addition, the clinic staff should keep the remaining suspension in the refrigerator until the next dose. The suspension, or the dose to be administered should be allowed to reach room temperature before administration.

Pharmacists must be aware of "hidden" ingredients when compounding suspensions for any patient. For example, Aromatic Elixir, NF, contains as much as 21% to 23% alcohol and is unsuitable for patients taking drugs in respect of which alcohol should be avoided.

A modern trend has been for pharmaceutical manufacturers to include instructions, for the compounding pharmacist, on how to make a suspension from the manufacturer's solid oral dosage form. It is usually preferable to use the manufacturer's formulation rather than develop a new one. The manufacturer, very likely, expended significant resources to develop and test a suitable

formulation. Of course, a particular patient may have special circumstances which require the compounding of a formulation that is different from the manufacturer's suggested formulation. It should be remembered that the manufacturer is offering a method for compounding a suspension for general consumption.

Cozaar tablets is an example of a product where the manufacturer provides the formulation and a method for the preparation of a suspension from the tablets. Each tablet contains 10 mg of the drug, losartan, which belongs to the drug class, angiotensin receptor blockers (ARBs). This drug is used to treat hypertension. The following method for the preparation of a suspension (200 mL containing 2.5 mg/mL) is from the Cozaar package insert, rewritten as numbered steps:

1. Add 10 mL of Purified Water USP to an 8 oz (240 mL) amber polyethylene terephthalate (PET) bottle containing ten 50-mg COZAAR tablets.

2. Immediately shake for at least 2 minutes.

3. Let the concentrate stand for 1 hour and then shake for 1 minute to disperse the tablet contents.

4. Separately prepare a 50/50 volumetric mixture of Ora-Plus™ and Ora-Sweet SF™.

5. Add 190 mL of the 50/50 OraPlus™/Ora-Sweet SF™ mixture to the tablet and water slurry in the PET bottle and shake for 1 minute to disperse the ingredients.

6. The suspension should be refrigerated at 2°C to 8°C (36°F-46°F) and can be stored for up to 4 weeks.

7. Shake the suspension prior to each use and return promptly to the refrigerator.

Recap Questions

1. Why is a wetting agent required when water is part of the formula of a suspension?

2. Why should the mortar be rinsed with several small amounts of dispersion medium? Why not use one large amount?

3. Do you think that Aromatic Elixir, NF is a suitable vehicle for compounding a suspension for a 4-year-old child?

4. Why, in your opinion, does the manufacturer not market the Cozaar suspension?

5. Why does the manufacturer stipulate the type of bottle to be used?

6. How is the manufacturer's preparation method different from the general method provided in this chapter?

SUSTAINED-RELEASE SUSPENSIONS

The earlier attempts at formulation of sustained-release (SR) suspensions had only limited success because these attempts were based on modifications of SR solid oral dosage forms. For example, wax-containing beads, and polymer-coated beads filled into capsules were popular at the time. Ethyl cellulose, which is insoluble in water, may have served as the coating polymer. After consumption by the patient, water slowly permeates the bead, through pores in the coating, dissolves the drug, and the drug solution leaches out of the bead. Since this technology was known, early SR suspensions were prepared by suspending ethyl cellulose–coated beads, or wax particles impregnated with drug, in water. The problem with this type of formulation was premature drug release; the drug leaked out of the beads into the dispersion medium in the container during storage. Some leakage from the beads could be considered acceptable as the "immediate release" component of the formulation. However, the leaked drug often crystallized out of solution within the container. For this reason, this type of preparation was considered an unacceptable formulation.

The concept of simply transferring solid dosage form SR technology to SR liquids was eventually abandoned and different approaches were taken for the development of the latter. With this approach, a great deal of success was achieved. For example, resin systems such as the Pennkinetic system have proved successful. This system uses an ion exchange resin complexed with the drug. The ion exchange resin is a solid, insoluble, high molecular weight polyelectrolyte and the complex with the drug forms a resinate. The resinate, or complex, is then coated with polyethylene glycol 4000 to make it plastic (flexible) and a rate-controlling polymer, such as ethylcellulose, on the exterior. A unique feature of these ion exchange resins is the fact that they can exchange their mobile ions (the drug) with ions of equal charge that are present in the medium.

The most common use of this technology is with a resin containing numerous sulfonic acid residues. These can be complexed with a cationic drug. Drug release is dependent on exchanging sodium ions or hydrogen ions for the drug. Since the drug-resin complex is formulated into a suspension where the dispersion medium is ion-free, drug release in the bottle is negligible during storage. If significant drug release occurred, it would amount to failure of the system. After consumption by the patient, drug release occurs in the acidic environment of the stomach. H^+-ions are exchanged for drug ions in the resin complex and, in this way, the drug is released. Examples of this type of suspension are Delsym and Tussionex Pennkinetic Extended-Release Suspension. These formulations contain, respectively, dextromethorphan, and hydrocodone with chlorpheniramine.

Another approach is to use liquid crystalline phases. A drug is complexed with a special combination of lipid ingredients and suspended in water. The lipid/drug, although in the liquid state, has some characteristics of a crystal, that is, the molecules are arranged in an orderly fashion. This type of formulation has been researched quite extensively.

Since the particles in a suspension must dissolve for the drug to be available for absorption, an injection consisting of suspended particles serves as an effective SR dosage form. The SR effect is enhanced if the injection is administered to a site low in water or biological fluid, for example, muscle tissue. Thus, intramuscularly injected suspensions serve as effective SR dosing systems. If the injectable suspension is prepared in oil in which the drug is insoluble, the SR properties are even better since the drug must first come into contact with aqueous fluids before it can dissolve. In view of the fact that tissue fluid volume is limited, the rate at which the drug dissolves is slow. Thus, the drug is slowly released from the particles for absorption into the surrounding muscle tissue.

Recap Questions

1. Why were resin systems successful where wax systems were not, for developing SR suspensions?
2. What is preferable to facilitate the efficacy of a SR injection: a high, or a low, water content of the tissues at the injection site?

PACKAGING AND STORAGE OF SUSPENSIONS

Since suspensions must be shaken before each use, the containers should have a space above the liquid to permit thorough mixing, that is, they should be packaged in bottles that have a volume greater than the fill volume. Also, the ease of pouring a somewhat viscous liquid should be taken into account and a bottle with a wider mouth should be selected. In the absence of specific information to the contrary, the medication should be assumed to be light-sensitive and protected from light.

Some of the best-selling suspensions in the US market (in terms of the number of units sold) are given in Table 6-1.

TABLE 6-1	Some Pharmaceutical Suspensions Available in the USA	
DRUG	**INNOVATOR BRAND NAME**	**THERAPEUTIC CLASS**
Acyclovir	Zovirax	Anti-retroviral
Amoxicillin/ Clavulanate K	Augmentin	Antibiotic
Amoxicillin	Amoxil	Antibiotic
Azithromycin	Zithromax	Antibiotic
Carbamazepine	Tegretol	Anti-convulsant
Clarithromycin	Biaxin	Antibiotic

SUMMARY POINTS

- Suspensions provide a convenient, pleasant-tasting liquid dosage form.
- Suspension categories are deflocculated and flocculated.
- The particles of a deflocculated suspension settle slowly as individual particles; a compact cake forms after a long period of standing, accompanied by crystal growth eventually.
- The particles of a flocculated suspension settle relatively rapidly in the form of flocs that are easy to disperse.
- Compounded suspensions may be prepared utilizing the drug powder, or tablets or capsules containing the drug.
- Some components of a suspension may be purchased pre-formulated and, therefore, the suspension does not need to be made from scratch.
- Some manufacturers of tablets and capsules provide instructions for the preparation of suspensions from these dosage forms.

What do you think?

1. If alcohol or glycerin is not a part of the formula, can we add this additional ingredient?
2. Suggest a modification of the above method, if you need to add alcohol to the powders to serve as a wetting agent and the formula also contains methyl paraben (which is poorly water soluble but soluble in alcohol).
3. Is it possible to have no settling in a suspension at all? Where must a suspension be kept in order to have no settling? (You are required to think "out of the box" for this one.)
4. It has been stated that agglomeration of particles in a suspension is undesirable. Why, then, are flocculated suspensions formulated?
5. Explain why having a slight positive charge, instead of a slight negative charge, on the particles of a flocculated suspension makes little difference to suspension properties.

Emulsions

7

PREVIEW

- What are emulsions?
- Emulsion formulation for compounding and manufacture
- Emulsion stability
- Emulsion products

An emulsion consists of two immiscible liquids. The one liquid is composed of small globules, referred to as the dispersed phase, and is distributed throughout the second liquid, termed the dispersion medium. When an emulsion is freshly made, the distribution of the dispersed phase is more or less even throughout the dispersion medium. With time, this distribution changes as discussed later in this chapter under "Stability of Emulsions."

The dispersed phase is also referred to as the internal phase, and the dispersion medium as the external, or continuous, phase. Any two liquids that are immiscible may be formed into an emulsion (with appropriate formulation additives and processing). In pharmacy one phase is usually water, or aqueous, and the other is oily but two organic liquids that do not mix can also be formed into an emulsion, in keeping with the above concept. This leads to (a) oil in water (denoted as "o/w") emulsions with an oily internal phase and an aqueous external phase; or (b) emulsions having an aqueous internal phase and an oily external phase, which are termed water in oil (w/o) emulsions. We will use these abbreviations throughout this chapter. Other

components, such as a drug or a perfume, may also be added to an emulsion. The salient features of emulsions are given in Mind Map 7-1.

Typically, oils are yellow-brown in color (and translucent to varying degrees), while water is clear. However, the formed emulsion is white and opaque (like milk or body lotion). This is due to the fact that the distributed droplets diffract light in a different way than each liquid on its own in the unmixed state. Because the external phase of an emulsion is continuous, an o/w emulsion may be diluted with water to form a diluted emulsion of good appearance, that is, the added water blends with the external phase. If oil is added to this type of emulsion, it cannot blend with the external phase (water) and appears as a separate phase. A w/o emulsion can, similarly, be diluted with an oil since oil is in the external phase.

If an oil and some water are shaken together very vigorously, they appear to distribute and may take on a slightly whitish color, resembling an emulsion. However, as soon as one stops shaking the bottle, the two phases, oil and water, begin to separate almost instantly. Such a formulation, if it were for external use (eg, as a lotion), will not be pleasant to use as the oil would separate from the water, will not spread, and will have an oily feel. If such a preparation contained a drug and was intended for oral consumption, the drug is likely to be preferentially dissolved in one of the phases. If the drug were largely dissolved in the oil phase and the phases tend to separate, then the dose that

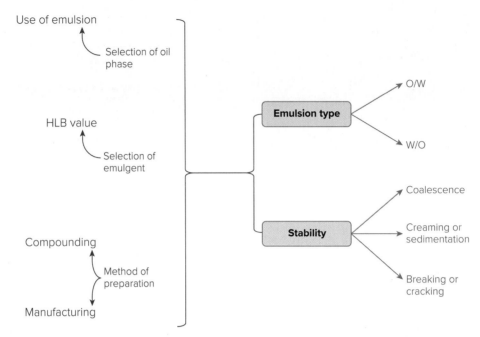

MIND MAP 7-1 **Emulsions**

the patient receives would depend on whether more oil, or more water, was consumed as the phases began separating. Obviously, this is unacceptable from a dosing perspective as well as from the esthetic perspective.

To prepare a useful emulsion, that is, one that is sufficiently stable that it may be dispensed and used by the patient before separation of the components, the addition of a third essential component, an emulsifying agent, is usually necessary. Depending on the different components used to formulate the emulsion (and their proportion in the formulation), the viscosity of the emulsion can vary greatly. Pharmaceutical emulsions may be liquid or semisolid. While semisolid emulsions are usually applied topically, liquid emulsions may be consumed orally, applied topically, or administered by injection. Many pharmaceutical formulations that are in the form of emulsions are not typically referred to by this term. The dosage form may also be described by another term (such as "lotion," "liniment," and "cream"), and the latter description has become commonly used. Some commercial vitamin "drops" are supplied in the form of an emulsion. Vitamins D and A are oils that may be better absorbed when emulsified. The emulsified formulation is also better tasting which improves patient acceptability.

PURPOSE OF EMULSIONS AND OF EMULSIFICATION

By the process of emulsion formation, the pharmacist is able to prepare relatively stable and homogenous mixtures of two immiscible liquids. In the absence of this method, it would be difficult to produce an elegant, patient-acceptable formulation of such ingredients, in most cases. An emulsion allows easy administration of a liquid drug in the form of minute globules dispersed throughout another liquid. The drug will tend to be less irritant to the digestive tract which comes into contact with

many small droplets, spread over a large area of the gastrointestinal tract, rather than a large volume in one area. Mineral oil, used as a laxative, is much less irritant when emulsified. Emulsification also allows the administration of oil in a form that is more palatable, digestible, and more easily absorbed. The o/w emulsion is more palatable since the external phase (water) is more directly in contact with the tongue. The oil drops that are suspended in the water are less accessible to the tongue and to the taste buds.

Emulsions that are to be applied to the skin may be o/w or w/o. For non-medicated emulsions, the emulsion type depends on whether a tissue softening, or emollient, effect is desired (in which case a w/o formulation is prepared), or whether a water washable preparation is required (o/w emulsion). For external medicated emulsions, the choice of emulsion type depends on the phase in which the drug is soluble. Generally, the drug is dissolved in the phase in which it is most soluble and that phase becomes the internal phase of the emulsion. It is usually best to distribute the drug within fine droplets that are dispersed throughout the external phase.

When the emulsion is applied to the skin, the droplets, and the drug, are spread over a large area of the skin. This allows better distribution of the drug. If the skin is sensitive, the emulsion is best compounded as described (drug in the internal phase) especially when the medicinal agent irritates the skin. In this case, it will be less irritating. The fact that the drug in the internal phase causes less irritation is analogous to the taste effect of emulsions, mentioned earlier (being in the internal phase, there is less contact with the tissue). Whether an ingredient is soluble in oil, or in water, dictates to a great extent where that ingredient will be **primarily** located in the formed emulsion. Frequently, however, the drug is soluble to some extent in the opposing phase as well. A drug that was added to the oil phase during formulation may be detected, to some extent, in the aqueous phase in these instances.

Recap Questions

1. What is meant by "immiscible"?

2. Why is the external phase termed "continuous" and why is the internal phase considered to be discontinuous?

3. How should emulsions be diluted, if the need arises?

4. From arachis oil and water, two types of emulsions can be formed. Name these two types of emulsions and describe the differences between them.

SELECTION OF EMULSIFIER

The first step, in the preparation of an emulsion, is to select the emulsifier which may also be referred to as "the emulsifying agent" or the "emulgent." These terms will be used interchangeably. The emulsifying agent must be carefully chosen. First, it should produce an emulsion of the desired type and maintain the stability of the emulsion throughout the shelf life of the product. In addition, it should be compatible with the other formulation ingredients and not interact with the therapeutic agent; it should be stable and not breakdown; it should not be a good substrate for micro-organisms; it should be non-toxic in the amount taken; and it should have little odor or taste.

Various types of materials have been used in pharmacy as emulsifying agents. The most important classes of emulsifiers and stabilizers for pharmaceuticals (with some representative examples) are given in the following sections:

Carbohydrates

Acacia, tragacanth, agar, chondrus, and pectin are examples of carbohydrates used as emulsifying agents. These are naturally occurring materials which form hydrophilic colloids with water. They usually produce o/w emulsions. Acacia is probably the most frequently used emulsifier for extemporaneous emulsions (as prepared in a compounding pharmacy, for example). Tragacanth and agar are commonly used as thickening agents in preparations where acacia serves as the emulsifier. Microcrystalline cellulose is used in many commercial suspensions and emulsions to increase the viscosity of the external phase.

Proteins

Gelatin, egg yolk, and casein are examples of proteins that have been used as emulsifying agents. These substances produce o/w emulsions. Mayonnaise is an everyday example of an emulsion which is emulsified with egg yolk. The disadvantage of gelatin is that the emulsion is often not viscous enough. The use of a secondary thickener may resolve this issue.

High-Molecular Weight Alcohols

Stearyl alcohol and cetyl alcohol are used as thickening agents and stabilizers for o/w emulsions used externally as lotions. Cholesterol and cholesterol derivatives are used to produce w/o emulsions and may be included in products for internal consumption. Different grades of cholesterol are available for different applications. Glyceryl monostearate is an ester of stearic acid that is commonly used.

Nonionic Surface-Active Agents

Surface-active agents or surfactants are a large group of emulsifying agents that may be divided into nonionic, cationic, and anionic surfactants, depending on their capacity to ionize in water and which ionic group retains the emulsifying capacity. As the name implies, non-ionic emulsifiers show no inclination to ionize under normal conditions, and these agents do not have a charge. They contain both hydrophilic and lipophilic groups. Thus, they can relate to both water and oils and may form a "bridge" between the two phases. The balance of the groups designates whether the surfactant will tend to be more lipophilic or more hydrophilic.

It must be emphasized that a chemical entity must be fairly well balanced with lipophilic and hydrophilic groups to be considered a surface-active agent: overtly lipophilic, or hydrophilic, compounds are not surface active. Within the range of compounds that have well-balanced groups and surface-active properties, some compounds are slightly more hydrophilic, and some slightly more lipophilic. Depending on their hydrophilicity or lipophilicity, surfactants have different properties. How can one assess a surfactant, by looking at its chemical structure, and determine whether it will be more lipophilic or more hydrophilic? If two chemicals are both more lipophilic than hydrophilic, their slight lipophilicity may not be the same. How can one evaluate the extent of the lipophilicity imbalance? Can this measure be related to the utility of the chemical as a particular subtype of surfactant?

William C. Griffin addressed these questions and, in landmark papers published in 1949 and 1954, respectively, outlined methods for determining numerical values which describe the balance/extent of hydrophilicity or hydrophobicity in surfactants.[1,2] The first paper describes experimental methods for determining this balance, while the second paper deals with a method of observing the chemical structure and assessing a numerical value that describes the chemical's balance of hydrophobic and hydrophilic characteristics.

Each type of lipophilic group is given a certain score. Likewise, each OH or each COOH group (and other hydrophilic groups) are also given a score. For example, a –COOH group has a value of 2.1, an –OH group 1.9, and a –CH3 group a value of –0.475. The final computation is the sum of (a) the total of the lipophilic score (negative) and (b) the total of the hydrophilic score (positive). The number thus obtained is the hydrophilic-lipophilic balance (or HLB). This value can be calculated for all non-ionic surfactants. The final score is a measure of the tendency of the molecule to be a little more hydrophilic, or a little more lipophilic. Devised while Griffin was at the Atlas Powder Company, initial estimations were for Atlas surfactants (which were later acquired by ICI Corporation and now reside with Croda, Inc.).

While theoretical scores with very high values can be computed, those up to a value of 20 are useful as surfactants. It has been found that certain values are associated with certain surface-active properties (see Figure 7-1). For example, high values such as 18 to 20 provide a solubilization effect. Compounds with values of 3 to 7 are useful w/o emulsifiers, and those with values of 8 to 16 are useful o/w emulsifying agents. This information guides the formulator by pointing towards broad categories of surfactants that might be useful for particular formulation types. Direction for the selection of specific emulsifiers is provided in the paragraphs that follow.

Examples of nonionic surfactants are given in Table 7-1. Common non-ionic emulsifiers include sorbitan esters (Spans®) which are more lipophilic, and the polyoxyethylene derivatives of sorbitan esters (Tweens®) which are more hydrophilic. From this characterization, and a consideration of Figure 7-1, it will be appreciated that Spans may have HLB values that are too low, while Tweens may have HLB values that are too high for some applications mentioned in this figure. However, Spans and Tweens may

be combined in a formulation to obtain the desired HLB value. For example, if a Span has an HLB of value 4 and a Tween has an HLB of 12, equal parts of each of these surfactants will result in a mixture having an HLB of (4 + 12)/2 = 8. Similarly, other proportions can be calculated to develop emulgent mixtures with various HLB values, as desired or required for the formulation to be prepared. The ability to adjust HLB values is important in consideration of the concept presented in the paragraph below.

Through trial and error, it has been found that certain oils work best if the emulsifier has a certain HLB value. For example, mineral oil requires an emulsifying agent with an HLB of 12 to form a good o/w emulsion. It is said that 12 is the "required HLB" for mineral oil. It is important to remember that the HLB is the property of the surfactant or emulsifying agent, and not that of the oil. The concept of required HLB makes it easier for formulators to select emulsifiers for certain oils. While many combinations may give the same HLB value, for example, 6.2, the ultimate selection will depend on the compatibility of the two emulgents with each other, and with the other ingredients in the formulation. To some extent, it will also depend on the personal preference of the formulator.

Anionic Surfactants

In anionic surfactants, the lipophilic portion is negatively charged, with a small cation to provide electrical neutrality to the molecule. Anionic emulsifiers include various monovalent, polyvalent, and organic soaps, such as triethanolamine oleate, and sulphonates such as sodium lauryl sulfate. Some anionic emulsifying agents are listed in Table 7-1.

Cationic Emulsifying Agents

In cationic agents, the organic chain that is active as an emulsifying agent is positively charged. It is associated with a small anion. Benzalkonium chloride, known primarily for its bactericidal properties, may be employed as a cationic emulsifier. Owing to the opposing ionic charges, anionic and cationic agents tend to neutralize each other and are, therefore, incompatible. Table 7-1 lists some cationic emulsifying agents.

Finally Finely Divided Solids

This includes clays (such as bentonite), magnesium hydroxide, and aluminum hydroxide. The finely divided powder locates at the interface of the oil and water and forms a tough film around the globule. These agents are versatile in that o/w or w/o

TABLE 7-1	Some Emulsifying Agents with HLB Values	
EMULSIFIER TYPE	NAME	HLB
Anionic	Triethanolamine oleate	12
	Sodium oleate	18
	Potassium oleate	20
	Ammonium lauryl sulfate	31
	Sodium lauryl sulfate	40
Cationic	Didocecyl dimethyl ammonium chloride	10
	Dodecyl trimethyl ammonium chloride	15
	Cetyl pyridinium chloride	26
Nonionic	Sorbitan tristearate (Span 65)	2.1
	Glyceryl monostearate	3.8
	Sorbitan monooleate (Span 80)	4.3
	Polyoxyethylene sorbitan monooleate (Tween 80)	15
	Polyoxyethylene sorbitan monolaurate (Tween 20)	16.7

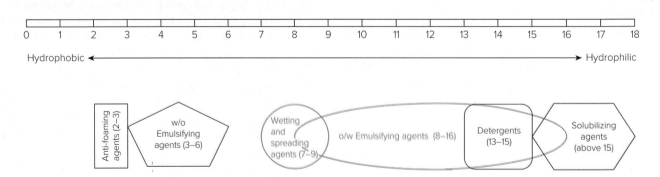

FIGURE 7-1 Surfactant function according to HLB values.

emulsions may be formed, depending on the relative amount of each phase. The powder is first blended with the phase that has the larger volume. This type of emulsion is called a Pickering emulsion, named for the scientist who first described them in 1907, SU Pickering, even though he may not have been the first to observe the phenomenon.

METHODS OF EMULSION PREPARATION

Emulsions may be prepared by several methods. On a small scale, for example, in a compounding pharmacy, emulsions may be prepared using a dry Wedgwood (porcelain) mortar and pestle. It may not seem obvious that a glass mortar and pestle cannot be used. However, many a pharmacy student has been frustrated trying to form an emulsion in a glass mortar (often selected because it was the correct size for the volume of emulsion to be prepared). The smooth surfaces of the glass mortar and pestle do not provide the friction needed to shear the oil into smaller droplets. A mortar and pestle with a rough surface will perform this function adequately. A mechanical blender or mixer, such as a Waring blender, may also be used. Sometimes, vigorous shaking in a bottle (the type used for dispensing liquid medications) provides sufficient shear that a good emulsion can be formed. (Although the glass bottle also has smooth surfaces, emulsion formation is dependent on the vigorous shaking and not friction between two equipment surfaces.) On an industrial scale, large mixing tanks may be used to form the emulsion through the action of a high-speed impeller. The design of the equipment is such that sufficient shearing stresses are applied to form the emulsion.

In the small-scale, extemporaneous preparation of emulsions, three techniques may be employed. They are the continental or dry gum method, the English or wet gum method, and the bottle or Forbes bottle method. An overview of each method is provided to highlight their differences before a detailed description of each method is given. Using the dry gum method, the emulsifying agent (usually Acacia) is mixed with the oil in a mortar using firm pressure on the pestle, until the mixture is smooth. The water is then incorporated into this oily, gum mixture. In the wet gum method, the emulsifying agent and the water are mixed together using a mortar and pestle to form a mucilage (the emulsifying agent is water soluble). Then, the oil is slowly incorporated to form the emulsion. The bottle method is reserved for volatile oils or less viscous oils and is a variation of the dry gum method but is prepared in the bottle. These methods are described in more detail below.

Continental or Dry Method

Using the following formula as an example, the dry gum method may be described:

Mineral oil	40 mL
Acacia	qs
Water	ad 150 ML

A primary emulsion, which is more stable, must first be made. The primary emulsion usually contains different proportions of ingredients compared to the final emulsion. It is also easier to first make the primary emulsion, and then to adjust, or dilute, this formulation to the final formula. To make the primary emulsion, four parts by volume of oil, two parts by volume of water, and one part by weight of gum are used. Hence, this method is also known as the 4:2:1 method. In the above case, 40 mL of oil, 20 mL of water, and 10 g of gum are measured to prepare the primary emulsion.

The Acacia is triturated with the oil in a completely dry Wedgwood or porcelain mortar until thoroughly mixed. After the oil and gum have been mixed, the water (two parts) is added slowly but all at once, and the mixture is rapidly and continuously triturated until the primary emulsion forms and the contents of the mortar become creamy white. When a crackling sound is heard, it signifies that the endpoint has been reached. Generally, about three minutes of rapid mixing is required to produce a satisfactory primary emulsion. However, the mixing time does depend on the type of mortar used (the roughness of its internal surface, and the optimal size and shape to allow proper mixing), and the suitability of the mixing action. Narrow, tall mortars do not work as well as shorter, squat mortars (of the same volume).

The emulsion is next gradually diluted with the addition of small amounts of water, each incorporated into the emulsion with mixing before the next addition of water. To the diluted emulsion, other formulation ingredients are added. For example, liquid formulation ingredients that are soluble or miscible with water (the external phase) may be mixed into the diluted primary emulsion. Solid substances, such as preservatives, stabilizers, colorants and any flavoring material, are usually dissolved in a suitable volume of water and added as a solution to the diluted primary emulsion.

Any substances that might interfere with the stability of the emulsion, or of the emulsifying agent, are added toward the end of the process, when the emulsion has been diluted. For instance, alcohol has a precipitating action on gums such as Acacia. Therefore, no alcohol or alcoholic solution should be added directly to the primary emulsion. After almost maximum dilution of the emulsion (according to the final formulation), the alcohol-containing ingredient is added, in small portions, and mixed after each addition. In this way, the alcohol content is not high in any portion of the emulsion. When all necessary ingredients have been added and mixed, the emulsion is transferred to a measuring cylinder. The mortar is rinsed with water, using small amounts repeatedly, and the rinsing is used to make the emulsion in the measuring cylinder up to volume. Rinsing is done to remove as much as possible of the emulsion from the mortar. The dry gum method can also be used with an electric mixer or blender.

English or Wet Gum Method

By this method, the same proportions of oil, water, and gum (as in the continental or dry gum method) are used but the order of mixing is different. Generally, a mucilage of the gum is prepared by mixing granular Acacia and twice its weight of water in a mortar. Using light pressure, mixing is continued until a smooth mucilage is formed. The oil is then added in small quantities, with rapid mixing, to emulsify the added oil at each step. The oil must be completely emulsified before the next addition of oil. After all of the oil has been added, the mixture is thoroughly mixed for several minutes to ensure uniformity. Then, the other formulation ingredients are added, after dilution of the primary emulsion, as with the continental method. The emulsion is then transferred to a measuring cylinder and made up to volume with water, as described above.

BOTTLE OR FORBES BOTTLE METHOD

The bottle method is useful for the extemporaneous preparation of emulsions from oils of low viscosity, such as volatile oils. Powdered acacia is placed in a dry bottle, two parts of oil are added, and the mixture is thoroughly shaken within the capped container. A volume of water, approximately equal to that of the oil, is measured and then added, in small portions, to the oil mixture in the bottle. The mixture is thoroughly shaken after each addition. This is continued until all the measured water has been added.

From the above description, it can be seen that this method is similar to the dry gum method, except that the proportions of oil to water to gum are 2:2:1, in addition to the fact that a bottle, instead of a mortar and pestle, is used. When all of the measured water has been added, an aqueous solution of the other ingredients may be added to the formed primary emulsion. Lastly, this is diluted to the final volume of the formulation with additional water. This method is not suitable for viscous oils because they cannot be thoroughly mixed in the bottle with the emulsifying agent. Viscous oils by definition do not flow easily and, hence, cannot be shaken adequately, using this manual method.

AUXILIARY METHODS

These methods are not intended for the formation of an emulsion. They are used for the improvement of an emulsion, by secondary processing, after the emulsion has been formed by some other technique. An emulsion prepared by either the wet gum or the dry gum method can generally be improved in quality by passing it through a hand homogenizer. In this apparatus, the pumping action of the handle forces the emulsion through a

very small hole. The effect of this action is to reduce the globule size. It also makes the sizes of the globules very uniform, and this makes the emulsion much more stable. The size of the hole may be adjusted by turning a screw. Initially, a wider aperture is used and, with successive passages of the emulsion through the apparatus, the aperture size is progressively decreased.

In industry, a large-scale mechanical device, similar in principle of operation, may be used to homogenize large volumes of emulsion. The emulsion is forced through a small aperture which reduces the size of the oil droplets. Milk, which is an emulsion, is homogenized in this way, that is, the oil droplets naturally found in milk are size reduced and the droplet sizes are made more uniform. The cream formation, at the top of the bottle, is less evident with modern containers of milk for this reason (creaming is a sign of emulsion instability). In pharmaceutical processing on a large scale, a colloid mill may also be used. This consists of a cone-shaped rotor that spins on its axis, and a stationary stator which fits over the cone (Figure 7-2). There is a very small gap between the cone and stator, which can be adjusted. By passing the emulsion between the rotor and stator while the former is spinning very fast, the globule size of the emulsion is rapidly reduced. Again, a relatively large gap is used initially and the gap is gradually decreased with successive passages of the emulsion through the apparatus. By comparison with a hand homogenizer where all of the emulsion must pass through a small hole, in the colloid mill the gap between the entire rotor and stator is the "hole" through which the emulsion must pass. Hence, the apparatus is very effective, and large volumes of emulsion may be rapidly processed.

IN SITU SOAP METHOD

As previously mentioned, soaps can serve as emulsifying agents. The name of this technique refers to the fact that the soap is created as the other ingredients are mixed, that is, the soap is made within the processing vessel or "in situ." Two types of soaps that can be formed are calcium soaps and soft soaps. The latter are made from monovalent cations, such as sodium. Calcium soaps form w/o emulsions. When equal parts of olive oil and calcium hydroxide solution, USP (limewater) are mixed, the oleic acid in the olive oil reacts with the limewater to form calcium oleate, an emulsifying agent which emulsifies the olive oil. Because the oil phase is the external phase, this formulation is ideal

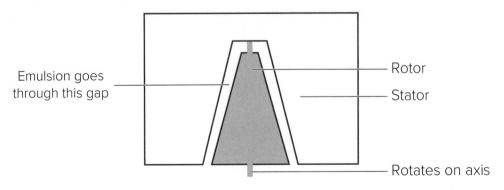

FIGURE 7-2 Section through a colloid mill.

Emulsion goes through this gap

Rotor

Stator

Rotates on axis

where occlusion and skin softening are desired. This is the case when the skin is itchy and dry, or when sunburned skin is being treated. This emulsion is a constituent of calamine lotion which contains, additionally, calamine and zinc oxide.

STABILITY OF EMULSIONS

Emulsions are inherently unstable systems because two immiscible phases are "forced together" using mechanical energy and the appropriate formulation ingredients. Over time, the oil and water will separate because it is not in their nature to be in the close relationship of globules of one phase distributed throughout the other phase. Several instabilities that can be discerned are related to this natural tendency to separate. These instabilities, in fact, represent different stages or levels of separation. There are, in addition, other instability phenomena that may be observed that do not relate to the tendency for oil and water to separate.

Creaming, Coalescence, and Breaking

When viewed under a microscope, an emulsion can be observed to consist of droplets dispersed in a liquid. In pharmaceutical emulsions, these are either oil droplets dispersed in water, or water droplets dispersed in oil.

Due to density differences, the globules in an emulsion will either settle at the bottom of the container, over time, or rise to the surface. Whether they fall or rise depends on whether the globules are more, or less, dense than the external phase. In a w/o emulsion, the water droplets are more dense than oil and, therefore, they tend to settle to the bottom of the container. On the other hand, oil droplets in an o/w emulsion will rise since oil is less dense than water. When droplets fall to the bottom of the container, the process is referred to as sedimentation. When the same effect occurs in the opposite direction, that is, the droplets rise, it is referred to as negative sedimentation or creaming. The latter term is derived from the phenomenon that occurs with milk, that is, the cream rises to the top over time. Creaming and sedimentation are illustrated in Figure 7-3. Creaming in milk is not so obvious in modern times due to homogenization of the milk. This simply means that the oil globules in the processed milk are smaller, and more uniform, than in milk in the natural

state. More than 50 years ago, homogenization was not widely practiced and creaming was easily observed in the glass bottles in which milk was sold.

The movement of globules within the emulsion occurs in accordance with Stokes' law, which describes the rate of settling of small particles in a fluid (Eq. [7-1]). The square of the diameter of the globules, and the density difference between the internal and external phases, is directly proportional to the rate of settling. The settling rate is inversely proportional to $18\times$ the viscosity of the external phase. The symbol "g" is the gravitational constant.

$$\frac{dx}{dt} = \frac{d^2(\rho_1 - \rho_2)g}{18\eta} \tag{7-1}$$

As the oil globules rise, they tend to aggregate, in small numbers initially. Over time, the aggregates become progressively larger. The aggregates move at a faster rate since the factor "d" in Eq. (7-1) is effectively increased. Aggregation and creaming are manifestations of instability but they are not serious instabilities since the creamed droplets can easily be re-dispersed by agitation of the container (shaking of the bottle). It is possible to redisperse the droplets because the emulgent is still in place around each globule. However, creaming brings globules closer together and the longer they remain in close contact increases the chances that they may fuse (two smaller globules forming one larger globule). The latter process is referred to as coalescence.

In an undisturbed emulsion many pairs, or small numbers, of globules will coalesce. The longer the emulsion is left undisturbed, the greater will be the number of these coalesced units. If the emulsion remains undisturbed, the process will continue, with the coalesced droplets further coalescing with other coalesced groups, or with individual droplets. If this process is allowed to continue, larger and larger droplets will form. Eventually, the emulsion will completely separate into an oil phase and water. When this occurs, it is referred to as cracking or breaking of the emulsion. In a typical, broken pharmaceutical emulsion, this will be seen as an oil layer floating on water, but closer observation will show a thin emulgent layer between the other two layers. Coalescence and breaking are illustrated in Figure 7-4. Cracking is a serious instability since the emulsion cannot easily be reformed (by shaking the bottle, for instance). This is because the emulgent has been removed from its location around each droplet. Another

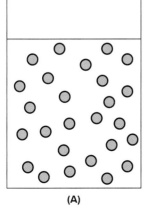
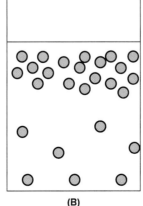
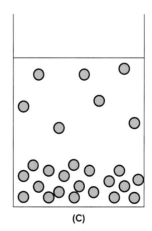

FIGURE 7-3 **Globules in an emulsion.** **(A)** Fresh emulsion. **(B)** Emulsion with creaming. **(C)** Emulsion with sedimentation.

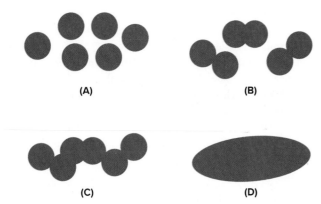

FIGURE 7-4 **Coalescence in emulsions.** (**A**) Aggregated globules. (**B**) Early coalescence. (**C**) Later coalescence. (**D**) Complete coalescence (breaking).

way to describe this effect is to say that coalescence continued until one very large drop of oil was formed!

Creaming is not considered a serious instability since it can be reversed. However, if the emulsion is left for a long time in the creamed state, there is a greater opportunity for coalescence to occur. The latter is irreversible, that is, those droplets that have coalesced into one larger droplet cannot be separated into the constituent small droplets simply by shaking the container. Continued coalescence leads, ultimately, to breaking of the emulsion. Therefore, continued creaming is a threat to emulsion stability because it can induce coalescence and finally cracking, even though creaming, itself, is not considered a serious instability. The difference between creaming and breaking is illustrated in Figure 7-5.

Miscellaneous Instabilities

While coalescence, creaming and breaking are the major instabilities that occur with emulsions, there are others that are observed fairly frequently and deserve to be mentioned.

Microbial Growth

An emulsion, especially its aqueous phase, is a good medium for the growth of microorganisms, fungi in particular. This problem can be alleviated by the addition of antimicrobial preservatives.

The parabens are commonly used as preservatives. While there are many parabens, propylparaben (propyl p-hydroxy benzoic acid) and methylparaben (methyl p-hydroxy benzoic acid) are probably the most commonly used. They are often used as a pair since each has a somewhat different efficacy spectrum, and they complement each other when used together.

Very small amounts of the preservatives are used but their solubility in water is poor and the solution may have to be heated to dissolve the preservative. If the emulsion contains small amounts of other liquids, the parabens may be dissolved in these if they are better solvents. For example, if the formulation has propylene glycol or ethanol (or can tolerate the incorporation of these additional ingredients), the preservatives may be dissolved in either of these liquids which are then slowly added to the emulsion with stirring. In this way, the preservatives can be easily incorporated. These liquids should not be added all at once or without vigorous stirring since these actions may result in the precipitation of the parabens.

In spite of adding amounts of preservatives that are known to be effective, microbial growth has still been observed to occur in emulsions. One of the reasons for this is the phenomenon described below. Suppose a concentration of 0.02% of a particular preservative is required (usually the percentage concentrations are low). Suppose the correct amount has been added to the water phase. Once the emulsion has formed, the concentration in the water phase (where fungi are most likely to grow) is reduced due to the fact that the preservatives are more soluble in oil and partitioned into the oil phase. Depending on the type of oil, the concentration of the preservative in the oil phase may be high. Thus, the aqueous phase becomes deficient and may not effectively counteract microbial (especially, fungal) growth. This situation is depicted diagrammatically in Figure 7-6 in which the depth of color of the aqueous phase is intended to depict the concentration of preservative.

Rancidity of Oil

Oils can become rancid over time. The term refers to their oxidation with the development of an "off" odor. This gives the bad odor and taste of oil-containing products that are stale. Rancidity can be reduced by the addition of antioxidants such as butylated hydroxy toluene (BHT) and butylated hydroxy anisole (BHA) which are commonly used.

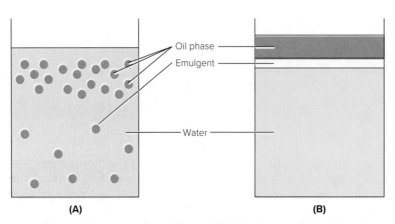

FIGURE 7-5 **Diagrammatic comparison of (A) creamed emulsion and (B) broken emulsion.** Note that each droplet of the creamed emulsion still has its associated emulgent (which may not completely surround the oil droplet as shown in this cartoon).

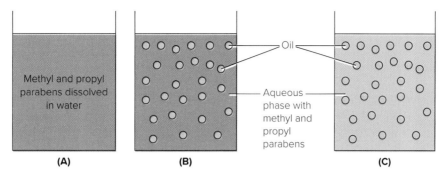

FIGURE 7-6 Distribution of preservatives in an emulsion: **(A)** Methyl and propyl parabens dissolved in water. **(B)** Addition of oil (emulsified). **(C)** Addition of oil with partitioning of preservatives into oil phase. Note: The intensity of the color of the aqueous phase of **A** denotes the preservative concentration. The situation with no redistribution of preservatives is shown in **B** (color intensity remains the same as in **A**). The lighter aqueous phase color in **C** denotes a lower preservative concentration.

NANOEMULSIONS

While typical oral emulsions or those for external use may have globule sizes ranging from about 1 μm to about 50 μm. The higher the globule size, the less stable is the emulsion. Therefore, while globule sizes larger than 50 μm are possible, they will not be very stable. Globules larger than about 5 μm are fairly easily observed with a light microscope. Injectable emulsions generally have globule sizes below 1 μm.

A preformed emulsion may be processed with special equipment to reduce the globule size well below 1 μm. The equipment forces the emulsion through very fine apertures. This creates very high shear to reduce the globule size significantly. Using this equipment, emulsions with globule sizes in the range of a few hundred nanometers, or less than a hundred nanometers in some cases, may be produced. The principle is effectively the same as the hand homogenizer discussed earlier. However, the aperture through which the emulsion is passed is much finer and the pressure used is much higher.

One such apparatus is the Microfluidizer. In this apparatus, the emulsion is forced through a Y-configuration in which the pathway has a width of a few hundred nanometers (100 nm is approximately 1/1000 the thickness of a human hair which has a diameter of about 100 μm). The splitting of the emulsion stream by the Y-configuration (and the subsequent recombining of the two streams) is said to be very effective in reducing the globule size. The company has a patent on this special configuration of the size-reduction chamber. Forcing the emulsion through such a small aperture, with the use of great force (up to 8000 psi for a bench top apparatus), generates heat with the result that the formed emulsion must be passed through cooling coils that are surrounded by cold water to reduce the temperature of the emulsion.

Nanoemulsions are much more stable than regular (or "coarse") emulsions. Emulsions with such small globule sizes settle much more slowly. They also have special properties and are said to penetrate biological tissues more readily. Thus, they may be used for drug delivery in situations where the drug is not easily permeable through the tissue in question. Pickering emulsions have been effectively used to prepare nanoemulsions in research studies. While nanoemulsions are emulsions with globules of a few hundred nanometers (and sometimes less), it is not true to say that microemulsions are emulsions with globule sizes in the micrometer range. The term, microemulsion, is a misnomer since the product is not an emulsion. They are composed of an oil phase, an aqueous phase, a surfactant and a co-surfactant (typically a medium-chain alcohol) but the dispersed phase may best be described as swollen micelles. In this sense, they are similar to colloidal dispersions. They appear to be clear because the very small micelles do not refract light and, in this sense, they resemble solutions. Thus, microemulsions may be said to be related to both solutions and colloidal dispersions.

EXAMPLES OF PHARMACEUTICAL EMULSIONS

Besides the use of topical emulsions to hydrate the skin, emulsions are used to formulate elegant products for oily drugs, and for oil-soluble drugs that are poorly absorbed. In the latter case, the drug solution in oil is converted into an emulsion for palatability, easy storage and handling, and to improve the bioavailability of the drug. These products may be formulated as oral liquids (including drops), topical creams and lotions, and injectable emulsions. The latter usually provides much better absorption of the drug, with reduced side effects. Table 7-2 lists some commercial emulsion products.

Recap questions

1. Stokes' equation is elsewhere described in this book in connection with suspensions. How is it possible that the same equation can apply to both suspensions and emulsions?

2. Explain, in theoretical terms, why nanoemulsions are more stable than regular emulsions.

3. If pharmaceutical emulsions have a long history and are sufficiently stable that the patient may remove a precise dose, why would one go to so much trouble and expense to produce a nanoemulsion?

TABLE 7-2	Some Commercial Emulsion Products		
FORMULATION TYPE	**TRADE OR COMPENDIAL NAME**	**ACTIVE INGREDIENT(S)**	**COMMENTS**
Oral Liquid	Acacia and Mineral Oil Emulsion, NF	Mineral Oil	Lubricant/ laxative
Oral Drops	Phazyme; Gas-X	Simethicone	Antiflatulant – disrupts gas bubbles, allowing easier expulsion
	D-Mulsion 1000	Vitamin D (cholecalciferol) 1000 IU	Vitamin D Supplement
Topical Cream	Differin Cream	Adapalene	Acne cream – retinoid action
	Nizoral Cream	Ketoconazole	Anti-fungal topical agent
Emulsion for injection	Diprivan	Propofol	Anesthetic
	Diazemuls	Diazepam	Anxiolytic-sedative

SUMMARY POINTS

- Emulsions consist of two immiscible liquids as a relatively stable formulation
- Emulsions allow convenient consumption of oils that would otherwise be irritant to the gastro-intestinal tract
- Pharmaceutical emulsions distribute oil as fine droplets in water, or water as fine droplets in oil
- Amongst a range of materials that can be used as emulsifiers, non-ionic surfactants are popular
- "HLB" describes the balance between the hydrophilic and lipophilic groups of the surfactant
- In the extemporaneous preparation of emulsions, the wet gum method, the dry gum method, and the Forbes bottle method are commonly used
- Coalescence, creaming and breaking are manifestations of emulsion instability with respect to the distributed phase; Stokes' law is an important theoretical underpinning to understand these effects

What do you think?

1. What do you think are the differences between the formulation of injectable emulsions and oral emulsions? Name at least two important differences that you can think of.

2. What do you think would be the difference in patient acceptability between unformulated cod liver oil versus cod liver oil emulsion, when administered to a 6-year-old child? What brings about this difference?

3. A student in your class thinks that a microemulsion has globules that are measured in micrometer dimensions whereas a nanoemulsion has globules measured in nanometer dimensions. Is this student correct? If not, how would you explain the difference to him?

4. Suppose you are working as a pharmacist at a compounding pharmacy. The pharmacy has compounded a few different oils into creams, as prescribed by dermatologist, Dr. Skin. You have just received a prescription for a cream which requires the incorporation of an oil that your pharmacy has not compounded before. The technician wants to use a formula that was previously used for emulsification, just switching the new oil for the old one. Do you think this is a good idea? Explain your answer.

REFERENCES

1. Griffin WC. Classification of surface-active agents by "HLB." *J Soc Cosmet Chem.* 1949;1(5):311-326.

2. Griffin WC. Calculation of HLB values of non-ionic surfactants. *J Soc Cosmet Chem.* 1954;5(4):249-256.

Granulation

8

PREVIEW

- Granulation, an important processing step in pharmaceutical technology
- The composition of granules
- Methods for the production of granules:
  - Fusion method
  - Low, and high shear wet granulation
  - Fluid bed granulation
  - Production of spherical granules
  - Dry granulation
- Granulation endpoint determination
- Continuous granulation

INTRODUCTION

Granules are small agglomerates of pharmaceutical powders, prepared by special processing methods. They usually contain a drug and may be used as a convenient, patient-acceptable dosage form. Examples of products where the granules are the final formulation include effervescent granules such as E-Z-Gas II (the CO_2 produced aids in gastrointestinal imaging), and Citro Soda® and Ural® which are urinary alkalizers sold, respectively, in South Africa and Australia. More often, however, granules are prepared as an intermediate material to be used in the formulation of the final dosage form. For example, granules can be prepared for filling into capsules or for the compression of tablets. In both cases, the use of granules has an advantage over the use of fine powders for these applications.

There is a basic problem inherent in the use of most powders in pharmaceutical processing that the granulation step rectifies. As explained in Chapter 5, Pharmaceutical Powders, fine powders are irregularly shaped and do not flow well. Particles that are more spherical flow better. In addition, powders may be light and fluffy (have a low bulk density) and exhibit a static charge. Fine particles also have a large surface area and moisture adsorption will be greater than it would be for larger particles, if the material is adsorbent in nature. Moisture makes the particles cohesive and retards flow. For these reasons, fine powders, generally, have poor flowability.

THE NEED FOR GRANULATION

Why is poor flowability bad for pharmaceutical processing?

In the case of tableting, the material to be compressed into tablets must flow from a hopper (storage container that supplies the material) to the dies of the tablet press where the tablets are compressed. The movement of material from the hopper to the die is through a series of pathways that get narrower and also have bends in them. Finally, the material flows into a die in which it is compressed into a tablet. The diameter of the die determines the diameter of the final tablet. Thus, the flowing powder has to finally pass into a relatively small-diameter receptacle, the die. Poor flow results in incomplete fill of the die. In the next step, the material in the die next comes under intense pressure as it is squeezed between two punches to form the tablet. If the die is incompletely filled, the tablets will have a lower weight than desired. Even more problematic is the fact that poor fill is usually accompanied by varying die fill. In practical terms, this means a tablet formulation that was intended to be compressed to a weight of 500 mg may have tablets weighing 300 mg, 340 mg, and 375 mg, as hypothetical examples. Clearly, such variability is unacceptable.

Similarly, with capsule filling, granules may produce, relative to powders, a more consistent capsule weight with a more uniform drug content. The process of filling capsules is different from the filling of dies for tablet manufacture and capsule filling does not have as serious an issue with weight variation, due to poor flow, as does tableting. For this reason, capsules are frequently filled with powders. Nevertheless, capsule formulations may also benefit from the use of granules to fill the capsule.

As mentioned in the next section on granule formulation, the tablets that are compressed from granules are intended to have several ingredients. If a powder blend is used to produce tablets, the powder mixture may, in the course of handling and processing, become a non-homogenous blend of the different ingredients. Each powdered ingredient has its own properties and behavior, including flow rate, and the ingredients of a mixture of powders may behave independently of each other. Assuming the blend is totally homogenous initially, each ingredient may flow at a different rate during passage to the die. Suppose that ingredient "S" is present in 20% concentration in the initial blend and it flows slowly relative to the other ingredients in the formulation. The initial tablets compressed from this blend will have less than 20% of component "S," due to this ingredient not reaching the die at the same rate as the other (faster-flowing) ingredients. As a consequence, the powder remaining in the hopper becomes progressively richer in ingredient "S." Therefore, tablets made at the end of the tableting run will be richer in this ingredient. If ingredient "S" is the drug, the variability in the flow rates of the individual components will result in tablets with variable drug content.

The above depicts a scenario in which tablets made at the beginning may be deficient in the drug, and those made at the end may have more of the drug than intended. This separation of ingredients based on flow rates is referred to as segregation. Since an industrial batch may consist of 1 million (or more) tablets, segregation by the end of the batch may be severe. Obviously, this is not a good situation. One solution to this problem is the use of granules for tableting.

The granule is a small aggregation of powder particles held together by a chemical binder. Each granule contains all the ingredients, in the correct proportion as required in the final dosage form. As the granule flows, its constituents remain together. Therefore, the granule reaches the die cavity largely intact, with the ingredients in the correct proportion and the problem of segregation of ingredients is largely removed. The granulation process creates agglomerates that are somewhat more spherical and this shape makes the granules flow better. In addition, the manufacturing process involves some amount of compression with the result that the granules have a greater density than the mixed powders. Materials that are more dense flow better than less dense materials.

In the process of preparing granules, a binder is added to the mixed powders. The function of the binder is to act as the "glue", holding the individual components together so that each granule functions as a unit. When pressure is applied to the granules in the tablet press, the binder also helps the individual granules to bond together to form the tablet. In relation to the latter function, it is said that the binder confers on the granules the property of "compactibility," that is, the ability to be compacted into a tablet. Due to the fact that much of the drug is in the interior of the granule, oxidation and moisture sensitivity are reduced in granules, in general. When an ungranulated mixture of powders containing a very sensitive drug is tableted, it is subjected to more atmospheric degradation. As the powder flows during the tableting operation, particles from the interior of the powder mass move to the surface and more of the drug is exposed to the atmosphere.

The taste of granules is also improved over the taste of the ungranulated mixed ingredients. Frequently, the drug is very bitter but present in the formulation in small quantities. In the granule, much of the drug is in the interior of the granule. Only the surface drug can be tasted, leading to less taste perception. In addition, the outer surface of the granule has a partial coating of the binder solution. The binder is frequently a fairly viscous polymer solution. When the granules are dried, the water in the polymer solution evaporates and some polymer residue remains on the surface of the granules, or of the tablet that is compressed from such granules. Upon administration to a patient, some of this polymer hydrates in contact with saliva to form a viscous solution once again. This solution, due to its viscosity, retards the diffusion of the drug to the taste buds on the patient's tongue, resulting in less taste perception. Of course, the granules may also contain flavors to enhance taste.

Recap Questions

1. List the reasons for the constituents of a powder mixture becoming segregated during the production of tablets.
2. How does granulation overcome the problem mentioned in question 1 above?
3. How do granules improve the taste of drugs?

COMPOSITION OF GRANULES

Granules for tableting contain all the ingredients required to be in the tablet. These include the active ingredient, or drug, and the excipients. In addition, the granules contain other excipients that are necessary for the optimal functioning of the tableting equipment or to facilitate the tablet production process. Over and above these, other excipients are needed to facilitate the production process. Excipients to aid tableting include the glidant and lubricant, while the granulating agent helps to form the granules. A lubricant also facilitates the filling of capsules and is included in granules intended to be filled into capsules. Granules intended to be provided to the patient as the final dosage form do not contain the excipients required to ensure good production of tablets. The lubricant, for example, is excluded from such granules.

Some ingredients, such as the drug, are included within the core of the granule (intra-granular ingredients), whereas other ingredients are extra-granular. Intra-granular ingredients are incorporated by blending the ingredient in question with the other intra-granule components before the granulation step. Extra-granular ingredients are added to the formed granules. The lubricant, magnesium stearate, is an extra-granular ingredient. A very brief description of the excipients used in granulation is provided below. They will be covered in more detail in the chapter on tableting where the functionality of each excipient is more relevant to the processes that will be discussed in that chapter.

Diluent

Many drugs, especially those recently developed, may have a very low dose. It is not uncommon for a drug to have a dose of 10 to 20 mg per tablet or capsule. It would be very difficult to reliably produce individual dosing units close to the weight range of these drugs. Instead, a diluent is added to increase the bulk of the material to be included in the dosage form, such as a tablet or capsule. If sufficient diluent is added to make a tablet of approximately 300 mg weight, such a unit is much easier to manufacture and handle. Of course, the issue becomes even more relevant when the dose is 1 or 2 mg, or even less.

Disintegrant

The disintegrant is required to assist in the breakup of the tablet when it is added to water or an aqueous medium. This process, known as disintegration, is an important step that helps the release of the drug. Depending on the constituents of the tablet formulation, some components may be insoluble or poorly soluble. Since the tablet is a compacted, hard dosage form, it may not immediately take water into its interior when placed in contact with an aqueous medium. Without a disintegrant, some tablets may remain whole for many hours after the tablet is swallowed. A disintegrant may also be included in a granulation that is not intended to be tableted or encapsulated, if rapid breakup of the individual granules, after consumption, is required. Many disintegrants work by rapidly swelling in the presence of water, thus pushing the tablet apart. A portion of the disintegrant may be added after the formation of the granules (extra granularly). This fraction helps the tablet to break up into large pieces, whereas the disintegrant added intra-granularly assists the individual granules to break up or de-aggregate.

Granulating Fluid

In the wet granulation process, which is described in more detail below, a wet mass has first to be created. This involves adding a liquid to the blended powders and mixing to distribute the liquid. The liquid used to create this wet mass is referred to as the granulating fluid, or granulating liquid, or granulating agent. The wet mass is then passed through a sieve which breaks it up into small, wet agglomerates or wet granules. The granulating agent, therefore, helps to form the wet granules.

Water is frequently used as the granulating agent, or a combination of ethanol, or isopropanol, and water may be used. Frequently, some percentage of alcohol is added to water to facilitate rapid drying of the wet granules, since alcohol vaporizes readily. The ability of a liquid to hold individual powder particles together depends on its surface tension. Water has a high surface tension and, generally, holds particles together better than alcohol which has a lower surface tension. Therefore, the addition of alcohol reduces the surface tension of the combination granulating fluid, compared to that of water alone. This factor must be taken into account when water is able to form a cohesive wet mass and the addition of alcohol is contemplated simply to facilitate drying. On the other hand, hydrophobic powders may resist wetting with water and the addition of alcohol may be beneficial in that it allows better wetting. The hydrophobic powders may be moistened with the alcohol first. This improves the ease of wetting when water is subsequently added.

Binder

In some instances, as mentioned above, the powders will form a cohesive mass with the addition of the granulating agent alone. In many instances, however, water may wet the powders effectively, yet the wet mass is not sufficiently cohesive to form good granules. If such wet material were to be passed through a sieve (required for granule formation), granules may form but they tend to break up into powders again very easily during the handling required to dry the granulation. In extreme cases, the wet granules break up as they fall from the sieve.

In such cases, it is necessary to add a binder to hold the components of the granule together. This requirement can also be stated as follows: A binder is needed to make the wet mass more cohesive. Usually, the binder is added as a solution in water or water-alcohol mixture, that is, the binder and granulating fluid are combined. The powdered binder may also be blended with the other powders, and the granulating fluid is then added to activate the binder. When this technique is used, the binder is less potent than is the case when the binder is first dissolved in the granulating fluid. Not all binders may be added dry and later activated; some require special techniques to form the binder solution. Examples of binders that are commonly used are given in Table 8-1.

The use of too much binder may result in the formation of excessively hard granules. The granule must break up when in contact with water and the active ingredient must dissolve. Excessive amounts of binder may retard the dissolution of the granule and, thus, the drug may not be readily available for absorption. When granules with an excess of binder are used in tableting, it may result in hard tablets which do not disintegrate (break up into pieces) readily, again retarding drug dissolution and, potentially, drug absorption. Disintegration is described more fully in Chapter 9, Tablets.

TABLE 8-1	Binders Commonly Used in Granulation	
BINDER	**COMMON SOLVENT FOR GRANULATION**	**COMMENTS**
Methyl cellulose	Water	Dispersed in hot water; then cold water added to dissolve
Hydroxypropyl cellulose	Water	Semi-synthetic polymer; delays dissolution in higher concentrations; viscosity increases with MW
Hydroxypropylmethyl cellulose	Water	Semi-synthetic polymer; delays dissolution in higher concentrations; viscosity increases with MW
Ethylcellulose	Alcohol	Semi-synthetic polymer; not water soluble; delays dissolution in higher concentrations
Polyethylene glycol	Water and alcohol	Synthetic polymer; higher MW grades are more viscous (better binders)
Polyvinylpyrollidone	Water and alcohol	Synthetic polymer; higher MW grades are more viscous (better binders)

The effect of the binder in the finished dosage form is the opposite of that of the disintegrant. It is possible to produce good quality, hard tablets that disintegrate readily due to the incorporation of appropriate amounts of disintegrate. This is especially true with modern, high-efficiency disintegrants. Nevertheless, excessive binder should not be used with the intention of compensating by the use of excess disintegrant.

Glidant

The glidant consists of very fine particles of a material that helps the granules flow better. Since the glidant particles are required on the outside of the granules, they are not incorporated during the initial blending of the powders since this would cause much of the glidant to be located within the interior of the granule. The glidant is added after the granules are made and is blended with the dried granules. For the reasons previously mentioned, a good flow is required in the production of tablets and capsules. In the preparation of granules in a compounding pharmacy, where the granules are the final dosage form, the addition of a glidant is usually not necessary. In the industrial production of granules as the final dosage form, however, a glidant may be added to the formulation to facilitate the filling of the granules into containers.

Lubricant

The lubricant, as the name implies, lubricates the granules. Lubrication is necessary when the granules are under intense pressure in the die of the tablet press. The granules must slip and slide past each other as the first step of the process that eventually forms the tablet. The lubricant is usually needed in granules for capsule formulations as well as there may be compression of the granules in the process of filling the capsules. When compounding granules in a pharmacy, a lubricant is usually not needed.

The methods by which granules are manufactured will be covered in the next few sections, one section being devoted to each type of granule manufacture. The different granulation methods are summarized in Mind Map 8-1.

Recap Questions

1. Why is a diluent needed in a granule formulation?

2. Why is a disintegrant needed—will the granule not dissolve as soon as it reaches water?

3. Why are glidants and lubricants added to the formed granules, at the end of the granulation process, rather than to the other powders at the beginning?

FUSION METHOD OF GRANULATION (SMALL SCALE)

The fusion method is used to make effervescent granules on a small scale in a compounding pharmacy. The ingredients of the granulation are the drug, diluent, flavor and sweetener, a base (usually sodium bicarbonate or sodium carbonate), and citric acid. Citric acid has a pleasant citrus taste. Frequently, a small portion of the citric acid is replaced with tartaric acid for flavor enhancement since tartaric acid has a sharp, tart flavor. The base and acid together are known as the effervescent couple, that is, in the presence of water, the base and acid react to form carbon dioxide and water.

Citric acid is specifically chosen as the acid component because it is a hydrated salt ($C_6H_8O_7 \cdot H_2O$). Upon heating above 55°C, citric acid releases its bound water. This water promotes the effervescent reaction which produces carbon dioxide and water, as mentioned. The foregoing is the basic principle of the fusion method. The steps involved in the production of effervescent granules by this method are as follows:

First, all the ingredients are weighed and blended using, for example, a mortar and pestle. Next, the mixed powders are transferred to a low, flat container that can be heated. A container that has a handle is useful. The container with the powders is placed on a hot plate and heated gently at about 55°C. A Bunsen burner is not suitable for this application because a

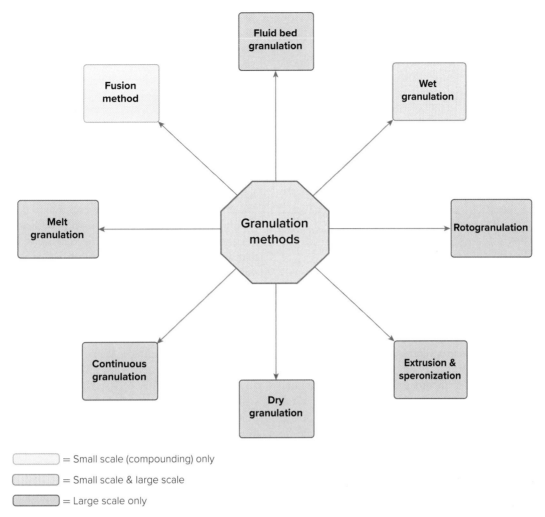

MIND MAP 8-1 Granulation methods

low, consistent temperature is not easy to maintain with this heat source. As the material is carefully heated, a spatula is used to compress the material from the top surface. It will be noticed that the material begins to get moist, as the heating and compression are continued. With continued compression, the powders become flattened and eventually a moist "cake" forms. It is important not to heat for too long since this would make the material completely wet.

Using the spatula, the cake is lifted up as a unit and turned over in the dish, so that the undersurface is now exposed. Heating with pressure from the spatula is continued. When the exposed surface becomes moist and has a compressed appearance, the heating is stopped. It is important not to overheat the material since heating releases the bound water. Each molecule of released water is capable of initiating the following effervescence reaction:

$$NaHCO_3 + C_3H_5O(COOH)_3 + H_2O \rightarrow$$
$$CO_2 + 2H_2O + Na^+ + C_3H_5O(COOH)_2COO^- \qquad (8\text{-}1)$$

It can readily be seen that the reaction releases two molecules of water which are, each, capable of producing the reaction again. Continued heating produces this chain reaction which goes faster the longer the heating is continued. Once a critical point is reached, the process cannot be stopped until all reactants

are consumed. However, the intention is to allow the chain reaction to proceed only to a point that produces sufficient moisture to dampen the mass of powders in the dish to facilitate the formation of granules. Thus, the heating is carefully controlled and stopped before the critical point is reached. It should be noted that citric acid is a tricarboxylic acid and one molecule of citric acid is capable of reacting with three molecules of sodium bicarbonate. Also, note that the reaction given above utilizes sodium bicarbonate as the base; an equivalent reaction could be written where sodium carbonate serves as the base.

The adequately moistened material is passed through a sieve, a little at a time, using a spatula. A non-metallic spatula is preferred in order to avoid metal-on-metal friction which carries the risk of contamination of the product. A number 10 or 12 sieve is suitable for this purpose but other sizes may be chosen. Lower numbers give coarser granules. The formed granules are spread out on a tray and allowed to dry at a temperature of less than 54°C. The dried granules are re-sieved through a somewhat finer sieve than that used for forming the granules, for example, if a no. 12 sieve was used to form the granules, the dried granules may be passed through a no. 14 sieve at this step. This step is performed to ensure that all granules are more or less of the same size, since granules may fuse during the drying process, forming larger agglomerates. The final granules are packaged in an airtight container. Any moisture let into the bottle during storage may initiate the effervescence reaction.

Recap Questions

1. In the fusion method, the water required for granulation is obtained from two sources. Name these sources.

2. Why are the moist granules dried at less than 54°C? Would a higher temperature not ensure faster and more complete drying?

3. Why are the dried granules passed through a sieve again?

WET GRANULATION

Wet granulation begins with the moistening of the mixed powders with the granulating fluid, or a combination of granulating fluid and binder. The latter is more common. Next, the wet mass is passed through a sieve, and the wet granules are collected and dried. The dried granules are re-sieved to produce the final granulation. Many of the steps are similar to the fusion method described above, without the step involving the heating of the powders. While the fusion method is used on a small scale (it is not easily adapted to large-scale manufacture), wet granulation is routinely conducted on both a small scale as well as in large-scale industrial manufacture. A relatively small production batch may be 100 kg, whereas the batch size could easily be 500 kg in weight.

The first step is to dry blend the powders. In a compounding pharmacy this could be done using a mortar and pestle, in which case the next step, formation of the wet mass, is done in the same vessel. The powders may also be blended using a tumbling action or by spatulation, as described in Chapter 5, Pharmaceutical Powders. On an industrial scale, a V-blender which is capable of achieving efficient mixing, could be used for the dry blending step. This equipment choice has the disadvantage that the material must be transferred to another piece of equipment for the formation of the wet mass. Similarly, a cone blender is efficient for blending of large amounts of drug powder but the blend would then have to be transferred to another device for wet massing. The additional work and the time involved with transferring the material to the second piece of equipment, on a large-scale, is obvious.

What may not be immediately evident is the fact that the two pieces of equipment would have to be cleaned, and the cleaning verified, before they can be used again in GMP production. The time involved in this step could be significant. For these reasons, equipment that can perform both operations, dry blending and wet massing, in the same piece are preferred. In an industrial setting, additional steps (which involve both additional personnel and time) are expensive. The remaining equipment types that will be described are all capable of dry blending as well as wet massing of the material in one container and, therefore, such equipment is more efficient. All mixers have a mixing element, or impeller, which is the device that actually performs the mixing. It is equivalent to the propeller in liquid mixing.

A planetary mixer is one type of equipment that could be used for both the dry blending of the powders as well as the formation of the wet mass. The planetary mixer is so named because it has an impeller that rotates on its axis while the impeller (together with the shaft that drives the rotation) also revolves around the mixing bowl. These movements are illustrated in Figure 8-1. These two mixing actions, rotation of the impeller and its revolution around the mixing bowl, resemble the movement of the planets which also rotate on an axis and revolve around the sun.

For effective mixing, two mixing actions are required of any mixing device. First, there must be intense localized mixing which is achieved in the planetary mixer by the rotation of the blade. Next, the blended material must be moved to another area of the mixing vessel and fresh material brought to the intense mixing zone. The mass movement of material, in the planetary mixer, is achieved by the revolution of the impeller around the mixing vessel, that is, the impeller moves to fresh material.

The large-scale, industrial planetary mixer depicted in Figure 8-2 is similar to planetary mixers used in the kitchen, for example, KitchenAid˚. While similar in design, the laboratory

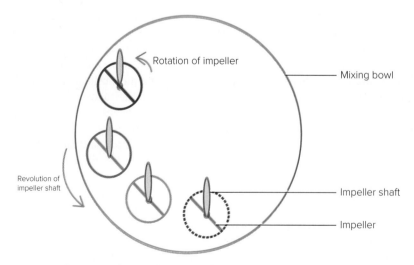

FIGURE 8-1 Top view of planetary mixer bowl, illustrating dual mixing movements.

plastic is used to push the wet mass through the sieve. This is done by moving the block back and forth over the screen. Although it may sound appealing to use a stainless steel block, it cannot be used since the metal-to-metal friction against the screen may cause metal particles to be shed into the granulation. Alternately, a mechanical granulator such as the oscillating granulator, or a Comil, may be used to screen the wet mass.

The oscillating granulator (Figure 8-3) consists of a wire mesh tightly stretched into a broad V-shape. A circular oscillator is in the center of the V-shaped mesh. The movement of the oscillator alternates between clockwise and anticlockwise. This back-and-forth motion of the oscillator pushes the wet mass through the sieve and is collected at the bottom for subsequent drying. The oscillating action reduces the possibility of large clumps of wet material remaining attached to the oscillator. The Quadro Comil (Figure 8-4) has a cone-shaped screen within a screen chamber. A cone-shaped impeller fits the screen closely. The wet material is fed into a feed chute (not shown in the figure) which is located above the screen chamber. The rapidly rotating impeller imparts a vortex flow pattern to the material. The product is forced outward to the screen surface by centrifugal acceleration. The closely fitting impeller

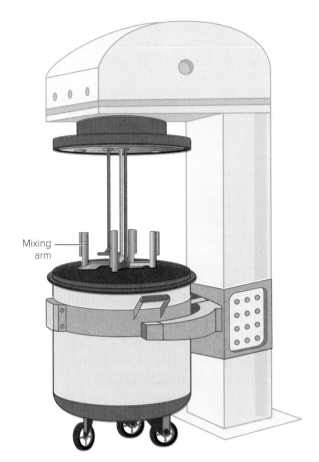

FIGURE 8-2 Large-scale, industrial planetary mixer. (Adapted from Aulton ME, Taylor K. *Aulton's Pharmaceutics: The Design and Manufacture of Medicines*. 6th ed. Elsevier Health Sciences; 2021.)

and industrial versions are made stronger to handle continuous use and are made of materials that are unlikely to react with the constituents of the wet mass. In addition, they are designed to be easily cleaned (as described in Chapter 16, Good Manufacturing Practices) and are manufactured to narrower tolerances with regard to speed of rotation and revolution.

The granulation process using a planetary mixer involves, first, the blending of the dry powders in the mixer. Next, the granulating fluid is slowly added with continuous mixing until the powder mass is moist but not wet. The two mixing motions mentioned above assist to keep the material uniform. Additionally, a scraper removes material adhering to the wall of the mixing bowl. Without the scraper, this material would have escaped continued mixing with the rest of the contents of the mixing bowl. At the end of the process, the material must appear damp and "crumbly" but not doughy. The wet mass is then passed through a sieve to form the granules. A doughy wet mass means that too much granulating fluid has been added, that is, it is over wet.

The wet mass may be passed manually through large screens that contain a mesh framed by stainless steel or plastic sides. The frame sizes may be of the order of 1.5 × 2 ft while the mesh size (aperture size) is selected for the desired particle size of the end product. A hand-held block, made from a hardwood that does not shed material into the product, or from a hard, nonreactive

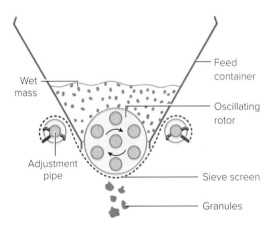

FIGURE 8-3 Oscillating granulator. Note that the adjusting pipe is used to set the tension on the screen which helps to produce good granules. (Adapted, with permission, from Aulton ME, Taylor K. *Aulton's Pharmaceutics: The Design and Manufacture of Medicines*. 6th ed. Elsevier Health Sciences; 2021.)

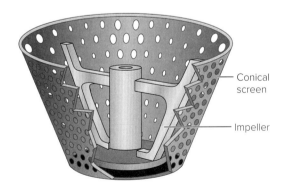

FIGURE 8-4 Quadro Comil. The cutaway figure shows the essential parts of the Comil which consists of a conical screen and an impeller. The wet mass is fed in from the top and the spinning impeller pushes the material through the screen, breaking it up into granules. The granules are thrown out in a vortex.

pushes material through the screen openings. The finished product is discharged through the bottom of the screen chamber.

The wet granules, formed by any of the wet granulation techniques described above, are spread on trays which are placed in an oven to dry. For large batches, many trays of granules are loaded onto special carts which are then wheeled into a drying room. The granules are dried at an elevated temperature, chosen to be below the temperature at which the drug will degrade, or melt. A melted drug may solidify, upon cooling, to a different polymorphic form which may alter its dissolution rate. The drying conditions should also not alter any excipient adversely. At the end of the drying cycle, the cart is wheeled out of the drying room and the trays removed. The use of the cart with wheels makes the process more efficient.

High shear granulators are a special type of granulator that work in a somewhat similar manner to planetary mixers except that a "high shear" is applied to the material being mixed. The high shearing force breaks up lumps. Why is the use of high shear important? When using low shear mixers, the material may appear to be uniform without actually being well mixed. Certain small volumes of the wet blend may be repeatedly moved around to different locations within the vessel, as high drug-load aggregates. Conversely, other small aggregates may be drug deficient. If these aggregates are not broken down, and the resulting smaller particles subsequently mixed with the rest of the material in the container, drug-rich and drug-deficient aggregates could remain intact despite prolonged mixing.

The situation depicted above is likely to lead to some tablets or capsules with a higher amount of the drug, whereas others will have a lower amount. This is unacceptable since consistent dosing of the patient is desired. This situation is unlikely to arise with a high shear mixer where the damp material is chopped repeatedly by a blade, in addition to the material being mixed by other actions. This leaves little opportunity for a clump of material to move around the container without being broken up. This mechanism ensures a very even distribution of all ingredients throughout the mass of material being mixed. In addition, the high shear granulator, by repeatedly applying a high shearing force to the material, creates dense granules which are advantageous both in capsule filling as well as in tableting.

The construction of the high shear granulator (Figure 8-5) is also similar to that of the planetary mixer in some respects.

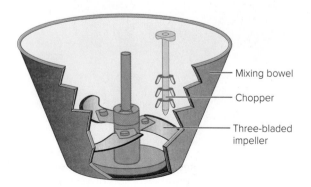

FIGURE 8-5 **High shear granulator.** (Adapted from Aulton ME, Taylor K. *Aulton's Pharmaceutics: The Design and Manufacture of Medicines.* 6th ed. Elsevier Health Sciences; 2021.)

- Mixing bowel
- Chopper
- Three-bladed impeller

It has a large, usually stainless steel, mixing bowl and an impeller for mixing. In addition, it has a series of chopper blades on a second shaft. The chopper is perpendicular to the vertical impeller in some models, while it is also vertically placed in other versions. While the impeller operates at a few hundred rpm, the chopper usually rotates at a few thousand rpm. The machine is operated as a closed system, that is, after the powders are added to the mixing bowl, a lid is placed over the bowl. The shafts of the impeller and of the chopper pass through this cover and these devices are within the covered container. The dry powders are mixed by the action of the impeller, and the chopper is not turned on during the powder blending stage. Next, the binder solution is pumped into the bowl at a predetermined rate and the chopper is turned on. As the wet mass is formed, the impeller mixes the material while the chopper breaks up lumps, and the combined action of both leads to the formation of dense granules. The wet material may then be passed through a granulator, such as an oscillating granulator or a Quadro Comil, to produce granules with a narrow size distribution.

GRANULATION ENDPOINT

When using the wet granulation technique, an important parameter to control is the amount of water or granulating fluid that is added. This is referred to as the granulation endpoint and is critical to the production of good granules. If the material is not wet enough, the powder will not be sufficiently cohesive and the granules will crumble and fall apart. Over wet material is also a problem since long strands of wet material, resembling spaghetti, will be formed upon passing the wet mass through a sieve. Naturally, when a binder/granulating fluid combination is used, over wet granules will also contain too much binder, accentuating the problem of an over-cohesive wet mass. The granulation endpoint is important with respect to both the making of granules in a compounding pharmacy as well as to industrial production. A relatively simple test is used when preparing granules on the small scale and this technique will be described first since it provides a visual picture that may help with understanding the issue.

First, it should be mentioned that the amount of granulating fluid given in a formula for compounding is considered an approximate amount. The formulator must use his or her judgment to recognize when sufficient granulating fluid has been added. Why should this amount be approximate? There are several reasons, including the temperature of the room (which affects the evaporation rate), and the particle size of the powders. As mentioned in Chapter 5, Pharmaceutical Powders, the particle size of a powder has a huge impact on its surface area. Since particles must become partially wet during granulation, the extent to which they do so, depends on their surface area since wetting is a surface phenomenon. Slight changes in particle size from batch to batch could affect the total surface area of a fixed weight of powder. Therefore, the extent to which the powder gets wet by a fixed volume of granulating fluid could be affected to a significant extent by the surface area of the powder.

To test, on a small scale, if the granulation endpoint has been reached, the pharmacist should attempt to form a ball of the wet material by compressing a small amount of wet mass between the fingers. If a good ball is not formed, it means that the material is not cohesive enough and more granulating fluid has to be added, followed by trituration. If a good, cohesive ball is formed, the next step can be performed. This involves holding the ball with the tips of the fingers of one hand so that approximately half of the ball is exposed. Then, the index finger of the other hand is used to tap the exposed half of the ball. If the ball splits in half with a clean break, it means that the granules are not over wet and the next step of the granulation (wet screening) may be performed. If the break is not clean but "strings" of wet material cling to the retained half of the ball, the granulation is over wet. On a small scale, it may be possible to simply allow the wet mass to air dry, with the repetition of the test. On a large scale, the remedy is not simple and the wet mass may have to be trashed.

In large-scale manufacture, a similar manual test was performed in years gone by. Skilled operators, with many years of experience, could quickly determine if the material is ready for granulation using the test described above. The need for a more scientific and exact determination was realized many years ago and several methods have been developed. These tests are done in process: While the material is being wet massed, electronic instrumentation takes readings and interpretation of such readings allows the operator to conclude whether the endpoint has been reached. The mixing operation does not have to be stopped in order to test the wet mass and this is a tremendous advantage in industrial production. While many advanced methods have been reported in the literature as methods in development or as research studies, two methods have found widespread use and will be briefly described.

A test that saw early development is the power consumption measurement. As more liquid is added, the wet mass gets increasingly more viscous and it becomes more difficult for the impeller to mix this material. The power consumption of the mixer (the number of watts used) increases. At the granulation endpoint, the power consumption is at its maximum. With over wetting, the wet mass begins to flow more like a liquid than a paste, and power consumption becomes less. When power consumption reaches a maximum, and just begins to drop, the endpoint has been reached and the operator will stop the process at this point.

The more popular type of device at the present time is one that measures the torque of the impeller. The torque required to continue mixing the material is a measure of the resistance of the wet material to mixing. The impeller is instrumented in these machines, that is, a small electronic unit is attached to the shaft of the impeller to take electronic measurements of torque. The resistance to the turning action of the impeller is determined (in Newton-meters abbreviated as Nm). As mixing continues, the torque increases to a maximum and then decreases. The point at which the torque begins to decrease (just after the maximum) is the point at which to stop adding granulating fluid.

Recap Questions

1. Explain what is meant by a "planetary mixer."
2. How does a planetary mixer differ from a high shear mixer?
3. What is the advantage of using high shear for granulation?

FLUID BED GRANULATOR

Fluid bed granulators are very efficient for manufacturing granules from powdered materials and for drying the wet granules. Both processes are done in one container as a single operation. The basic apparatus is a tall, cylindrical chamber, extending to the upper floor of the building in large-scale industrial equipment. The powders are loaded into a circular bowl with a mesh to retain the powders. The bowl is then pushed under the tall chamber and sealed (Figure 8-6). The fluid bed granulator has ancillary equipment (not shown in the figure) to provide rapid airflow through the apparatus. The air flows from the bottom through the wire mesh and powder bed, and into the tall chamber. The air is exhausted through the top after passing through filters to catch any powder particles entrained with the air. The equipment allows for fine adjustment of the airflow rate and it also has the capacity to heat the air, the temperature of which can be accurately controlled. Sensors measure the airflow rate upon entry into the apparatus and at the point at which the air exits the apparatus. The temperature of the air can also be measured at these points, in addition to the ability to read the temperature of the bed of granular material.

The principle of operation of the fluid bed granulator is as follows. When air is blown into the apparatus at a low flow rate, it flows through the powder bed without lifting the powder much. At a very high airflow rate, the powder would simply be thrown against the filters in the upper part of the chamber. At the optimum airflow rate, the particles are lifted off the mesh,

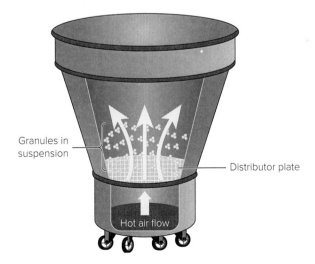

FIGURE 8-6 Fluid bed granulator.

rise up the chamber and fall back again, to be lifted by the air once more. This circulation is brought about by the very specific design of the chamber which is in the shape of a tall cylinder, narrower at the bottom and wider at the top.

Air comes into the apparatus at a fixed flow rate (measured in cubic feet per minute or cfm) and exerts a lifting force equivalent to the air pressure. At the bottom of the apparatus where its diameter is narrow, the air pressure is high and the powdered material is lifted up from the bowl. As the air reaches the broader part of the apparatus, the air pressure falls and its ability to lift the particles is progressively less. When the air pressure is insufficient to support the particles they fall to the bottom of the apparatus. The reason for the different air pressures is the fact that air is brought into the apparatus at a fixed rate (the preselected number of cfm). This fixed volume of air per minute, results in a high pressure when the cross-sectional area of the vessel is small. When the part of the apparatus with a larger diameter (greater cross-sectional area) is reached, the same airflow results in a lower pressure. At the broadest part of the apparatus, the air pressure is insufficient to lift the granules further and they fall to the lower part of the container under the influence of gravity. Here, they experience a high air pressure and are lifted by the air once more. This circulation of the material continues as long as the airflow rate is adjusted to be neither too high nor too low.

The filters, that are located at the top of the chamber, are available in different mesh sizes. An optimal mesh size prevents most of the powdered material from escaping the chamber, without clogging and limiting airflow out of the container. These filters (in the form of bags) are automatically shaken at preset intervals to allow adhering powder to fall back into the chamber to be mixed with the rest of the material.

The granulation process starts with the loading of the powdered material onto the mesh on the bowl of the apparatus. The bowl is attached to the chamber and locked into place. Sufficient airflow is set so that the powder rises and falls, as described above. Next, a granulating fluid is sprayed onto the particles that are suspended in the air, or "fluidized." The liquid wets the particles and causes them to adhere to one another. The rate at which the granulating fluid is sprayed onto the powder has to be strictly controlled so that the powder does not become over wet. Over wet clumps of powder would stick to each other, forming larger and larger agglomerates. At the correct spray rate, the clumps grow to a small size but no further.

To prevent over wetting, spraying is intermittent, for example, spraying of granulating fluid may take place for 10 seconds, with 15 seconds of drying, before the next spraying event. Since the inlet air is warm, drying will take place when no liquid is sprayed onto the granules. These numbers are hypothetical and the actual cycle of spraying and drying will be chosen by the operator, depending on many factors such as the batch size, the size of the fluid bed granulator, the nature of the granulating fluid, and the rate of spraying (mL per minute). The intermittent spraying and drying allows the forming granules to partially dry before the next addition of granulating fluid. This prevents continued agglomeration and the formation of large particles. At the correct rate and extent of wetting, with appropriate drying steps in between,

small agglomerates form and dry fairly rapidly, preventing the formation of large agglomerates. The resulting products fall within a narrow range of particle sizes. The last step, before collecting the product, is the final drying which is longer than the intermittent drying steps. In this way, a dry, powdered starting material is wet granulated and dried in one container. The fluid bed granulator is very efficient; a large industrial batch may be obtained in hours compared to days for a typical wet granulation process with tray drying.

The fluid bed apparatus may be used for the drying step only, granulation being achieved, for example, in a high shear granulator. In fact, the fluid bed dryer (without the spray nozzles for applying granulating fluid) was developed before the fluid bed granulator. Fluid bed dryers are very efficient for drying since the granules, in the fluidized state, are completely surrounded by air and can be dried from all surfaces of the granule. This is in sharp contrast to the tray dryer where only the top layer of granules is in intimate contact with the drying air. Thus, in addition to rapid drying, drying is also more complete with the fluid bed dryer, with no damp areas in a container of dried granules. This is in contrast to the tray dryer where drying may not be uniform. In addition, pre-dried air could be used to improve the ability of the fluidizing air to dry the granules.

The industrial-scale fluid bed dryers and granulators are computer controlled and the operator sits at a keyboard to type in changes, as needed. The apparatus provides data on essential functional parameters to enable the operator to control the process. The information is provided at short time intervals, the length of which is selected by the operator. From the data on airflow rates and temperature, at various points within the apparatus, the operator is able to control aspects of the process. For example, the difference between the inlet temperature and the outlet temperature gives an indication of the rate of drying of the granules. The binder solution that was sprayed onto the granules evaporates, and as it does so, it absorbs the latent heat of vaporization, cooling the air in the process. If the difference between these temperatures is large, it means that the liquid is drying too fast, with the possibility that it does not have the opportunity to interact with the powdered material sufficiently before it starts to dry. It is important to realize that the nature of the material being fluidized is constantly changing as the process continues. Therefore, it is reasonable that the operational parameters may also have to be changed to maintain a controlled state of fluidization.

Recap Questions

1. List the ways in which fluid bed granulation is different from other forms of wet granulation.
2. What are the advantages of fluid bed granulation in the pharmaceutical industry?
3. What is the advantage of using pre-dried air in a fluid bed granulator?

MELT GRANULATION

In melt granulation, the binder in powder form is mixed with the other powders constituting the formula. Thereafter, the binder is activated by heating the powders to the melting point of the binder or slightly above this temperature. This is usually done in a jacketed mixing vessel, such as a jacketed planetary mixer. The powders are mixed with the molten binder which makes the mixture cohesive. It is important that the whole mass of material be kept heated until a uniform mixture is obtained. If this is not the case, the binder will solidify before becoming well distributed. For this reason, it is not practical to melt the binder separately and pour molten binder over the powders while mixing in a container that is not heated.

Hydrophilic polymers, such as polyethylene glycol and polyvinylpyrrolidone, are used where immediate-release tablets are to be prepared and the polymer should not delay disintegration and dissolution of the tablet. For sustained-release preparations, a hydrophobic matrix is created to retard the penetration of water and to provide a slow rate of drug release. For this purpose, fatty acids and alcohols, glycerides, and waxes may be used.

The temperature range at which the binder melts is usually 50°C to 100°C. Below this range, the tablets produced from the granulation will soften and become distorted, or stick to each other, in hot geographical areas. If the melting temperature for the binder is very high, the combined powders would have to be heated beyond this temperature, increasing the probability of drug degradation. Melt granulation is similar, in one respect, to the addition of dry binder to the powdered ingredients of the formulation with the subsequent addition of water with mixing. In both cases, the binder is inactive initially and it is activated by subsequent processing. In the case of the dry binder, this processing step is the addition of water, and in the case of melt granulation, it is the heating of the material.

The major advantage of the melt granulation process is the fact that no water or other granulating fluid (which frequently is a mixture of alcohol with water) need be added. This is an advantage with drugs or excipients that are sensitive to water. An important example of excipients that are sensitive to even small amounts of moisture is the components of an effervescent mixture. Hence, melt granulation, incorporating hydrophilic polymers, may be used for preparing effervescent granules, if the polymer melts at less than 55°C. If the granules are the final dosage form, the issue of tablet softening during handling, mentioned above, does not arise. A major disadvantage of melt granulation is the fact that the material has to be heated to a fairly high temperature which can cause adverse effects in many drugs. Therefore, the technique is limited mainly to those drugs that are stable at 50°C to 100°C.

SPECIALIZED SPHERICAL GRANULATION

The wet granulation techniques described up to this point produce granules that are more spherical in shape than the starting materials. The latter may be highly irregularly-shaped particles or crystals that may be flat, cuboidal, or elongated. However, the formed granules are not completely spherical in shape and are still irregular in outline, that is, they have a rough surface. They may be described as resembling the spherical shape more closely than the starting materials. A spherical shape is preferred for pharmaceutical processing. In addition, a smooth surface is desirable. When coating small particles to produce sustained-release medication, for example, the coating is applied more evenly to spherical particles that are smooth. Two specialized techniques for producing granules that are very close to the spherical shape will be briefly described.

Extrusion and spheronization is one of the techniques that may be used to produce spherical, or nearly spherical, granules or beads. When this technique is used, the powdered material is first wet massed using, for example, a planetary mixer. The wet material is then transferred to an extruder. While extruders are manufactured in different configurations, Figure 8-7 shows a single screw extruder. The wet material is fed into a hopper which distributes the material to the horizontal chamber which has a large screw-type of impeller within the metal case of the chamber. As the impeller turns, it forces the material forward and it becomes compressed. Finally, the material is forced through a die plate with circular holes. Long strands of wet material (referred to as spaghetti) form and eventually fall into a collection vessel, breaking into shorter strands as they do so.

The strands or "spaghetti" are transferred to the spheronizer (Figure 8-8) which has the shape of a large pot with a circular loose bottom. When the spheronizer is turned on, the bottom rotates at a preset speed. The bottom has grooves that cross each other at 90° in a regular pattern. As the bottom spins, the spaghetti break up into small pieces, or rods, which rotate with the bottom of the spheronizer. The friction experienced by each rod changes it to an elliptical shape, and then the ellipses round up to spheres. With the correct extent of spheronization and an appropriate formula, well-shaped spheres are formed. If spheronization is continued for too long, or the formula is too tacky, or too wet, the spheres may agglomerate into larger and larger balls.

The spheronized product can be transferred to a fluidized bed coater. First, the beads are subjected to the drying air only. When they are sufficiently dry, the spray nozzles are turned on to coat the beads with a sustained-release coating. Then, the coating is dried and the product is discharged from the vessel. The combination of spheronization and fluid bed coating produces a very elegant product in which the drug release rate can be very closely controlled.

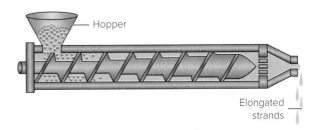

FIGURE 8-7 Screw extruder.

(A)

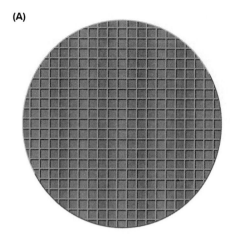

(B)

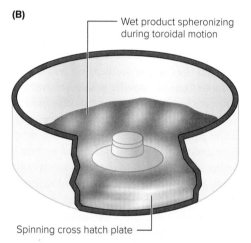

Wet product spheronizing during toroidal motion

Spinning cross hatch plate

FIGURE 8-8 Spheronizer. (A) Cross hatch plate. **(B)** Cut-away view of spheronizer in operation: the pellets being formed rotate in a rope-like configuration. (**B**: Adapted from Aulton ME, Taylor K. *Aulton's Pharmaceutics: The Design and Manufacture of Medicines.* 6th ed. Elsevier Health Sciences; 2021.)

The rotorgranulator is similar in construction to the spheronizer: it has a rotating bottom (base plate) that is notched in a similar fashion to the spheronizer. The stationary walls of the "pot" are referred to as a stator. The entire vessel is covered and has an inlet (in the cover) for the addition of granulating fluid. The powders are transferred into the vessel, the rotor turned on, and the granulating fluid sprayed onto the rotating powder. Due to centrifugal force, the wet powder particles are thrown toward the periphery of the rotor (as they are in spheronization). Air that is mechanically forced into the vessel through the gap between the rotor and stator (at the bottom of the "pot") helps to keep the wet material fluidized. As the rotor spins, the granules grow in size and also become more spherical. The pattern of the rotating material within the container is rope-like, that is, the rotating particles give the appearance of a twisting rope. However, there are only individual particles in the container. This appearance is similar to the appearance of the material in an open spheronizer.

Once the granules have formed, the spraying of the granulating liquid is discontinued and the material is dried by continued rotation of the base plate and circulation of the drying air. Once dry, a coating solution is sprayed onto the rotating beads to produce sustained-release material. The entire process, starting with powders and ending with coated sustained-release beads is completed in one vessel. It is also possible to start with spheres containing no drug and to layer a drug powder mixture onto these spheres with the aid of a binder. The product of this operation is a larger sphere with a shell of drug around the original sphere. With subsequent coating with the appropriate materials, sustained-release beads may be formed. Again, all of this is done in one container, as one operation.

DRY GRANULATION

Dry granulation, as the name implies, is a process whereby granules are formed without the addition of granulating fluid. There are two methods of achieving granulation by dry techniques: slugging and roller compaction. The former method is not used to a great extent in modern pharmaceutical technology and will be briefly described. More attention will be placed on roller compaction which is widely practiced in the pharmaceutical industry.

Slugging involves the formation of large-diameter, thin tablets, or "slugs." The material used to form the tablets is not very compressible and, for this reason, a high compression force has to be used to create the compacted tablet. Also, the tablets may not be perfectly formed in that they may have chips and cracks. These thin tablets are then subjected to mechanical crushing and passage through a mesh to from the dry granules. A large amount of fine powder may be formed during the crushing step. This is added to the powder still to be made into slugs and is used up in this way. Sieving is also done to remove very large particles which can be re-crushed.

It should be noted that the lack of compressibility of the powdered material is the reason to form granules in the first place. Granules are more compressible than the powders from which they are formed. Where powders are compressible without the need for granulation, such material is referred to as being "directly compressible." These are materials with special characteristics which confer direct compressibility, or they are materials that are processed to achieve the direct compression property. Direct compression is discussed in Chapter 9, Tablets. Most materials, however, are not directly compressible and, therefore, need to be converted into granules before tablet production.

As mentioned, roller compaction is far more popular, at the present time, than slugging as a method to produce dry granules. The process is also known as chilsonation, a term which is not used frequently at present. The process starts with the feeding of the powdered material into a large, conical hopper which has a worm screw to force the material under pressure out of the hopper (Figure 8-9). This mechanical device is needed since the powders are not free-flowing and will not flow well under the influence of gravity alone. The material that leaves the bottom of the hopper (under the influence of the worm screw) enters the space between two rollers which rotate in opposite directions (one clockwise; the other counterclockwise). This arrangement forces the powdered

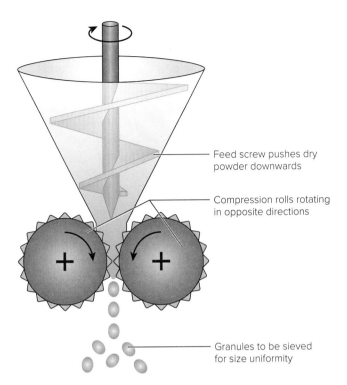

Feed screw pushes dry powder downwards

Compression rolls rotating in opposite directions

Granules to be sieved for size uniformity

FIGURE 8-9 Roller compactor. (Adapted from Aulton ME, Taylor K. *Aulton's Pharmaceutics: The Design and Manufacture of Medicines.* 6th ed. Elsevier Health Sciences; 2021.)

material through the space between the rollers. This space is set to a narrow gap which causes the material to be squeezed between the rollers. The compaction experienced by the powders causes them to bond together, though not very strongly.

The material that comes through the rollers has the appearance of a thin pancake that is not holding together very well, that is, it breaks up into pieces as it comes out of the gap between the rollers. The material then enters a granulator that forces it through a mesh. The resultant product, which falls into a receiving container, is granular in nature with a relatively narrow size range. The major advantage of roller compaction (dry granulation) is the fact that no water or heat is used to create the granules. Many chemical reactions require water as the medium and several reactions will not occur at all in the dry state. Therefore, this technique has a tremendous advantage. Heat, which is required to dry a wet granulation, also causes many changes including the melting of drugs with subsequent recrystallization into a different polymorphic form. The latter may have less desirable characteristics, such as a lower solubility, than the original polymer. Since no heat is applied in roller compaction, this technique has further advantages.

Recap Questions

1. What is the major advantage of using melt granulation?
2. What is the potential disadvantage of using melt granulation?

3. Why must the polymer melt at less than 55°C when using melt granulation for making effervescent granules?
4. Describe the need for spherical granules.
5. Name two types of apparatus that can be used for spherical granulation.
6. Why is dry granulation useful in the pharmaceutical industry?

CONTINUOUS GRANULATION

Granulation has been a batch process until fairly recently. Batch processes involve manufacture of the batch from instructions contained in a batch record, testing of the quality of the product, review of the batch record for possible deviations in procedure, review of test results, release of the batch if it conforms to requirements, cleaning of the equipment, and cleaning verification. This is repeated for each batch that is produced in a GMP environment (see Chapter 16, Good Manufacturing Practices). For high throughput products, for example, over-the-counter pain relievers, it may be appropriate to have continuous production for a week, for example, with subsequent tear down of the equipment for cleaning. In the context of this chapter, continuous production will be discussed with wet granulation as the example. Continuous production would be an enormous saving in time and money but can only be done if the accuracy of production, and of the final product, and the safety of patients, can be assured. At the present time, testing is largely done at the end of the production of a batch. If all test criteria are within pre-set limits, the batch passes; if not, it fails. Frequently, failed batches have to be trashed. With continuous processing, extensive in-process testing is conducted. This is different from the limited in processing testing that is done at the present time with batch products. Using advanced testing methods, it is possible to check that the batch is within predetermined quality standards, *while the batch is being produced.* Process analytical technology (PAT) utilizes functional tests, carried out in the course of batch manufacture, so that adjustments can be made, if necessary, during processing to ensure a quality product.

SUMMARY POINTS

- Granulation is an important technique in pharmaceutical processing; it provides material that can easily be tableted or filled into capsules.
- Conventional wet granulation can be conducted by low shear techniques.
- High shear wet granulation provides a more dense, uniform product that provides better assurance of consistent drug distribution throughout the granulation.
- Fluid bed granulation affords the convenience of one-container processing for granulation and drying; the process is also much faster that wet granulation followed by tray drying.

- Melt granulation utilizes heat to melt tacky materials to facilitate granulation without the use of water.

- Special techniques are used to produce spherical granules that can be coated very evenly with materials for sustained release, or for other purposes.

- Dry granulation uses neither heat nor water and offers tremendous advantages for processing drugs that are sensitive to these factors.

What do you think?

1. In the fusion method of granulation, why is the material dried at a temperature of less than 54°C?

2. If granulating fluid, which is tacky, is sprayed onto fluidized particles in the fluid bed granulator, why do the particles not coalesce into large balls of material?

3. In the midst of a fluid bed granulation process, the operator notices that the outlet air temperature is very slightly lower than the inlet air temperature. What is the significance of this observation?

4. If very fine particles are used in a fluid bed granulator, does this pose a risk of contamination of the atmosphere? What can be done to limit such contamination?

5. Can a hydrophobic polymer be used for making effervescent granules by the melt granulation process? Explain your answer.

6. For the granulation of a newly discovered drug (properties not yet fully characterized), which granulation technique would you recommend using? Give reasons for your answer.

Tablets

PREVIEW

- History and relevance of tablets
- Overview of tablet production methods and equipment
- Constituents of tablets with examples of each excipient type
- Direct compression and its relevance
- Problems encountered during tablet production
- Specialized tablets
- How is the quality of tablets evaluated?

INTRODUCTION AND HISTORY

Tablets may be defined as solid pharmaceutical dosage forms containing drug substances, usually prepared with suitable excipients by compression or molding methods. Molding methods involve moistening the drug and diluent mixture with water or some other solvent and, by means of a spatula, spreading the wet material over the surface of dies in a metal plate (marked "A" in Figure 9-1). This process fills the dies with the wet material. The dies may be visualized as a series of regularly spaced holes in the metal plate. A set of pins, shaped to accurately fit the dies, is attached to a second plate (marked "B" in Figure 9-1). When plate A is placed onto the pins and pressed down, the molded tablets are pushed out of the dies. The holes and pins shown in the diagram are round but they may be square-shaped, producing square tablets in the latter case. The wet, molded tablets are left to dry on the top of the pins. The dried, molded material is packaged and supplied to patients. This technique is not used as an industrial production technique but may be used in a compounding pharmacy. Most tablets are prepared by compression techniques and this production method will be the focus of this chapter. The compressed tablet is one of the most popular dosage forms.

There is evidence that tablets were used well over 1000 years ago. Rhazes, or al Rhazi, who lived in Persia in the 9th century, is credited with the first manufacture of tablets. These tablets were not the sophisticated dosage forms we know today. Although

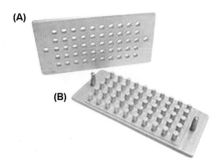

FIGURE 9-1 Apparatus for making molded tablets. "A" is the plate onto which the wet powdered material is spread; **"B"** is the second plate containing the pins.

simple, the basic principle underlying their production is the same as that of modern tablets. In manuscripts written in the latter half of the 10th century, tablet molds made of wood, ivory, or grinding stone are described. At least 1000 years ago, the weight of tablets was controlled. With regard to more recent history, Brockedon is credited with the introduction of tablet fabrication to England in 1843. About 1872, John Wyeth and coworkers designed a machine that greatly reduced the cost of compression, so that tablets could be made commercially available. They are thought to have been the first to use the term "compressed tablets." By 1894, tablets to treat almost every known disease were sold in the European and American markets.

The general manufacture of compressed tablets, however, assumed considerable proportions only at the beginning of the 20th century when many new machines were devised and a considerable amount of research was done on methods of production. The compressed tablet has continued to increase in popularity and has largely replaced the pill and other solid dosage forms such as powders, cachets, and granules. Many new tablet forms, with specialized actions, have been devised. An example of the latter is the development of orally disintegrating tablets (ODT) which are described in more detail later in this chapter.

The compressed tablet offers several advantages over the solid dosage forms mentioned above, some of which are as follows:

1. Precision of dosage

2. Convenience of administration

3. Masking of unpleasant tastes by appropriate methods, including the addition of flavors and the coating of the tablet

4. Stability of chemical and physiological activity of the drug

5. Stability of the dosage form over extended periods of storage

6. Relatively low cost (due to mass production) for a sophisticated, quality-controlled dosage form

A round tablet, intended to be swallowed by an adult, should usually not exceed about 1/2 in (or 12.5 mm) in diameter. The volume of the dose of the drug (ie, its bulkiness) may decide the size of the tablet to be made and, if necessary, the therapeutic dose may be given as two tablets. Most often, however, the dose is small and occupies a very small volume since many newer drugs are very potent. As a result, a diluent has to be used to increase the bulk of the material to be compressed.

During much of the 20th century, the manufacturer's main concerns were that the tablet should look elegant and that it should contain the desired amount of the active ingredient. To confirm the latter, effort was expended to develop assay methods. Little attention was paid, however, to what occurred once the tablet was taken by the patient. It was only from about the 1960s that serious consideration was given to the rate of drug release, and the pattern of drug release from the dosage form. Three formulations may each contain the same drug in the same quantity and, furthermore, the formulations may release approximately 100% of the drug in 1 hour. However, one formulation may release the drug rapidly in the beginning and slower later, the second formulation may release the drug slowly in the beginning and rapidly later, while the third formulation may release the drug at an even rate throughout the 1-hour period. Each of these formulations displays a different pattern of drug release which may be expressed by different mathematical equations. Only one of these may be the desirable release pattern for a specific drug.

It was also recognized, during this period, that the ability of the body to absorb the active ingredient from the tablet is of tremendous importance. For example, with very rapid initial release, the body's drug absorption mechanism may be overwhelmed. The drug that is not absorbed immediately may be degraded by the prevailing physiological conditions, for example, an unfavorable pH. In addition, the process of producing a tablet, that is, the conversion of a powdered active ingredient into a compressed, solid dosage form in which the active ingredient is interspersed between other ingredients, may have a profound effect on the bioavailability of the medicament.

Well-formulated and -manufactured tablets should possess the following properties:

1. They should meet the predetermined specifications for tablet quality. These include chemical characteristics such as the content of the active ingredient, as well as physical characteristics, including hardness and freedom from defects such as chips, cracks, and mottling.

2. They should be able to withstand the vigorous production process as well as subsequent handling during packaging, shipping, and dispensing.

3. They should have an aesthetic appeal to ensure good compliance with the dosage regimen and should have a shape and size that is appropriate for the route of administration. Most tablets for oral administration are round, while those with a larger dose may be elongated or capsule-shaped for easier swallowing. Vaginal tablets are typically diamond-shaped for easier insertion, especially when using an applicator.

4. During the shelf life of the product, tablets should have good chemical and physical stability. The need for the correct dose, even toward the end of the shelf life of the product, may be readily appreciated. It is equally important that the tablets should not soften and break up during handling, or become excessively hard, during this period. In the latter case, slow drug release may be evident.

Mind Map 9-1 summarizes several aspects of tablet production and testing.

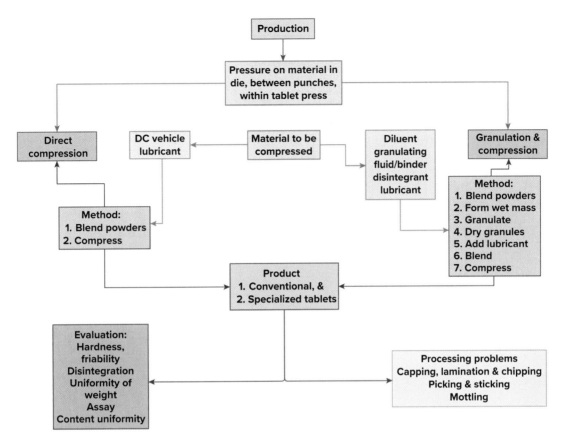

MIND MAP 9-1 Tablets

PRODUCTION OF TABLETS

The methods by which compressed tablets are produced in the pharmaceutical industry will be discussed. All tablet production equipment contains an essential mechanical unit, referred to as a punch and die set (Figure 9-2). This consists of an upper, and a lower, punch and a die. These components are matched to each other and have ground, polished surfaces of stainless steel or some other unreactive material. The tablet is formed by pressure on the punches while the tips of both punches are within the die, and with the granules filling the rest of the space in the die cavity (Figure 9-3). This basic unit is part of a fairly complex piece of machinery referred to as a tablet press.

TABLET PRESSES

Machines built to compress tablets are referred to as tablet presses (or tableting machines) and they consist of the following basic components:

1. A hopper is used for storing the material to be compressed.
2. A mechanism for feeding the material to be compressed into the dies. This consists of a feed frame in most industrial production machines. In small research and development machines, which have only one punch and die set (see below), it may consist of a feeding shoe which has a much lower filling capacity than a feed frame.

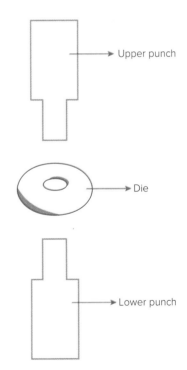

FIGURE 9-2 A typical punch and die set. Note the heads of punches are not shown in detail.

3. Punches and dies as referred to above. The size and shape of the die and the concavity of the punches determine the size and shape of the tablets produced.
4. A mechanism is used to apply pressure to the punches.

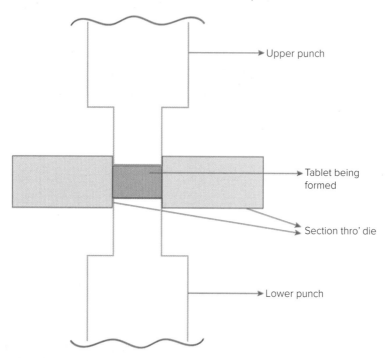

FIGURE 9-3 Formation of a tablet within the die.

5. Cams are used for guiding the punches as they move within the tablet press, the head of the punch residing in the cam.

6. Control mechanisms that enable the consistent production of uniform tablets. These include the speed at which the dies are filled and at which tablets are produced, the amount of pressure applied to the tablets, and even the height to which formed tablets are raised when ejected from the die. All tablets must comply with predetermined specifications (eg, tablet weight and hardness are controlled).

When a very small amount of the drug is available for research studies, tablets may be compressed on a single-punch machine which contains one set of punches and a die. This machine requires a much smaller minimum quantity of material to function than a rotary press which has multiple sets of punches and dies. The punches move up and down in order to bring about compression of the tablet but no other motion is needed. When a larger output is required, a "rotary tablet press" is used. This machine is so named because the punches and dies rotate in the machine, in addition to the up-and-down motion of the punches during compression.

Small-scale research and development rotary tablet presses may contain 4 to 8 sets of punches and dies, whereas larger research, or small-scale production, equipment may contain 16 sets of punches and dies. The larger the machine, and the greater the production output, the more sets of punches and dies the machine contains. Large-scale production equipment usually contains 33, or more, sets of punches and dies. Apart from the number of punches and dies, there are other differences between a multi-station and a single-station tablet press with regard to both the structure of the machine and the mechanism of tablet production. There are, also, differences in the tablets produced.

To avoid differences in the product made from very small-scale research and development equipment, on the one hand, and large-scale production equipment, on the other hand, the compaction simulator was developed. This single-punch, computerized equipment can mimic the action of any large-scale production machine. Adjustments are effected by keyboard strokes to set electronic parameters in order to simulate a specific large tablet press. Thus, the small quantity of product from the compaction simulator can reliably be expected to resemble the product from a large rotary tablet press.

The multi-station rotary press will be described in order to give the pharmacist an appreciation of the way tablets are made in an industrial production machine, some of the problems that might occur, and defects that may be present in tablets. The purpose of this description is to allow the pharmacist to be aware of manufacturing issues that they may come across in daily practice so that they could answer patient's questions. It also puts the pharmacist in a position to have a meaningful discussion with a manufacturing company, or its representative, when product defects or other issues are noticed. Likewise, when a pharmacist at a large hospital is entrusted with the task of choosing between competing brands, he or she would have some technical knowledge with which to assess the quality of the competing brands. This may be very important when the competing brands are the innovator's and a generic product, or two generic products.

A photograph of a multi-station rotary press is shown in Figure 9-4, while the diagrammatic representation of this equipment in Figure 9-5 will facilitate an understanding of its mechanism of operation. A head carrying a number of sets of punches and dies revolves continuously. The dies are contained in a circle around the periphery of a steel plate, also referred to as the die table (A). The punches and dies move in a circular fashion and are brought to each "service" (ie, die filling, compression, or ejection) in turn. The tablet granulation flows from the hopper (not shown), through a feed frame which has interconnected compartments (B), into the dies. The dies, located in the steel plate, revolve under the feed frame.

The compression cycle starts when the heads of the lower punches enter the pulldown cam (C) and are allowed to go to their lowest point. This allows the dies to overfill with the material that

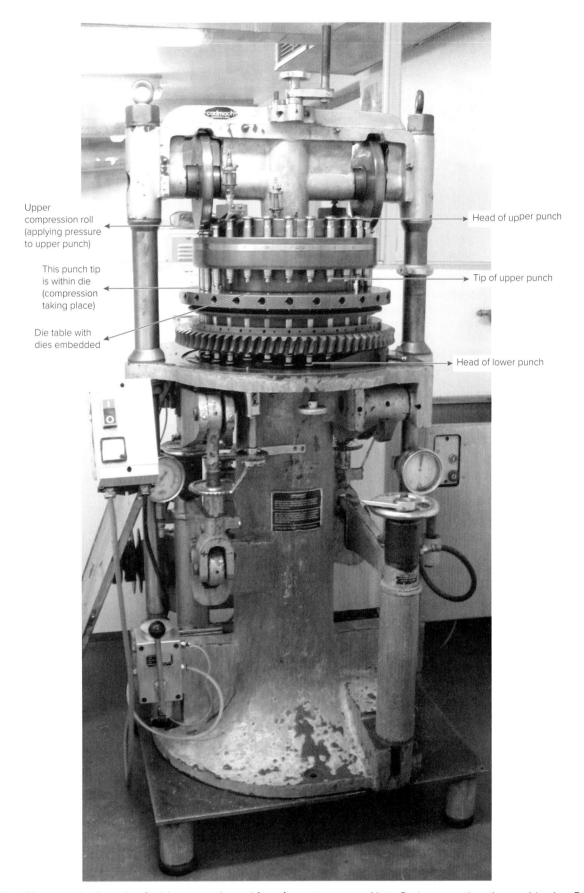

Upper compression roll (applying pressure to upper punch)

This punch tip is within die (compression taking place)

Die table with dies embedded

Head of upper punch

Tip of upper punch

Head of lower punch

FIGURE 9-4 **Photograph of mechanical features of a multi-station rotary press.** Note: During operation, the machine has Perspex covers to keep out contamination and for the safety of the operator. (Reproduced, with permission, from Mishra S, Banerjee J, Panakkal JP. Fabrication of nuclear fuel elements. In: Tomar BS, Rao PRV, Roy SB, Panakkal JP, Raj K, Nandakumar AN, eds. *Nuclear Fuel Cycle*. Singapore: Springer; 2023:81-116.)

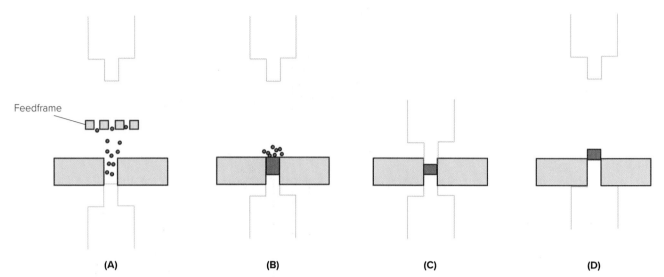

Feedframe

(A) (B) (C) (D)

FIGURE 9-5 Steps in the compression cycle of a tablet. A. The lower punch moves to its lowest travel and granules flow from the feed frame into the die cavity while the upper punch remains raised. B. The head of the lower punch moves over the weight controlling cam (not shown), causing the lower punch to be raised to a level that accords with the required tablet weight. This action pushes excess granules out of the die and a mechanism sweeps these granules away. C. The lower punch rises while the upper punch is lowered simultaneously. This action squeezes the granules between the punches, within the die. D. The lower punch rises to bring the formed tablet flush with the die table while the upper punch also rises. Note: 1. Components are as labeled in Figure 9-3. 2. Several punches and dies are arranged in a circle in the tablet machine but only one set is depicted as it moves in a circle through the various stages needed for compression. 3. With further rotation of the die table after the completion of step D, the tablet strikes a plate attached to the front of the feed frame and is pushed off the die table down a chute into the collecting receptacle and the depicted punches and die return to position A to begin another cycle.

is in the feed frame. The lower punches then pass over a weight-controlled cam which pushes the lower punches up, reducing the fill in the dies to the desired level. A blade (D) on the feed frame removes the excess granulation (that was pushed up) and directs this material around the turret (the central metal column) and back into the front of the feed frame. This method of die filling (overfilling and removal of excess) promotes a uniform fill of the die and, therefore, an accurate weight for the tablets.

The upper punches then move under the upper compression guide roll (E), while the lower punches move simultaneously over the lower compression guide roll (F). This step provides the required compression pressure to form the tablet. Since this mechanism applies pressure to the powder in the die from both the top and the bottom, the trapped air has a better chance of escaping. Many tablet presses also have a pre-compression step. This step occurs before the main compression step, described above, and involves the passing of the upper and lower punches, respectively, under and over smaller guide rolls (G and H) which apply pressure to the material in the die. The extent of pressure is less than that of the main compression rolls. This pressure reduces the volume of the particulate material but it is insufficient to form a tablet. When the pre-compression pressure is relieved, however, the air in the powder blend escapes. Next, the main compression is applied to form the tablet. This method (pre-compression followed by the main compression) allows more efficient removal of air from the powder mixture or granules compared to the use of the main compression only.

Each type of material to be compressed may require a different compression pressure. The change in the compression pressure is achieved by adjustments to the lower compression guide

roll. By mechanically lowering the lower compression guide role (F), the applied pressure is reduced. This is due to the fact that the lower punches are pushed upwards to a lesser extent by the adjusted lower roll during compression. To increase compression pressure, the lower compression guide role is raised which causes the lower punches to rise further up into the die during compression.

After compression, the upper punches move up removing the compressive force. Next, the lower punches rise to bring the tablet flush, or slightly above, the surface of the dies. The height to which the tablets rise may be adjusted. The raised tablet strikes a plate on the front of the feed frame which forces the tablet off the die table and down a chute to a collecting receptacle. Thereafter, the heads of the lower punches re-enter the pulldown cam (C) causing the lower punches to drop to their lowest point, enabling the dies to be overfilled once more when the dies move under the feed frame, at the beginning of the next compression cycle.

Recap Questions

1. Tablets are a 20th-century innovation. Is this statement true or false?

2. Apart from compressed tablets, what other types of tablets have been produced for drug administration? Which is the more popular type?

3. Name two advantages of compressed tablets over powders and granules.

PROPERTIES OF MATERIAL TO BE COMPRESSED

Materials to be compressed into tablets must have the following *essential* characteristics:

1. Fluidity or the ability to flow freely
2. Cohesiveness or compactability
3. Lubrication

Fluidity is necessary for the transport or flow of the material through the hopper into the feed frame. As particles move under the force of gravity through progressively smaller openings (from the hopper to the die cavity), they experience pressure from the material above, and alongside, the particles under consideration. These pressures may not be equal in all directions. Depending on the size and geometry of the passageway, this may give rise to bridging or rat holing, phenomena which have been described in Chapter 5, Powders. In the worst cases, cessation of flow might occur.

The weight of the tablets is determined by the volume of the die cavity, that is, the size of the cavity formed by the lower punch at a fixed height within the die. This cavity forms the receptacle for the particulate material to flow into and its size is fixed for a particular tablet by adjustment of the height to which the punch rises at the weight-controlling cam/weight adjustment ramp. Consequently, the cavity must be filled completely each time a tablet is compressed, during a particular tableting run. If it is not, tablets of varying weight will result, the under-filled dies producing lighter tablets. Overfilling of the die cavity and subsequent removal of excess material is a better way to ensure complete die fill than a simple filling of the die in one attempt. Secondary tablet properties such as hardness and thickness may also vary with inconsistent die fill. This is due to the fact that different volumes of material present more, or less, resistance to the fixed compression pressure of the punches.

When poor flow from the hopper occurs, it can be controlled by vibrators. However, this solution may introduce another problem: separation or de-mixing. This is due to the fact that the material to be compressed usually has some variation in particle size and vibration causes separation of particles of different sizes. Actually, the smaller particles "percolate" between the larger particles and flow faster than the large particles. If

vibration persists, the separation of particles according to size, in the feed frame and hopper, continues and the small particles get further ahead. This process is referred to as segregation and leads to variation in the fill weight of the die.

A greater proportion of small particles in the die leads to higher fill weight since there is less air space in the die. With the above situation, heavier tablets will be produced early in the tableting run (Figure 9-6). Later, toward the end of the production run, there are more large particles filling the die. Due to more air spaces in the die, lighter tablets result. The production of tablets of variable weight is the overall result, which is undesirable. If the active ingredient is the component that separates out, it may also lead to changes in the content uniformity of the tablets. Since drug substances frequently do not compress well, the hardness of the tablets may also vary.

Materials for tableting should also have the important characteristic of compactability. This is the ability of the material to form a stable compacted mass when pressure is applied. In consideration of the above, the desirable properties of materials to be compressed may be summarized as follows:

1. The material should contain particles which approach a spherical shape.
2. The particle size of the material should represent a normal distribution curve with a small percentage of both coarse and fine particles, and with the majority of particles in a narrow range between these extremes.
3. The material should have a uniform distribution of all the ingredients in their respective percentages.
4. The material should be compactible, or possess compactible components, in sufficient quantity, to confer physical strength and form to the tablets.

When the dose of the active ingredient is small, diluents are largely responsible for determining these properties. Conversely, when the dose is sufficiently high that the drug forms the major part of the tablet, the drug will determine the overall properties of the material to be compressed. Since most materials have only some of these properties, other materials have to be added to confer certain characteristics (such as compactability). Alternately, the material has to be formed into granules. Granules approach a spherical shape and flow well, especially with the aid of glidants. They also possess compactible components, including the

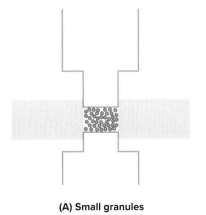
(A) Small granules

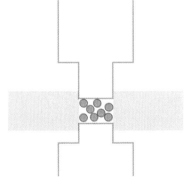
(B) Large granules

FIGURE 9-6 Airspaces within the die cavity related to the size of granules. Note the large air spaces when large granules are used.

binder. Granulated material, possessing these properties, can be successfully tableted. In addition, the granule has a mix of materials, of large particle size and small, and of all components of the tablet in the correct proportion. Since the granule flows as a unit, these components reach the die cavity in the correct proportion. A few materials inherently possess the above properties, and these materials may be successfully tableted without the modifications brought about by granulation. Such materials are referred to as being "directly compressible" and are described more fully in a later section of this chapter.

The different categories of ingredients incorporated into tablets, to provide them with the desired characteristics, were discussed in general terms in Chapter 8, Granulation. This was done in the context of providing a basic understanding of how to make granules. In this chapter, examples of ingredients in each of these categories will be discussed. In some cases, the differences in the properties of the tablets, as a result of the choice of a specific ingredient, will also be mentioned. Granulating agents and binders were described in more detail in Chapter 8 since they are integral to the formulation of good granules. They will not be described in detail in this chapter.

DILUENTS

Table 9-1 lists some common diluents used in tablet formulation, classified according to whether, or not, the diluent is soluble in an aqueous medium. The solubility of the diluent may have an impact on the dissolution rate of the drug, particularly if the drug is poorly soluble and/or has a slow rate of solution. In other instances, the solubility of the diluent may have little impact on the dissolution rate of the drug, especially if the drug is very rapidly soluble. In addition, when very rapid disintegration is achieved, the drug may be able to dissolve according to its solubility characteristics, with little hindrance from the diluent. Rapid disintegration may be achieved with the addition of certain modern disintegrants which are described in more detail in the section on disintegrants, later in this chapter, and also by the use of low compression forces to produce soft, highly porous tablets.

When a new therapeutic agent is formulated into a tablet, the compatibility of the diluent with the drug must be considered. For example, calcium salts used as diluents for the broad-spectrum antibiotic, tetracycline, have been shown to interfere with the drug's absorption from the gastrointestinal tract (GIT). Some diluents may be acidic, or basic, in nature and may respectively react with basic, or acidic, drugs. Calcium carbonate, for example, is basic and should not be used with acidic drugs. Some diluents, such as lactose, contain a fairly high amount of water and are unsuitable for use with water-sensitive drugs. In spite of this, lactose is a commonly used diluent which is stable, dissolves readily in water, and does not react with most medicinal substances (except for moisture-sensitive drugs, as noted). Its rapid solubility facilitates quick release of the active ingredient. Its high melting point means that it will not soften during compression during which there may be intense pressure at the points of contact of irregularly shaped particles, resulting in an increase in temperature at the contact points.

TABLE 9-1	Some Commonly Used Diluents
DILUENT	**COMMENT**
A. Soluble Diluents	
Lactose	One of the most commonly used diluents in wet granulation. Dissolves readily.
Sucrose	Forms hard tablets which harden further with age. Not suitable for diabetics; use has declined.
Mannitol	Sugar alcohol. Provides very smooth, "melting" effect; useful for lozenges and ODT. High amounts per day can cause bloating and loose stools.
Sorbitol	Sugar alcohol. Provides very smooth, "melting" effect; useful for lozenges and ODT.
B. Insoluble Diluents	
Calcium carbonate	Serves as a diluent as well as a source of calcium. Used in antacid tablets.
Calcium sulfate	Serves as a diluent as well as a source of calcium.
Dibasic calcium phosphate	Serves as a diluent as well as a source of calcium. Forms hard tablets. Available as anhydrous and dihydrate forms.
Tribasic calcium sulfate	Serves as a diluent as well as a source of calcium.
Starch	One of the older diluents; replaced by modified starches and other newer diluents.
Modified starches, eg, Starch 1500	A range of chemically modified starches, with improved characteristics, available commercially. Starch 1500 is used as a diluent, direct compression ingredient, and also as a binder in wet granulation.
Microcrystalline cellulose	Long cellulose chains subjected to scission at appropriate points to maximize the crystallinity of the shorter strands (improves compactibility). Widely used as a direct compression ingredient as well as a conventional diluent.

GRANULATING FLUID

The granulating fluid is the liquid that is added to the powders to form the wet mass. The latter should be cohesive but not tacky, a state that is achieved by adding sufficient, but not too much, granulating fluid. Excessive granulating fluid makes the wet mass tacky or "doughy" in consistency.

Some materials are so hydrophobic that they will not wet easily with water. For this reason, the powders may be first moistened and mixed with another liquid agent, called a wetting agent. An example of a wetting agent is alcohol. The alcohol displaces air and makes the powders more amenable to subsequent wetting with water.

BINDERS

After wetting the powders with the granulating fluid, the resulting wet mass, in many instances, is insufficiently cohesive to form good granules. In other instances, adequate granules may be formed but these granules do not form good tablets under compression. This is due to the granules lacking sufficient compactability. What is required, in both cases, is the addition of a binder. The binder increases the cohesiveness of the powder, thus forming good granules. In addition, the binder contributes to better compactability when the granules are compressed. The portion of the binder located on the surface of the granules may be especially important in this regard. Typically, the binder and granulating fluid are combined, usually as a solution of the former in the latter. As mentioned in Chapter 8 (Granulation), the addition of the binder as a powder and subsequent activation with the granulating fluid is frequently less effective than using a binder/granulating fluid solution. Cellulose derivatives, such as hydroxypropyl methyl cellulose (HPMC), *with a low degree of substitution,* may be used as a binder. The degree of substitution refers to the extent to which OH groups on the cellulose backbone have been replaced with methoxy or hydroxypropyl groups. There are different types of HPMC, varying by the extent of each substitution type. For example, the E grade has 28% to 30% methoxy substitution and 4% to 12% hydroxypropyl substitution. This grade has a low viscosity and is suitable to use as a binder. A high viscosity grade will bring about a sustained-release effect. Some commonly used binders are listed in Table 8-1.

DISINTEGRANTS

When a tablet contacts water, it is intended that the tablet should break up into large pieces, and that the pieces then break up into finer granules. Thereafter, the granules break up into their constituent particles, or prime particles. This overall process, as described above, is referred to as disintegration. Disintegration is depicted schematically in Figure 9-7. Obviously, when the tablet is in contact with an aqueous body fluid, such as gastric fluid, disintegration is also expected to occur. An excipient, known as the disintegrant, is added to tablet formulations to promote the disintegration process. The function of the disintegrant is essentially the opposite of that of the binder.

In the absence of a disintegrant, some disintegration of the tablet may still occur, although at a slower rate. The potential for disintegration to occur, in the absence of a disintegrant, depends on the nature of the other constituents of the tablet, especially the diluent in low-dose tablets. In the presence of insoluble diluents in such a tablet formulation, very little or no disintegration may occur. Conversely, with soluble diluents, the dissolution of the diluent promotes breakup of the tablet. It should be noted that some tablets are specially formulated not to disintegrate.

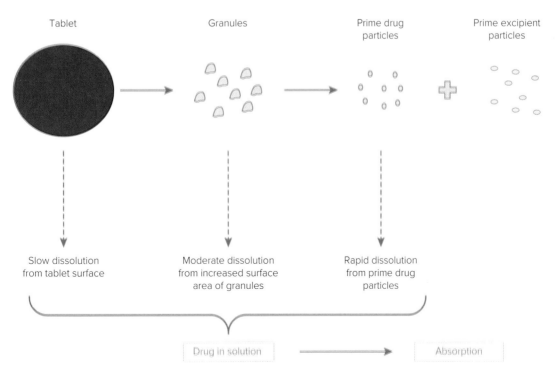

FIGURE 9-7 Diagram of disintegration process.

Such non-disintegrating tablets do not contain a disintegrant, apart from other formulation changes that may be incorporated to ensure that disintegration does not take place.

Starch was a very commonly used disintegrant but has been replaced, to some extent, by the availability of other disintegrants. These include modified starches, such as pre-gelatinized starch and clays, for example, kaolin, bentonite, or Veegum. The latter is the trade name for a complex consisting of magnesium, aluminum, and silicate. Microcrystalline cellulose, generally used as a direct compression vehicle, has effective disintegrant properties. Other gums that are used as disintegrants include guar gum and locust bean gum.

The most common mechanism of disintegrant action is the swelling of the disintegrant which pushes apart the tablet constituents and is responsible for disrupting bonds holding the tablet together. Other disintegrants cause the wicking of water into the tablet. Their high affinity for water draws water into the matrix (interior) of the tablet. Usually, a wicking agent is used in combination with a swelling disintegrant. Thus, the wicking agent draws water into the core of the tablet where it causes the swelling of another disintegrant, effectively disintegrating the tablet. An example of a wicking agent is alginic acid which has a strong affinity for water although it is insoluble in water. Its high sorption capacity, especially when used in conjunction with a swelling disintegrant, leads to rapid disintegration. Purified wood cellulose is also a good wicking agent. The water that is drawn into the tablet may also cause the swelling of other components of the tablet, contributing to the disintegration effect. Some commonly used disintegrants are shown in Table 9-2.

TABLE 9-2	Some Commonly Used Disintegrants
DISINTEGRANT	**USUAL CONCENTRATION RANGE (%)***
Starch	5-20
Pre-gelatinized starch	5-15
Avicel	5-20
Alginic acid	5-10
Guar gum	5-10
Kaolin	5-15
Bentonite	5-15
Veegum	5-15
Acid-base mixture	3-20
Low substituted HPMC	2-8
Super Disintegrants	
Sodium Starch glycolate	2-8
Croscarmellose sodium	2-5
Crospovidone	2-5

*Note that this is the usual concentration range for use as a disintegrant. For other functions, such as a diluent function, the concentration may be different.

Effervescent mixtures were considered efficient disintegrants at one time. Water drawn into the tablet, after consumption, came into contact with the effervescent mixture and CO_2 was liberated within the tablet. The rapid increase in the volume of gas, within the tablet, literally pushes it apart. This effect was more efficient than that of some of the older disintegrants, such as starch. However, with the advent of the so-called "super disintegrants," effervescent mixtures are no longer considered to be very efficient.

Super disintegrants, as the name implies, are highly effective at producing tablet disintegration. They are used in lower concentrations than typical "conventional" disintegrants. Three of the most popular super disintegrants are croscarmellose sodium, crospovidone, and sodium starch glycolate. They have a rapid, and high, swelling capacity, thus bringing about efficient disintegration. It is important to pay careful attention to the name of the excipient. For example, povidone is used as a binder in tablets. Crospovidone which is the cross-linked derivative is insoluble, but swells, in water and is used as a disintegrant. These are very different functions from ingredients which have similar names.

LUBRICANTS, GLIDANTS, AND ANTI-ADHERENTS

What was previously termed a "lubricant" in the literature actually describes three separate functions, namely, lubricant, glidant, and anti-adherent. The term is sometimes still used loosely when a glidant or anti-adherent is meant.

Lubricants

A first function that the lubricants play is a role within the die cavity when the punches apply force to the material to be compressed. The moving metallic parts (punch surface against die wall) experience friction which has to be overcome by the use of a lubricant. This aspect of the lubricant's activity is similar to any mechanical device's need for a lubricant, such as oil, to reduce friction between moving parts. The lubricants used in tablet compression are usually in powder form and are blended with the material to be compressed. A second function of the lubricant is to lubricate the particles within the die cavity during compression. At this phase of the compression cycle, the particles must slip and slide, one against the other, under high pressure. Without a lubricant, friction between the particles would be high and the temperature would rise to an unacceptable level, especially at the points of contact between adjacent particles.

A third function of lubricants is during ejection of the tablet. While the punches in a rotary tablet press move up and down in the vertical direction, the compression force exerted on the tableting components within the die causes these components to be squeezed outward in a radial fashion. For this reason, the newly-compressed tablet (prior to ejection) would experience a tight fit within the die. Therefore, when the lower punch raises the tablet to eject it from the die, a great deal of friction is experienced between the edge of the tablet, along its circumference, and the die wall. The lubricant reduces this friction. When the amount of lubricant is insufficient, a "grunting" sound will be heard as the tablet press strains to eject the tablet. In addition, the edges of insufficiently lubricated tablets will also have striations ("burn marks") due to the friction experienced during ejection.

There are two types of lubricants: hydrophobic and hydrophilic. The hydrophobic type has been in use for longer and has been well studied. The prime example of a hydrophobic lubricant is magnesium stearate. Hydrophilic lubricants are used in those instances where all the components of the tablet are desired to be soluble, or at least hydrophilic. An example of such an application is in the production of effervescent tablets where the tablet is required to be dissolved in a glass of water before consumption by the patient. Insoluble magnesium stearate would appear as scum on the surface of the liquid and may remain as an insoluble residue in the drinking glass, after consumption of the liquid. The former effect occurs because the highly hydrophobic lubricant resists wetting by water, and therefore floats on the surface. Since magnesium stearate is the best-known and the most widely used example of a hydrophobic lubricant, its use in the production of tablets will be described.

When considering magnesium stearate and its lubrication action, two important factors must be taken into consideration. First, lubrication is a surface phenomenon. The magnesium stearate particles, which are generally smaller than the particles of the tableting material, coat the larger particles after mixing. While the particles are small, magnesium stearate from different manufacturers, and different grades from the same manufacturer, may be produced in different particle sizes. For a given weight of magnesium stearate, the smaller the particle size, the larger the number of particles. Therefore, when magnesium stearate is mixed with the tableting constituents, the smaller particle size grade will distribute better, and coat the tableting components more evenly, than a larger particle size grade. The fewer particles of the latter do not coat the particles of the tableting components efficiently, simply because there are too few particles to adequately cover the large surface area of the other tablet components.

The second factor to take into account is the fact that a particle of magnesium stearate consists of numerous plates of magnesium stearate, stacked one upon the other. This is referred to as a laminated structure. A single magnesium stearate particle can be represented by a deck of playing cards. When magnesium stearate is mixed with other particles, layers of the magnesium stearate particles "slough off." The analogy of individual cards sliding off the top of a deck of cards may also be useful. The longer the mixing is allowed to continue, the more layers will slough off (or more "individual cards" will come off the deck). These individual layers of magnesium stearate coat the tableting particles. This means that longer mixing times (which create more separated layers of magnesium stearate) will result in a greater coating of the tableting components with a hydrophobic material. This leads to greater lubricating efficiency. However, the coating of a hydrophobic layer on the tableting components also has the capacity to delay disintegration and dissolution.

The time for mixing magnesium stearate with the tableting components is, therefore, critical. For this reason, magnesium stearate is added at the end of the process of blending the tableting components in a direct compression formulation, after all the other components have been adequately blended. (Direct compression has been mentioned previously and is described in more detail in the next section.) Or, it is added after the formation and drying of granules, if granules are to be compressed to form the tablets. In addition, it is mixed for a short time. The short mixing period ensures that a limited amount of sloughing off of magnesium stearate occurs. This releases sufficient magnesium stearate layers to partially coat the tableting components to provide good lubrication. It is not long enough to result in an extensive, or complete, coating of individual tablet particles with the hydrophobic material, which would result in delayed water permeation into the tablet. In addition, another negative effect occurs if the particles are nearly completely coated with magnesium stearate.

Consider two particles that are nearly completely coated with magnesium stearate and are also under compressive forces within the die. As these particles approach each other, it is the coating on each of these particles that will make contact. The wax-like magnesium stearate bonds very poorly. Many bonds of this type, within a tablet, result in a soft tablet which easily breaks apart when handled. When magnesium stearate is mixed for a short time, the partial coating of the particles is sufficient to provide good lubrication under compression (Figure 9-8). However, there are still a large number of particle-to-particle

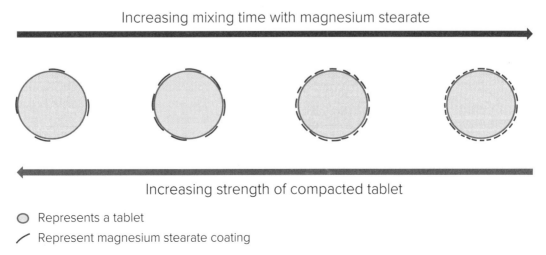

Increasing mixing time with magnesium stearate

Increasing strength of compacted tablet

◯ Represents a tablet

╱ Represent magnesium stearate coating

FIGURE 9-8 Extent of magnesium stearate coating related to strength of compacted tablet.

contacts, upon compression, since there is incomplete magnesium stearate coating around the particles. This leads to harder tablets. Obviously, it is important to maintain the same (short) mixing time for every batch of the product that is produced in order to have consistent lubrication.

With the use of soluble lubricants, the mixing time does not have to be short, as it is with magnesium stearate and other hydrophobic lubricants. Soluble lubricants do not slough off layers as is the case with magnesium stearate. In fact, in the author's experience, longer mixing times are better. Table 9-3 lists some commonly used lubricants.

Glidants

Glidants are excipients that are added to the tablet formulation to facilitate the flow of material from the hopper through the various components of the tablet press and, finally, into the dies. Glidants carry out their function by the following major mechanisms:

1. Reduction in friction
2. Reduction in static charge
3. Absorption of moisture

Friction, static charge, and the presence of moisture reduce the flow properties of powders. Since the glidant has a lower coefficient of friction than the granulation, it reduces the overall coefficient of friction of the blended material. Silicon dioxide is a very popular glidant (trade names, Aerosil and Cab-O-Sil) that may be obtained in different particle sizes. Silicon dioxide also reduces the static charge that may develop from the process of grinding tablet components, or from vigorous mixing.

In addition to adsorbing moisture, silicon dioxide, because of its fine particle size, has a tendency to round out irregular particles. This is achieved by deposition of the fine silicon dioxide particles in the hollows of tableting component particles and this effect decreases the interlocking tendency of these particles. Talc is also a reasonably good glidant, but its popularity has waned with the advent of silicon dioxide. It is important to note that the glidant may improve flow by a few percent, whereas the properties of the tableting particles themselves are the major determinant of good flow. Stated differently, a very poorly flowing tableting mixture cannot be made to flow well by the addition of a glidant.

Anti-adherents

In many instances, fine particulate material will stick onto a container. For example, after most of the powder leaves a metal hopper, a thin layer of powder on the hopper may be noticed. Frequently, the drug is of a finer particle size than the other tableting components and may preferentially adhere to the hopper. This effect may be sufficiently serious to lower the drug content of the compressed tablets. Anti-adherents aid in decreasing this phenomenon. Starch is an example of an anti-adherent, as is silicon dioxide.

Recap Questions

1. Why is it important to check the grade of a pharmaceutical ingredient, in addition to its name, before incorporating the ingredient into a formulation?
2. Do all disintegrants function in the same way? Does it make sense to combine disintegrants?
3. Why is it important to mix magnesium stearate for a short time?
4. Why is it important to have the same particle size of magnesium stearate from batch to batch of pharmaceutical products?

TABLE 9-3	Some Commonly Used Lubricants
LUBRICANT	**USUAL CONCENTRATION RANGE (%)**
Hydrophobic Lubricants	
Magnesium stearate	0.2-2
Calcium stearate	0.2-2
Zinc stearate	0.2-2
Stearic acid	0.2-1
Glyceryl monostearate	1-3
Hydrophilic Lubricants	
Glyceryl behenate	1.5-3
Sodium stearyl fumarate	1-2
Boric acid	1
PEG 4000	1-5
PEG 6000	1-5
Sodium lauryl sulfate	1-5
Magnesium lauryl sulfate	1-2
Sodium benzoate	1-4

DIRECT COMPRESSION

Direct compression, as the name implies, involves the production of tablets by compressing the ingredients directly, that is, without first granulating them. Many crystalline chemicals, including potassium chloride, sodium chloride, and ammonium chloride, are directly compressible because they possess the required cohesive and flow properties. The above materials exist in the form of cuboidal crystals which have large flat faces. Under pressure in the die of the tablet press, the flat faces of two adjacent crystals come together, are compressed, and form a strong bond. Some other crystal types also bond well. In addition, many crude drugs compress well, without prior granulation. The crushed, dried leaves or roots of plants are frequently able to be compressed readily. The equivalent to the commercial product, Senokot tablets (used for constipation), may be made by directly compressing senna leaves.

TABLE 9-4	Some Commonly Used Direct Compression Excipients	
TRADE NAME	CHEMICAL NAME	COMMENTS
Avicel	Microcrystalline cellulose	Good flow properties, some lubrication effect, relatively high moisture content
Emcompress	Dibasic calcium phosphate	Available as anhydrous and dihydrate forms. Larger particle size grades (approx. 200 µm) used in direct compression. Produces hard, insoluble compacts; only disintegrates upon addition of disintegrant
Fast Flo Lactose	Lactose	Spherical lactose particles
Lactopress Spray Dried 250	Spray dried lactose	Particle size range up to 250 µm
SuperStarch 200	Partly pregelatinized maize starch	
Advatab	Proprietary blend	Developed for orally disintegrating tablets; smooth, melting mouth feel
Lubritose Mannitol	Mannitol	

If a material possesses sufficient binding properties but does not flow well, a force-feeding device may be used. In a typical feed frame, as described earlier in this chapter, the flow of material occurs under the influence of gravity only. The force feeder has, usually, two rapidly spinning impellers that mechanically push the material to the dies. Although they are compressible, poor flow may be an issue with many of the crude drugs.

When a drug is required in a very small quantity, the nature of the diluents determines the properties of the tableting mixture. Hence, the small amount of drug can be mixed with a large amount of the directly compressible diluent, for successful tableting. Several manufacturers specifically developed so-called "direct compression excipients" for this purpose. Among the earliest of these were microcrystalline cellulose (Avicel') and dibasic calcium phosphate dihydrate (Emcompress'). Spray-dried lactose and spray-dried mannitol are materials consisting of spherical aggregates which flow well and have good compression characteristics. Some direct compression ingredients are listed in Table 9-4.

SPECIALIZED TABLETS

Chewable Tablets

Chewable tablets are preferred by those who experience difficulty swallowing. They are, therefore, useful for pediatric, and geriatric, patients. These tablets are also convenient for any patient to take: they may be taken at any time or place, even when water is not readily available.

Since chewable tablets are intended to be pleasant to take, palatability is a major concern when formulating such tablets. It must be taken into account, especially, when new ingredients are added to an existing formulation. Mouthfeel, as distinct from taste, is also very important. While these tablets may be fairly hard, the granules resulting from chewing them should not be hard or gritty. Therefore, the choice of binder, and its concentration, are important. Polyvinylpyrrolidone (PVP) and methylcellulose may be used as they impart a smooth feel to the

tablet, and produce non-gritty granules when used in reasonable concentration. Mannitol is often used as the base because it has a pleasant "melting" and cooling effect, although chewable tablets are not intended to disintegrate rapidly. For this reason, a disintegrant is usually not added. The melting effect of mannitol is due to its rapid solubility whereas the cooling effect is due to its negative heat of solution. Mannitol is relatively expensive and it may be partially substituted with sorbitol, which is somewhat cheaper, or by lactose which is considerably cheaper. The melting feeling may also be enhanced by the addition of glycine.

Multivitamin chewable tablets have become popular in recent years, whereas antacid chewable tablets have been available for a long time. Since the latter frequently contain calcium compounds which may have a chalky or gritty mouth feel, it is important that the formulation contain ingredients, such as mannitol, to compensate for this characteristic.

Orally Disintegrating Tablets (ODT)

As the name implies, ODT are tablets that disintegrate rapidly in the mouth without chewing and without the need to take any liquid to facilitate disintegration. The resultant mixture of saliva and powder is intended to be swallowed. The drug is absorbed from the GIT, as would be the case for a swallowed tablet. The FDA defines ODT as follows:

A solid dosage form containing medicinal substances which disintegrates rapidly, usually within a matter of seconds, when placed upon the tongue.

The FDA recommends, further, that the tablet weight not exceed 500 mg and that the in vitro disintegration time, as tested by the USP apparatus, not exceed 30 seconds (see section "Evaluation of Tablets," later in this chapter). ODT are not intended for drug absorption through the mucosal lining of the mouth as is commonly, but incorrectly, assumed by patients. The drug particles contained in the tablet are usually coated for taste masking. This coating is intended to dissolve as soon as the drug particles are swallowed, to enable dissolution and absorption of the drug. The formulator, therefore, has a very narrow path to tread: too little coating would result in some dissolution in the month and the patient tasting the drug, whereas too much coating, delays drug release.

The major difference between ODT and chewable tablets is the fact that the former do not have to be chewed: the tablet disintegration is so rapid that chewing is unnecessary. Chewing should also be discouraged since it could rupture the coating around the drug particles, if such coating is used, leading to taste perception of the drug. ODT are usually more pleasant to take because of a lack of grittiness in the tablet residue. This is brought about by the use of rapidly dissolving excipients. If very bitter drugs are incorporated into chewable tablets as coated drug particles, the chewing action would disrupt the coating, resulting in the patient experiencing the bitter taste. The fact that ODT are more palatable and convenient to take is not simply a minor advantage. These properties lead to better patient compliance and, therefore, to improved therapeutic efficacy. The ability to take ODT discretely is seen as a big advantage, especially when the consumer is in a formal situation, such as a meeting.

Sugar-Coated Tablets

There are various types of coated tablets and one of the basic types, in terms of functionality, is the sugar-coated tablet. The major purpose of sugar coating is to make the tablet more aesthetically pleasing. The heavy coating that is applied rounds out the angular edges of the tablet and also covers any imperfections such as chips or blemishes. In addition, the taste and odor of the drug are masked. Sugar coating consists of several coats, many of which are applied in multiple layers. The coating is done in a conventional coating pan (Figure 9-9). The tablets to be coated are placed into the pan which rotates at a speed set by the operator. At the correct speed, the rotating action of the pan causes the tablets to ride up the wall of the pan and then

to tumble back to the bottom. The coating solution of sugar (sucrose) is ladled onto the tablets and, as the tablets rotate, the coating solution spreads from one tablet to the next. A stream of air is blown onto the tablets to facilitate drying. An exhaust (in the form of a vacuum pipe which enters the front of the pan) removes moisture-laden air, so that drying may continue at a faster rate. These pans have been in use for a very long time and may be distinguished from modern vented coating pans in that the latter have perforations in the pan. To facilitate drying, vapors of the coating solvent are drawn out of the pan through the perforations (using an external vacuum).

The tumbling action prevents the tablets from sticking together in clumps, bound by the coating solution. For this reason, the pan should also rotate at the correct speed. At a very low speed, the tablets remain at the bottom of the pan with the tablets in the uppermost layers of the tablet bed rotating and exchanging position with the tablets in the next layers. The lowest layers of the bed will not reach the uppermost position in the tablet bed and will not be coated. On the other hand, at a very high speed, the tablets are thrown outward due to centrifugal force and stick to the side walls of the pan. This results in the tablets rotating with the pan, without any tumbling action, defeating the purpose of rotating the pan. On the other hand, tumbling of the tablets (as described above) causes the coating solution to spread from one tablet to the next and brings fresh tablets to the surface of the tablet bed. For tumbling to take place, the correct rotation speed is critical.

The first coat is the sealing coat which commonly contains shellac in a non-aqueous solvent. Because the remaining coats are water-based, they would dissolve the tablet constituents if a sealing coat were not used. Thus, the first coat has to be non-aqueous and must contain a sealant, while the remaining coats

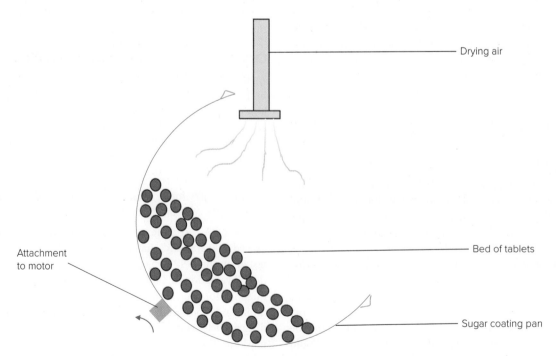

FIGURE 9-9 Conventional coating pan. Note: 1. The sugar solution is ladled or poured onto the bed of tablets. The rotation of the pan causes the tablets to tumble and roll over one another, spreading the coating solution. Heated air facilitates drying. 2. The motor is not shown.

may be aqueous. The sealant prevents rapid ingress of water into the tablet from the remaining aqueous coats. The formulator has to be judicious in selecting the amount of shellac to be added to the tablets: too little would not provide the waterproofing layer, while too much may delay drug release. On the other hand, as shellac ages it may cross-link, that is, bonds may form between two adjacent polymer strands. When cross-linking occurs, it may also delay drug release. In some instances, a thin coating of ethyl cellulose has been used as the sealing coat.

The next coat is referred to as the grossing coat, or the sub coat, and consists of a very heavy sugar syrup. This quickly builds up the volume of the tablet and rounds off the angles and sharp edges. The end product after the grossing coat is a larger tablet without the straight sides, around the circumference of the tablet (Figure 9-10). However, the surface may be rough due to the large amount of sugar (in the form of syrup) that was rapidly deposited onto the surface, and the rapid rate of drying the syrup.

The grossing coat is applied in many layers, with drying between each addition of coating solution. Also, starch or another dusting powder is sprinkled onto the tablets after the drying step. This ensures complete drying before the next layer of coating solution is added. This precaution ensures that the tablets do not become overwet, which may cause sticking of tablets to each other. As dusting powder may build up in the coating pan, periodically the tablets are emptied from the pan and residual dusting powder is removed. If this step is not undertaken, dusting powder would be picked up from the bottom and sides of the pan, with the next addition of coating solution, resulting in clumps of powder potentially adhering to the tablet surface and giving it a very rough appearance.

The next coat that is applied is the smoothing coat. The coating solution, for this coat, has a lower amount of sucrose and, when dried, the tablets have a much smoother appearance. This coat is, also, applied in several layers. Next, a finishing coat, which has even less sucrose in the coating solution is applied. This solution is much less viscous and, because of the lower sugar content, dries to a very smooth finish. Finally, a wax coat may be applied in a special drum that has canvas sides. The wax that is initially applied to the empty drum coats the canvas. This serves as the source of the coating material for the tablets that are subsequently added to the drum. The wax is picked up as the tablets move about the drum and this action also polishes the tablets.

Conventional tablets may be marked with identifying symbols or letters in a very simple manner. The tablet punch may contain, for example, a raised letter "X" on the surface of the punch. Every tablet that is compressed with this punch will show the letter X as a depression on the surface of the tablet. This is referred to as debossed lettering (embossed means the letters are raised off the surface). Just as sugarcoating covers any chips or imperfections on the tablet, any debossed lettering

would also be covered. For this reason, any lettering or identifying symbols that are required must be printed onto the coating, using ink.

Gelatin-Coated Tablets

After the capsule tampering incidents (see Chapter 10, Capsules), attempts were made to produce solid dosage forms that could easily be swallowed and which had the slipperiness of gelatin, when wet, without the potential for deliberate tampering. The result of these efforts was capsule-shaped tablets that were coated with gelatin. The elongated shape means that the width of the tablet is less than the circumference of a round tablet of equivalent weight. Therefore, with the length of the tablet-oriented to the length of the esophagus, a high-weight tablet could be easily swallowed. The fact that wet gelatin is slippery facilitates the swallowing process.

Since aqueous gelatin solutions are to be applied to the tablet, it follows that a sealing coat is also necessary. The gelatin coat is thinner than the sugar coat and does not increase the tablet mass appreciably, as is the case with sugar-coated tablets. However, it is thick enough to cover debossing and any desired symbols or lettering would have to be printed on the surface of the coated tablet using ink, as it is done with sugar-coated tablets.

Film-Coated Tablets

As the name suggests, the coating layer, in these tablets, is very thin. The coating may be colored and used as a means for identification of the tablet. Early coating materials were applied as solutions in organic solvents. Since the solvent vaporized fairly rapidly, drying was rapid but the level of residual solvents had to be determined due to toxicity concerns. Today, fine particle suspensions are frequently used for film coating, both to eliminate residual toxic solvents in the dosage form as well as for environmental protection. Upon drying, the particles of the coating material are in close proximity to each other on the surface of the coated tablet. After "curing," these particles fuse with each other forming a complete coating on the surface of the tablet. For Aquacoat ECD (an aqueous dispersion of fine-particle ethyl cellulose), heating the tablets at 60°C for 2 hours is the recommended process for curing.

In either case, coating with solutions in organic solvents or with ultrafine suspensions in aqueous media, the coating pans are required to be more efficient than the older sugar coating pans. Film coating pans have spray nozzles (the number depending on the size of the pan) to efficiently spray the coating solution, at a controlled rate, onto the tablets. The spraying is usually intermittent, and the time between spray applications allows the coating to dry on the surface of the tablet. In addition, the vapors have to be rapidly removed from the coating pan and this is achieved with the use of vented

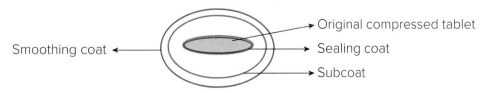

FIGURE 9-10 Layers of a coated tablet. Note that the finishing coat and wax coat are not shown.

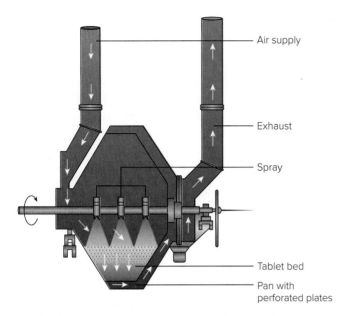

FIGURE 9-11 Example of a vented coating pan (HI-Coater).

- Air supply
- Exhaust
- Spray
- Tablet bed
- Pan with perforated plates

coating pans. These pans are available in several designs, one of which is depicted in Figure 9-11. Extraction through the vented drum removes vapors rapidly for faster drying. Film coating is very efficient and can be done rapidly (in several hours or one day compared to the few days that are required for sugar coating). The coating is very thin and, therefore, any debossing can still be seen after the tablet is coated.

Enteric-coated Tablets

Enteric coating is a form of film coating in which the coating materials are insoluble in the acidic contents of the stomach. These materials are dissolved or suspended in a suitable solvent for the coating procedure. Modern enteric coating materials are very fine suspensions in water. When a tablet containing an acid-sensitive drug is enteric coated, gastric acid does not come into contact with the drug upon consumption of the tablet. Therefore, the drug will not be degraded. When the tablet passes into the small intestine, the less acidic (almost neutral) contents encountered in this region of the GIT dissolve the coating material. The drug is then released and will be available for absorption in the small intestine.

Recap Questions

1. What is the major advantage of direct compression?
2. What is meant by a "force feeder" in the context of tablet compression?
3. Which method of coating adds the most weight to tablets?
4. Are orally disintegrating tablets the same as buccal tablets? Give reasons for your answer.
5. An enteric-coated tablet has a similar appearance to a film-coated tablet. Is this statement true or false?

PROCESSING PROBLEMS IN TABLETING

During the course of tablet production, various problems can occur which may affect the quality of the tablets produced. In some cases, the fault lies with the formulation whereas, in other cases, the problem is with processing, or with the compression equipment or its maintenance. Sometimes, a combination of different issues results in defective tablets. Some of the defects that may arise are the following.

Capping, Lamination, and Chipping

"Capping" is a term that describes the partial or complete separation of the top, or the bottom, from the main body of the tablet. Lamination refers to the separation of the tablet into two or more distinct layers. Chipping occurs when small pieces, or chips, come off the tablet. These flaws are usually visible immediately but, in some instances, they only become apparent a few days after compression. Subjecting the tablets to the stress of a friability test (see next section) is the quickest way to reveal the problem which may be caused by a poor formulation. For example, the formulation may contain insufficient compactible materials, or it may contain an excessive amount of fines. The latter tend to trap excessive amounts of air. When the compression pressure is released, the trapped air expands rapidly, causing capping. On the other hand, poorly maintained punches and dies may also lead to capping, lamination, or chipping.

Picking and Sticking

Each of these conditions involves adhesion of material to the punch faces. When picking occurs, small, localized portions of the tablet face are missing or spots have been "picked" off the face. This may be due to an imperfection on the punch face, or it may be due to a granulation that is insufficiently dried. This problem can also be seen with debossed lettering where the angles of an enclosed space, such as found in the letters, "B" or "A," are too sharp. In this case, the enclosed areas within the letter are removed. Sticking occurs when there is adhesion to the whole face of the punch. The result is a tablet with a dull, rough appearance. If the condition is not corrected, it worsens progressively as more tablets are compressed. Sticking is usually due to the granules being insufficiently dried or containing too little anti-adherent. Rough or pitted punches could also result in sticking.

Mottling

Mottling is a condition in which there is an unequal distribution of color on the surface of the tablet. Consider a tablet containing a blue dye. When mottling occurs there are light, and dark, patches of blue on the surface of the tablet. This occurs when the dye is not well distributed within the granules, leaving lighter, and darker, granules. When these granules are compressed, it leads to lighter, and darker, patches on the tablet. Mottling can also occur in a white tablet when there are patches of white and an off-white, or cream, color. This happens in tablets that are intended to be white, yet some components are of a slightly darker color, or become darker with age.

EVALUATION OF TABLETS

Extensive research into the formulation of tablets, and developmental work into manufacturing processes are meaningless unless appropriate test methods are developed to judge the quality of the product. These test methods must be able to consistently evaluate the most important criteria that are identified as useful for ensuring the quality of the tablets. For each test criterion, there must be a specification, that is, the minimum and maximum values of the test results that are acceptable. The specifications are prepared and agreed upon before the manufacturing of the batch occurs. In this way, the specification cannot be "adjusted" to suit the observed test results. While many tests are used in the industry to judge the suitability of manufactured tablets, only a limited number will be briefly described. The intention is to give the practicing pharmacist an idea of how the quality of tablets is evaluated.

Hardness

Manufactured tablets must have the ability to withstand the shock of handling, packaging, and shipping. For a specific formulation, excessively hard tablets (ie, with hardness values above the upper limit of the specification) may not disintegrate as quickly as desired. This does not mean that a tablet of a different formulation with a similar hardness will not disintegrate appropriately; the ingredients of the latter formulation may allow a hard tablet to disintegrate acceptably. The test involves placing a tablet between the jaws of a hardness tester and then applying increasing pressure across the diameter of the tablet. The value of the applied pressure, at the moment the tablet breaks, is an estimation of tablet hardness. From the description of the test, it will be understood that the instrument is actually measuring resistance to crushing.

Friability

As tablets are handled, they may undergo chipping as well as abrasion. The latter causes powder to come off the surface of the tablets. More serious effects of friction and shock are capping or breaking of the tablets. A friability tester (or friabilator) is the device that is used to measure the friability of tablets. The unit consists of a plexiglass drum and a motor that rotates the drum (Figure 9-12). Twenty tablets are used for this test and, as a result of the design of the plexiglass drum, the tablets are raised to a height of 6 in during the rotation. The tablets are then dropped from this height to the bottom of the plexiglass drum. The drum rotates at 25 rpm and after 4 minutes of this treatment (100 revolutions) the tablets are removed, dusted, and weighed. The difference between the initial weight and the final weight is the loss in weight that the tablets experience due to the treatment in the friabilator drum. A loss in weight of no more than 1% is generally acceptable.

Disintegration Time

Disintegration is the process which results in the breakup of the tablet when it is placed into water or aqueous medium. The majority of tablets react to the presence of water by disintegrating which allows for faster release of the drug. There are some exceptions, that is, tablets specially formulated not to disintegrate. Some sustained-release tablets are formulated in this way. The drug may be slowly released from the whole tablet without disintegration occurring. The ability of a batch of tablets to disintegrate within the required time may be assessed using a disintegration tester.

The disintegration tester (Figure 9-13) consists of a rigid basket-rack assembly, connected to a mechanical device which raises and lowers the basket-rack assembly smoothly 29 to 32 cycles per minute. The basket-rack assembly has six glass tubes arranged in a circle and held in place by two plastic plates with holes in them to accommodate the tubes. Three bolts hold the two plates in position. A rod at the center is connected to the mechanical device which lowers and raises the basket-rack assembly. The lower plate has a woven stainless steel wire cloth covering its lower surface which prevents the tablets from leaving the glass tubes. The size of the holes in the wire cloth, the dimensions of the glass tubes, as well as many other parameters for the apparatus, are specified in the United States Pharmacopeia (USP).

The basket-rack assembly is suspended in the aqueous medium in a 1000-mL low-form beaker. The volume of the

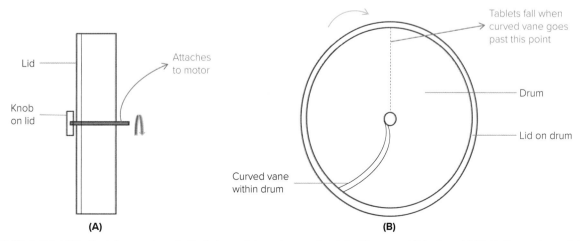

FIGURE 9-12 **A Friability Test Apparatus. A.** End view of drum (approximately 38 mm or 1.5 inches thick). **B.** Front view of drum. Note: Drum is rotated for 4 minutes at 25 rpm by a motor (not shown).

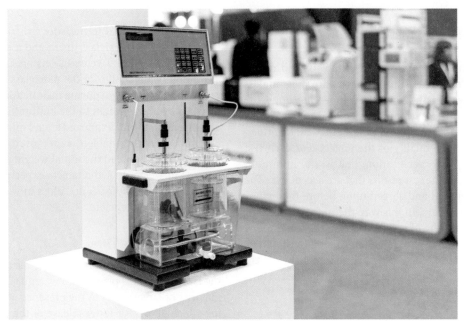

FIGURE 9-13 Disintegration tester. (Used with permission from Surasak_Photo/Shutterstock.)

liquid in the beaker is such that the wire cloth, at its highest point, is at least 15 mm below the surface of the liquid. At its lowest point, the wire cloth is at least 25 mm above the bottom of the beaker. At no point is the basket-rack assembly totally submerged. The beaker is maintained at 35°C to 37°C by a water bath into which the beaker is placed.

The general method is to introduce one tablet into each tube. The basket-rack assembly is then suspended in the beaker and attached to the mechanical device. The beaker contains the pre-warmed (37°C) aqueous medium specified in the USP. Next, the apparatus is operated for 15 minutes. The basket-rack assembly is then removed from the liquid and examined. The tablets pass the test if all six have disintegrated, that is, no tablet residue remains above the wire cloth. If one or two tablets have not disintegrated, the test is repeated with another 12 tablets. At least 16 of the total 18 tablets should have disintegrated within 15 minutes for the batch of tablets to pass the test. The time limit mentioned in this example is the general specification. The specifications for the test may vary for different types of tablets, or for specific formulations, as described in the USP. For example, variations of the basic test procedure are described for enteric-coated tablets.

Uniformity of Weight Test

The uniformity of weight test, as described below, is a quality control test that companies perform after the manufacture of each batch of tablets. In addition, the test is usually used as an in-process test that is conducted at regular intervals, for example, every 20 minutes during tablet production. Typically, the operator will remove sufficient tablets that have just been produced, for in-process tests which include hardness and uniformity of weight. This testing helps to ensure that the product is within specifications and, if it is not, adjustments can be made to the tablet press settings.

For the uniformity of weight test, 20 tablets are individually weighed and the weights recorded. The average weight is then determined. There are two separate specifications for this test. First, the calculated average weight should not differ by more than a given percentage from the theoretical weight. For example, for a tablet of theoretical weight of 300 mg, the company's internal requirement may be that the calculated average should not deviate by more than 3%. Second, no individual tablet should vary in weight by more than a stated percentage. For the 300-mg tablets used in the above example, the percentage deviation for the individual weight may be no more than 5% (as an example of the company's requirement). Table 9-5 shows an example of weight variation calculations for two competing tablet brands of the same drug. These two specifications, taken into consideration together, give an assurance that the tablet weight is not variable beyond a reasonable level.

The in-process testing allows the operator to make adjustments to the weight control setting on the tablet press; that is, if the weight is slightly low (but still within acceptable limits), the operator can adjust the weight of subsequent tablets to be slightly higher, and vice versa. Since the tablets are within acceptable limits, no tablets need be rejected. If the tablet weight is outside the preset limits, the adjustment can still be made but all tablets produced since the last acceptable test results were obtained must be rejected. The last acceptable test results, in this example, would have been obtained approximately 20 minutes earlier.

Assay

For the assay, twenty tablets are randomly selected from the batch. The tablets are powdered in a mortar, using a pestle. Next, an amount of powder, equivalent to the theoretical weight of one tablet, is removed (300 mg in the above example). This powder is tested for its drug content by an appropriate chemical test. The result is reported as a percentage of the theoretical drug content. For example, if the tablet has a labeled drug content of 200 mg, and was found by chemical testing to contain 198 mg, the assay result will be reported as 99%. Variations of the general procedure, described above, are given in the USP for specific products.

TABLE 9-5	Examples of Weight Uniformity, Friability, and Assay Results*	
	BRAND A	**BRAND B**
Tablet Weight (mg)		
	303, 307, 308, 297, 298, 299, 300, 307, 306, 305, 307, 299, 298, 296, 298, 299, 302, 305, 307, 289	303, 303, 302, 297, 298, 299, 300, 302, 304, 303, 301, 299, 298, 299, 298, 299, 302, 303, 302, 282
Average	**301.5**	**299.75**
3% of Theoretical Wt.	9	9
Min Ave Wt.	291	291
Max. Ave Wt.	309	309
Complies	YES	YES
Individual Wt. Assess. Variation		
5% of Theoretical	15	15
Min Individual Weight.	285	285
Max Individual Weight.	315	315
Complies	YES	NO
Friability		
Initial Weight	6100	6080
Final Weight	6050	6000
Difference	50	80
% Weight loss	0.82	1.32
Passes Friability Test?	Yes	NO
Assay		
Assay value (%)	98	101
Acceptable Range (%)	90 to 110	
Within limits?	Yes	Yes

*Figures shown in red are not within limits.

Content Uniformity

The assay provides the average drug content of a fixed number of tablets, 20 in the example given above. The result showed that the tablets, on average, contained 99% of the labeled drug content in the above example, which is a good result. Suppose that there were two tablets, in the 20 randomly selected for the assay, that each had a drug content that was very different from the average. If one tablet contained 150 mg, and the other 250 mg, of drug, the average drug content of these two tablets is 200 mg. This hypothetical example demonstrates that it is possible to get an average value that is close to the theoretical value with two tablets having, respectively, a very high, and a very low, drug content. If these tablets were among the randomly selected 20 tablets, it is possible to obtain the good assay value noted above. Such a good result is obtained in spite of the sample containing two tablets which vary excessively in drug content.

From the foregoing, it can be seen that the assay would not be able to detect the described anomaly. A content uniformity (CU) test has the potential to do so. There are two methods prescribed in the USP for conducting a CU test. One of these tests applies to tablets containing less than 25 mg of drug, or to tablets in which the drug weight is less than 25% of the tablet weight. A 200-mg tablet that contains 30 mg of drug is an example of the latter. The second test that is described is for tablets containing 25 mg or more of the drug, or tablets in which the drug content is 25% or more of the tablet weight. An example of the latter is a 60-mg tablet which contains 20 mg of the drug.

For the CU test of the first type, 30 tablets are set aside. Ten tablets are tested individually for their drug content by an appropriate chemical analysis. The results are analyzed by statistical test methods detailed in the USP. These statistical methods will not be described in this chapter. In certain specified cases where the results do not meet, but are relatively close to, the prescribed criteria, additional individual assays, using the remaining 20 tablets, are allowed. The results of the second round of testing are also analyzed using prescribed statistical criteria, in order to determine whether the tablets pass or fail the CU test.

For the second test type, the individual weights of 10 tablets are determined from 30 tablets that are randomly selected and set aside for testing purposes. The individual weight of each tablet is used in conjunction with the assay value to obtain an estimation of the drug content of the individual tablet. As an example, if one tablet weighed 290 mg and the assay (of the 20 tablets as described in the section, Assay, above) was 198 mg (ie, using the value mentioned above), the drug content of the test tablet is determined as follows:

$$\text{Drug content (tab 1)} = \frac{290 \text{ mg}}{300 \text{ mg}} \times \frac{198 \text{ mg}}{1} = 191.4 \text{ mg}$$

The drug content of the other nine tablets is similarly determined. Next, the statistical test methods mentioned above are applied. Again, the remaining 20 tablets that were set aside may be used for additional testing, if needed, applying the same criteria.

As may be gleaned from the above description, the second test method assumes that tablet weight may be used to estimate drug content. This is the case when either of the following two criteria are met:

1. The drug content per tablet is not very low (25 mg or higher).
2. The drug content makes up a reasonable proportion of the tablet mass (25% or higher).

Recap Questions

1. Explain what is meant by "capping"?
2. How can lettering on a tablet cause picking?
3. Twenty tablets were found to weigh 10.125 g. After a friability test, the weight of the tablets was found to be 9.953 g. Do these tablets pass the friability test?
4. Excessive friability of tablets is undesirable from a quality-control perspective. How do you think a patient may notice excessive friability? In other words, what observation is the patient likely to make?
5. If an assay has been conducted on a batch of tablets and the results are favorable, why is it necessary to perform a CU test?

SUMMARY POINTS

- While the earliest tablets were produced more than 1000 years ago, tablets only came into widespread use in the 20th century.
- A tablet is a convenient dosage form that is quality controlled and relatively cheap to manufacture.
- Excipients used in the manufacture of tablets include diluents, binders, disintegrants, lubricants, glidants, and anti-adherents.
- Tablets are usually manufactured on high-speed rotary presses which contain many sets of punches and dies, while single-station presses may be used for research studies.
- Die filling, pre-compression, compression, and ejection are the major steps in tablet production.
- Some formulations may be directly compressed, that is, they may be tableted without first forming granules; direct compression excipients are sold commercially, after research to develop a high-performing excipient.
- Specialized tablets have unique properties and include chewable tablets, ODT, buccal and sublingual tablets, sustained-release tablets, and coated tablets.
- An overview of the quality control of tablets may allow the pharmacist to answer patient questions.

What do you think?

1. A student says that he can see why a liquid dosage form needs to be formulated, but cannot understand why solid dosage forms need to be developed. After all, an adult can just swallow the solid, powdered material. How would you respond to this student?
2. How does over-filling of the dies and subsequent removal of excess material lead to more uniform tablet weight?
3. Grade A of magnesium stearate contains 100 particles for a certain weight of the material whereas Grade B contains 200 particles for the same weight. Which grade of magnesium stearate, grade A or grade B, is likely to offer the best distribution of magnesium stearate in a mixture of powders, when used in the same concentration? Make a drawing to illustrate your answer.
4. Enteric-coated tablets may be formulated to release the drug at different (less acidic) pH values, for example, 6.8, 6.2, 5.8. Why do you think different pH values are chosen for different tablets?
5. A patient who has a degree in statistics tells you, the pharmacist, that he thinks low-dose tablets (eg, 1 mg) may have close to zero drug in some tablets, and much more (eg, 2 mg) in other tablets, resulting in the correct average drug concentration. He has noticed, he tells you, that some tablets have no effect on him, whereas others have a strong effect. How would you respond to this patient?

Capsules 10

PREVIEW

- Introduction, historical development, and refinement of capsules after tampering incidents
- Overview of the production of gelatin and the manufacture of gelatin capsule shells
- Different pharmaceutical materials that are suitable for filling into capsules
- Filling, finishing, and quality control of capsules in the pharmaceutical industry
- Small-scale filling of capsules
- How does the formulator determine how much material to fill into a capsule?
- Liquid, semisolid, and multicomponent capsules
- Non-gelatin capsules, and capsules not intended to be swallowed
- The role of capsules in double-blind clinical studies
- Soft gelatin capsules

INTRODUCTION

Hard gelatin capsules are a common oral dosage form, probably second only to tablets, in terms of the number of units manufactured. The elongated shape of the capsule allows it to be easily swallowed. The slipperiness of gelatin, when wet, also facilitates swallowing. The hard gelatin capsule consists of two pieces, a body and a cap. The body is the longer piece that is filled with the active ingredient and excipients during manufacture. The cap is shorter than the body but its diameter is slightly larger. The cap fits over the body, closing the unit to prevent the spilling of its contents. Mind Map 10-1 provides a graphic overview of the production of capsules and their utility.

Mothes and Dublanc, working in France, were the first to develop a capsule and obtained a patent in 1834. Their capsule was not the two-piece gelatin capsule which is in use today; it was a one-piece, elongated, hard gelatin capsule. The small hole at the top of the capsule, resulting from the manufacturing process, was used to fill the capsule through a small, narrow funnel. A drop of gelatin was then used to seal the hole. While this was a relatively simple dosage form that was not mass-produced and, additionally, was cumbersome to fill, it began to become popular. Others copied this idea and soon there were many capsule manufacturers and products in the European and American markets. Initially, the patent holders did not attempt to enforce their patents but allowed these companies to continue production until they were fairly well established in the marketplace. Mothes and Dublanc then claimed royalties for the use of their

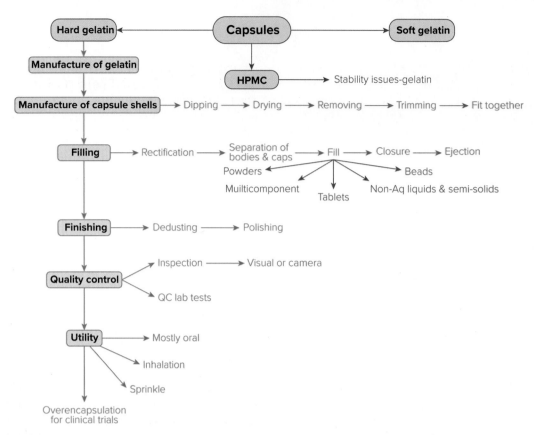

MIND MAP 10-1 Capsules

patent, threatening legal action if the request was not complied with. Since the companies concerned, presumably, did not want to lose the business they had developed, they willingly paid the required royalties. The fact that Mothes and Dublanc did not immediately assert their patent rights may have been an ingenious business plan that allowed capsule manufacture to flourish.

The safety of capsules was called into question after a series of bizarre incidents in the Chicago area in 1982. Several people died mysteriously and suddenly in what became known as the "Tylenol murders." The only link between these people was the fact that they had all taken Tylenol Extra Strength capsules shortly before their deaths. The consumed capsules came from seven different pharmaceutical factories yet the victims were all from the Chicago area. This led police to rule out sabotage at a factory but instead to focus on whether tampering occurred with the capsules sold from individual pharmacies in Chicago. It is believed that the perpetrator purchased packs of capsules from the different pharmacies, opened the capsules, laced them with potassium cyanide, and closed the capsules again. The perpetrator is then thought to have returned the packs of capsules to the pharmacy shelves. Since the person responsible for this crime was not apprehended, the motivation for the murders is still unclear.

The fact that capsules could be opened and closed easily, with no visible evidence of interference, allowed this crime to take place. After the shock of these events, strategies to prevent such an incident were given much consideration. First, effort was expended, and legislation passed, to make packages for over-the-counter (OTC) products tamper evident. If a package had been tampered with, there should be clear evidence, such as a broken seal, so that the potential risk was obvious to a consumer wishing to purchase that package. Tamper-evident packaging is discussed in Chapter 14, Packaging. Many of the pharmaceutical resources were also devoted to producing a capsule-shaped tablet that was gelatin coated. Such a tablet has an elongated shape which, together with the slipperiness of gelatin, allows for easy swallowing. It has the user-friendliness of a capsule without the major disadvantage of being easy to tamper with. This type of tablet is described under specialized tablets in Chapter 9, Tablets. Additionally, banding, which is described in a later section of this chapter, makes the individual capsule, itself, tamper evident. If the banding was removed, for the purpose of tampering with the capsule, it would be readily apparent.

Efforts to prevent the spilling of the contents of capsules led some manufacturers to develop capsules that snap closed and lock, so that they may not easily be opened inadvertently. Among the first patents for this type of capsule were those by RP Hobbs in 1894, which described the formation of a ring around the inside of the cap and a corresponding depression in the body, and that by M. Pollock in 1914, which described notches in the cap and body that engaged when the capsule was closed.[1] Neither of these patents was exploited, probably because the need for a locking capsule was not perceived as acute. Spot welding, in which droplets of gelatin were used to fuse cap and body at certain points along the edge of the cap, did not become popular because they lacked aesthetic appeal. In 1963, Eli Lilly produced "Lok-Caps" that had indentations inside the cap which caused a friction seal.

Most modern manufacturers of capsule shells have incorporated a locking system. Shionogi's Posilok system has a circular

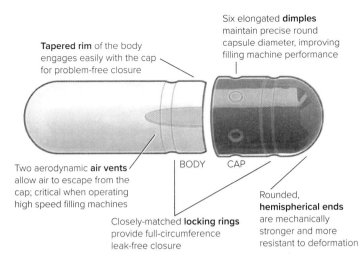

Tapered rim of the body engages easily with the cap for problem-free closure

Six elongated **dimples** maintain precise round capsule diameter, improving filling machine performance

Two aerodynamic **air vents** allow air to escape from the cap; critical when operating high speed filling machines

BODY   CAP

Rounded, **hemispherical ends** are mechanically stronger and more resistant to deformation

Closely-matched **locking rings** provide full-circumference leak-free closure

FIGURE 10-1 Capsugel's coni-snap locking system.

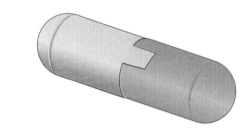

FIGURE 10-2 Telescoping of a capsule.

groove on the body and a corresponding ridge close to the dome of the cap. Capsugel's Coni-Snap system has an elevated ring on the inside of the cap which fits a circular groove around the body and also has several additional features (Figure 10-1). The body has a tapered rim for easy fitting of the body into the cap in a high-speed, fully automated capsule manufacturing machine. Without the tapered rim, the potential for "telescoping" is increased. This occurs when cap and body are misaligned during the closing of the filled capsule. The cap may cause a tearing of the body, with a portion of the body outside the cap, and the body pushed into the cap further than usual (Figure 10-2). The inner surface of the Coni-Snap cap also has six elongated dimples for a tight fit when the capsule is closed. In high-speed filling machines, the body is placed into the cap rapidly which, ordinarily, does not allow air in the cap to escape. Escape of air subsequent to capsule closing may result in opening of the capsule and loss of contents. The Coni-Snap capsule has two air vents on the rim of the body to allow air to escape as the capsule is being closed.

PRODUCTION OF GELATIN

Gelatin is obtained from the skins and bones of animals by extraction, after treatment with either an acid or a base. The acid-treated material has somewhat different properties from the base-treated material. The usual source of the raw materials

is pigs and cattle. It is possible to purchase porcine gelatin or bovine gelatin and, most recently, even fish gelatin.

The skin and bones used to make gelatin are first chopped up into small pieces and then treated with either acid or base, while being gently heated. This treatment continues for several days and the purpose is to digest the tissues and to dissolve the salts contained in the material. The resultant product consists of some pieces of undigested skin and bone fragments, collagen solution, salts, and fat. After coarse filtration to remove the undigested skin and bone fragments, the solution is centrifuged to remove the fat and some of the salts. The remaining collagen solution is subjected to heating under mildly acidic conditions to denature the collagen. A collagen unit consists of three polypeptide chains.[2] Each chain is coiled into a helix, and the three chains are coiled around each other to form a triple helix. Denaturation involves breaking the bonds that stabilize the helix, then disentanglement of the polypeptide chains, and, finally, the dissociation of the chains into smaller components. The resulting product is referred to as gelatin and the solution is subjected to extraction to separate the gelatin from the remaining collagen that has not been denatured. The extract consists mainly of gelatin and salts, and it is turbid because of the latter. This solution is filtered through a resin bed which adsorbs the salts. The resultant solution is clear and may be concentrated by removal of some of the water. The concentrated solution is darker in color and, by appropriate treatment, may be decolorized and then further dried to produce solid gelatin. The latter is either ground and supplied as a powder, or supplied as thin sheets. The powdered material is used in the production of both soft and hard gelatin capsules.

MANUFACTURE OF HARD GELATIN CAPSULE SHELLS

The gelatin is dissolved in hot water and other agents, such as colors and opaquant extenders, may be added to the solution. An opaquant extender is a substance, such as silicon dioxide, that makes a material opaque. A small amount of sodium lauryl sulfate (less than 1%) is usually also incorporated in the gelatin solution as a surfactant to serve as a wetting agent. The capsule bodies are manufactured by dipping a series of pins, affixed to a rectangular plate, into the hot solution of gelatin. The wetting agent helps the pins to be evenly wet by the gelatin solution, so that capsule components of consistent thickness are formed. The plate is attached to an arm to enable the pins to be dipped, and withdrawn, from the gelatin solution. Upon withdrawal of the pins, excess gelatin solution flows off the pins and back into the container of gelatin. The pins spin, and the entire plate rotates slowly and intermittently, to ensure that the layer of gelatin on the pins is of even thickness and that a blob of gelatin does not form at the end of the pins. At the same time, cold air is blown onto the pins to aid in drying.

The next step, in which a pair of jaws grip the gelatin capsule body and remove it from the pins, is referred to as stripping (Figure 10-3). The capsule body is placed into a collet which may be considered a tube into which the body of the capsule fits. The collet has a fixed length and the open end of the capsule

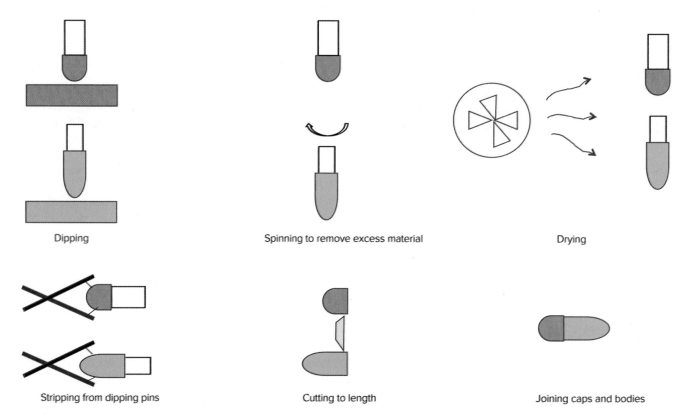

Dipping

Spinning to remove excess material

Drying

Stripping from dipping pins

Cutting to length

Joining caps and bodies

FIGURE 10-3 Diagram of capsule shell manufacturing.

body protrudes from the collet. The collet spins and a knife is brought to the edge of the collet to trim the body of the capsule to the correct length. By a similar process, capsule caps are produced simultaneously and, at this stage, a cap is located in its collet opposite to the collet containing the capsule body. (The cap is wider and is made by dipping a larger-diameter pin into the gelatin, and the cap is also shorter; the collet holding the cap reflects these dimensions.) The two collets are now brought together and the capsule body is pushed out of its collet and inserted into the cap (Figure 10-3). The capsule is then ejected and is provided in this form (closed) to the manufacturers of capsule products.

Recap Questions

1. Compare hard gelatin capsules and tablets in terms of their physical form.

2. In which major ways were the first capsules developed by Mothes and Dublanc different from modern two-piece capsules?

3. How did the Tylenol scare result in improved pharmaceutical products?

4. Mention the steps involved in the transformation of bones and skin into gelatin.

5. Why are the caps and the bodies of capsules placed into collets during the process of manufacturing capsule shells?

MATERIAL TO BE FILLED INTO CAPSULES

The solid materials that can be filled into capsules are powders, granules, pellets, beads, and small tablets. The most common fill material for hard gelatin capsules is powder. Immediate-release capsules may also be filled with granules, beads, and pellets which create less dust than powders during the filling operation. These materials are not as prone to segregation, and flow better, compared to blended powders, and may be used to advantage especially when the drug powder blend flows poorly. For sustained-release multi-particulate systems, beads and pellets are coated to retard drug release. A capsule may contain a blend of several populations of beads or pellets, each coated to a different extent with a release-retarding polymer. Each population displays a unique release profile and is combined with other populations in a fixed proportion to produce the desired release profile for the capsule. Similarly, small tablets filled into capsules are generally used for sustained-release purposes. Each of a small number of tablets (generally less than 10) may be coated with different levels of sustained-release coating, for similar reasons as described for beads. Mini tablets have diameters in the 2 to 3 mm range and are becoming increasingly popular for filling into capsules. More mini tablets can be filled into a capsule than small tablets. While liquids may be filled into hard gelatin capsules, this process is very different from powder filling and will be described in a separate section.

CAPSULE FILLING PROCESS

There are several types of capsule-filling machines that are commonly used in the pharmaceutical industry. Some of these are fully automated, while others are partially automated and require the presence of an attendant at all times to complete the manual steps. In fully automated equipment, these steps are performed by the machine. Several processing steps are common to all types of capsule-filling machines. The semi-automated filling of capsules will be described, as an illustration of the general process. Central to this process is the "filling ring" which is actually a double ring that can be separated into an upper ring and a lower ring. The bottom ring has holes into which the bodies of the capsules fit; the caps, which have a larger diameter, cannot fit into these holes (Figure 10-4A). The upper ring has holes that are wide enough to accommodate the caps. In high-speed, fully automated capsule-filling machines, the filling ring is replaced by several filling blocks, arranged in a circle.

The capsule filling process can be divided into four major steps, namely, rectification (orienting the capsule in the correct direction for placement into the filling ring), separation of the caps and bodies, filling of the capsule bodies with powder or other material, and closing of the capsules and ejection of the capsules from the filling ring. These steps are described below:

Rectification

The empty capsules (with caps attached to the bodies) are filled into the hopper of the filling machine where they are present in random orientation. The capsules must pass through narrow vertical channels and then into the filling ring. The channels orient the capsules so that they are correctly aligned to fit into the two-piece filling ring. The correct orientation is when the capsules pass through the narrow channels with their bodies facing downward. The channels are just wide enough to allow capsule bodies to flow freely, but provide friction at the cap end of the capsule. An interesting feature of the capsule filling process is the manner in which the rectifying unit aligns the capsules. At the top of the channels, there are blades to help with this alignment. If a capsule, flowing downward through the hopper, arrives at the top of the channel with the cap facing downwards (and therefore unable to enter the channel), blades at the top of the channels push the capsule out of the way. Similarly, horizontal capsules are pushed out of the way of other capsules. Only the correctly oriented capsules (bodies down) may enter. These capsules flow down the channels of the rectifying unit and into the two-piece filling ring. In high-speed, fully automated capsule-filling machines, the capsules are filled into two-piece filling blocks, one machine having several blocks. A single-filling block is shown in Figure 10-4B with capsule bodies in the lower half of the block and caps in the upper half.

Separation of the Caps from the Bodies

The two-piece filling ring is placed on the turntable, below the rectification unit, prior to the addition of capsules to the hopper. Rectification causes the capsules to enter the two-piece filling ring, body first (Figure 10-5). Because of the different sizes of the holes in the lower, and the upper, rings, the capsules will

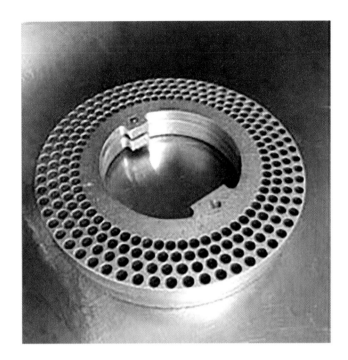

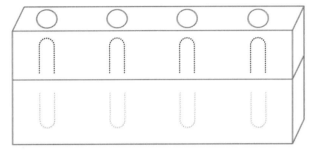

FIGURE 10-4 **(A) A two-piece filling ring. (B) A single rectangular filling block.** Note: The two rings are placed one on top of the other; the top ring will hold the caps, the bottom ring the bodies, of capsules. It is similar for the filling block.

be located with their bodies within the lower ring, while the caps will be within the upper ring. A vacuum is drawn at the bottom of the lower ring to assist the capsules to fall into the holes and to seat firmly. The situation is similar in a high-speed fully automated capsule-filling machine. The capsule bodies are located in the lower filling block whereas the caps are in the upper filling block. For ease of illustration, the capsule positioning is shown only for the filling blocks (Figure 10-4B) but a similar positioning of capsule bodies and caps occurs in the two-piece filling ring.

The upper fill ring is then separated from the lower fill ring. The caps remain in the upper fill ring and become separated from the bodies which are retained in the lower fill ring. The continued application of a vacuum to the lower fill ring, during the separation of the upper fill ring, assists in the retention of the bodies in the lower fill ring. The opening of the capsules at this step allows for the bodies to be filled with the powder or other fill material. In essence, the caps fit tightly in the upper ring and stay with it when the two halves of the fill ring are separated. Similarly, the bodies fit tightly into the lower fill ring and remain so seated when the caps are removed with the upper fill ring.

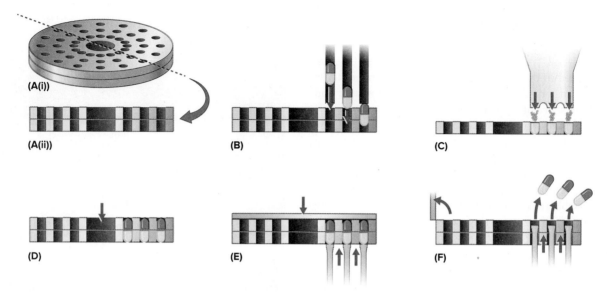

FIGURE 10-5 Diagram of capsule filling process. Note: **(A(i))** is a representation of the top view of the two-piece filling ring shown in more detail in Figure 10-4A. Figure **(A(ii))** is a section through the two-piece filling ring as indicated by the broken red line in **(A(i))**. In **(B)**, the rectification and loading of capsules into the two-piece filling ring is shown. In **(C)**, filling of the capsule bodies with powder is shown. The bodies are seated in the lower fill ring, while the top ring has been removed. In **(D)**, the top ring (with the caps of capsules) is fitted onto the bottom ring. In **(E)**, with the stop plate in place, pegs push the bodies of the capsules into the caps. In **(F)**, the pegs move further into the filling ring. With the stop plate moved out of the way, the capsules are ejected.

Filling of the Bodies with the Powder Fill Blend

The lower fill ring is placed on a turn table and the powder hopper is moved into place above it. Powder from the hopper is fed by means of an auger into the capsules. The auger is a large vertical screw which forces powder downwards as it turns. The feeding end of the hopper is just above the capsules. The turn table turns slowly, so that each row of capsules in the filling ring is successively filled. Since fill is volumetric, the slower the rotation of the turntable, the greater is the chance of complete capsule filling. As the ring turns, excess powder is scraped off its surface.

Closing of Capsules and Ejection from Filling Ring

The hopper is moved out of the way and the upper ring is reattached to the lower ring. The joined upper, and lower, rings are moved from the turntable to the closing station of the capsule-filling machine. Here, the filling ring is placed, in the vertical position, onto pegs which match the holes in the lower ring. A solid stop plate is brought in front of the rings (touching the top filling ring). Pneumatic pressure then forces the pegs into the lower filling ring (now held vertically). This action pushes the bodies into the caps, while the stop plate prevents the capsules from being ejected from the upper ring. In some capsule machines, the pegs are pushed manually into the lower filling ring by the operator applying pressure to the plate to which the pegs are attached. The stop plate is then moved out of the way, and the pegs are pushed in again by pneumatic pressure or manually. With no stop plate to impede their movement, the capsules are ejected through the top ring.

As opposed to the semi-automated filling machine described above, there are high-speed fully automated machines available and in common use. The manual steps described above, for example, separating the two halves of the filling ring, re-joining the two halves of the filling ring, and moving the filling ring to the closing and ejection station, are all performed automatically in the fully automated machine. Such a machine does not require the constant attention of an operator.

An alternate way to fill the capsules in industry involves the dosator principle. In this mechanism, a hollow tube containing a piston dips into a powder bed (Figure 10-6). The force of the tube entering the bed causes powder to move into the tube (compare with the punch method of hand-filling capsules, as described below). The piston then moves down slightly to compress the powder into a loose plug. (A plug is a semi-cohesive volume of powder in which the powder particles stay together and are transferred as a unit, provided little disruptive pressure is applied to it.) The dosator is then removed from the powder bed and is positioned over an empty capsule body. The piston moves down to eject the powder, in the form of a plug, into capsule body.

The temperature of the production room as well as its relative humidity are noted at regular intervals, as specified in the production batch record. The capsules are also regularly inspected visually, during the course of production, for obvious faults such as the denting of capsules, incomplete closure, etc. These may be remedied, when observed, by simple adjustments of the capsule machine. The weight of the filled capsules must be checked periodically during production, as specified in the batch record. This is done by the operator removing, for example, 10 capsules every 30 minutes to manually obtain the individual weights of the capsules, from which the average weight can be determined. The newer trend is to use a weight checker which automatically weighs the capsules fed into its hopper. Within the machine, the capsules are mechanically transferred individually to weigh

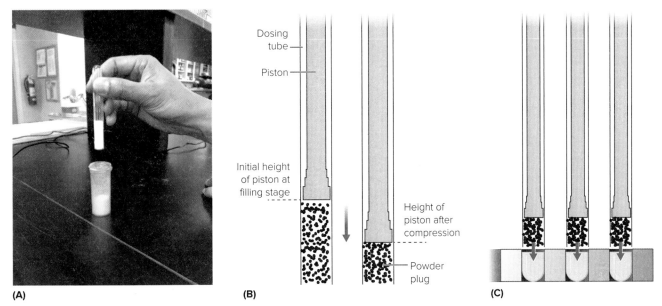

FIGURE 10-6 Capsule filling using a dosator. (A) The photograph shows the principle of the dosator method: an open tube inserted into a powder bed will retain the powder when the tube is lifted out of the bed. **(B)** In the dosator, a piston moves down (after the tube is filled) to compress the powder into a plug within each tube. **(C)** The plugs are fed into capsules in the filling ring (or filling block) by further downward movement of the pistons.

stations and their weight determined. Using this machine, the periodic weight checking can be done automatically with a much larger sample of capsules. Interestingly, the weight checker can be used to weigh every capsule in a production batch and this is routinely done with high-potency capsules. The weight-checking device can be an add-on to a high-speed, fully automatic capsule filler, for a seamless filling and check weighing operation. Capsules that are out of a narrow weight range, specified by the operator, are rejected and passed to a separate container.

The powder to be filled into capsules should have certain properties:

1. It should flow well to ensure accurate and consistent fill weight of the capsules. The addition of a glidant such as silicon dioxide helps.

2. Some lubricity is necessary, for example, when the capsules move under the hopper tip there is friction between the powder attached to the capsules and the hopper. For this purpose, a small amount of magnesium stearate is usually added to the powdered materials. As with tablet production, the magnesium stearate is added last to the blended powders and mixed for a short time.

3. The particles of the various components should be of approximately the same size to prevent segregation during flow. The exceptions are the glidant and lubricant which usually have much smaller particle sizes.

The above properties are needed for both the auger and dosator filling methods but are more important for the dosator. Once the dosator removes powder and lifts out of the powder bed, it is essential that powder flows into the hole that was formed by the dosator. This allows efficient filling to occur at the next filling cycle. Since there is tamping of the powder

within the dosator, a lubricant is critical for the tamping step as well as for the ejection of the plug. In addition, the material must have some compactibility, to enable plug formation, in the dosator process. The obvious advantage of the dosator process is a greater fill weight of the capsules due to the tamping process.

FINISHING AND QUALITY CONTROL OF CAPSULES

After being filled, capsules pass through a de-duster in which the capsules flow over a vibratory screen on their way to a collecting receptacle. A gentle vacuum is applied to the underside of the screen. While the vibration of the screen loosens any powder particles adhering to the outside of the capsules, the vacuum removes the powder. In a more elaborate capsule polishing apparatus, soft brushes remove adhering powder particles and also impart a shine to the capsules. Stiff bristles would scratch the soft capsule surface and give the capsules a dull appearance. In some models, the capsules pass between two conveyor belts. The lower one, moving at a faster speed, conveys the capsules forward toward a collection container for the finished capsules, while the upper belt moves slowly in the opposite direction. The upper belt has a soft cloth attached to it which has a polishing action on the capsules.

Finished capsules are also inspected visually for defects. This is done while the capsules move on a broad conveyor belt which is set up such that the capsules rotate slowly as they are conveyed forward. An inspector observes the capsules and rejects those that are faulty. Some of the faults that may be observed are empty capsules (ie, capsules that do not contain powder), broken or dented capsules, telescoped capsules, and capsules that have two caps on one body. As this is a tedious process, automated systems that visually inspect capsules, using strategically-placed cameras, are preferred. Defective capsules are rejected by the apparatus. (Note that equipment that checks the weight of every capsule, in process, will detect and reject empty capsules, capsules with two caps, and broken capsules with the powder spilled out, since the capsule weight will be out of the acceptable range.)

Apart from these end-of-batch inspections and the in-process controls (such as capsule weight determination) which were described under "Capsule Filling," every batch of capsules is subjected to rigorous testing by the quality control (QC) department. Only after review, and approval, of the test results is a production batch released for human consumption. The more important of these tests are the assay, uniformity of dosing units, disintegration, and dissolution. These tests will not be described as they are similar to the tests for tablets, described in Chapter 9, Tablets.

Recap Questions

1. What disadvantage does powder filling have compared to the filling of beads and pellets into capsules?
2. What is the difference between immediate-release pellets and sustained-release pellets, in terms of pharmaceutical processing?
3. What is the purpose of separating the upper and lower rings, if they are to be joined again a little later?
4. What is the purpose of *in process* weight checks?
5. Name two quality control tests that are performed after a batch of capsules has been manufactured.

SMALL-SCALE FILLING OF CAPSULES

A pharmacist may be called upon to compound capsules for a variety of reasons, for example, when the patient requires a dose that is not manufactured by the pharmaceutical company. Such a situation may arise, for example, when a drug is supplied as 10 mg and 20 mg capsules but the physician determines that the patient needs a 15-mg dose. Capsules may be compounded when the active pharmaceutical ingredient (API) can be purchased but a similar pharmaceutical product is not available, or when a commercial product is temporarily unavailable.

Hand-filling equipment, that may be used to fill a small number of capsules in a pharmacy, follows the same principles as the semi-automated capsule filling described above. The unit is usually rectangular or square (not a ring). After manually filling empty capsules into this apparatus with the bodies in the lower half and the caps in the top half, the two halves are separated. Powder is filled and leveled over the lower plate, containing the capsule bodies, using a spatula (Figure 10-7). The upper half of the rectangular, or square, plate is then fitted onto the lower half again. The capsules are closed and ejected in an analogous manner to that described for the semi-automatic machine. While

the manual equipment is small, and relatively cheap, capsule filling can be quite efficient, with several hundred capsules being filled within an hour. On the other hand, if only a few dozen capsules are required, a completely manual, non-mechanical, method may be used. This is referred to as the "punch" method of filling capsules.

Utilizing this method, the powders to be filled into the capsules are first weighed and blended, using the small-scale blending methods described in Chapter 5. The blended powder is then spread out in a layer of approximately even thickness. The thickness of the powder layer should be approximately one-quarter to one-third the length of the body of the selected capsule. (The determination of fill weight and capsule size is described in a separate section below.) The body of one capsule is manually separated from the cap. Holding its closed end, the body is inverted and pressed onto the powder bed. When the open-end makes contact with the powder bed, the body partially fills with powder. This action is referred to as "punching." The body is repeatedly punched until it is filled with powder. A spatula may be used to ensure that the powder surface is flat at the open end of the body. The cap is placed on the body and the capsule is then weighed. By subtracting the weight of the empty capsule, the fill weight is obtained. If the fill weight is lower than required, punching is continued in order to increase the fill weight of the capsule. Once the fill weight is correct, the first capsule has been filled and the filling of additional capsules can continue. The filling technique must mimic, and the extent of fill must approximate, that of the first capsule.

For low-potency drugs, the weight of capsules is checked periodically, for example, every tenth capsule. In the case of potent drugs, the weight of every capsule must be determined. For these capsules, an alternative filling method may be better: weigh the powder required to fill each capsule on a separate weighing paper, and use the weighing paper to pour the powder into the capsule. It is possible to make a block of high-density plastic material with holes to precisely fit a particular capsule size. The empty bodies of capsules can be fitted into this block and then each capsule filled individually and sequentially. Once all the bodies have been filled, the caps can be fitted to the bodies, prior to the removal of the capsules from the block. The holes should not be very deep so that the cap can easily be fitted to the protruding portion of the body, and the filled capsule easily lifted out of the block. The diameter of the holes should be sufficiently large that the capsules are not squeezed when fitting the bodies into the holes, or during removal of the capsules from the block.

With any filling method, there may be some powder particles adhering to the outside of the capsules. While this detracts from the appearance of the capsules, a more serious issue is the possibility of contamination. This could occur, for example, if food preparation takes place immediately after touching a capsule to administer a dose, in the case where the adhering particles had not been removed after capsule filling. The powder on the outside of the capsules may be removed by adding the compounded capsules to a plastic bag containing table salt (NaCl) and tumbling to mix the capsules with the salt. The fine powdered material adhering to the outside of the capsule is

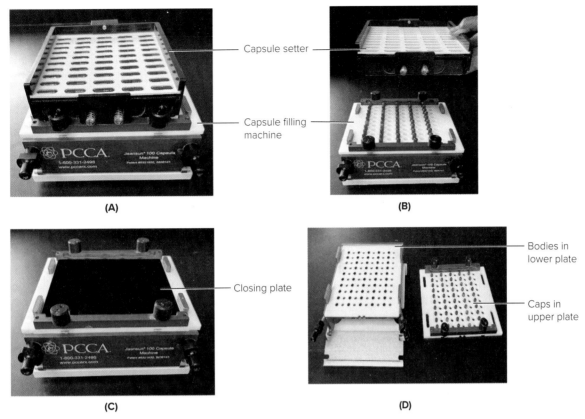

FIGURE 10-7 Hand filling equipment. (A) Capsule setter loaded with capsules is placed on capsule filling machine. The capsule setter has two plates at the bottom (not visible in photo). The plates are pressed in, from front to back, to drop the capsules from the capsule setter into the two white plates of the capsule filling machine. This process rotates the capsules longitudinally into the correct orientation as the capsules are dropped into the plates. **(B) The empty capsule setter is lifted off the capsule filling machine.** The blue caps of the capsules can be seen protruding from the upper plate while the bodies of the capsules are in the lower plate (not seen in photograph). **(C) The closing plate is placed on top of the caps and locked into place by twirling the four black knobs.** The closing plate and the top plate of the capsule filling machine are lifted, using the blue upright pieces for leverage. **(D) The two plates are shown side-by-side. The top plate houses the blue caps while the bottom plate has the red bodies of the capsules.** In subsequent steps (not shown), powder is filled into the bodies of the capsules, the top plate with caps is returned to the machine. With the black closing plate in place, a third plate of the capsule filling machine, located below the bottom of the capsule bodies and accessible from the sides, is lifted to insert the bodies of the capsules into the caps. Finally, the filled capsules are ejected from both plates.

removed by adsorption onto the larger salt particles. The capsules are then separated by adding the salt/capsules mixture to a coarse sieve and gently shaking. The salt particles, together with adsorbed powder, pass through the sieve. The capsules may then be bottled and dispensed.

CAPSULE FILL WEIGHT

It is possible that the dose of the drug is so large that it would not fit into a reasonably-sized capsule. In such a case, two capsules would have to be used. Generally, however, the dose of the drug is much lower, and the formulator must decide on the size of capsule shell to use, taking into account the following factors:

1. Filling a very low weight (eg, 3 mg) of the drug into a capsule is not very accurate.
2. It is considered good practice to completely fill the body of the capsule with the powder.

Considering the first factor, it would be better to combine the 3 mg of drug with 47 mg of a diluent, such as lactose, because 50 mg of blend can be filled into a capsule with much greater accuracy. The reason for the second factor, the complete filling of the capsule body, is as follows: when translucent capsules with partially filled bodies are shaken, the powder spreads out as a layer over the interior surface of the capsule and its appearance is not elegant. Shaking occurs during transport, and also when the capsule is handled by the pharmacist and the patient.

Capsule shells are made in a range of sizes with different nominal capacities, as provided by the manufacturers (Table 10-1). These capacities are given in terms of volume units (eg, 0.3 mL or 0.5 mL), while the dose of the drug is usually specified by weight (eg, 10 mg or 20 mg). Therefore, to determine the extent to which a given dose will fill a specific capsule, the volume of the dose is required, and this may be obtained from the density of the drug (volume is equal to mass divided by density).

TABLE 10-1	Capsule Size Chart*									
Nominal Size	000	00el†	00	0el	0	1	2	3	4	5
Volume (mL)	1.37	1	0.91	0.78	0.68	0.5	0.36	0.27	0.2	0.13

*Sizes are somewhat approximate as there is slight variation between manufacturers and capsule type.
†el = elongated

Given the wide variety of drugs that a pharmacist may be required to compound, the dose of the drug can vary widely. Since the density of the drug can also vary, there is a wide range of volumes that a single dose of drug may occupy and a limited range of capsule sizes available. For this reason, it is usually not possible to precisely fill a capsule with the drug alone, even with higher-dose drugs. The volume of a high-dose drug may be greater than a particular capsule size, but less than the next (larger) capsule size. A diluent would be needed to fill the volume of the larger-sized body. On the other hand, most modern drugs have a low dose. This necessitates the inclusion of a large amount of diluent to make up the remaining volume of the body. While the capsule formulation, whether low dose or high dose, requires the incorporation of a glidant and a lubricant, the amounts that are included in the formulation are small and do not make a practical difference to the extent of fill of the capsule body.

In addition, the filling of capsules involves some amount of tamping and volume reduction and this factor has, also, to be taken into account. It is obvious that tamping occurs with the dosator, and the punching, methods of capsule filling. The former is an industrial method, while the latter is used on a small scale. However, even with the auger method of industrial capsule filling, there is some degree of tamping of the material.

In the industrial development of capsules, pre-formulation research is conducted as a prelude to the development of the final capsule formulation. Such research includes the determination of the density of the material as well as the resultant density after some degree of tamping. Such determinations could be conducted for the various ingredients used to fill the capsules, especially the drug and diluent, and for blends of fixed proportion. Using such techniques, the volume of a particular blend of powder, tamped to a specific extent, can be accurately determined and this information helps in the choice of an appropriate capsule size. In compounding, such extensive research is not practical for each formulation that is developed. However, a simple method may be used to estimate fill weight. This helps with the choice of capsule size as well as the proportion of ingredients to be used.

The first step is to develop an approximate formulation based on the amount of the drug and other ingredients that are required. This formula should include some diluent, chosen based on past experience and its compatibility with the drug, relevant information being sought from the literature. The individual ingredients (for the number of capsules to be prepared) are weighed and added to a measuring cylinder of sufficient capacity. The covered measuring cylinder is raised and tapped onto the workbench 25 times from a distance of approximately 1 in. The volume of the powder in the measuring cylinder is then read.

This volume (eg, 28 mL) is then divided by the number of capsules to be filled (eg, 60), to give a fill volume of 0.47 mL per capsule. The capsule size chart (Table 10-1) is then reviewed to find the next higher-volume capsule. As can be seen, from the table, size 1 capsules have a volume of 0.5 mL. Therefore, the fill volume has to be increased by 0.03 mL per capsule, with the addition of the same diluent used for the primary formulation. Hence, 1.8 mL of the diluent has to be added to the measuring cylinder (0.03 mL × 60 = 1.8 mL). In practice, the diluent is carefully added to the measuring cylinder until the top surface of the powder reaches 29.8 mL (28 + 1.8 mL).

The powder in the measuring cylinder is then weighed. The difference between this weight and the original weight of the powder is the weight of the additional diluent added. This weight is needed so that a record of the complete formula can be maintained as a part of the pharmacy's record-keeping process. This record would also be useful if the same formulation is made again.

The method of tapping the measuring cylinder, to simulate tamping during the punch method of filling capsules, is based on the tapped density procedure described in Chapter 5, Pharmaceutical Powders. The tapped density apparatus generates a practically complete tamping of the powder. Punching produces only partial tamping of the powder which the method described above attempts to simulate. The number of taps, 25, is an arbitrary figure which may be varied with the compounder's own experience. As the tapping continues, the level of the powder in the measuring cylinder can be observed to go down, that is, the continued tamping of the powder can be observed.

Recap Questions

1. If a pharmaceutical manufacturer produces capsules of drug X, why would a compounding pharmacy be required to make capsules of drug X?

2. What is meant by "punching" when used in the context of compounding capsules?

3. Why is it necessary to completely fill the body of the capsule with powder?

4. How are capsules polished on a small scale?

5. Describe one undesirable effect that may occur if capsules are not "polished"?

LIQUID AND SEMISOLID FILLING OF CAPSULES

Solid materials such as powders, granules, beads, and other multi-particulates, as well as small tablets, have been filled into hard gelatin capsules for many years. Soft gelatin capsules filled with liquids are considered a separate dosage form, distinct from hard capsules and have been extensively used in the vitamin and supplement market for many years (see section, Soft Gelatin Capsules, later in this chapter). A relatively new innovation is the filling of liquid formulations of drugs into hard gelatin capsules. Since gelatin is soluble in water, it is only possible to fill non-aqueous organic liquids into capsules, with the following exception. Some research studies have reported the coating of the interior surface of capsules with oil, or another water-immiscible liquid, and then filling an aqueous solution of the active compound into the capsules. The rationale for such studies is that the oil would prevent contact between the water and the gelatin. For practical reasons, non-aqueous solutions are most commonly used as a fill material for this application.

For absorption to occur, the vast majority of drugs must be in solution. Many newer drugs, however, are poorly soluble. If a poorly water-soluble drug can be dissolved in a non-toxic, non-irritant organic solvent, the solution may be filled into hard gelatin capsules for administration to the patient. The advantage is that the consumed drug is in solution upon dissolution of the capsule shell in the gastrointestinal tract (GIT). If the drug can be made to remain in solution, in contrast to precipitating out of solution in the presence of water, drug absorption and bioavailability may be enhanced. There are many techniques to keep drugs in solution. The following is a brief description of a few of these methods.

The solvent in which the drug was dissolved for incorporation into the capsule may continue to solubilize the drug after dilution with a specific volume of aqueous fluid. Upon further dilution, the concentration of the drug may be so low that it remains in solution. This may be the case with some modern, low-dose drugs. The fact that the drug was in solution when it was exposed to the gastrointestinal (GI) fluids is advantageous. If the drug will not remain in solution, upon further dilution with GI fluids, micellar components may be included in the capsule. Micelles are formed upon dilution with GI fluids and the drug is kept in solution.

Another approach is to dissolve the drug in an oily liquid and to also incorporate emulsifying agents into the oil that is filled into hard gelatin capsule shells. When the gelatin capsule shell dissolves, the oil will mix with the GIT contents and be emulsified. Since the emulsification process depends on the natural mixing of stomach contents, without any mechanical production process, this type of dosage form is referred to as a self-emulsifying drug delivery system (SEDDS). Further mixing of the GIT contents brings an oily solution of the drug, in the form of fine oil droplets of the emulsion, to the absorptive surface of the GIT. The drug can be absorbed by diffusion from these fine oil droplets.

Bile that is secreted in response to the presence of oil, digests the oil and releases the drug molecules, providing an additional mechanism for absorption. Bile salts, present in the bile, also serve to solubilize poorly soluble drugs, making them more readily absorbed. Analogous to SEDDS, self-micro-emulsifying drug delivery systems and self-nano-emulsifying drug delivery systems may also be formulated. The smaller the oil droplet, the greater is the possibility of the droplet being engulfed by the absorptive cells of the GIT. Within the cell, the drug is released from the oil droplet.

Returning to the topic of capsule filling, it is relatively easy to make the conversions necessary for the filling of liquids into hard gelatin capsules in modern, high-speed fully automated capsule-filling machines. Some of the high-end machines are equipped for filling powders, tablets, mini tablets, or liquids and it is simply a question of changing to the required mode of operation of the machine. Therefore, the filling of liquids into the capsule is not a major difficulty and the fundamental problem with liquid-filled hard gelatin capsules is the fact that the liquid may leak out of the capsules. This occurs between the cap and the body and may become worse due to handling and transport of the capsules. Therefore, to make this a practical dosage form, the joint between the body and the cap must be sealed to prevent leaking of the liquid. This is achieved by the so-called "banding" of the capsules. While some machines apply one band, the Qualicaps machine applies two thin, partially-overlapping bands of gelatin around the joint between the cap and body of the capsule. While both bands cover the joint—one is applied more to the cap, and the other more to the body, of the capsule.

A gelatin solution with plasticizers and other excipients is prepared and maintained at a warm temperature. The horizontally-oriented capsules are rotated about the long axis of the capsule, while the bands of gelatin are applied. The capsule is then moved to a heating station which helps to dry the bands of gelatin. This seal prevents the leaking of the solution out of the capsules. Other polymer solutions may be used as substitutes for gelatin solution, or to confer other functionalities on the capsules. In addition, hydroxypropyl methylcellulose (HPMC) capsules may be used for the same purpose. In this case, it would be preferable to use HPMC solution, instead of gelatin, to form the bands. NyQuil Cold and Flu Liquicaps and Motrin IB Liquid gels (ibuprofen) are examples of liquid-filled hard capsules.

Semisolids may, similarly, be filled into hard gelatin capsules for the same utility. If the semisolid is hydrophobic in nature, for example, a fatty material, it will dissolve hydrophobic drugs. An advantage, of using a semisolid instead of oil, is the fact that the potential for leaking from the capsule is reduced. The semisolid, consisting of one, or a mixture, of components may be filled into the capsule while warm and less viscous (liquid) which facilitates the filling process. As the solution cools, its viscosity increases and the tendency for leaking becomes less. There are several semisolid lipid materials that enhance the absorption of drugs, as exemplified by the Gelucire® family of excipients. These materials are claimed to enhance the bioavailability of drugs. A liquid material that is similarly used to enhance bioavailability is Vitamin E TPGS, also known, simply, as TPGS.

MULTICOMPONENT CAPSULES

The above descriptions cover single components filled into capsules, whether they are solids (such as powders or beads), liquids, or semisolids. It is also possible to fill more than one component into a single capsule where these components are all compatible and of the same type. For example, a small tablet and powder may be added to capsules, without any special processing, if they are compatible with each other. It is also possible, with special processing, to combine physically, or chemically, incompatible components into a single capsule by forming individual compartments, one for each component, within the capsule. This is done by an injection molding process. In this form, the components do not react with each other during the shelf life of the product. After consumption of the capsule by the patient and dissolution of the capsule shell, all the contents of the capsule will be spilled out into the GI tract and mixing actions will tend to separate the components.

The advantages of such systems, which are in the research phase, are several. Besides the fact that incompatible ingredients may be included in one dosage form, different drugs may be incorporated in the form of secondary drug delivery systems, each having a different rate of drug release. For example, an immediate-release powder may be contained in one compartment, a sustained-release small tablet may be contained in a second, and enteric-coated beads may be in a third compartment. In addition, it is also possible to have solids and liquids within the same capsule, each within a different compartment. Multiple, low-dose drugs, each treating a different condition, may be contained within one capsule. This would improve compliance since the patient requiring multiple therapies would have a smaller number of dosage forms to consume. Combination products have fixed doses of each drug. This may not be suitable for all patients.

NON-GELATIN CAPSULES

Gelatin is obtained from animal sources by a process that was described at the beginning of this chapter. Vegetarians and vegans may object to the consumption of material from animal sources. In addition, some people who are not vegetarians may be uncomfortable taking a product from a particular animal source. For example, there may be cultural objections to products derived from pork, or from beef. In addition, there were concerns with bovine spongiform encephalopathy (BSE), commonly known as "mad cow disease." Since BSE is endemic to certain countries, the sourcing of the gelatin as well as the method of manufacture has to be carefully controlled. Gelatin to be used in capsule manufacture has to be certified to be free from BSE.

Another concern, with the use of gelatin in pharmaceutical products, is the fact that it is very sensitive to fluctuations in environmental moisture conditions. Gelatin is only stable in the narrow relative humidity (RH) range of 35% to 65%. Below 35% RH, the capsules become brittle and may crack or break easily. Above 65% RH, the capsules absorb moisture and become soft and easily deformed during handling, or with mechanical

processing. Therefore, capsule filling requires a relatively narrow RH range in the production suite.

A major problem may also be observed during storage of capsules. The gelatin capsule shell consists of long strands of gelatin which hydrate readily upon the addition of the capsule to water. Subsequently, the capsule shell dissolves and releases its contents to the surrounding medium. Ordinarily, the dissolution of the capsule shell is relatively rapid and does not represent a delay in the release, and subsequent absorption, of the drug. However, gelatin is sensitive to the presence of aldehydes, formaldehyde being a prime example of this class of chemical compound. Aldehydes may be present as contaminants in excipients used in the pharmaceutical formulation of the capsule product. Even trace amounts of aldehydes can react with the capsule shell, causing cross-linking of the gelatin strands. The crossed-linked gelatin is poorly soluble in water and delays dissolution of the shell and, therefore, release of the active ingredients.

When gelatin capsules which have been exposed to aldehydes are subjected to a dissolution test, a strange phenomenon may be observed. The gelatin shell hydrates and, to the observer, appears to have dissolved. However, the contents of the capsule retain the shape of the capsule, and do not become dispersed in the dissolution medium, even after prolonged exposure to the medium and the rotation of the paddles of the dissolution apparatus. What, in fact, has happened is that the gelatin has become hydrated, but not dissolved. If the capsule shell was colorless, a swollen, hydrated, clear layer, or pellicle, of gelatin would now surround the contents of the capsule (powder or beads, for example). This phenomenon is referred to as "pellicle formation" and, obviously, retards the release of the drug to an unacceptable level. Under unsuitable storage conditions, for example at temperatures that are higher than recommended, the gelatin can also be affected with the result that the dissolution of the capsule shell is delayed. Such an effect may actually be seen during stability testing under accelerated storage conditions (40°C/75% RH) (see Chapter 15, Dosage Form Stability).

To overcome these objections, alternative materials for capsule manufacture were needed and were developed from plant sources, as well as from synthetic and semi-synthetic polymers. HPMC has been extensively researched for this purpose and capsules consisting of this material have been manufactured and sold commercially on a large scale since 1998. This material is a cellulose derivative, formed by replacing some OH groups with either methoxy or hydroxypropoxy groups. Depending on the proportions of each of these substituents, HPMC variants may be produced with differing properties.

Some problems were experienced with the first generation of capsules made from this material, which is also known as hypromellose. HPMC capsules (commonly known as Vegetarian capsules) have been extensively used in the vitamin and herbal supplement markets for a long time. Historically, new excipients are not adopted for use in drug products very rapidly. The major reason for this is, generally, thought to be the fact that drug product manufacturers are loath to take the risk of rejection by the FDA in their New Drug Application. Additionally, there is the potential risk and expense of a product recall. If a problem with the new excipient was not previously observed but is now seen after widespread use of the new product, it may justify such a recall.

Once the first drug manufacturer incorporates the new excipient into a product, without significant problems, other manufacturers are likely to adopt the excipient. This has been the case with HPMC capsules as well. In addition, HPMC capsules have not been without some issues. In the remainder of this section, some of the problems associated with first-generation HPMC capsules, and the improvements that have been made in the second-generation product, will be described. Comparisons between HPMC and gelatin capsules will also be made.

HPMC is soluble in cold, but not in hot, water. Therefore, the basic manufacturing method, used for gelatin capsules, of dipping pins into a hot gelatin solution and then allowing the pins to cool, does not work for HPMC. For this reason a gelling agent, commonly κ carrageenan, was used for the manufacture of the first generation of HPMC capsules. In addition, a gelling promoter, for example, KCl, was used in conjunction with the gelling agent. Calcium and potassium salts speed up the rate of gelation, promoting, in conjunction with the use of the gelling agent, faster formation of the HPMC capsule shell. However, variable dissolution results were observed with these capsules. In addition, large differences in the weight of the empty capsule shells were observed. Since the capsules have been widely used in the health supplement market, it provided the opportunity to obtain test data.

The second generation of HPMC does not use chemical gelling. A thermal gelation process was developed and used to obtain the solid capsule shells. The process can be summarized as follows: the pins are heated prior to dipping them into a cold solution of HPMC. After removing the pins from the cold solution, the heating is continued in order to obtain rapid solidification of the material. With the omission of the gelling agent, variations in dissolution rate appear not to be a problem in the second-generation HPMC capsules. In addition, the variability in the weight of empty capsule shells was greatly reduced.

Gelatin capsules have a higher moisture content than HPMC capsules (12%-15% compared to 2%-9%). At low RH values, gelatin loses moisture to the environment and becomes brittle. At less than 35% RH, gelatin capsules become difficult to use in manufacturing processes because of the brittleness. In cold climates, the RH is low on cold winter days and the manufacture of capsule products may not be easy. Even in an air-conditioned production suite, difficulties may be experienced with the handling of gelatin capsule shells. On the other hand, HPMC capsules, due to their low moisture content, do not lose moisture easily at low RH values. HPMC capsules only become brittle when their moisture content falls below 2.5%. Since HPMC does not easily become brittle, HPMC capsules are easier to work with at low RH values. Since HPMC only becomes brittle at extremely low RH conditions, the problem of brittle HPMC capsules is usually not encountered. At moderate RH values, such as those usually encountered in production suites, gelatin and HPMC have approximately equal strength. At very high RH values, gelatin absorbs moisture and becomes soft.

Because of their low moisture content, moisture-sensitive drugs are much more stable when formulated in HPMC capsules, that is, the moisture content of the capsule shell does not influence drug stability. Environmental moisture has little impact on moisture-sensitive drugs in HPMC capsules that are sealed. The banding of capsules is described in the section, Liquid and Semisolid Filling of Capsules, above. While the purpose of the seal is primarily to keep the capsule contents from leaking out, the seal may also prevent ingress of substances at the joint between the cap and body of the capsule. As a separate matter from the sealing of capsules, there is a smaller tendency for the contents to leak out of the capsule because HPMC capsules have a smaller gap between the cap and the body. The fact that HPMC capsules are smoother than gelatin capsules contributes to the good seal in that there are less "bumps" between cap and body.

HPMC capsules commonly display a lag period during dissolution testing, that is, a delay before detectable drug release occurs. This lag period is seen in both first- and second-generation HPMC capsules. Capsugel Corporation, the manufacturer of V-Caps brand (first-generation HPMC capsules) and V-Caps Plus brand (second-generation HPMC capsules), claims that moisture has first to be absorbed into the capsule shell, due to the low moisture content of HPMC, before dissolution of the shell can begin, that is, the low moisture content causes the lag in dissolution. This lag may be significant for drugs that are required to be rapidly released from the capsules and absorbed by the body. In addition, HPMC capsules are more permeable to gases and caution should be exercised when filling easily oxidized drugs into these capsules.

Non-gelatin capsules may be produced in the form of any of the specialized capsules mentioned in various sections of this chapter, that is, inhalation capsules, locking capsules, sprinkle capsules, and multicomponent capsules.

Recap Questions

1. How is the liquid fill material prevented from leaking out of the two-piece capsule?
2. What is the major advantage of a multicomponent capsule?
3. Name one advantage of using HPMC, over gelatin, capsules.
4. Name one disadvantage of using HPMC, over gelatin, capsules.

CAPSULES NOT INTENDED TO BE SWALLOWED

While the vast majority of capsules are intended to be swallowed, there are certain instances of pharmaceutical hard capsules that are not intended for consumption in this manner. The most common example of this is probably a capsule containing powder for inhalation. This capsule is used in conjunction with a device that releases the powder, which is then inhaled through the device. A sprinkle capsule is a capsule that may be swallowed whole, or the capsule may be opened and the contents sprinkled over soft food, such as applesauce, which is then consumed by the patient. This provides a convenient and palatable way of taking the drug, especially for children or patients who have difficulty swallowing. Sprinkle capsules will be discussed briefly before providing somewhat more detail on inhalation capsules.

The contents of sprinkle capsules are typically beads or pellets that are coated for sustained release. The capsule may contain different populations of beads, each coated to a different extent and providing a different release profile. Depakote (divalproex sodium 125 mg) and Topamax (topiramate 50 mg) are examples of drugs that are supplied as sprinkle capsules. Depakote is used to treat bipolar disease whereas Topamax is used to treat certain types of seizures. The food may be warm but not hot (to prevent potential melting of the coating material). The soft food should be eaten immediately and without chewing. This is a very palatable way to take the medication. The restriction on chewing is to prevent the crushing of the beads. In connection with this, the FDA has stipulated that the beads should be no larger than 2.5 mm in diameter, with some allowance for oversized beads (no more than 10% may be up to 2.8 mm). The reason for this requirement is that there is a greater tendency to chew larger particles.

As sprinkle capsules became more popular, manufacturers used capsule shells that were in common use. Since locking capsules were available, they were used for sprinkle capsules. However, some patients experienced difficulty opening these capsules. This was especially true for geriatric patients who, together with children, are the major users of sprinkle capsules because of the ease of swallowing. As a consequence, capsule shell manufacturers developed special capsule shells for sprinkle capsules. These had a locking mechanism to prevent spilling during processing, shipping, and handling but were easy to open. An example is the ConiSnap sprinkle capsule made by the Capsugel company.

An important and increasingly popular application of capsules that are not swallowed is the inhalation capsule. It is a capsule which contains powder that is released from the capsule, for inhalation by the patient. The first inhalation product containing powder in a capsule was Lomudal, manufactured by Fisons plc, a British pharmaceutical company which is no longer in business. The capsules were inserted into a handheld device, the spinhaler. The patient or caregiver (many patients were children) exerted pressure on the device to pierce the capsules (the mechanical pressure was transferred to pins for this purpose). Inhalation through the device caused the capsule to spin, allowing the drug, sodium cromoglycate, to leave the capsule and to be inhaled by the patient. This product was used for the prophylaxis of asthma.

The Spiriva Handihaler functions in a similar manner in terms of the device. It contains tiotropium bromide for the control of chronic obstructive pulmonary disease (COPD). The Foradil aerolizer has a device that operates on a similar principle. Formoterol fumarate is the medication for long-acting control of asthma. The Onbrez Breezhaler (Novartis) also uses a device and a capsule containing the drug. The latter is punctured upon the application of pressure, by the patient, onto two buttons on the device.

All of the above devices work on the principle of puncturing the capsule with pins, followed by the inhalation of the powder by the patient. It is, therefore, important that the capsule is able to be punctured easily and cleanly, to allow the powder to leave the capsule shell. On the other hand, the capsule shell should not be so brittle that it fractures into pieces, in order to prevent capsule shell particles being inhaled. In addition, if the patient attempts to puncture the capsule multiple times, by repeatedly pressing the buttons, the tendency for the capsule to shatter becomes greater. Consequently, there may be a greater probability that the patient will inhale capsule shell particles. However, it should be noted that the delivery system has a mechanism to filter out larger particles which are, therefore, unlikely to be transported into the oral cavity. This mechanism is described in more detail in Chapter 19, Pulmonary Drug Delivery.

Those capsule shell particles that do get transported in the airstream will probably end up in the mouth where they may be allowed to dissolve, or they can be swallowed. If very fine particles of the capsule shell are inhaled, they will dissolve, because of their aqueous solubility, at the point at which they are deposited (eg, the trachea). A second concern, regarding the capsule shell, is that it should not become so soft and pliable that it cannot be pierced by the needles. With respect to both problems: fracturing, and swelling and softening, the RH under which the capsules are stored is important.

When using the Rotahaler, the patient twists the bottom half of the device to remove the body of the capsule from the cap. With this system, the drug is available from the opened capsule body. Upon the patient's inspiration, the drug is inhaled. This system avoids any potential issues with the piercing of the capsule. All that is required, for release of the drug, is that the capsule opens correctly when subjected to the opening action of the device (which consists of twisting one part of the device relative to the other).

While the shattering of the capsule may not be a common event, and is unlikely to have serious consequences when it does occur, it is undesirable to have shattering capsules. Since HPMC capsules have less dependence on RH for their stability, they will have less tendency to shatter, or to soften and swell, and may, therefore, be better for pulmonary drug delivery applications.

CAPSULES IN DOUBLE-BLIND CLINICAL STUDIES

A double-blind study is a clinical study in which neither the patient nor the clinic staff knows the identity of two (or more) products being compared. The two products may be a drug product and a placebo (a dosage form resembling the drug-containing product but containing no drug). The comparison may also be between an innovator's product and a generic, or between two generic products. Alternately, the two products under comparison may be a newly-developed test formulation, and the company's standard formulation, of the same drug at the same dose. The study may also utilize two different products, containing different drugs, to compare their efficacy. When two small tablets or capsules are being compared, for any purpose, they may be inserted into identical, opaque capsules. This process has been referred to as "over encapsulation."

Since the capsules are not see-through, neither the patient, nor the clinic staff, can identify the product to be taken by an individual patient. Thus, patients and clinical staff are not influenced, in their evaluation of efficacy or of side effects, by the identity of the product taken by the individual patient. For example, if the patient knows that he or she has received the drug (and not the placebo), the patient may "experience" more side effects. Analogously, clinical staff may be biased toward seeing improvements in the patient's clinical condition, if they know that the drug, and not the placebo, was consumed. Typically, the clinical pharmacist at the clinical test facility is the only person to have the "key" to identify the clinical test products at the test facility, in case of a medical emergency. Scientists and medical personnel in the clinical department at the sponsor company also have the key, in order to evaluate the test results.

SOFT GELATIN CAPSULES

Soft gelatin capsules, also known as "softgels," are considered a different dosage form from hard gelatin capsules. The capsule shell is made from a different mix of gelatin and other ingredients, such as plasticizers. While each company has its proprietary formulation, soft gelatin capsules, generally, contain more water and a plasticizer (and therefore less gelatin) than hard gelatin capsules. The composition differences confer a softer feel to the soft gelatin capsule. Soft gelatin capsules are utilized in the pharmaceutical industry for liquid ingredients. Solid drugs may be dissolved in an appropriate non-aqueous solvent and the solution filled into the capsule, in the same way as liquid drugs are filled. In addition, suspensions of finely powdered drugs in non-aqueous liquids may also be incorporated into soft gelatin capsules.

The liquid that is filled into soft gelatin capsules must not be aqueous because of the dissolution of the capsule shell that would occur. The filling liquid may be an oil, or another organic liquid, that is non-toxic, non-irritant, and compatible with the capsule shell. Liquid polyethylene glycols (PEGs), such as PEG 400, are commonly used as the solvent for drugs or vitamin products. Soft gelatin capsules are commonly used in the vitamin and supplement industry, for example, for encapsulating oily solutions of vitamins D and E. Vitamin E in so-called "snip capsules" are used to supply vitamin E solutions for topical application.

A solution of the API in a hydrophobic material may take the form of a SEDDS, as described in the section, Liquid and Semisolid Filling of Capsules. The formulation and mechanisms of drug release and absorption, described under this section, apply to SEDDS in soft gelatin capsules as well. Soft gelatin capsules limit contact with oxygen compared to the measuring of a dose from a bottle of solution. For this reason, easily-oxidized API, such as certain vitamins, may be conveniently formulated in this dosage form. However, the soft gelatin capsule is more permeable to oxygen than a hard gelatin capsule. The oil-soluble vitamins, such as vitamin D and vitamin E, are supplied as patient-friendly softgels containing the oily solutions.

The first step in the production of soft gelatin capsules is the manufacture of the gelatin solution that is used to form the capsule shell. This is done by first hydrating the required amount of gelatin in warm water overnight. The next morning, the water/gelatin mixture is heated further, with stirring, to dissolve the gelatin. This step may take several hours. Glycerin which serves as a plasticizer is added and the solution stirred further. Sorbitol may also be used as a plasticizer. Colorants and opaquant extenders may be added to the solution, as desired. Without the opaquant extender, the soft gelatin capsule will be transparent.

The production of soft gelatin capsules by the rotary die process, the most commonly used manufacturing method, will be described. This method involves the continuous formation of two sheets of gelatin (which eventually form the two halves of the capsule), the filling and the sealing of the soft gelatin capsules. The production of soft gelatin capsules by this method (Figure 10-8) consists of the following steps:

1. Using the hot gelatin solution, two sheets of gelatin are first formed.

2. By passing each of these sheets, while still warm, over a die with indentations, depressions are made in each sheet.

3. The two sheets are brought into close contact, with the depressions on the one sheet matching the corresponding depressions on the other sheet.

4. The filling liquid is injected into the cavities, formed in step 3, by an array of jets simultaneously filling one row of cavities.

5. Pressure is applied around the periphery of each cavity, forming a seal between the two sheets and cutting the sheets along the periphery of the cavity.

6. The capsules formed in step 5 fall into a collecting vessel and are subjected to the finishing process as described below.

These steps are described in greater details as follows. The two sheets of gelatin are formed on either side of the filling machine by allowing gelatin to flow onto a large roll and using a spreader to form a layer of even thickness on the roll. The formed sheets (one on each side of the filling machine) move like a conveyor belt to the central area of the equipment. The sheets of gelatin begin to dry as soon as they leave the roller on which they were formed. In the central area, the capsules are formed between two large cylindrical dies. The dies have indentations on them. The gelatin sheets, which are still warm and less viscous than they will finally be when cold, flow onto each of these dies. To enable this functionality, the temperature of the gelatin solution, when the process starts, is critical. The dies are in close proximity to each other and each spins in the opposite direction to the other. The gelatin sheet over the die follows the depressions on the die. The dies are arranged such that the depressions on each coincide with the depressions on the other. At the closest point on the cylindrical dies, the two sheets touch, so that the corresponding depressions form a receptacle made of gelatin. Before the sheets completely close around the depression, jets inject a metered volume of liquid fill material into each partially formed capsule, which is then fully sealed by further rotation of the dies. The edges of each depression on the die are slightly raised, so that when the two rolls touch, the gelatin sheets are cut, resulting in the formation of the individual soft gelatin capsules (Figure 10-8).

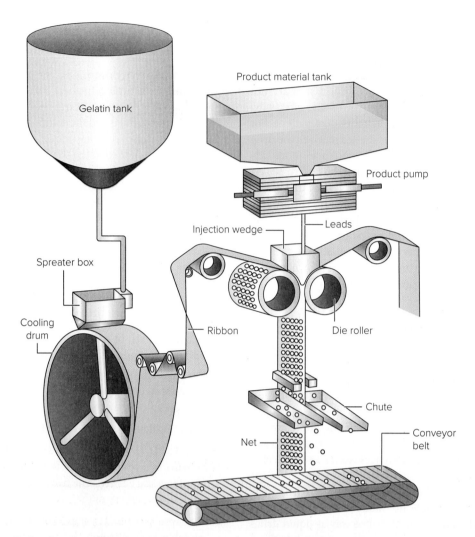

FIGURE 10-8 Soft gelatin capsule production. Note: the piping and ancillary structures needed for the formation of the second ribbon (on the right) are not shown for simplicity. If a bi-colored softgel were required, then a second gelatin tank [containing of a differently colored gelatin solution] would be used. The "net" is the residue of the ribbons, once the softgels have been formed.

Finishing of the capsules involves transporting them through a drying tunnel or a tumble dryer where heat is applied to facilitate the loss of moisture. This results in the capsules becoming firmer but they are still tacky at this stage. Both drying devices result in minimal contact between capsules, limiting the potential for them to stick to each other. The capsules are then transferred to trays and stored in a low-humidity drying room for sufficient time to complete the drying process and to achieve an equilibrium moisture content.

A major advantage of soft gelatin capsules is the fact that the liquid fill is injected as a metered dose. This means that the volume of liquid filled into each soft gelatin capsule is accurate. Since it is relatively easy to make a solution of known concentration, the drug concentration per capsule can be very consistent. In this respect, soft gelatin capsules have an advantage over powder-filled hard gelatin capsules or tablets. Even with liquid suspension fill material, the uniformity of dosing units can be very good. In addition, the soft gelatin capsule is made in-house (unlike hard gelatin capsule shells which are purchased) and this may provide greater control to the pharmaceutical manufacturer, over raw materials and formulation variations. In

addition, confidentiality is maintained and technology know-how is developed in-house. On the other hand, soft gelatin capsule manufacturing equipment is very expensive. The cost may be prohibitive to many smaller manufacturers who may be forced to outsource soft gelatin capsule manufacture, thus eliminating some of the advantages mentioned. In contrast to this, if a manufacturer is already producing hard gelatin capsules (with a powder fill, for example), it is easy to convert many modern capsule-filling machines to accommodate a liquid fill. While a banding machine is not cheap, it is much less expensive than soft capsule manufacturing equipment. Therefore, the banding of hard gelatin capsules may be a cost-effective option to a capsule manufacturer wishing to incorporate liquids.

Most soft gelatin capsules are administered orally but they may be administered by other routes as well. Gyno Daktarin ovules are an example of a soft gelatin capsule that is inserted vaginally for the treatment of fungal infections.

As is the case with hard gelatin capsules, attempts have been made to produce soft gelatin capsules with non-animal constituents. Dietary supplements in "vegetarian softgels" are available commercially. The most commonly used shell material appears to be HPMC, sometimes described in the product literature as "cellulose" or "cellulosic derivative." Gum acacia and starch are two ingredients that appear as promising materials for soft capsule shells, and some formulations have been patented.

Recap Questions

1. Why is the RH, at which inhalation capsules are stored, important?
2. Mention two methods by which currently used devices make the powder contents of a capsule available for inhalation.
3. Sprinkle capsules were developed for geriatrics, among others. What problem did some geriatrics have with the use of the first generation of sprinkle capsules?
4. Why are capsules useful in double-blind clinical trials? Can translucent capsules be used for this purpose?
5. What is the difference in the shell material of hard and soft gelatin capsules?

SUMMARY POINTS

- The manufacture of soft, and two-piece hard, gelatin capsules is described.
- Gelatin is produced by modification of collagen obtained from animal bones and skin.
- Caps and bodies of hard gelatin capsules are made by dipping pins into hot gelatin solution, cooling to solidify and then trimming.
- Filling of hard gelatin capsules involves the rectification of the capsules, opening of the capsules, filling powder into the bodies, and then re-joining the caps and bodies.
- The finished capsules are polished and subjected to quality control testing.
- For aesthetics, capsules are completely filled, using a diluent to make up the rest of the volume of the body of the capsule.
- Liquid and semisolid materials, which may improve the bioavailability of poorly soluble drugs, may be filled into capsules and sealed by banding.
- Capsules may also be used for pulmonary delivery: the contained powders are released by a device, and then inhaled through the device.
- Soft gelatin capsules, commonly used for vitamins and health supplements, are formed and filled in one operation; the shell contains a plasticizer, more water, and less gelatin.
- Opaque capsules are useful for double-blind clinical studies to mask the identity of the drug and a comparator.

What do you think?

1. What is the reason for filling liquids into hard two-piece capsules?
2. What makes a softgel softer than a two-piece hard gelatin capsule?
3. What is the difference between collagen and gelatin?
4. "In systems that perform check weighing of every capsule, the final visual inspection becomes easier." Do you agree or disagree with this statement? Give reasons for your answer.
5. What is the difference between granules and spherical pellets with regard to the filling of hard gelatin capsules?
6. What would be the impact of high RH conditions on the following situations involving capsules?
   a. High-speed powder filling into capsules
   b. The pharmacist handling the capsules during dispensing
   c. A patient using an inhalation capsule in a device that punctures the capsule
7. What is the major disadvantage of providing multiple drugs, for different conditions, within the same multicomponent capsule?
8. *From the perspective of the ease of determining the fill weight only,* which of the following is easier to compound:
   a. Several different formulations of high-dose drugs (eg, 40 mg or 50 mg); or
   b. Several different formulations of low-dose drugs (eg, 1 mg or 2 mg)
   Give reasons for your answer.
9. For the delivery of drugs by inhalation, capsules that shatter are undesirable. What counseling points will you make in order to reduce the incidence of shattering capsules?

REFERENCES

1. Jones B. The history of the medicinal capsule. In: Podczeck F, Jones B, eds. *Pharmaceutical Capsules*. 2nd ed. Pharmaceutical Press; 2004:1-22.
2. Jones RT. Gelatin: manufacture and physico-chemical properties. In: Podczeck F, Jones B, eds. *Pharmaceutical Capsules*. 2nd ed. Pharmaceutical Press; 2004:23-60.

BIBLIOGRAPHY

1. Podczeck F, Jones B. *Pharmaceutical Capsules*. 2nd ed. Pharmaceutical Press; 2004.
2. Capsugel website. www.capsugel.com. Accessed 25 June 2017.
3. Qualicaps website. https://qualicaps.com. Accessed 28 June 2017.

Modified-Release Oral Dosage Forms

11

PREVIEW

- Why modified-release dosage forms are needed
- Nomenclature used to describe modified-release dosage forms
- Matrix systems and the distinction between different types
- Coated modified-release systems
- Gastro-retentive dosage forms, differentiated according to the mechanism of retention
- Osmotic delivery systems—historical development and the major types
- Chronotherapy—significance, dosage form development, and utility
- Mathematical modeling of drug release from modified-release dosage forms
- Colonic drug delivery

INTRODUCTION

Dosage forms for oral delivery have traditionally been formulated to release the drug rapidly, that is, the product is not formulated to delay the release of the drug. Such dosage forms are referred to as "immediate"-release dosage forms. These formulations do not actually release the drug immediately since several steps must, generally, take place before a drug is released from a dosage form, especially one that is solid. These processes are described in Chapter 9, Tablets. Rather than a literal meaning, this term is used to denote formulations which do not have an intentional formulation mechanism to delay the release of the drug. Examples of immediate-release dosage forms are aspirin tablets, acetaminophen capsules, and ibuprofen tablets. Conversely, dosage forms may be intentionally modified, by means of formulation interventions, to produce a slower rate of drug release. Such formulations are referred to as modified-release (MR) dosage forms. There are basically two types of MR dosage forms recognized by the FDA and USP: extended-release (ER) and delayed-release (DR) dosage forms.

ER Dosage Forms

Extended-release products are formulated in a way that causes drug release to be extended for a significant length of time, although release begins soon after drug administration. The release is usually sufficiently extended that the dosage form may be administered twice, or even once, a day to produce significant drug effects for a major part of the day. In a few cases, drug administration may be at even longer intervals.

DR Dosage Forms

Delayed-release products are intentionally modified so that drug release *begins* sometime after drug administration, that is, there is a lag period when no drug (or an insignificant amount) is released. Drug release, thereafter, is usually rapid but may be formulated for MR after the lag period.

Many terms were used previously to denote MR dosage forms. These included: delayed release, modified release, sustained release, controlled release, extended release, timed release, and prolonged release. Some of this terminology was designed to illustrate a particular release technology that had been developed by the pharmaceutical company. In other cases, the term may have been coined to distinguish the product from the competition for marketing purposes. The variety of terms that were in use led to confusion among consumers. Several of these terms were used interchangeably, in the literature, leading to further confusion about their exact meaning. There has been an effort, more recently, to standardize terminology. In this chapter, the terms MR, ER, and DR, as defined above, will be used. The United States Pharmacopeia (USP) recommends that all other terms, and their acronyms, should not be used in describing MR drug products.

The first aim of this chapter, apart from clarifying terminology, is to explain the need for such formulations. MR dosage forms were first developed in the early 1950s. These formulations consisted of pellets that were coated with a material that slowed down drug release. Such coated pellets were filled into capsules which served as the dosage form taken by the patient. Certain antihistamine-containing formulations were among the earliest commercial dosage forms of this type. One of their major advantages, as claimed in initial advertising, was the fact that less frequent dosing was needed. This was an advantage to the patient who may have been taking medication, for example, four times a day. With the development of these dosage forms, the patient could now take one capsule in the morning and one at night. With the further enhancement of product design, a single capsule could be taken to deliver an entire day's drug supply.

The above description places emphasis on the number of doses per day taken by the patient, where each involves the swallowing of a tablet or capsule. The fewer the number of doses, it is implied, the greater the patient convenience.

When a medication is convenient to take, it is more likely that the patient will take the medication regularly, as prescribed, leading to better therapeutic outcomes. However, MR medication has far greater advantages than simply patient convenience and compliance. The major advantage of this type of medication can be observed in the resulting drug blood level profile.

When conventional medication is taken, the blood levels of the drug generally rise rapidly. This occurs because the drug is released rapidly and, consequently, is rapidly absorbed (if the chemical properties of the drug permit). As a result, the blood levels of the drug, a short time after consumption, may be significantly higher than is required for therapy and this could result in side effects (Figure 11-1). On the other hand, the blood drug levels usually also decline rapidly. Hence, the blood levels, a few hours after administration, may be below that required for a therapeutic effect. This occurs, especially, in the period shortly before the next dose is taken. Upon consumption of this dose, the blood levels again rise to higher level than required—only to fall, once more, to a sub-therapeutic level. This rise and fall in a seesaw fashion is characteristic of rapid-release dosage forms that are administered repeatedly and their blood level-time profile is distinctly different from the profile of MR dosage forms (Figure 11-1).

With MR dosage forms, the drug levels may still go up and down, but the swings are smaller and occur less frequently. The net effect is to have more consistent blood levels, showing smaller variations, that is, the blood level-time profile is more flat. This is shown in Figure 11-1 which also shows the idealized profile. The modeling of blood level profiles after specific dosing is explored in more detail in Chapter 17, Introduction to Bioavailability.

Most MR dosage forms are oral liquids, injections, and solid oral dosage forms. Of these major formulation types, solid oral dosage forms are by far the most numerous and are illustrated in Mind Map 11-1. This category includes tablet and capsule dosage forms and is the focus of this chapter. MR of liquids is dealt with in Chapter 6, Pharmaceutical Suspensions, whereas a description of MR injections is included in Chapter 12, Injections.

The formulation types used for solid oral MR can be divided into the following major categories: matrix dosage forms, coated dosage forms, and osmotic systems. While the dosage form may contain additional mechanisms to modify the release of the drug, the primary mechanism can, usually, still be classified as one of the above mechanisms. For example, there are tableted dosage forms with a coating through which a laser-cut hole is responsible for drug release. The tablet core contains osmotic materials and osmosis is the driving force which expels the drug through the laser-cut hole. Hence, the system is classified as osmotic although a coating is also present. There are also formulations which are truly dual mechanism. For example, small particles or beads may be coated with a material to reduce the rate of drug release. These beads may then be embedded in a matrix of MR materials. In such a case, the mechanisms, coating and matrix formation, are each responsible for modifying drug release to a significant extent.

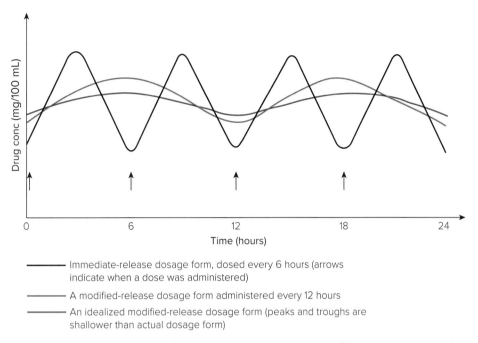

FIGURE 11-1 Plasma level-time profile for an immediate-release dosage form, a modified-release dosage form, and an idealized modified-release dosage form. Note that this is a snapshot of plasma profiles some time after dosing has begun when plasma levels have become consistent.

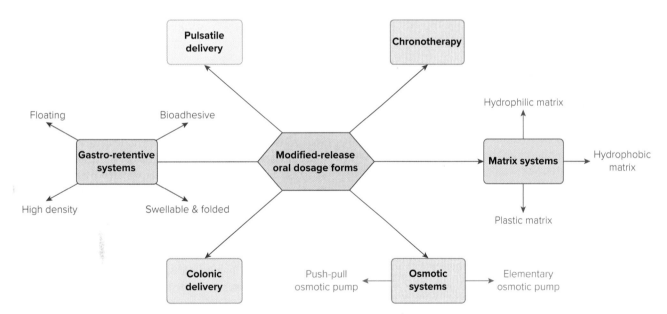

MIND MAP 11-1 Modified-release solid oral dosage forms.

MATRIX SYSTEMS

A typical tablet matrix system is depicted in Figure 11-2. The core of the tablet consists of a mixture of drug and the matrix material. The former is embedded in the latter which modifies its release from the tablet. While many materials will form a matrix, the matrix will not necessarily modify the release of the drug. For example, a drug and lactose blend could form a matrix, upon compression, with the drug embedded within the lactose matrix. However, this matrix does not reduce the rate of drug release. When the tablet is placed into water, water penetrates the tablet, via pores in the matrix, and comes into contact with disintegrants. The disintegrant swells and the tablet disintegrates, exposing the drug in the interior of the tablet. Because water is brought into the interior of the tablet rapidly, drug dissolution can readily occur. Rapid drug release may also occur because this matrix material dissolves fairly rapidly, releasing the drug into the aqueous medium for dissolution. It is possible that both mechanisms, tablet disintegration and matrix dissolution, operate simultaneously. Lactose behaves in this way because of its nature, that is, it allows water to permeate the matrix and it also dissolves fairly quickly.

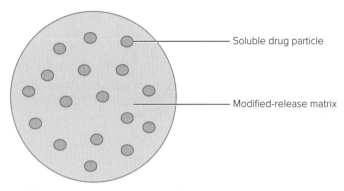

FIGURE 11-2 **A typical matrix tablet.**

Other materials, with different properties, will function differently. Only certain matrix materials will form MR matrices. In such cases, the matrix impedes the penetration of water into the tablet for dissolution of the drug. In addition, the matrix material may retard the diffusion of the dissolved drug, via the pores in the tablet, to the aqueous medium surrounding the tablet. The group of matrix materials that retard drug release is not uniform. There are different types of materials that function in this manner, each acting by a different mechanism. Thus, MR matrix dosage forms may be classified into hydrophobic matrices, plastic matrices, or hydrophilic matrices, each with a different nature. Hydrophilic matrices are also referred to as "gel-forming matrices" because they hydrate in the presence of water, swell, and form a gel.

Hydrophobic Matrix Tablets

These materials are fatty or waxy and the entry of water into the tablet, via pores, is slow since the matrix is hydrophobic. The water that enters the tablet will dissolve the drug with which it comes into contact and a drug solution is formed within the matrix. Analogous to the slow entry of water, the rate at which the drug solution leaves the tablet is also slow.

Tablet Preparation

Tablet preparation involves, first, the preparation of drug-loaded particles and, second, the compression of such particles into tablets. To prepare the particles, the various fats and waxes are melted together and the drug is dispersed into this melt. Examples of hydrophobic matrix materials include carnauba wax, stearyl alcohol, cetyl alcohol, cetostearyl alcohol, and glyceryl monostearate. Sometimes these ingredients are used in combination in the matrix. The enzyme, lipase, pH-adjusting substances, or wicking agents may be added to the molten fat for the reasons described later in this section.

The molten material is allowed to cool to form a solidified mass which is then ground to the required particle size. In an alternative method, the liquid may also be spray-congealed to form particles which have a narrower size distribution than in the first method. Spray congealing is analogous to spray drying discussed in Chapter 9, Tablets. The molten material is first sprayed, by means of a suitable device, which creates droplets of the desired size. When these droplets meet cold air, within the apparatus, the liquid congeals into solid particles. Unlike spray drying, there is no drying step since there is no moisture (or

other solvents) to be lost; instead, the molten material congeals during cooling.

The particulate material, however prepared, is then compressed into tablets or the particles can be filled into capsules. From this description, it can be concluded that the matrix may have the drug embedded within the matrix material itself.

An alternative method to prepare the materials for compression is as follows. A granular form of the waxy material (which is available commercially) may be blended with the drug powder and other excipients. This mixture is then used for directly compressing tablets. Direct compression is the easier, more cost-effective method of tableting, compared to granulation and subsequent tableting. However, some waxes are not available in granular form and cannot easily be size-reduced since they are generally soft materials, or they soften with heating. Consequently, grinding the material, which produces heat from fiction, cannot be used. The fluid energy mill, as the name implies, operates on the principle of the energy imparted by a fluid (a gas) to rapidly move the coarse material. Collisions of one particle with another, or with the side walls of the vessel, cause the particles to shatter. Little heat is generated and this mill may be used for size reduction of waxy materials. Since the materials are soft, during compression they "flow" around drug particles. Hence, even with this method, the drug may be virtually embedded within the matrix material.

Some examples of hydrophobic matrix tablets are given in Table 11-1.

Drug Release

Drug release from a fatty matrix tablet involves the penetration of water through pores into, and the diffusion of drug, out of the tablet, as previously mentioned. This process can be assisted by the gradual erosion of the fatty material, from the outer surface of the tablet, as time passes. Erosion refers to the process whereby pieces of the matrix material break away from the tablet's surface. If the matrix fatty material contains fatty acid esters that can be hydrolyzed, then pH and the presence of enzymes greatly affect the rate of drug release due to enzymatic breakdown of the fat. Enzymes may be available in the physiological environment of a consumed tablet. In some instances, a lipase enzyme may be added to the fatty matrix to promote drug release. Water is needed for enzymatic activity and the described effect will only occur in an aqueous medium.

Since water penetration is slow, the drug contained in the depths of the tablet may not easily be reached by water. Hence, incomplete drug release generally occurs with fatty matrix tablets. The utilization of the enzymatic breakdown technique may be important when incomplete release is pronounced. In some formulations, wicking or channeling agents, which are hydrophilic materials, are added in small proportion to the matrix to assist the entry of fluid. These agents promote more complete drug release because they draw water into the interior of the tablet.

Plastic Matrix Tablets

The tablets, which are formed from the drug and an inert plastic material, can be produced by several methods:

TABLE 11-1	Examples of Commercial Extended-Release Tablets
TRADE NAME	**DRUG**
Actoplus Met XR	Metformin hydrochloride; pioglitazone hydrochloride
Adalat CC	Nifedipine
Altoprev	Lovastatin
Ambien CR	Zolpidem tartrate
Belviq XR	Lorcaserin hydrochloride
Biaxin XL	Clarithromycin
Calan SR	Verapamil hydrochloride
Cardura XL	Doxazosin mesylate
Cipro XR	Ciprofloxacin; Ciprofloxacin hydrochloride
Concerta	Methylphenidate hydrochloride
Covera-HS	Verapamil hydrochloride
Depakote ER	Divalproex sodium
Sinemet CR	Carbidopa; Levodopa
Seroquel XR	Quetiapine fumarate
Roxicodone	Oxycodone hydrochloride
Toprol-XL	Metoprolol succinate
Tenuate Dospan	Diethylpropion hydrochloride
Tegretol-XR	Carbamazepine
Uroxatral	Alfuzosin hydrochloride
Ultram ER	Tramadol hydrochloride
Viramune XR	Nevirapine
Wellbutrin SR	Bupropion hydrochloride
Xanax XR	Alprazolam
Xigduo XR	Dapagliflozin; Metformin hydrochloride
Zyban	Bupropion hydrochloride

Granulation with an Organic Solvent

The drug powder and the powdered plastic material are intimately mixed together and then a suitable organic solvent is used to moisten the mixture which is then granulated. This method is likely to produce a drug in plastic solution to some extent.

Dissolution of Drug and Plastic Material

For this step, a suitable organic solvent is used to dissolve the plastic material. Next, the drug is dissolved in this organic solution. In some instances, a mixture of organic solvents is needed to effectively dissolve the plastic as well as the drug. Then, the solution is partially evaporated leaving a thick paste which may be granulated through a sieve of suitable dimensions. The dried granules consist of a solid-in-solid solution of drug in plastic. These granules are suitable for compression. This preparation method is most likely to lead to a larger percentage of the drug being present in a plastic solution than the previous method, granulation with an organic solvent.

Direct Compression

The drug powder and the plastic particles are mixed together intimately, and then directly compressed. The simplicity of the process makes it the most elegant. A problem that may be encountered is the fact that the plastic powder may consist of much larger particles than the drug powder, which could lead to segregation of the two powder types. The obvious solution, of grinding the plastic to a suitable size, cannot be used in many instances. This is because the plastic material would soften, and form lumps, due to the heat generated during grinding. One solution is to pre-granulate the drug powder to make larger drug particles. Then, the granulated drug particles are mixed with the plastic particles. Using this method, there is less potential for powder segregation.

Direct compression is most likely to lead to a significant proportion of the drug particles located between plastic particles in the tablet matrix. However, heat is momentarily generated in localized areas during compression, and this could cause partial melting of some of the plastic material during the tableting process. Some of the drug could dissolve in this molten plastic. Thus, even the direct compression tableting process may facilitate the dissolving of a small portion of the drug in the plastic material but the amount of solid solution formed is expected to be relatively small.

During the compression process, the plastic particles adjacent to a drug particle may not melt but only soften due to the heat of friction. Under continued pressure in the die of the tablet press, these particles deform and "flow" around the harder drug particle. As the material cools, the plastic particles (now wrapped around the drug particle) fuse with one another. This process continues throughout the material in the die cavity, forming the matrix. Since the deformation is incomplete, there will be some drug particles not engulfed by the matrix material. Therefore, the process results in some of the drug located within pores in the tablet, that is, in the spaces between fused plastic particles. In addition, a portion of the drug is dissolved within the plastic material itself.

A modification of the basic direct compression method has been utilized to increase sustained-release efficacy. This involves placing the compressed tablets into a closed system and exposing them to solvent vapors for a controlled length of time. This may be achieved by simply spreading the tablets on a tray and placing an organic solvent (in which the plastic is soluble) in a small, open container within the oven or other closed system. A small elevation of the temperature promotes vaporization of the volatile solvent. The vapors that are produced filled the entire space within the oven and reach the tablets, penetrating pores in the tablet matrix. This causes partial dissolution of the plastic material, especially on the surface. The dissolved plastic might fuse with an adjacent plastic particle, resulting in the formation of a more complete film of plastic on the surface. This has a greater barrier effect on water penetration into the tablet and drug particles would, also, be surrounded more completely. Some of the drug may also dissolve in the plastic solution, forming a drug-in-plastic solution. These effects of exposure to solvent fumes lead to slower dissolution, that is, to a more efficient MR product.

Depending on the method of preparation, the product may consist of drug particles dispersed in the pores between plastic particles, or a solution consisting of the drug dissolved in the plastic material, or a combination of these forms. The advantage of a drug in plastic solution is the fact that water takes longer to penetrate and dissolve the drug and longer for the drug solution to leave the matrix, that is, it shows greater efficacy as a sustained-release product. The vapor treatment of directly compressed plastic matrix tablets takes only slightly longer than direct compression itself, yet it creates more drug-in-plastic solution. Thus, it enhances the prolongation of drug release and improves the MR effect greatly. The fusion of numerous plastic particles within the tablet to form a more complete fused matrix creates a more tortuous path for fluid entering, and solution leaving, the tablet. Vapor treatment, overall, creates a much better ER dosage form.

Hydrophilic Matrix Tablets

The materials that form hydrophilic matrices consist of nondigestible hydrophilic polymers that are capable of swelling to form a gel layer. When the tablet is placed into water, the entire surface becomes wet, and the polymer located superficially swells to form a gel layer. It is important to recognize that the gel layer is on the surface of the entire tablet. This layer is important because it retards the release of the drug by the mechanism that is described below.

Upon administration of the tablet, it passes into the stomach fairly quickly and makes contact with the digestive fluids. The tablet absorbs water, from the gastric fluids, to form the gel layer. The gel is at the tablet/GI fluid interface and retards further penetration of water into the tablet. Such penetration is necessary for the entry of water into the tablet to dissolve the drug. Subsequently, the drug solution should diffuse out of the tablet. Water penetration into, and solute diffusion out of, the tablet is retarded by the gel barrier. In this way, the presence of the gel slows down or retards drug release from the tablet. For an effective ER medication, the polymer must be capable of hydrating quickly and of rapidly forming the gel barrier for the reasons explained below. Additionally, the gel barrier must be of sufficient viscosity to be effective since a low-viscosity gel impedes water penetration minimally.

The gel is the barrier to water penetration; in the absence of the gel, water penetration is rapid. Therefore, it is important that the gel barrier forms rapidly. From the moment of immersion of the tablet into an aqueous medium, until the gel barrier forms, the rate of drug loss from the surface of the tablet is rapid. If the gel barrier forms rapidly, the period of rapid water entry and rapid drug solution exit is very brief, and the initial drug loss is not significant. The drug released from the tablet enters the aqueous environment surrounding the tablet from where it may be absorbed into GI tissues. The viscous barrier protects the tablet from rapid drug release, resulting in correspondingly slow absorption. In many instances, the drug solution must pass into the small intestine before absorption can occur, despite the tablet being in the stomach.

Once the gel layer is formed, it controls the rate of drug release and continues to do so as long as the integrity of the gel barrier is maintained. However, the gel barrier is not static and changes to it and to the tablet occur over time. More water is progressively absorbed by the outer region of the gel barrier, causing it to become progressively thinner or less viscous (Figure 11-3). Consequently, the outer layers of the gel barrier are removed by erosion (breaking off of small bits of the gel barrier) and any motion of the tablet in its aqueous environment in the gastrointestinal tract (GIT) will facilitate such erosion.

It is important to bear in mind that the interior of the tablet would still be dry at this stage. (In a sense, this is a demonstration of the effectiveness of the gel barrier since water does not rapidly penetrate the tablet to reach deeper layers.) As the outer layers are removed, as described above, water is able to penetrate further into the tablet. As the water penetrates slightly

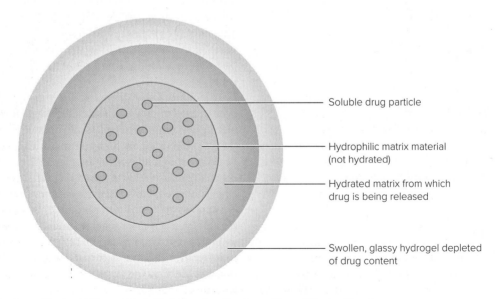

FIGURE 11-3 A hydrated hydrophilic matrix tablet showing the formation of the gel barrier.

deeper into the tablet, fresh hydrophilic polymer now becomes hydrated. In this way, the gel barrier is constantly changing with the removal of its outer layer and the expansion of the gel barrier further into the interior of the tablet. This process occurs at all surfaces of the tablet and increasing water penetration occurs in a three-dimensional manner. The gel barrier is maintained in this dynamic fashion: as the outer layer is removed, a new layer forms toward the interior of the tablet, the processes occurring simultaneously. As long as a gel barrier is maintained, in spite of these changes, drug release from the tablet is extended. This happens because the gel controls the rate of two phenomena:

1. The penetration of water into the gel from the surrounding aqueous fluids
2. The diffusion of drug solution out of the tablet (through the gel) to the external medium

The extent to which drug release is prolonged can be modified by certain factors. Increasing the molecular mass of the hydrophilic polymer extends the release time since the gel barrier is more viscous and water permeation is slower. In addition, the erosion of the gel barrier is also slower since the viscous material takes longer to become more hydrated, and thin enough to erode. The percentage of polymer (of a fixed molecular weight) that is used in the formulation is inversely proportional to the release rate, that is, the higher the percentage of polymer, the slower is the release rate.

Hydrophilic matrix tablets may be prepared by the wet granulation, or direct compression, techniques. The choice is influenced by the polymer selected and its concentration. When relatively high polymer concentrations are used, the tablet contains a large proportion of the polymer and can, usually, be directly compressed. When most of the tablet is made up of the polymer (eg, when the drug weight is low), another problem must be considered: the dissolution rate may be too slow to be useful. In such cases, an inert ingredient, such as lactose, may be used as part of the matrix to effectively reduce the hydrophilic polymer concentration. By careful adjustment of the lactose and polymer concentrations, a tablet with the appropriate release profile can be produced.

When wet granulation is used, the granulating agent is typically a solvent in which the matrix material (hydrophilic polymer) is insoluble. A suitable binder, which must be soluble in the granulating agent, should be used. The binder must possess sufficient binding power to allow the formation of good granules. The binder/granulating agent combination could, for example, be polyvinyl pyrrolidone (PVP) in ethanol, or polyethylene glycol in ethanol, provided the hydrophilic polymer is not soluble in ethanol. It is important not to add water to a hydrophilic matrix since the material is likely to form a cohesive mass that is very difficult to manipulate or to break up into granules.

In a matrix dosage form, the matrix serves to retard the release of the drug through various aspects of its nature. For this reason, drug release is referred to as being "matrix-controlled." For example, water moves into the matrix through very narrow pores. The size of these pores may control the rate at which water migrates into the interior of the tablet, where it dissolves the drug. The pore size also controls the rate at which drug solution may diffuse out of the tablet. These water channels are curved

and twisting, and the extent to which they have this property is referred to as the "tortuosity" of the matrix. Pore size and tortuosity are properties of the matrix.

Recap Questions

1. Give two examples of materials that act as a hydrophobic matrix.
2. What is the effect of including a lipase enzyme in a hydrophobic matrix tablet?
3. What effect does pH have on drug release from a hydrophobic matrix?
4. Name the ways in which a plastic matrix material can be made into a tablet.
5. Why does water, added to a mixture of drug and hydrophilic matrix constituents, result in the formation of a cohesive mass that is difficult to process further?
6. What is a "gel barrier"?

COATED SYSTEMS

Dosage forms such as tablets, capsules, and beads may be coated with different types of pharmaceutical material, for different purposes. The coating of a dosage form may, or may not, significantly modify the release of the drug contained within that dosage form. It must be emphasized that every coating does not provide modified drug release. It is possible to coat a tablet, for aesthetic purposes, or for some other reason, with minimal effect on drug release. Coating may be used to cover slight imperfections on the tablet surface, thus improving its appearance. On the other hand, a coated tablet may look more attractive than the uncoated one, even when there is no imperfection on the tablet. In addition, coating may be used to mask the taste of the contained drug. For example, the bitter taste and "burning" mouth sensation of ibuprofen is masked by coating of the tablets. Beads may similarly be coated to mask the taste of the contained drug. In such cases, the coating material is soluble and dissolves upon contact with water. It is only required to delay drug release until the dosage form is swallowed.

If the nature of the coating material, however, is such that the permeation of water through the coating is retarded, the release of drug from that dosage form will be slower. As a result of such a coating, water enters the dosage form very slowly and the dissolution of the drug within the dosage form is correspondingly slow. The dissolved drug must also leave the dosage form by passing through the coating material, in the reverse direction to water entry. The coating material also causes this process to be slow since drug diffusion can only occur through pores in the coating.

Selecting the appropriate coating materials, and their amounts, is of tremendous importance to effective coating. In addition, numerous physical parameters related to the coating process (as discussed in Chapter 9, Tablets) have an impact on the successful production of an elegant coated product, whether the dissolution rate from such a product is rapid or sustained. For the production of a pharmaceutically elegant product, with the appropriate dissolution rate, all parameters, whether relating to formulation or processing, must be optimal.

Special coatings are chosen for their ability to retard drug release. In such cases, the coating material is typically made up of a mixture of substances, the major portion of which is insoluble in an aqueous environment. An insoluble coating material may also contain a small amount of water-soluble material. The latter rapidly dissolves when the coated dosage form is placed into water. The dissolution of these small portions of coating on the surface of, for example, a coated bead creates small pores for the penetration of aqueous media into the bead.

Most often, the drug, contained within the bead and surrounded by the coating, is rapidly soluble. The water entering the bead, after creating pores in the coating, dissolves the drug. The drug solution leaves via the pores. In this case, the drug contained in the pellets (or beads), within the shell of coating, can be considered a "reservoir" of drug and the coating controls the rate of drug release. This type of system is referred to as a reservoir system, as opposed to a matrix system, described earlier, in which the matrix controls drug release.

Coated systems may consist of tablets, or multi-particulate systems (beads or pellets). It is unusual for the major release-modifying mechanism to be the coating of a tablet. Coating may be used in conjunction with a matrix formulation to provide enhanced retardation of drug release or to improve the aesthetics of the tablet. Coating, as the major mechanism to modify drug release, is typically utilized in multi-particulate systems. Multi-particulate systems consist of many small units. These units are then incorporated into the final dosage form. Most often they are filled into a capsule the shell of which dissolves fairly quickly, upon consumption by the patient, to release the contained units. However, the multi-particulates may also be compressed into a tablet. In this case, the coating is distorted, or even fractured, to an extent and the particle shape is altered (made less spherical) as a result of compression forces. Notwithstanding these changes, the entire dosage form has MR properties.

The few dozen particles contained within the capsule have a much larger surface area than the capsule itself. Similarly, the surface area of a sufficient quantity of particles to be combined into a

single tablet is much larger than the surface area of the tablet itself. Thus, the release of each milligram of drug within a single, coated particle requires much more release-modifying coating material, than is the case for each milligram of drug in a coated tablet or a coated capsule. Even though the beads have a correspondingly larger surface area for dissolution, than is the case for tablets, retardation of drug release in pellets can be achieved to an extent that is usually better than it is for tablets. For this reason, multiparticulates function more effectively for drug release modification by coating than is the case with a whole tablet.

Small tablets may be coated in a fluid bed coater whereas larger tablets are coated in a coating pan (Chapter 9, Tablets). Spherical particles may be formed in a fluid bed granulator, then dried, and coated in a continuous process in the same apparatus as described in Chapter 8, Granulation. Briefly, non-pareil seeds, consisting of sugar, may be suspended in a fluidized bed, within a fluid bed coater, and drug particles successively layered onto the non-pareils, dried, and then coated with several release modifying coats. Spherical granules may also be produced by the process of extrusion-spheronization or roto-granulation. These processes are described in Chapter 8, Granulation.

Whatever the technique used for the production of spherical particles (beads, pellets, or granules), they may be coated for MR. Most commonly, the fluid bed coater is the equipment used for coating and the nature and proportion of coating materials determines the extent of MR. The process of coating must be carefully monitored to prevent spraying the coating liquid too rapidly. If the latter occurs, it could cause sticking of the multi-particulates to each other, becoming progressively larger agglomerates. On the other hand, if the coating material is sprayed too slowly, the droplets of coating may dry before they can reach the surface of the bead or particle. This dried coating material is not effective in modifying the release of the drug.

The drying rates of the material are, naturally, also affected by the rates at which air is pumped through the machine, the temperature of the air, and its initial moisture content. Since the coating materials are polymers, their inclusion with the solvent increases the viscosity of the solution. Since the solution must be pumped into the equipment, its viscosity should not be too high. There are many other factors affecting effective coating and the above is only intended to give the reader a glimpse of the intricacies of the process. Some of the commonly used coating materials for MR are given in Table 11-2.

TABLE 11-2	Examples of Modified-Release Coating Materials	
TRADE NAME	**CHEMICAL NAME**	**COMMENTS**
Ethocel	Ethylcellulose (EC) powder	A range of viscosity grades producing different rates of drug release.
Surelease	Aqueous EC dispersion	Very fine particles, upon drying, form a continuous membrane. Different grades produce differing extents of MR.
Opadry CA	Cellulose acetate dispersion	Very fine particles, upon drying, form a continuous membrane. Used for osmotic pump manufacture.
Eudragit	Methacrylic-acrylic acid copolymer	Different grades are anionic or cationic, and are soluble at different pH values, providing enteric coating that can be targeted for release in different parts of the GIT.

A novel coating method, phase separation-coacervation, involves dispersion of particles in a clear solution of coating material. By various means, a portion of the coating polymer can be brought out of solution to form a viscous gelatinous layer, without precipitation of the polymer as solid particles, while the remaining polymer solution remains less viscous. One of the mechanisms to achieve this effect is by the slow addition of a controlled amount of non-solvent to the polymer solution, with continuous stirring. After the formation of the coacervate, multi-particulates are added to the container and the viscous polymer is caused to wrap around the individual particles, with continued stirring. With further processing, such as continued stirring while reducing the temperature, the coating around the multi-particulates is converted to a solid. Coacervate-coated particles are used in oral medication for taste masking and for modified-release. Since such particles are also used in injectable formulations, coacervation is described in more detail in Chapter 12, Injections.

GASTRO-RETENTIVE DOSAGE FORMS

Any solid dosage form that is swallowed usually reaches the stomach in a few seconds, in the absence of any pathology that delays swallowing. Once in the stomach, a conventional tablet may disintegrate and release the medication which may then be absorbed in the stomach. Alternately, the released medication may pass into the small intestine, for absorption in this region of the GIT. Small granules or coated beads, released from a capsule, also pass unhindered into the small intestine where the majority of the drug is released and absorbed. When large enteric-coated non-disintegrating tablets are taken, passage of the whole (un-disintegrated) tablet depends on stomach emptying which may take several hours. Stomach emptying is described in Chapter 3, Oral Route of Drug Delivery. Essentially, the migrating motor complex (MMI) helps to drive larger-sized material from the stomach into the intestine, during the unfed state. In particular, the "housekeeper wave" (a segment of the MMI) rapidly propels any residual particulate matter (including un-disintegrated tablets) into the small intestine. Here, the enteric-coated tablet disintegrates after the dissolution of its coating material in the intestine which has a pH that is favorable for this purpose. As a consequence, the drug is released for absorption.

Consider the situation where a research group wished to make a product that was effective over 24 hours with one dose (ie, once-a-day administration). Assume that the drug, once absorbed, is fairly rapidly metabolized and/or excreted as unchanged drug. To enable effectiveness over the intended period, such a drug should be absorbed over an extended period of 12 hours or more. To allow such a long absorption phase, drug release from the dosage form should also occur over an extended period. As described in Chapter 3, Oral Route of Drug Delivery, the time for the passage of material through the small intestine averages about 3 hours. Thereafter, the food material passes into the colon, a region of the GIT that is not as efficient as the small intestine for absorption. Therefore, a large non-disintegrating tablet would reach the colon, perhaps, 7 or 8 hours after it is swallowed. This period is too short to allow

for the required extended drug release and subsequent absorption in the small intestine. If the dosage form consisted of multi-particulates, these would reach the colon even sooner.

A second issue is that the period over which release occurs should be longer than 10 hours. This would allow absorption to occur over a slightly longer period, thus satisfying the requirements for extended absorption outlined earlier. However, if the dosage form were simply formulated to release over a longer period, it would reach the colon before drug release is complete, that is, the rate of movement of the dosage form through the GIT hinders the successful production of a once-a-day dosage form. Without the development of special technology to address this issue, an effective once-a-day dosage form cannot be made for many drugs.

For drugs that are rapidly metabolized and/or excreted, then, a longer duration of action in the body may be attained by delaying the passage of the drug through the GIT. This can be achieved by developing a product that is retained in the stomach for a longer duration than naturally occurs under normal physiological conditions. The fact that the dosage form is not rapidly emptied into the small intestine affords a longer time for absorption to occur from the slowly releasing dosage form. Such a formulation also delays the passage of the dosage form to the colon. Therefore, the problem can be resolved by maintaining the dosage form within the stomach, where it can slowly release the drug to pass unhindered into the small intestine for absorption. This type of formulation is important in another situation, besides MR, as described below.

Some drugs have a very short absorption window, that is, there is a very short portion of the GIT (usually a short segment of the small intestine) that is capable of absorbing these drugs rapidly or effectively. The absorption window is frequently a section of the duodenum close to the pyloric valve. The better absorption that occurs in this region may be due to the presence of loose junctions (between adjacent cells), or an active transport mechanism may be present. For ease of description, the situation with a conventional, non-disintegrating, dosage form will first be described. If such a dosage form (containing a drug with a short absorption window) is administered, it may start releasing the drug soon after it reaches the stomach, and continue releasing the drug for a significant time thereafter, during the passage of the dosage form through the GIT. The drug that is released, while the dosage form is in the stomach, passes into the small intestine and will be absorbed through the absorption window.

Once the dosage form, itself, is transferred into the small intestine and passes the absorption window, any drug released from it continues to flow with the food material towards the large intestine, and further, without significant absorption. Beyond the absorption window, the dosage form may release the drug slowly, as it was designed, but effective absorption will not occur. Thus, a small non-disintegrating tablet administered on an empty stomach may pass rapidly into the small intestine. Soon, it will move beyond the absorption window and further drug release will not result in effective absorption of the drug.

The following situation may occur with an immediate-release disintegrating tablet containing a drug with a short absorption window. The tablet disintegrates into large granules in the stomach, and these disintegrate further into prime particles from which the drug will dissolve (as described in Chapter 8, Granulation). The drug that is in solution will pass into the small intestine and may then be absorbed through the absorption window. Depending on the length of time required for these steps to occur, some of the material (granules and prime particles) may pass the absorption window with a similar outcome to that described above for whole tablets: the material may pass the absorption window and significant drug release may only occur after passing the absorption window and this drug will not be effectively absorbed. A well-known example of a drug that behaves in this way is riboflavin which has a very short absorption window in the proximal duodenum, that is, it can only be absorbed effectively for a short distance after passing out of the stomach. Other examples of drugs with a short absorption window are levodopa, ranitidine.HCl, and metformin.

If reasonable absorption of a short–absorption-window drug cannot be assured for an immediate-release dosage form, a conventional MR dosage form makes no biopharmaceutical sense since the ER dosage form would pass the absorption window, and further drug release would lead to insignificant absorption. A special type of MR dosage form, as described below, can be effectively used both for ER beyond 12 hours and also for drugs with a short absorption window.

Retaining a non-disintegrating tablet of a short–absorption-window drug in the stomach for a longer duration would be beneficial in that it would increase the probability of effective absorption of such drugs. As the drug is released from the non-disintegrating tablet, it passes into the small intestine where it is absorbed in the absorption window. The rate of drug release from such a tablet can be controlled so that the absorption mechanism (in the absorption window) is not overwhelmed. If extended absorption of the order of 12 hours is required through the entire small intestine (and an absorption window is not the issue), a similar formulation approach can be used.

Another application of the described gastro-retentive dosage forms is for optimal utilization of a drug that is required for local action in the stomach. Such a drug is not required to be absorbed, or to exert an action, in any other part of the GIT. Maintaining the dosage form of such a drug in the stomach for a longer period will be advantageous, for similar reasons. Examples of such drugs include calcium supplements and drugs used to treat *Heliobacter pylori* (H. pylori).

Furthermore, drugs that are acid soluble but poorly soluble at alkaline pH may also benefit from retention in the stomach. Such drugs could be slowly released from the dosage form to form a solution in the acidic stomach fluids. In terms of the solubility of such drugs, the pH of the small intestine is unfavorable. When these drugs pass into the small intestine *in small quantities*, the drug has a better chance to remain in solution and, therefore, to be absorbed in the small intestine because the small quantity of drug in solution does not exceed its limited solubility at the higher pH of the small intestine. An example of such a drug is furosemide.

Gastric retention may be significantly increased by creating a non-disintegrating tablet that floats on the liquid contents of the stomach. Since the tablet floats, it will escape passage into the small intestine when stomach emptying occurs. Tablets or other units float on the surface of stomach fluids and the fluid is replenished so that the stomach does not become completely empty. The fact that the tablet is floating prevents the propulsive movements of the stomach from pushing it out into the small intestine. This is one mechanism to achieve gastric retention, providing a longer time for drug release and absorption to occur. This technique has been successfully applied in many studies. While the fluid content of the stomach does become very low in the fasting state, patients taking these medications are advised to ensure that they drink water repeatedly throughout the day.

Other techniques, apart from floating tablets, exist for maintaining the dosage form within the stomach and delaying its passage into the small intestine. These include bio-adhesive systems in which the dosage form adheres to the stomach wall, delaying its passage into the small intestine. In addition, there are systems which have a high density that causes them to fall to the bottom of the liquid in the stomach. This is in contrast to floating systems that have a low density which keeps them buoyant. The high-density systems are also not easily moved by the propulsive motions of the stomach, because they are located at the bottom, adjacent to the wall of the stomach, and resist propulsion into the small intestine. This results in a longer residence time in the stomach. Systems that expand greatly and/or have a shape that does not readily permit movement into the intestine have also been developed.

Naturally, the drug contained in a retained dosage form, irrespective of the retention method, must be stable in the acidic contents of the stomach for extended periods. In addition, such a drug must not irritate the stomach. Eventually, all dosage forms must disintegrate or dissolve to clear the material from the stomach. If mechanisms to clear the dosage form from the stomach did not work, within a reasonable period of time, it could serve as a trigger to promote vomiting or diarrhea, processes which the body utilizes to expel foreign matter from the stomach. These processes are brought into effect if the residence time in the stomach has been very long. Hence, the formulator must ensure that the formulation will disintegrate or dissolve after a reasonable time.

The formulation and development of the different types of gastric retentive systems will now be described.

Floating Systems

Floating systems may be created by incorporating gas-forming ingredients into polymers that swell upon hydration. Most often, the released gas is CO_2 which, in combination with the polymer, forms a gel that floats on the stomach contents. An example of a swellable polymer is hydroxypropyl methylcellulose and the most common gas-forming ingredients are effervescent mixtures. Examples of the latter are sodium carbonate and bicarbonate, in combination with acids such as citric acid or tartaric acid. The liberated CO_2 bubbles become trapped within the gel mass that forms in the presence of water. Due to its viscosity, the gas bubbles do not readily escape the polymer. The combination of hydrated gel with bubbles of CO_2

dispersed in it has a density less than that of water and, therefore, it will float. This is the first mechanism that was utilized to create a floating dosage form. Currently, there are other mechanisms utilized to create floating dosage forms and some of these are much more complex. Alternative mechanisms to create floating devices will not be described in this introductory text.

Floating drug delivery systems have certain limitations which include the following:

1. A high level of stomach fluid is required. This allows the device to float correctly. For this reason, patients are advised to consume adequate quantities of water. This may present a problem when the stomach is empty or approaches this condition. Water consumed, in this state, is emptied rapidly and it may be difficult to maintain sufficient water in the stomach, for an adequate time, to allow the floating device to operate correctly.

2. The supine position is not advisable. When the patient is in this position for long periods, for example when sleeping, the floating dosage form may more easily be swept away by contractile waves. Where possible, the patient should not take this type of medication shortly before bedtime.

Bio-adhesive Systems

Bioadhesive systems contain materials that will adhere to biological membranes when moistened. This allows the dosage form, typically a matrix tablet, to adhere to the stomach lining. It is important that the tablet adheres soon after administration in order to prevent expulsion of the dosage form by peristaltic action. On the other hand, bioadhesion should not occur so quickly that the tablet adheres to the lining of the mouth or the throat while it is being taken. This is usually achieved by applying a thin coating (of non-adhesive material) over the bio-adhesive material to prevent premature adhesion of the dosage form before it reaches the stomach. The coating dissolves rapidly after the tablet reaches the stomach, exposing the bioadhesive material which becomes hydrated and tacky, allowing bioadhesion.

From this position, the dosage form slowly releases its drug load. As the material continues to hydrate, its outer layers become thinner and, with the constant movement of the stomach contents, these layers are slowly eroded and removed. Eventually, all of the tablet mass becomes completely eroded and bioadhesion ends. As mentioned, prolonged retention of any mass in the stomach can stimulate the body's expulsion mechanisms: vomiting or diarrhea. The stomach lining is covered by a viscous layer of mucus and it is important to realize that bioadhesion actually occurs with the mucus layer, and not the stomach lining itself. Since the lining and the mucus are in close proximity, the mucus may be considered a part of the stomach lining. In addition, some mucin types are transmembrane and contribute to anchoring the mucus to the stomach lining. Hence, the adhesion is typically described as occurring to the stomach lining. The constant turnover of mucus prevents extremely strong adherence to the lining, which is beneficial because of the need to expel the dosage form after a length of time. However, if the turnover of mucus is too fast, it may result in inadequate adherence of the dosage form to the lining of the stomach.

Swellable Systems

While these systems swell, upon contact with water, buoyancy is not necessarily involved in the gastro-retentive mechanism. Instead, the large size and shape of the drug-containing unit does not predispose it to expulsion into the small intestine. Such shapes include a large, flexible disc or a flexible ring (shaped more like a rubber band than a doughnut). The unit may be folded and placed into a capsule that is consumed by the patient (Figure 11-4). The capsule shell disintegrates in the stomach contents to release the specially-shaped unit which then unfolds. Non-floating systems that swell to a larger size, or unfold, must do so rapidly to avoid being propelled into the small intestine before the change can occur.

High-Density Systems

When conventional tablets or small pellets contain a sufficient quantity of a high-density material, such as bismuth subnitrate, barium sulfate, ferrous oxide, titanium dioxide, or zinc oxide, the dosage form, as a whole, attains a higher density. Obviously, the toxicity of these ingredients must be determined before inclusion into the dosage form. Even the use of ferrous oxide-containing products for extended periods could lead to iron toxicity. These dosage forms tend to sink to the bottom of the gastric fluids and remain there, escaping much of the churning of digestion as well as the propulsion of liquid and low-density materials through the pyloric valve. In addition, small particles may be trapped in the folds of the stomach lining. There appears to be a minimum density that is required for optimal retention by this mechanism. This value appears to be about 2.5 g/mL.

The floor of the body of the stomach is also at a lower point than the entry to the duodenum. Small tablets as well as multiparticulates that are not retained in the folds of the stomach, presumably, fall to this lower point and are retained in the body of the stomach. As mentioned previously, particle size controls the passage of materials into the small intestine during most of the digestive phase. When the housekeeper wave is in operation, larger particles (and tablets) are swept through the pyloric valve into the small intestine. By sinking to the bottom of the fluid contents, small particles escape the constant propulsion of materials into the small intestine during digestive movements in the fed state. Likewise, they may be less affected by the strong wavelike propulsive action during the inter-digestive phase.

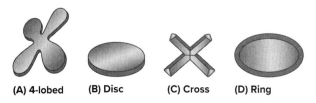

(A) 4-lobed   (B) Disc   (C) Cross   (D) Ring

FIGURE 11-4 Gastric-retentive systems which depend on size and shape.

Recap Questions

1. Why do some coated systems allow rapid absorption of the drug while others do not?
2. What is the major advantage of coating materials in a fluid bed coater?
3. What is the basic purpose of gastro-retentive systems?
4. Name three product formulation mechanisms by which a dosage form may be retained in the stomach for longer than usual.
5. Describe one mechanism that allows a floating device to float.

OSMOTIC SYSTEMS

Osmotic systems may be used in medication for oral drug administration or in implantable drug delivery devices. Only oral delivery systems will be discussed in keeping with the focus of this chapter. In external appearance, such systems resemble an ordinary coated tablet. Since they consist of an inner core containing the drug and osmotic agents (or osmogens) and operate on the principle of osmotic pressure "pumping" out a drug solution, they are referred to as osmotic pumps.

The inner core is coated with a semi-permeable membrane. This membrane allows the penetration of water into the inner core but not the diffusion of drug out of the core. A tiny hole is cut into the coating using laser technology or a mechanical drill. When this system is placed in an aqueous environment, the core absorbs water and expands. The expansion is due to the greater volume of material (water and original materials) now present within the core, in the form of a solution. The liquid within the core is under pressure because the coating restricts expansion. This pressure results in drug solution being pushed out through the delivery port(s).

Osmosis is the net movement of water across a selectively permeable membrane due to a difference in solute concentrations on either side of the membrane. The osmotic pressure is created by the soluble material, or osmogen, included in the systems. Table 11-3 provides the osmotic pressure of various substances that may be utilized for their osmotic properties. The most common osmogens that are currently used are potassium chloride, sodium chloride, and mannitol. Generally, a combination of osmogens is used to achieve the desired osmotic pressure. The proportion of each osmogen is calculated from data, such as that given in Table 11-3. In connection with such a calculation, it is important to realize that a soluble drug, itself, has an osmotic pressure which contributes to the driving force utilized by this mechanism.

Osmotic pumps release the drug at a rate that is independent of pH and the hydrodynamics of the dissolution medium. For this reason, there is a close correlation between drug release in vitro and in vivo and, in addition, there is little change in the drug release rate due to the specific location of the osmotic pump along the length of the GIT. For these reasons, the

TABLE 11-3	Osmotic Pressure of Some Osmogens
OSMOGEN	**OSMOTIC PRESSURE (ATM)***
Sodium chloride	356
Potassium chloride	245
Sucrose	150
Xylitol	104
Sorbitol	84
Dextrose	82
Citric acid	69
Tartaric acid	67
Potassium sulfate	39
Mannitol	38
Lactose	23
Fumaric acid	10

*Relates to saturated solution

osmotic pump offers favorable characteristics for drug delivery to the GIT. The first osmotic pump (the Rose-Nelson pump) was developed in Australia in the 1950s for use in farm animals. Several modifications and improvements to this initial pump have been made over the years. The two types of osmotic pumps that are most commonly used, the elementary osmotic pump and the push-pull system will be discussed.

The Elementary Osmotic Pump

Developed by Dr. Felix Theeuwes in 1974, the elementary osmotic pump was a simplification of the Rose-Nelson pump. The drug and osmogen are combined as a tablet which is then coated with cellulose acetate (Figure 11-5). A small hole is drilled through the cellulose acetate membrane. The semipermeable membrane which is present around the entire tablet allows water to be drawn in through the large surface. The soluble drug and osmogen, dissolved in water, create a saturated solution in the interior of the tablet. As the membrane is not flexible, it cannot expand. Hence, the increasing volume of water within the tablet increases the hydrostatic pressure which forces the saturated solution of drug through the laser-cut hole, in the coating, to the outside of the tablet. The osmotic pump releases the drug at an almost constant rate. This rate is proportional to the rate of inflow of water multiplied by the solubility of the materials within the tablet.

Push-Pull Osmotic Pump

The push-pull osmotic pump is a modification of the elementary osmotic pump. The push-pull osmotic pump is capable of delivering both highly water-soluble, as well as poorly water-soluble, drugs. The release rates are constant for both drug types. In physical appearance, the system resembles a conventional bilayered, coated tablet. The upper layer contains the drug combined with a polymeric osmotic agent as well as other tablet excipients. In the presence of water, this polymeric agent has the

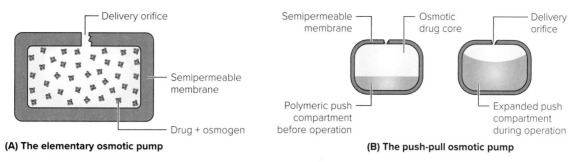

FIGURE 11-5 (A) Elementary and **(B)** push-pull osmotic pumps.

ability to form a suspension in situ. The second layer contains greater amounts of osmotic agents, as well as coloring agents, and other tablet excipients. The tableting process bonds the two layers together into a single core.

A tablet press capable of double compression is needed for the production of this type of dosage form. After the first layer is compressed, the newly-formed tablet is not ejected from the die. Instead, the die, containing the first layer, rotates with the die table and reaches a second feeder on the tablet press (see Chapter 9, Tablets, for a description of tablet press operation). This feeder contains the granular material for the second tablet layer which it feeds into the die cavity. After compression, the two-layer tablet is then ejected from the die. For purposes of this description, this two-layered tablet is considered the core. The core is then coated with a semipermeable membrane. Next, a small hole is drilled through the membrane by a laser or a mechanical drill. This is done on the side of the tablet that contains the drug.

When the tablet is placed into an aqueous medium, water is drawn into it by the osmotic agents present in both layers. The water that is drawn into the drug layer forms either a suspension or a solution, of the drug within the tablet. Suspensions will form with insoluble drugs, whereas solutions will form with soluble drugs. More water is drawn into the non-drug layer, because of the higher content of osmogens. This causes the layer to expand. As a result, it applies pressure onto the drug layer. This pressure pushes the drug suspension or the drug solution out through the small orifice.

PULSATILE DRUG DELIVERY SYSTEMS

Some drugs require immediate release from the dosage form to provide rapid, intense drug action. Other drugs require a slow, constant release from the dosage form in order to provide near-constant drug levels in body fluids. In each case, the drug release pattern is chosen to provide optimal therapy for the specific disease condition being treated, and also taking into account the properties of the drug. The latter include the solubility and partition coefficient of the drug which have an impact on the ease with which the drug can be absorbed. For some disease conditions, neither of the above-described release profiles is ideal. Ideal therapy may require no drug release for a certain time, followed by a rapid release of the drug thereafter. The no-drug release period is also known as the lag time.

An example of a product with a lag time is given in the section on chronotherapy below.

Any formulation that exhibits a lag time and then one, or more, distinct releases of the drug (ie, a pulse of drug) is referred to as a pulsatile dosage form. Two pulses of drug may be required in order to supply the drug to different parts of the GIT (spatial distribution). On the other hand, the pulses may be purposefully designed to provide the drug at different times (temporal distribution). It is possible that a dosage form designed for temporal distribution also unintentionally releases the drug in different parts of the GIT. This may occur, especially with coated beads which have a natural tendency to distribute along the length of the GIT. Enteric coating is an example of a technique to create spatial distribution of the drug.

Pulsatile drug delivery may be utilized to provide slow drug release over an extended period, such as 12 hours. This may be done by preparing, for example, three populations of drug-containing beads where each population is coated to a different extent with a coating solution that retards the release of the drug. The thickness of the coating may be increased progressively from population b to d, as depicted in Figure 11-6. The thickness of the coating in each case is chosen very carefully so that drug release occurs with different lag times after dosing. It is possible to provide both different lag times for drug release, as well as different release rates after the lag time. For example, beads may be prepared with a 4-hour lag time and then a fast release of the drug. Alternatively, there may be a 4-hour lag time followed by extended release of the drug over an additional 4 hours.

The amount of coating for each population is decided from the results of in vitro dissolution testing. For example, coated beads may be required to produce a cumulative 30% to 40% drug release in the period from 0 to 4 hours, 50% to 70% in the period from 4 to 8 hours, and 80% to 100% drug release in the period from 8 to 12 hours. This is an example of beads with a lag time followed by extended release of the drug. If the beads release more drug than the predetermined range, the extent of coating can be increased, and vice versa. The release of drug from each population of beads produces a somewhat overlapping profile. These profiles are shown in Figure 11-7. When the overall profile (of the three populations) is considered, it provides for a steady drug release over the period under consideration. A major use of pulsatile dosage forms is in chrono-therapeutics, which is described in the next section, whereas colonic delivery, which may be considered a special case of pulsatile drug delivery, is described in the last section of this chapter.

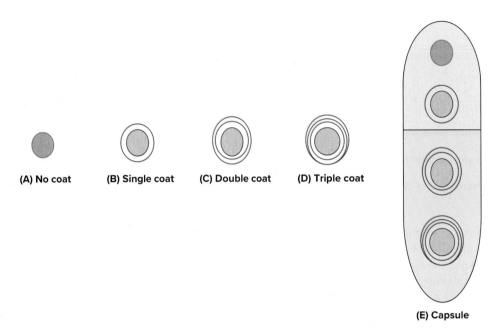

FIGURE 11-6 **Coated beads for a pulsatile delivery system, showing (A-D) pellets with different coating levels, and (E) a capsule filled with different pellet populations.** Many beads of each type are filled into one capsule.

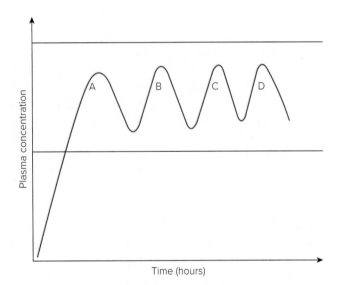

FIGURE 11-7 **Blood level-time profiles for a pulsatile drug delivery system.** The letters on the curve illustrate release from the correspondingly labeled pellets in Figure 11-6.

CHRONOTHERAPY

Many body functions fluctuate in intensity during the 24-hour cycle of each day. A specific body function may be more intense in the morning and less intense in the evening, or at some specific point during the night. The production of hormones or enzymes, for example, may vary in this way. This is a natural rhythm of the body, according to the time of day. The results of such biochemical changes allow one, for example, to be alert during the morning and sleepy at night. With reference to blood pressure, a reading of 120/80 mm Hg implies two consistent levels. The values of the systolic and diastolic pressures actually rise and fall throughout the day in a regular pattern. This is over and above any temporary changes due to emotional states, etc. This regular cycle of biological change has been built into our genetic system over millennia and is known as the circadian rhythm. Any upset of this rhythm may lead to an abnormal state of physiology.

Just as the body secretes varying quantities of hormones at different hours of the day and night, a patient with a particular illness may also need a drug in varying amounts, during the 24-hour cycle. When medication is delivered in varying amounts according to the time of the day, in accordance with the changing needs of the body, this mode of therapy is referred to as chronotherapy. The changing needs of the body are brought about by the circadian rhythm. Analogously, drug absorption at different times of the day may also differ due to physiological changes brought about by the circadian rhythm.

Using the changing blood pressure during different times of the day as an example, the rationale behind the development of a chronotherapeutic antihypertensive medication will be described. In general, blood pressure rises in the morning and falls at night. The rise in morning blood pressure may be fairly large, relative to the night-time blood pressure. For this reason, it is referred to as a surge. For patients who do not have hypertension (ie, their blood pressure is not elevated), the surge in morning blood pressure is inconsequential. On the other hand, the surge can be problematic for hypertensives. Morning surges have been correlated with an increased number of heart attacks (myocardial infarctions), stroke, and other cardiovascular events. The problem is considered worse from 6 AM to 12 noon. For this reason, these morning hours have sometimes been referred to as the morning risk zone.

Propranolol has long been used in the treatment of hypertension. There are conventional (immediate release) tablets and a long-acting version, Inderal LA. Considering the higher occurrence of cardiac events in the morning risk zone, it would be ideal to make available to the body a high dose of this drug early in the morning. This high level of medication, from 6 AM onwards, covers the patient's needs upon waking and has the potential to prevent a heart attack. How can this medication be conveniently administered to the patient so that a high level of the drug is available in the morning hours?

If a conventional tablet were given at bedtime, say 10 PM, the highest blood levels would be available long before the 6 AM period, and blood levels would then decline fairly rapidly. The only way to get high drug levels with an immediate-release dosage form is to administer the tablet very early in the morning, for example, at 4 AM which is impractical since the patient's sleep has to be interrupted to do so. The long-acting dosage form, Inderal LA, is also not a good choice for this purpose for two reasons. First, the peak blood concentration occurs about 6 hours after administration and goes down slowly for the next 12 hours. Thereafter, drug levels go down rapidly. Interestingly, this dosage form is considered a 24-hour medication, FDA-approved for once-a-day administration, in spite of this pattern of drug release. Given this release profile, it is uncertain whether Inderal LA would provide sufficiently high drug levels in the later hours of the morning if dosed at 10 PM, as previously assumed. For example, the drug level at 11 AM is expected to be very low and likely insufficient to prevent cardiac events. Ideally, drug levels should still be high at this time.

Second, a higher percentage of the drug is metabolized, compared to a conventional tablet. This is due to the fact that the slow release of the drug from the dosage form permits liver enzymes to break down a higher percentage of the drug, making less drug available to the systemic circulation. With an immediate-release dosage form, on the other hand, the enzymes are overwhelmed by the large amount of drug released, resulting in less drug metabolism. Consequently, a higher amount of the drug is actually delivered into the systemic circulation with an immediate-release drug.

Innopran® is a propranolol-containing product that was specifically developed to reduce heart attacks in the morning risk zone. It is intended to be administered at bedtime, for example, at 10 PM. The product has practically no release for about 4 to 5 hours (lag time), then drug release gradually increases, reaching a maximum level at about 12 to 14 hours after dosing. The drug levels are high during the morning risk zone to reduce cardiac events. This pattern of drug release is achieved with a capsule dosage form containing several populations of beads, prepared as described below.

The beads are formed by coating the drug and binder onto an inert base, such as non-pareil (sugar) seeds. The drug layer is built up gradually with each successive addition of the drug and the binder. The latter aids in the drug adhering to the sugar seed. After each addition, the bead is allowed to dry before the next aliquot of drug is added. When sufficient drug has been added, a sealing coat is applied. This coat prevents the drug from leaching off the bead as the next, drug-retarding, coats are applied. Between the coating layers, the beads are allowed to thoroughly dry before the next coat is applied. When sufficient coating has been applied, the beads are subjected to final drying. The entire process (drug layering, coating, and drying) may be conducted in a fluidized bed dryer. Each population of beads is coated to a different extent with drug release-retarding polymer. Predetermined quantities of each population of beads are filled into capsules, which are the final product supplied to patients. When a capsule is taken, the shell dissolves, the beads disperse in the gastrointestinal fluids and each bead releases its drug content according to the level of polymer coating that it received.

Recap Questions

1. In terms of the range of drugs that can be included, which is the more versatile system: the elementary osmotic pump or the push-pull osmotic pump?
2. Is a pulsatile dosage form developed for spatial or temporal drug delivery?
3. Could propranolol be administered by injection in the early hours of the morning (before 6 AM) to provide the desired drug cover to cardiac patients?

MATHEMATICAL MODELING OF DRUG RELEASE

The drug release pattern from a dosage form can be determined using a dissolution test as described in Chapter 711 of the USP. The data can be fitted to different rate equations to determine the best fit. In this way, the rate at which the drug is released can be mathematically modeled. The release rates can be plotted (percent drug release vs time) to yield a distinct shape. Each graph, and its equation, is associated with a theory of the release mechanism. A few basic mathematical models will be described, with special reference to sustained-release medication, to provide an understanding of the basic concepts. Many more models have been described in the literature for both sustained-release medication as well as immediate-release medication. This limited treatment of the topic is in keeping with the basic nature of this book.

First-Order Release Profile

In this profile, the rate at which a drug is released from the dosage form is dependent upon the amount of drug (raised to the power 1) remaining within the dosage form at any point in time. This means that drug release will be rapid initially (when 100% of the drug is available). Conversely, when 50% of the drug remains in the tablet, the drug release rate will be significantly lower. This type of release is described by Eq. (11-1).

$$\log A = \log A_0 + Kt/2.303 \qquad (11\text{-}1)$$

where A_0 is the initial amount of drug in solution, typically zero,

A is the cumulative amount of drug released at time t,
K is the first-order rate constant,
t is the time.

From dissolution data and a knowledge of the amount of drug originally within the tablet, the amount of drug remaining within the tablet at any time point may be calculated. For example, if the concentration of the dissolution solution is determined to be 2 mg/100 mL at 1 hour after the start of the dissolution experiment and the volume of the dissolution medium is 900 mL, then 18 mg of drug have been released. If the tablet contained 100 mg originally, then 82 mg of the drug remain within the tablet at 1 hour and the release rate is proportional to the log of this value. When the log of the cumulative amount of drug released is plotted versus time, it yields a straight line with a slope of $K/2.303$.

Zero-Order Release Profile

Zero-order release is described by Eq. (11-2). If a drug is released according to this profile, the release rate is constant. Theoretically, the release rate is proportional to the amount of drug remaining in the dosage form, raised to the power zero. Irrespective of the amount of drug present in the dosage form, this term equals 1. This means that the rate of drug release is independent of the amount remaining in the dosage form. Whether the dosage form has its initial drug load (100%) or only 10% remaining, the rate of drug release is the same. This is in sharp contrast to the first-order release profile where the release rate is constantly decreasing.

$$A_t = A_0 + K_0 t \qquad (11\text{-}2)$$

where A_t is the amount of drug released at time t,

A_0 is the initial amount of the drug in solution (most often = 0),
K_0 is the zero-order release constant, and
t is time.

The amount of drug remaining in the dosage form at any time, t, can be calculated from the results of a dissolution experiment, as described above for first-order release. When the amount of drug released is plotted as A_t versus time, a straight line results. This line has a slope of K_0. The zero-order release profile is ideal since the drug is released at a constant rate throughout the release period. For a sustained-release tablet, if 10% of the drug content of the tablet is released in the first hour, the amount released in the last hour is also 10%. This means that a constant amount of the drug is supplied to the body for absorption. This release profile provides the best conditions for consistent absorption and, after an initial adjustment phase, blood levels of the drug can be expected to be relatively constant. Naturally, there are biological factors that influence the blood level at any point in time; it is not only the release rate from the dosage form that has an impact. Because a zero-order release profile presents the best opportunity, from a drug formulation perspective, for the most consistent (or zero order) *absorption*, it is considered the ideal release profile. Frequently, the zero-order release profile cannot be achieved with practical dosage form. At best, a portion of the release profile is zero order. The latter is an extremely desirable profile to have for MR dosage forms.

Higuchi Release Profile

Dr. Takeru Higuchi developed an equation to take account of the many factors that influence drug release from ER matrix tablets. As mentioned above, this involves the penetration of water into the tablet (through tortuous channels), dissolution of the drug, and diffusion of the drug in solution form out of the tablet through the same tortuous channels. The channels are described as tortuous, meaning that they have numerous, sharp bends in them. These channels take on this irregular shape since they are formed by the spaces between tablet particles. The dissolution of the drug depends on its solubility and the volume of water available for its dissolution in the channel adjacent to a drug particle. This channel is located in the interior of the tablet. Likewise, the exit of the drug in solution from the interior of the tablet depends on many factors. These include the tortuosity of the channels, and the amount of drug already dissolved in the water in a specific channel. The equation that Dr. Higuchi developed is very complex but, many factors can be combined into one constant, the Higuchi constant. Upon so doing, the equation is vastly simplified, and the amount of drug released at any time is equal to the product of the Higuchi constant multiplied by the square root of time (Eq. [11-3]).

$$A = K \cdot t^{1/2} \qquad (11\text{-}3)$$

Drug release is rapid initially and then slows down progressively. Toward the end of the release period, drug release gets progressively slower and reaches a "plateau." As Eq. (11-3) indicates, a plot of the amount of drug released at time, t, versus the square root of time will result in a straight line. Hence, this equation is also referred to as the "square root of time" equation. The line has a slope of K, the Higuchi constant.

The problem with the Higuchi profile is the fact that the release rate in the initial period is very rapid and that, toward the end of the release profile, it is extremely slow. In some situations, the initial rapid release may be viewed in a positive light: it provides the drug rapidly for the initial pharmacological effect. However, the slowing down of drug release in such an extreme manner, as occurs toward the end of the release profile, cannot be justified under any circumstances. Even the rapid initial release is only beneficial for MR drugs that are taken occasionally, for example, an antihistamine product which is only taken when the patient experiences allergic symptoms. A drug product of this type could provide rapid relief of symptoms, due to the initial rapid drug release, and then continued relief over a prolonged period. For MR medication that is taken on a daily basis, the initial "burst" effect is undesirable. For this type of medication slow, consistent release of the drug over the entire release period is desired because it results in steady uptake of drug and more consistent blood levels.

Recap Questions

1. In your own words explain what is meant by a "first-order" release profile.
2. What is the major advantage of zero-order drug release?
3. Why is the Higuchi profile also called the square root of time profile?

COLONIC DRUG DELIVERY

The colon may be afflicted by several disease conditions which can have a major impact on a patient's lifestyle. These diseases include Crohn's disease, ulcerative colitis, and irritable bowel syndrome (IBS). These are all conditions which affect a section of the GIT. They may be treated by dosage forms administered via either the oral, or rectal, end of the GIT. Rectal dosage forms are more difficult to develop and produce, may have less patient acceptance in several countries (including the United States), and may, therefore, result in lower patient compliance. By contrast, the methods utilized for orally-administered dosage forms are easier to develop and manufacture commercially. Manufacturing includes processes such as tablet compression and coating. While these techniques are not necessarily easy to perform, they are well-known and encountered routinely in the pharmaceutical industry. They are usually cheaper to produce and enjoy greater patient compliance than the typical rectally delivered dosage form, intended for the same purpose.

In keeping with the title of this chapter, only orally-administered dosage forms used to treat these conditions will be discussed. There are several marketed formulations (some examples are given in Table 11-4), and their development may be considered to be an extension of oral MR. These products have proven to be a boon to patients. Rectal dosage forms for these conditions are discussed in Chapter 24, Rectal and Vaginal Drug Delivery, since their development is in line with other dosage forms discussed in the latter chapter.

When rectal administration is used for colonic delivery, it places the medication at, or close to, the site of action. Conversely, oral administration, for this purpose, involves passage of the dosage form through a large part of the GIT before it reaches the intended area of therapy. An oral dosage form must enable most of the dose to reach the colon. The drug should not be destroyed by the harsh conditions in the GIT, nor should it be metabolized during its passage. It must also not be absorbed significantly in any earlier segment of the GIT.

Absorption elsewhere in the GIT limits the effective amount of drug available for its action in reducing disease symptoms in the colon. The desired drug effect is brought about by a topical action in the colon, or by absorption into colonic tissues; systemic absorption in the colon is not required for the treatment of colonic diseases. Hence, if any absorption occurs in the small intestine, it not only reduces the amount of drug available to the colon but may also lead to unwanted effects. (As explained later, colonic delivery for systemic effects may be desirable for other disease conditions.)

Drugs suitable for colonic delivery fall into two categories:

1. Those that are needed for local effects within the colon. These drugs are used to treat colonic dysfunction such as the conditions mentioned above.

2. Drugs needed for systemic action. Some drugs needed for systemic action are better absorbed in the colon. This may appear contradictory since most drugs are better absorbed in the small intestine (as they should since the latter is the organ specifically designed for absorption). There are, however, some drugs that are better absorbed in the colon and this route may effectively be used to treat non-colonic diseases. This group includes the anti-anginal drugs, such as isosorbide dinitrate. In addition, drugs that degrade in the stomach acids (eg, peptides such as insulin), and those that undergo extensive hepatic first-pass metabolism (eg, corticosteroids) may benefit from the dosage forms releasing their drug content in the colon.

Features of the Colon That Affect Drug Delivery

The features of the colon that influence drug delivery are very briefly summarized below:

Transit Time

Healthy subjects have a very long colonic transit time (about 52 hours, on average). As the dosage form passes from one end

TABLE 11-4	Some Marketed Colon Delivery Products				
TRADE NAME	DRUG NAME	DOSAGE FORM	ROUTE	TECHNOLOGY	PATHOLOGY
Canasa	5-aminosalicylic acid	Suppository	Rectal	Fatty base	Ulcerative colitis
Anucort-HC	Hydrocortisone acetate 25 mg	Suppository	Rectal	Fatty base	Ulcerative colitis
Asacol	Mesalazine	Tablet	Oral	DR	Ulcerative colitis & Crohn's disease
Pentasa		Capsule	Oral	Pulsatile (beads)	
Colal-Pred	Prednisolone	Capsule	Oral	Pellets	
MMX	Budenoside	Tablet	Oral	Multimatrix	
Uceris		Tablet	Oral	ER	
Clipper		Tablet	Oral	enteric coated, ER	
Azulfidine	Sulfasalazine	Tablet	Oral	DR	

of the colon to the other, the drug is slowly released. This is a very long time for drug absorption to occur. Transit times may be shortened by some disease states such as Crohn's disease and ulcerative colitis, the average transit time for the latter being approximately 24 hours. The transit time may also be affected by the presence of food residues.

Fluid Volume

The colonic fluid volume is approximately 13 mL, with a range of 1 to 44 mL. This volume may be insufficient for the dissolution of some dosage forms and, therefore, presents a challenge to adequate and consistent drug delivery.

Viscosity of Contents

The colon has a high water-absorbing capacity and is capable of absorbing 90% of the water entering it. Due to this action, the colonic contents have less water than is present in the contents of other parts of the GIT. The low water content produces the high viscosity of colonic material.

pH

In general, the pH is higher in the colon compared to the small intestine. However, the pH of the colon may be lowered due to the consumption of large amounts of carbohydrates. These complex molecules are broken down into polysaccharides by digestive mechanisms located in the proximal segments of the GIT. Polysaccharides reaching the colon are fermented by colonic bacteria, resulting in the formation of short-chain fatty acids. The latter lower the pH of the colonic contents. Since the dissolution of drugs is affected by the pH of the medium, diet may have an indirect effect on drug dissolution in the colon.

Enzymes

The colon contains over 400 species of aerobic and anaerobic microorganisms which produce numerous enzymes, including those that metabolize drugs and deactivate some harmful metabolites. These microorganisms are able to ferment certain carbohydrates (which are not digested in the proximal regions of the small intestine) as well as proteins. This characteristic is interestingly utilized in drug delivery, as explained under the Formulation Factors section below.

Drug Solubility

Since the colon has a low volume of water, the choice of drug used for colonic delivery is significant. In the first instance, the drug may not efficiently dissolve in the colonic liquid. On the other hand, there is an interplay between drug dissolution rate and drug absorption rate. For example, a drug may not be very soluble and, therefore, will not fully dissolve in the volume of aqueous fluid available. This drug may, nevertheless, display a high bioavailability, provided its absorption rate is high. By way of example, suppose only 20% of the drugs are able to dissolve in the available liquid in the colon. If the dissolved drug is rapidly absorbed, the colonic fluid will then have a low concentration of this drug, enabling further dissolution to occur. As this process continues, the drug will be efficiently absorbed and the resulting bioavailability is higher than would be estimated from solubility data alone. The rapid absorption of the drug in the small volume of liquid can be considered to "clear" the liquid of its drug content, enabling further dissolution of the drug to occur.

Formulation Factors

Dosage forms, such as tablets intended for colonic delivery, may be coated with certain polysaccharides which resist the acidic conditions of the stomach as well as the enzymes present in the upper GIT. The coated dosage form, or the coated sub-units of a dosage form (such as beads), therefore, pass unscathed into the colon. Here, the colonic (anaerobic) bacteria ferment these polysaccharides, resulting in the breaking down of their coating. As this occurs, the drug contained in the dosage forms is released for absorption by the colon.

This is a convenient way to manufacture colonic delivery systems and this technique has been utilized in the development of drug products. Polysaccharides used for this purpose include pectin (the first polysaccharide to be utilized in this way), guar gum, and chitosan. The drug may also be embedded in a matrix of the polysaccharide material which then serves not only to release the drug preferentially in the colon but also acts as a MR mechanism.

A drug may be chemically linked to another moiety so that the entire molecule, thus formed, is pharmacologically inactive. When the link is broken, the active drug is released once more. This is the basis of the prodrug approach to drug delivery. In this approach, the link is chosen such that it is preferentially broken only in a particular part of the body. This may be a region where the drug's activity is required, or where the drug is effectively absorbed. If release of the active drug is desirable in the colon only, the drug may be linked by a bond that can only be broken by colonic bacterial enzymes. This ensures that the prodrug is transmitted intact through the GIT, and the drug is only released when the bond is enzymatically cleaved by colonic bacteria. Azo conjugates are commonly used in the prodrug approach. The utility of this method depends on the drug compound having a nitrogen atom that is capable of forming an azo bond.

Sulphasalazine is the oldest drug used to treat ulcerative colitis. It consists of 5-amino salicylic acid (mesalamine) and sulfapyridine joined by a diazo bond. Without this derivatization, a large part of the mesalamine would be absorbed in the jejunum and little would reach the colon where it is needed to treat ulcerative colitis. The azo bond in sulphasalazine is cleaved enzymatically by azoreductases, produced by colonic bacteria to release its constituents as shown in Figure 11-8. Thus, mesalamine can be absorbed in large quantities in the region where it is needed. A newer derivative is olsalazine sodium which consists of two 5-amino salicylic units joined by a diazo bond. When this bond is cleaved in the colon, two mesalamine units are released, as also shown in Figure 11-8. Thus, the latter compound is more potent. In addition, it does not have the side effects of sulfapyridine, which are mainly dermal manifestations of allergy and increased skin sensitivity to sunlight. Where an active moiety is linked to an inactive component, for the release of the active component after consumption, in a specific region of the body, the process is referred to as the prodrug approach.

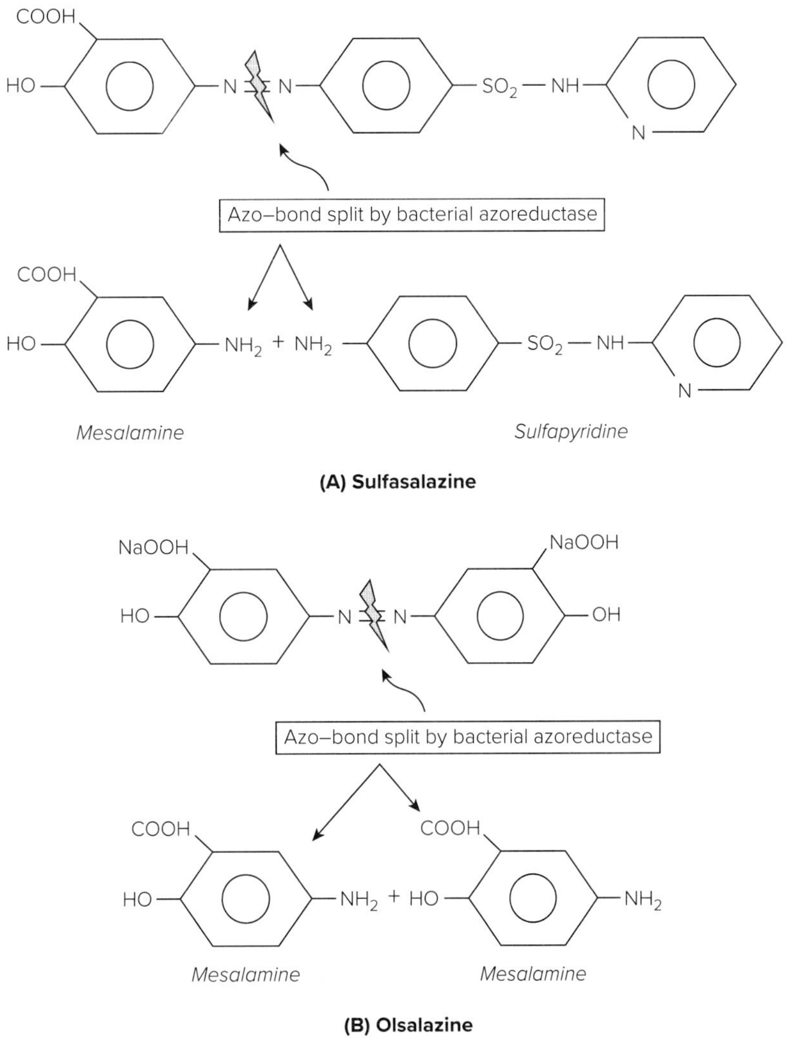

(A) Sulfasalazine

Mesalamine   *Sulfapyridine*

Mesalamine   *Mesalamine*

(B) Olsalazine

FIGURE 11-8 Chemical structure and enzymatic cleavage of (A) Sulfasalazine and (B) Olsalazine.

Some types of colonic delivery products use neither the technique of enzymatically-labile coating nor the prodrug approach. Instead, such formulations use the approach of releasing the drug in the ileum, rather than the colon, for transmittal through the ileo-cecal valve to the colon where the drug activity is needed. The rationale is that during the short travel from the ileum to the colon, drug degradation and absorption would be insignificant. Some marketed colonic delivery products are listed in Table 11-5.

TABLE 11-5 Some Marketed Osmotic Pumps

PRODUCT NAME	DRUG	SUPPLIER
Cardura XL	Doxazosin mesylate	Pfizer
Adalat OROS	Nifedipine	Bayer
Procardia XL	Nifedipine	Pfizer
Glucotrol	Glipizide	Pfizer
Invega	Paliperidone	Janssen
Ditropan XL	Oxybutynin chloride	Janssen
Concerta	Methylphenidate	Janssen

Recap Questions

1. What are the two routes of administration for colonic delivery products?
2. How do polysaccharides consumed in the diet affect the pH of colonic contents?
3. How can enzymes be usefully utilized in colonic delivery?
4. Why should a drug to treat ulcerative colitis not be absorbed in the upper GIT?

SUMMARY POINTS

- MR dosage forms have been developed with a specific clinical purpose.
- The formulation of MR products must take into account physiological factors that affect drug release, stability, and absorption.

- MR oral products include matrix tablets, coated multi-particulates, gastro-retentive systems, osmotic systems, and orally administered colonic delivery formulations.
- Drug release from MR dosage forms may be mathematically modeled, and the respective equations allow pharmaceutical scientists to predict how much drug will be released at any specific time after administration.
- Osmotic systems approach zero-order drug release.

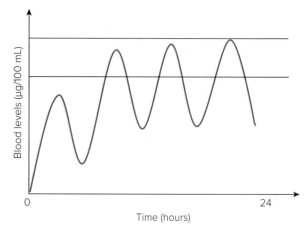

FIGURE 11-9 **Blood level vs time plot for question 10.**

What do you think?

1. Clinical studies of a newly formulated hydrophobic matrix tablet reveal that drug release is slightly slower than desired. Name two formulation techniques that can be used to increase the rate of drug dissolution from the tablets.

2. With reference to question 1 above, describe the design of an experiment that could prove that the formulation techniques that you recommended improved drug dissolution from the matrix tablet.

3. A hydrophilic matrix tablet is prepared from hydroxypropyl methyl cellulose, using ethylcellulose dissolved in ethanol as the binder to form granules for compression of the tablet. Does this binder contribute to the modified-release effect of the matrix? Explain your answer.

4. Assume you are a pharmacist practicing at a hospital. How would you answer if your pharmaceutical technician asks you the following question: "If a drug is rapidly absorbed in the proximal part of the small intestine, rapid drug delivery will result, and this is an advantage. Why should special formulations be used to slow down drug release and absorption?

5. As a research project, a pharmaceutical scientist substitutes a newly-available hydrophilic polymer for the previously-used polymer in his company's hydrophilic matrix tablet. If the previously-used polymer took 6 minutes to hydrate and become viscous, what is the impact of the new polymer which takes 22 minutes to hydrate and become viscous? Explain.

6. Make a series of color drawings to illustrate the appearance of a hydrophilic matrix tablet at 4 hours, 8 hours, and 12 hours postadministration. The tablet is intended to release the drug over 12 hours. Make comparative drawings to show the release of drug from a non-disintegrating plastic matrix tablet which also releases the drug over 12 hours.

7. How is the small hole formed in an osmotic pump? What do you think would be the impact of the hole getting blocked? Is it conceivable that the hole could get blocked during normal use?

8. Osmotic systems demonstrate strong agreement between in vitro dissolution and in vivo drug release.

Explain the advantage of this statement with respect to the development of osmotic systems for commercial use.

9. If you coated tablets and beads with the same thickness of coating material, for aesthetic reasons, explain which formulation would require more polymeric coating material. Assume both formulations contain the same amount of the drug.

10. If a single dosage form (taken at $t = 0$) gave the profile shown in Figure 11-9, what is the type of controlled-release dosage form?

11. Consider two methods to treat a condition localized in the colon:
    a. An orally administered colonic delivery dosage form, and
    b. The same drug, in the same dose, administered as a regular dosage form which releases the drug for absorption in the small intestine and subsequent circulation through the cardiovascular system to the colon. Are the two methods of drug delivery equivalent? Explain.

12. Controlled-release drug delivery may involve temporal or spatial control of the release of the drug. How would you categorize a dosage form which contains the drug embedded in pectin?

13. What is the physiological reason for the reduction in water content of the colonic contents?

14. If an antibiotic that the patient takes kills all the flora of the GIT, what impact could this have on the delivery of orally-administered colonic delivery products?

BIBLIOGRAPHY

http://www.insitevision.com/about.html. Accessed September 24, 2017.

Murphy C, Pillay V, Choonara YE, et al. Optimization of a dual mechanism gastrofloatable and gastroadhesive delivery system for narrow absorption window drugs. *AAPS PharmSciTech.* 2012;13(1):1.

Injections

12

PREVIEW

- Why injections are needed and how they contribute to appropriate therapy
- The different types of injections and a brief accounting of how they are made
- The therapeutic benefits of some of the extended-release injections available
- Sterilization methods
- A brief overview of relevant quality control tests for injections

INTRODUCTION

This chapter describes the formulation, production, testing, and utility of formulations intended to be injected into the body. Most often the formulations are supplied in the liquid state but they may also be supplied as dried powders, to which a suitable solvent is added, for the reconstitution of the liquid formulation. In general, the injection route of drug administration is used under the following circumstances:

1. When a rapid drug effect is needed: This may occur in an emergency situation, for example, EpiPen (epinephrine) for

the reversal of anaphylactic shock; or when an initial, rapid antibiotic effect is needed; or for rapid relief of pain.

2. Conversely, when a very long drug effect is desired: A long-acting medication may be injected intramuscularly, this leaves a reservoir or a "depot" of the injection material in the muscle from which the drug is slowly released. This results in slow absorption, providing drug effectiveness over a period of weeks to months. Considering the long duration of action, "extended release" (ER) for injections has a different timeframe than that for oral dosage forms.

3. When the patient is unconscious: Such a patient cannot take oral medication; an injection is useful for the treatment of an unconscious accident victim, for example.

4. When the drug is poorly absorbed or ineffective by other routes of drug administration: Most peptide drugs display very low bioavailability when administered orally and are usually poorly absorbed by alternate routes as well, whereas an injection provides acceptable therapy. However, the development of such drugs into non-injectable formulations is a very active area of pharmaceutical research, especially when the drug is intended for chronic use. Such a formulation would avoid the pain and inconvenience of repeated injections.

5. An injection may be used to administer a drug to an uncooperative patient: This has utility under very limited circumstances, due to legal restrictions concerning personal liberties and consent. However, it does find significant utility in mental institutions, for example.

The bird's eye view of injection preparation may give the impression of a relatively simple process: prepare a solution or suspension, package it in specialized containers, and sterilize it. This view is deceptive as each of these steps is complex. In addition, stability considerations must be taken into account. Injection production is a rapidly expanding technology that is influenced by discoveries in several related fields. Injections, in addition to being sterile, must be relatively pyrogen free. Pyrogens are endotoxins produced by gram-negative bacteria. If injected intravenously, especially in higher amounts, it will cause a fever and a reduction in blood pressure. As a result of these factors, the formulation and development of injections is complex.

The difficulty with respect to preparing the solution is that many drugs are insoluble, or very poorly soluble, in water. Hence, special additives, called solubility enhancers, must be used. Several new solubility enhancers have been developed in recent years. In some systems, an alternate solvent, or a co-solvent system is used. The latter is a mixture of solvents to be used in specific proportion. Solubility enhancers are a sub-group of surfactants with a specific range of hydrophilic-lipophilic balance. These additives must be non-toxic and have a very low irritation potential to the body, as is the case for all additives used in injection technology. Irritation at the injection site is a particular concern. While ingredients used for any dosage form should be non-irritating, this is a particularly stringent requirement for injections due to the invasive nature of the dosage form.

Furthermore, in many cases, drugs are unstable in water or when exposed to the atmosphere. To address the first concern, a sterile powder (Powder for Injection) may be presented in a sealed container. Upon the addition of sterile water for injections (WFI), the injectable solution, or suspension, is formed. The powder may be prepared, as a freeze-dried powder. This technology is complex and has seen several advancements in recent years. Where the powder is sensitive to oxygen, the dry powder is packaged under nitrogen and sealed to inhibit the entry of oxygen (and moisture) from the atmosphere.

When a suspension is used, the particles must be of a fine size and possess specific properties, such as easy dispersibility in a liquid medium after an extended period of standing. Powder technology has improved tremendously in recent years, enabling the formulation of better suspensions. However, this advance has, also, made the injection production process more complex since the powders are produced specifically for, and as a part of, the injection manufacturing process. Recent advances and better understanding of the requirements for good injections have vastly improved their quality. An important requirement is the limitations on foreign particulate matter in the final product. The enhanced knowledge of, and compliance with, the requirements for good injections has increased the difficulty of manufacturing such products. In addition, the extent and sophistication of quality control needed to deliver an acceptable product has also increased.

The USP recognizes five types of injections, based on their physical state. These are listed below with the naming convention for injections of each type given after each description. As used in this section, [DRUG] denotes the name of the drug, for example, Amoxicillin. Mind Map 12-1 summarizes the types, routes of administration and sterilization methods for injections.

1. Liquid preparations that are drug solutions or consist of liquid drug – [DRUG] Injection.

2. Dry solids to which a suitable sterile vehicle is added to form the injectable solution – [DRUG] for Injection.

3. Liquid formulations that are emulsions containing the dissolved or dispersed drug – [DRUG] Injectable Emulsion.

4. Liquid preparations that are suspensions of solids in a suitable liquid medium – [DRUG] Injectable Suspension.

5. Dry solids that require the addition of a suitable liquid to form an injectable suspension – [DRUG] for Injectable Suspension.

ROUTES OF INJECTION

The most common routes of injection are as follows:

Intravenous (IV)

This injection is given into a vein, usually one that is superficial and therefore easily accessible. It is a very common route, used for many different types of drugs in small volume (a few mL) in which case drug effects are rapidly noticed; or fluid replacement/parenteral nutrition which is administered in large volumes, such as 1 L.

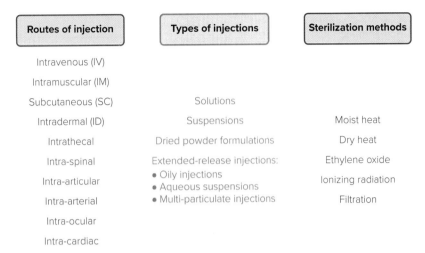

MIND MAP 12-1 **Types, routes of administration, and sterilization methods for injections**

Intramuscular (IM)

This injection is given into a muscle, usually a large muscle such as the ventro gluteal or deltoid. Aqueous solutions injected intramuscularly have a slower pharmacological effect than the injection delivered intravenously. It may, therefore, seem surprising that an EpiPen injection, which is used to reverse anaphylactic shock, is given intramuscularly. However, epinephrine administered intravenously will have an extremely rapid effect which could cause the heart to stop beating. The intramuscular injection has a slower, yet sufficiently rapid, effect. Thus, the assertion that IV injections of aqueous solutions are more rapid than similar IM injections is still valid. The reason for the slower absorption is the fact that the drug must diffuse through dense muscle tissue to reach capillaries for systemic absorption. The rate of absorption is also related to the particular muscle into which the injection is given due to the relative density of the muscle and the blood flow rate to that muscle. More dense muscle results in slower absorption, and faster blood flow to a particular muscle results in quicker absorption in that muscle. As an example, absorption from the gluteus maximus is slower than that from the deltoid muscle. Absorption from suspensions injected intramuscularly will also be slower than absorption from solutions, primarily due to the rate of drug dissolution from the suspended particles.

Subcutaneous (SC)

This injection is given under the skin and is also known as a hypodermic injection. Various types of insulin injections, with varying duration of action, are given by this method. A drug in solution must diffuse toward the veins located in the subcutaneous region in order to permeate them. If the drug is administered in suspension form (as is the case for some insulin formulations), dissolution of the drug must first occur from the suspended particles before diffusion and absorption can occur. Thus, there are several steps in the absorption process and the rate of absorption subcutaneously will be slower than an intravenous injection.

Intradermal (ID)

These injections are given into the skin. Usually, a very short needle is used to reduce the possibility of entering the subcutaneous area. This route is used for diagnostic agents and vaccines. The forearm is commonly used for the administration of allergy test substances by this route because of its accessibility and because the skin is thinner in this region.

Intrathecal

These injections are administered into the intrathecal space, surrounding the spinal cord, which contains spinal fluid. A common use of this type of injection is for the administration of an anesthetic to alleviate pain during childbirth.

Intra-spinal

This injection is given within the spinal column.

Intra-articular

These injections are given into a joint for the relief of inflammation and pain, and they have an extended duration of action. They are useful for patients with arthritis, for example. Since the injection, itself, causes short-duration pain, it is usually administered with, or after, a local anesthetic. Care must be taken to deliver the injection within the joint capsule.

Intra-arterial

This route, which involves injection directly into an artery, is not routinely used. One reason for this is the fact that arteries are less accessible, being situated deeper within tissues. Veins are more superficial and are therefore more accessible.

Intra-ocular

Intra-ocular (into the eye) injections are avoided, unless absolutely necessary, because of the danger of damaging the retina. They are given by ophthalmologists for serious eye diseases that cannot be treated adequately with topical formulations. These diseases often lead to blindness and oral medication is of practically no use. For a description of some of the conditions that are treated with intra-ocular injections, see Chapter 23, Ophthalmic Drug Delivery.

Intra-cardiac

Intra-cardiac injections are rare and are used in an emergency to reinstate the beating of a heart that has stopped.

> ## Recap Questions
>
> 1. Mention three reasons why injection formulation is not as easy as would initially appear.
> 2. What is the major difference between IV injections, and I/M injections when the latter contains suspended particles?
> 3. Why are intra-spinal and intra-ocular injections not given routinely?
> 4. Distinguish between subcutaneous and intradermal injections.

GENERAL FORMULATION CONSIDERATIONS

Pharmaceutical injections may take the form of a drug in an aqueous solution (usually with other excipients), a drug dissolved in a non-aqueous solution (usually an acceptable oil), a drug suspended in an aqueous or oily vehicle (usually with a suspending agent), and a drug in one of the phases of an emulsion. Oily injections are not intended for intravenous administration for the following reason: Upon admixture with blood, the oil will be broken up into large drops and these may occlude small blood vessels, especially those in the pulmonary circulation. Pulmonary embolism, which is the result of this event, can cause rapid death. In the case of an O/W emulsion, the droplet size of the oil must be verified to be 1 μm, or less, to prevent blockage of small blood vessels. In addition, the drug may be supplied as a dry powder to which a suitable vehicle is added at the time of injection. Typically, the added vehicle is WFI and, where a more complex vehicle is required, the manufacturer will supply this vehicle in a separate vial.

All pharmaceuticals for human consumption must be prepared under Good Manufacturing Practices (GMP) conditions, as described in Chapter 16, Good Manufacturing Practices. However, the requirements of current GMP are more rigid with respect to the manufacture of injections. Injectables are required to be sterilized and, frequently, they are sterilized as the last, or terminal, step of the production process. This fact must not be construed as freedom to work in a manner that is not scrupulously clean. A clean environment and clean equipment are required to reduce the micro-organism load, to the absolute minimum, before sterilization occurs. All personnel working in the manufacturing area must pay strict attention to personal hygiene, wash up thoroughly (according to written procedures), and follow gowning procedures before they enter the manufacturing area.

SOLUTIONS

Solutions are manufactured in scrupulously clean mixing tanks of a capacity that is typically in the hundreds of liters. The active ingredient and excipients are dissolved in the liquid medium which, most commonly, is WFI. If the drug is poorly soluble, solubilizing agents are included to increase the solubility, or the rate of solution. Since solubility is also affected by pH in the case of ionizable drugs, in accordance with the Henderson-Hasselbach equation, the pH of the solution is also adjusted. The pH must be within the acceptable range for the tissue into which the solution is to be injected. In addition, the aqueous solution should be isotonic and osmotic agents may be added for this reason. Examples of excipients that are usually added to aqueous injections are given in Table 12-1. In the pharmacy curriculum, the "pH-partition theory" is typically described in a Physical Pharmacy course, and "isotonicity" in the Calculations course. These topics will not be described in this chapter. Drugs for injection into certain tissues, such as muscle, may also be dissolved in oils, if soluble. This type of formulation is described under the "Extended-Release Injections" section in this chapter.

Manufacturing

Manufacturing may be done by two techniques: "conventional" production of an injection solution or suspension, filling into vials, followed by terminal sterilization; and compounding with sterilized ingredients and sterile equipment, using aseptic techniques. The first step of the manufacturing process is the preparation of the components used in both the manufacturing and the packaging of the injection.

Washing of Vials and Equipment

The FDA recommends an area with the classification class 100,000 (ISO 8) cleanliness for equipment cleaning. This class is less stringent than the one for final injection production. When terminal sterilization is used, thorough cleaning is needed to reduce the microbial load for the final sterilization and, also, to reduce endotoxins within the product.

For aseptic manufacturing, all equipment and primary packaging materials (vials, closures, etc.) must first be thoroughly cleaned and then sterilized. Preparation of materials for sterilization involves repeated washing cycles, with adequate rinsing in between. This removes foreign particulate matter, and reduces the bioburden and the endotoxin load. Well-designed equipment is easily disassembled, cleaned, sanitized, and sterilized, and then easily re-assembled. As described later, manufacturing of the final product also involves the pumping of the injection liquid through tubes and the final filling of vials through needles. Tubes and needles may be difficult to clean. In such instances, it may be cheaper to use disposable components that are used for one batch only. While this may sound counterintuitive, the cost incurred is mainly for the required cleaning verification. The verification process involves experimental work to demonstrate that the cleaning procedure is effective in adequately cleaning the equipment and demonstrating that it is free from all constituents of the batch, especially the drug, before the next batch is made. Cleaning verification is time-consuming

TABLE 12-1	Some Common Excipients Used in Injections	
Category	**Examples**	**Usual Concentration (%)**
Antimicrobial preservative	Benzalkonium chloride	0.01
	Benzethonium chloride	0.01
	Benzyl alcohol	1-2
	Chlorbutanol	0.25-0.5
	Phenylmercuric nitrate and acetate	0.002
	Methyl p-hydroxybenzoate (methyl paraben)	0.2
	Propyl p-hydroxybenzoate (propyl paraben)	0.02
Antioxidants	Ascorbic acid	0.01
	Butylhydroxyanisole (BHA)	0.02
	Butylhydroxytoluene (BHT)	0.02
	Sodium metabisulfite	0.2
Buffers	Citric acid + salt (eg, sodium citrate) (pH 2.5- 6)	1-5
	Acetic acid + salt (eg, sodium acetate) (pH 3.5-5.7)	1-2
	Phosphoric acid salts (pH 6-8.2)	0.8-2
Tonicity adjustment	Dextrose	Up to 5.5
	Sodium chloride	Up to 0.9
	Mannitol	Up to 5
Chelating agent	Ethylenediaminetetraacetic acid (EDTA) salts, eg, NaEDTA	0.01-0.075

and, therefore, expensive. A detailed description of cleaning verification is beyond the scope of this chapter.

The quality of water to be used, in the various cleaning steps, is described in an FDA guideline. "Purified Water," as defined in the USP, must be used for the initial washing and rinsing steps, while WFI, as defined in the USP, must be used for the final rinsing step. The latter is used for the preparation of injectable solutions and, therefore, it makes sense to use it in the final rinse. All detergents should be avoided, if possible. This is because trace amounts of detergent may remain, even after extensive rinsing, and may contaminate the product. The time between washing, drying, and sterilizing should be minimized since residual moisture, even in trace amounts, can support microbial growth and endotoxin production.

Siliconization

Siliconization refers to the application of a thin film of silicone to the primary packaging components of an injection, for example, the syringe parts. Treatment of the syringe, in this manner, enables easier, smooth action. Silicone oil is available in different grades which differ with respect to their viscosity. Lower viscosity grades spread more evenly. Siliconization also treats the surface of glass, sealing microcracks and leaving a smoother surface. In addition, it facilitates the complete emptying of vials and syringes.

Parts of the primary packaging that are in direct contact with the medication, are usually siliconized. These parts include vials, syringe barrels, stoppers, and syringe needles. This decreases the residual volume of the injection after administration is complete. Since an injection must be administered at the recommended dose, the residual volume is compensated by an over-fill at the time of the filling of the syringe. Since the residual volume is less with siliconization, the required over-fill is also less, resulting in less drug loss.

Where the injectable formulation is sold as a liquid-filled syringe (ie, in the primary packaging), siliconization of the barrel is required to make it easier to eject the dose. The siliconized barrel moves with less applied force. The smooth functioning of the barrel is particularly important in auto-injectors and may also be important for injections that are self-administered daily, for example, insulin injection. Silicon oil, spread evenly over the syringe barrel results in less force needed to eject the injectable liquid. The silicone oil must be compatible with the drug and its volume should be such that it does not detach from the wall of the syringe. Excess silicone oil will detach from the syringe wall since only a specific volume, dependent on the surface area of the barrel, will attach to the wall and remain there as a thin film. Stopper siliconization assists with stopper insertion into a vial and, hence, makes processing easier. The fact that stoppers do not stick to each other during processing, when a large number of stoppers are present in one part of the filling apparatus, is also due to siliconization.

Syringe needles are siliconized to facilitate needle insertion into the skin which also reduces pain. Silicone oil may be sprayed onto glass surfaces to be treated or wiped on (mechanically) with a cloth. It may also be applied as an oil in water emulsion. In the latter case, the water and emulsifying agents are driven off by heating the vials to 250°C to 300°C. This process is referred to as "baking" of the silicone onto the glass. Covalent bonding occurs between the added silicone oil molecules and the molecules of silicone on the glass surface. These bonds are of the type Si-O-Si. Uneven distribution of silicone oil results in the barrel moving easily sometimes, and only with difficulty at other times. Such a situation represents a more serious problem with auto-injectors.

Compounding the Solution

For the vast majority of injectable formulations, the preparation of the bulk solution (ie, the large volume prior to subdivision into small individual containers) involves simple dissolution of soluble ingredients in WFI. This relatively simple procedure, as mentioned earlier, is complicated by several factors the most important of which is the need to minimize contamination by organisms and particulate matter. The solution consists of one or more soluble active ingredients and several excipients, including osmotic adjusting substances, buffers, and possibly bacteriostatic agents.

At a very basic level, the procedure is similar to the compounding of a small-volume oral solution, a procedure with which students may be familiar. The mixing conditions depend on the solubility of the added ingredients. If all ingredients are highly soluble, a simple propeller mixer may be sufficient to bring about complete dissolution of the ingredients. If poorly soluble ingredients (or those that have a slow dissolution rate) are used, special impellers which confer improved mixing may be needed. These impellers may also be needed if very high concentrations of soluble ingredients are required in the formulation.

To avoid the formation of a vortex in the liquid, the impeller may be placed off-center. A vortex results in minimal mixing but significant air entrapment. The latter causes problems during the pumping of liquid for filling operations. Any foam that is pumped into a final container makes it difficult to provide an accurate volume. To reduce vortex formation, baffles may be attached, at an angle, to the wall of the container. The baffles are flat elements made of the same material as the container, which is frequently stainless steel.

The nature and quantity of the ingredients in a formulation may also necessitate the use of an elevated temperature so that dissolution is completed in a reasonable time. It is imperative that the drug, and all ingredients, are stable at the processing temperature. From the above, it is clear that a pharmaceutical scientist, before developing the procedure for manufacturing an injectable formulation, would have to determine the solubility of all ingredients in the formulation and, possibly, also their heat stability. This information may be obtained from reference books such as the *United States Pharmacopeia*, the *Merck Index or Martindale*, the *Extra Pharmacopeia*; or from online resources such as the US National Library of Medicine's website (https://pubchem.ncbi.nlm.nih.gov/) or Drugbank (https://www.drugbank.ca/drugs). In the case of a new drug, the company would most likely have such information in its development files. Alternately, the company's Pre-formulation Department will determine solubility, rate of solution, and heat stability experimentally.

When heat is necessary, jacketed mixing tanks are usually utilized. These are double-walled, with the product within the inner wall and hot water circulated between the walls. The mixing required for solution formation will also stir the solvent, preventing localized overheating. If a higher temperature is required within the mixing vessel, steam is pumped into the heating jacket.

After complete dissolution of all ingredients, the pH of the solution is determined and, if necessary, adjusted using a compatible pH adjuster (either basic or acidic). The solution is then made up to volume with WFI. Thereafter, cold water may be circulated through the jacketed vessel to cool the solution to room temperature. This is required for several reasons including the fact that some components may be stable to heat for a short time and, therefore, their heat exposure must be reduced. In addition, the liquid must be dispensed into individual containers, usually by volume, which is affected by the temperature. It should be noted that it may take many hours, or more than a day, to cool a large volume of solution to room temperature by simply removing the heat source.

Filling

In this step, the bulk solution is pumped through pipes to the individual containers and the precise dose is transferred into the individual, primary containers. The latter may be a single dose vial, a rubber-stoppered multidose container, or a prefilled syringe.

The next step in the manufacturing sequence, as described above, is sterilization or "terminal sterilization" since it is the last step. Sterilization methods are discussed in the next section. However, it should be noted that the exact sequence of the filling step in the overall production sequence depends on the method of sterilization that is used. If the solution is to be sterilized by filtration, then equipment sterilization would precede filling.

Many filling systems depend on a piston and cylinder pumping mechanism. The first movement of the piston draws liquid into the cylinder of the pump. The stroke of the piston (ie, the distance that it moves up or down) can be set by the operator. This determines the volume of liquid drawn into the cylinder and, consequently, the volume of liquid that is pushed out of the cylinder into the final container when the piston moves in the opposite direction. The precision of the filling step is critical since it determines the fill volume in the final container. If the latter is a single dose container, the quantity of liquid within it influences the actual volume of liquid injected and, thus, the dose of drug that the patient receives. It is important to realize that the volume of liquid drawn into the cylinder is not necessarily the volume delivered into the final container. This is due to the fact that there may be a dead volume in the system, that is, a certain small volume of liquid that is not ejected from the cylinder during filling. Compensation for dead volume can be made by a slight overfill of the cylinder, brought about by a small increase in the distance that the cylinder travels on the filling stroke.

While effort is expended in controlling the nominal fill volume of the final container, it should be kept in mind that it is, correspondingly, the dispensed volume out of the single-dose container (accounting for the dead volume of this container) and the injectable volume from the syringe (accounting for its dead volume) that are the parameters that determine the volume of the injection. This determines the dose that the patient receives. This consideration is complicated by the fact that in any filling operation, a range of fill volumes would be obtained in the various vials, that is, no filling procedure is 100% accurate. In contrast to the filling of single-dose injection containers, the error in the filling of multidose containers is less significant. For the filling of single-dose injectable containers, it is not average fill volume that is most important, but the volume at the lower end of the fill range. The patient may be receiving an inadequate dose after consideration of the dead volume. This is particularly important with narrow therapeutic-index drugs. The latter term is explained in Chapter 17, Introduction to Bioavailability.

The injectable liquid is dispensed into an open container, and then sealed, leading to an additional contamination risk. When the period between filling and sealing is kept as short as possible, the risk is reduced but not eliminated. Since it is the bulk liquid that is filtered, prior to filling, any subsequent contamination cannot easily be removed. The contaminants could be microbial or air-borne particles. The latter may be difficult to detect by visual inspection. Every injection in a batch (not only a representative sample) undergoes such an inspection. The operator views each vial against an appropriate background in a lightbox, which facilitates the viewing of particulate matter. A white background makes it easier to see black particles, and vice-versa. A representative sample from each batch is also subjected to a series of quality control tests which includes sterility testing. These methods (visual inspection and sterility testing) can only provide detection of contamination after the fact.

Microbial contamination during filling may be offset by terminal sterilization, when the product utilizes this form of sterilization. However, microbial load must still be minimized, as far as possible, in the preparation of the containers, the compounding of the solution, and in the filling process. Where terminal sterilization cannot be used (eg, if the drug is unstable at the sterilizing conditions), caution must be exercised to prevent contamination during any processing that is performed subsequent to sterilization of equipment or components.

Recap Questions

1. Mention four types of injectable products.
2. What is the purpose of siliconization?
3. Solubility is an important consideration in injection formulation. Name two sources of information on drug solubility.
4. Why is it important to wash vials thoroughly in spite of terminal sterilization?

SUSPENSIONS

An injectable suspension may be formulated simply because the drug is too insoluble to formulate as a solution. In other cases, suspensions are specifically prepared for extended-release applications. The dispersion medium may be either a vegetable/semi-synthetic oil, or an aqueous vehicle. Suspensions are intended principally for injection into muscles and, to a lesser extent, for injection into the subcutaneous region. After injection, the small volume of liquid spreads, to a limited extent, within the muscle tissue and becomes slightly diluted with tissue fluid. Dissolution of the drug in this fluid and absorption into the tissues precedes absorption into the bloodstream. The rate of drug absorption is dependent upon the dissolution rate of the suspended particles at the site of injection and the suspension formulation may not necessarily be an extended-release injection. In other instances, the drug is formulated in such a way that drug release from the suspended particles is slow and an extended-release profile is obtained. The latter topic is covered in the section of this chapter dealing with extended-release injections.

Many of the characteristics and stability behavior of injectable suspensions are similar to that of other forms of suspensions which are dealt with in Chapter 6, Pharmaceutical Suspensions. For example, the settling behavior of the suspended particles is described in this chapter. Stokes' Law is applicable just as it is relevant to injectable suspensions. Also similar to oral or topical suspensions is the need for a suspending agent and, potentially, an antioxidant. Sometimes, there is also the need for a surfactant to ensure adequate wetting of hydrophobic particles during the production process. In addition, a surfactant may be used to retard crystal growth. Unlike regular suspensions, injectable suspensions must be isotonic, sterile, and free from pyrogens. Because the suspension is directly injected into tissues, buffers are also required in the formulation. In addition, the range of ingredients that may be incorporated is limited to those that have been proven to be safe for injection. The irritation potential of ingredients, especially irritation at the injection site, is a factor that is getting increasingly more attention.

Injectable suspensions are usually not made by suspending drug particles in a dispersion medium, with the intention of finally sterilizing the formulation. Such terminal sterilization may induce drug degradation and, more generally, may cause crystal growth in a suspension. Typically, suspensions are, therefore, made from sterile solutions of the drug, which are then mixed with sterile non-solvents, causing precipitation of the drug to create sterile particles. The process is discussed further in the section, "Dried Powder Formulations" below. Betamethasone acetate suspension, USP, insulin zinc suspension, USP and penicillin G procaine are examples of injectable aqueous suspensions that are not depot formulations. Aqueous injectable suspensions that are depot products are described in the section on extended-release products and some examples are listed in Table 12-2.

It is important that the injectable suspension be syringeable. This characteristic refers to the ability of the injection to be passed through a reasonably-sized needle. A suitable needle is one of 18 to 21 gauge, that is, the diameter of the needle must be

TABLE 12-2	Examples of Commercial Aqueous Suspension Products			
TRADE NAME	ACTIVE	COMPANY	TYPE	INDICATION/FREQUENCY OF INJECTION
Abilify Maintena	Aripiprazole	Otsuka	For suspension	• Schizophrenia • Bipolar 1 disorder maintenance—once a month (both)
Zyprexa Relprevv	Olanzapine pamoate	Eli Lilly Co.	Suspension	Schizophrenia—every 2 or 4 weeks*
Invega Sustenna	Paliperidone palmitate	Janssen Pharmaceuticals, Inc	Suspension	Schizophrenia—maintenance: monthly
Trelstar	Triptorelin pamoate	Allergan	For suspension	Palliative treatment of advanced prostate cancer— every 4, 12, or 24 weeks*
Depot Provera	Medroyprogesterone acetate	Pharmacia and Upjohn Co. (Pfizer)	Suspension	Adjunctive therapy for endometrial or renal cancer— maintenance: monthly

*Multiple strengths available for different durations of action.

in the 300 to 600 μm range. One reason why a suspension may not be syringeable is the fact that the suspended particles are too large to pass through the needle. A less obvious reason relates to the nature of the interior of the needle. By microscopy, it can be shown that the interior surface is rough. Therefore, even if the particle size is significantly less than the internal diameter of the needle, particles may be trapped by the rough surface and particle buildup develops, preventing other particles from passing through.

As inferred, it is very important that the formulator develop an injectable suspension that is stable over the lifetime of the product. One of the issues that could occur is the formation of a cake of drug particles in the vial, upon standing for a long period. Such a cake is difficult to redisperse at the time of injection. Another problem is the maintenance of syringeability throughout the shelf life of the product. An injectable suspension that demonstrated good syringeability upon manufacture may not easily pass through the bore of the needle after storage for an extended time. The reason for this is the fact that agglomerates of particles, or crystal growth, during standing, may have caused the formation of larger particulates, even if cake formation did not occur. Though the particles were able to be drawn up into the syringe initially, the somewhat larger particles, created during storage, agglomerate more easily on the interior surface of the needle, as described above.

Agglomerates may be able to be dispersed by shaking the vial before drawing the injection into the syringe but the formation of large crystals cannot be dealt with so easily. If the cake cannot be redispersed easily with shaking, or large agglomerates, that do not quickly disperse on shaking are present, or large crystals are visible, the injection should not be administered from that vial.

Temperature variations during storage may be responsible for crystal growth. At the time of manufacture, a small amount of drug is in solution (even a poorly soluble drug has some degree of solubility). A somewhat elevated temperature, encountered

during the shelf life of the injection, may cause an additional, small quantity of the drug to dissolve from the suspended particles. If the temperature then falls, some of the dissolved drug may precipitate out of solution, onto existing crystals, to form larger crystals than were initially present. It should be remembered that a range of particle sizes exists and that deposition may occur on crystals which are at the larger end of the size range. Drugs whose solubility varies greatly with temperature are more likely to display this behavior than those displaying a smaller temperature effect on solubility. Dissolved drug that precipitates may also play a role in "bridging" two particles.

Polymorphic changes when the dissolved fraction of drug recrystallizes, during storage, could also be responsible for precipitation, if the polymorph is less soluble than the initial form of the drug. Since the rate of drug release is dependent upon the size of the particles, crystal growth may materially affect the rate of drug release. This is because an equal weight of large particles has a smaller total surface area compared to that of small particles and dissolution is a surface phenomenon (see Chapter 5, Pharmaceutical Powders). After injection, dissolution of the alternative polymeric form is also slower.

Hence, it is necessary, first to create particles of a suitable size and, second, to include in the formulation substances that will retard crystal growth. Most injectable suspensions contain a low concentration of particles, for example, 5%. A notable exception is penicillin G procaine which has a high concentration of the active and is viscous. Injectable suspensions may be presented in the following formats: a ready-formed suspension in water or in oil; or a powder that is suspended upon the addition of a suitable vehicle (WFI with added buffers, etc., most commonly).

Emulsions

Emulsions are not used to a great extent for the formulation of injectable drugs because of the difficulty of forming, and maintaining, the droplet size at 1 μm or less. The exception is total parenteral nutrition (TPN) emulsions which are commonly used. When a patient, who is unable to take food orally, is confined to bed for an extended period (usually more than 5 days), the administered intravenous feed must contain some oily component. This is needed for the provision of calories and essential fatty acids, for the maintenance of the health of the patient. The oil is usually sunflower or safflower oil which consists of triglycerides containing unsaturated fatty acids. Such formulations contain oil as small droplets of 1 μm or less. The co-administration of drugs into the venous line used for TPN administration may increase the coalescence of the oil globules, with attendant serious problems. Special precautions have to be taken when drugs are added to a TPN intravenous line.

DRIED POWDER FORMULATIONS

Preparation of Sterile Drug Powder

Sterilization is often the last step of the overall process of injection formulation and is referred to as "terminal sterilization." Since terminal sterilization is an acceptable process that is commonly used, it would seem logical that powder products could be prepared by filling the powder into vials which are sterilized; or, alternately, by forming the powder made into a suspension which is filled into vials and sterilized. However, this is not the usual way of producing such products because the powder may not be chemically stable at the high temperatures used in terminal sterilization, and the particle size may grow during this process. Consequently, the drug powder is usually created as a sterile powder that is aseptically transferred to sterile vials or is processed by alternate methods that do not require terminal sterilization. The method of producing the sterile powder is described below.

The basic method involves the preparation of a drug solution (frequently in a non-aqueous solvent) and sterilizing this solution by filtration. A sterile non-solvent is then added to the solution of the drug, with stirring, while ensuring that all equipment that has product contact is sterile. When a sufficient quantity of the nonsolvent has been added, the drug crystallizes out of solution. The rate of addition of the nonsolvent, the temperature at which the process is carried out, as well as the stirring rate, are critical process parameters that affect the shape and size of the particles that are formed. The crystals are allowed to settle, the solvents decanted and the residual crystals are washed and dried at low temperature, all processes being carried out aseptically.

Generally, powdered formulations must be filled into individual sterile vials under aseptic conditions. This is done on a weight, or a volume, basis. If the material is free-flowing, it can be fed from a hopper, by means of an auger, into individual containers. This is similar to the way powder is fed from a hopper to a tablet press (see Chapter 9, Tablets). Alternatively, a filling wheel may be utilized. This has cavities, whose volume is adjustable, along the rim of the wheel. The cavities are first filled and the powder is then transferred to the vials (volumetric method). Freeze-dried powders are the exception with respect to filling since a solution is first allowed to flow into the vials and this solution is then converted to powder form within the individual vials.

Powder for Injection

Upon addition of the required amount of solvent, usually WFI, to a vial containing the powder, a solution forms with minimal agitation. Apart from the drug, the powder may contain excipients required to make an acceptable injection solution. These include buffer components, antimicrobial substances, and antioxidants. The drug may be prepared as sterile powder as described in the previous section, or as a freeze-dried formulation, as described below. An example of the former is Thiopental Sodium for Injection, USP. An example of a freeze-dried product is Methohexital Sodium for Injection. Some reconstituted injection solutions must be further diluted before injection. Methohexital sodium for injection is an example of a formulation that can be used at full strength, after reconstitution, for some indications. The labeling also gives instructions for diluting the reconstituted solution to prepare multiple strengths of the injection, each for a different indication. Both Thiopental sodium and Methohexital sodium are anesthetics.

Powder for Suspension

Powders to be reconstituted and resuspended are similar to powders for solution with the notable differences that the powders do not dissolve, and that suspending agents are included in such formulations. It is also imperative that the formulation contain any component that is required to maintain particle size for the duration of the intended shelf life. Surfactants may retard crystal growth during storage. Polysorbate 80 is a frequently added surfactant. An example of an injectable suspension that is presented as a dry powder is Ampicillin trihydrate for Suspension.

Freeze-Dried Formulations

While solutions may be sterilized by terminal sterilization most freeze-dried solutions, on the other hand, are not. They are compounded, sterilized by filtration (as described in the section on sterilization below), transferred aseptically into individual sterile containers, and then freeze-dried. Since sterilization, in this process, is not the last step, it cannot be referred to as terminal sterilization.

The basic principle of freeze drying is the fact that ice can be converted to water vapor directly (ie, without the formation of liquid water) under the appropriate temperature and pressure conditions. This is illustrated in Figure 12-1 which is the phase diagram of water. Each area represents a single phase of water, that is, solid, liquid, or vapor. Each line represents the temperature and vapor pressure conditions under which two phases can coexist: solid and liquid along the line LA, liquid and vapor along the line VA, and solid and vapor along the line SA. The point A is the triple point of water, that is, the point at which all three phases can coexist. It occurs at a temperature slightly above zero and at a vapor pressure of 610 Pa. It is important to recognize the fact that it is the vapor pressure of water, and not the absolute pressure, that is in consideration. For points along SA, ice can be directly transformed into water vapor. For example, at the point marked X in the diagram, a slight application of heat will transform ice into water vapor. When the first aliquot of ice has changed to water vapor, the vapor pressure increases. Therefore, for further sublimation of ice, this water vapor must

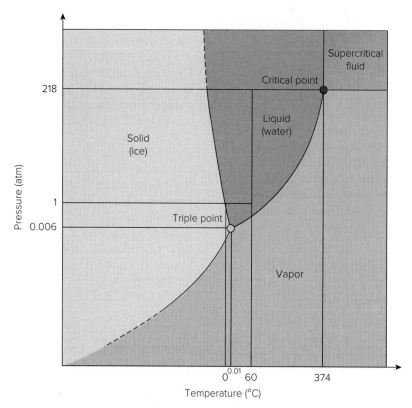

FIGURE 12-1 Phase diagram of water. (Modified from Dembek M, Bocian S. Pure water as a mobile phase in liquid chromatography techniques. *Trends Anal Chem.* 2020;123:1-13.)

be removed. This is done by means of a vacuum pump with a condenser installed between the vacuum pump and the freeze-drying chamber.

While the triple point of water has a temperature slightly above 0°C, the presence of solutes in an injection solution will depress the freezing point by several degrees. It is usual, therefore, to freeze the solution many degrees less than zero. Typically, −20°C to −40°C is used to ensure that the formation of water does not occur. In addition, all water cannot be removed from the product in this way. Therefore, freeze-drying is considered primary drying and a second step, or secondary drying, must be undertaken to remove the remaining water. The latter constitutes approximately 5% of the initial water.

The formulations for freeze-drying are, in many respects, similar to the formulation of solutions and suspensions for injection, with a few notable differences. While the addition of sodium chloride to liquid formulations for injection, to adjust tonicity, is typical, it is not always possible for freeze-dried products. Alternatively, a smaller amount of sodium chloride may have to be added. In either case, the resulting solution for injection, after reconstitution, is not isotonic. The major reason for not adding the required amount of salt for isotonicity is that salt tends to decrease the collapse temperature. The latter is the temperature at which the loose, fluffy cake of solids, formed by freeze-drying, collapses. A collapsed cake is considered an inefficient product for the reasons mentioned below, and the presence of salt allows collapsing to happen more easily.

Generally, the volume of the dried powder is close to the volume of the liquid initially in the vial. Since all the liquid is

removed at the end of the process, what remains is a loose network of particles with much airspace in between. When a solvent is added to this powder prior to injection, this formation of solid particles leads to rapid dissolution of the material. This is due to the large surface area exposed, and rapid dissolution is desired. Conversely, when the cake collapses, the dissolution rate is slower. Added salts also inhibit crystallization of other components.

The incorporation of buffers must, also, be carefully considered for the following reason: as ice forms, only a limited amount of the buffer component can be trapped in the ice crystals and the remaining buffer stays in the liquid. Hence, the residual liquid becomes progressively more concentrated in the buffer components. This is, roughly speaking, analogous to boiling off some water from a solution to leave the remaining solution more concentrated. More important than the mere concentration of buffer salts, is the fact that one component may become more concentrated than the other buffer component. This occurs because one of the buffer components may be less soluble, than the other component, at a lower temperature. This component precipitates out of solution and is trapped in the ice. The liquid component then becomes progressively more concentrated in the other buffered component and its pH changes.

In the phosphate buffer system, which has been studied extensively, it is the dibasic sodium phosphate (Na_2PO4) component which precipitates more rapidly because it is less soluble. The accumulation of mono-basic sodium phosphate ($NaHPO_4$) in the solution, makes it more acidic and deleterious to protein actives. The acetate, citrate, and Tris buffer systems show only small pH shifts upon freezing. In addition, high concentrations of sodium chloride result in a similar effect: with ice formation, the remaining solution becomes increasingly more concentrated in sodium chloride resulting in high osmotic pressure which affects materials of biological origin. For this reason, the incorporation of sodium chloride must be done judiciously, using the least amount necessary, but compatible, with the formulation.

In general, crystalline components improve the efficiency of freeze-drying. However, for the freeze-drying of actives of biological origin, amorphous excipients are preferred because they tend to stabilize the freeze-dried formulation. Examples of amorphous excipients include disaccharides such as sucrose and trehalose. The amorphous material tends to inhibit crystallization of buffer salts but, to be effective, this material must remain amorphous after freezing and throughout the shelf life of the product.

The solution to be freeze-dried is first sterilized by filtration and then filled, by aseptic transfer, into previously washed, sterilized, and de-pyrogenated glass vials. Special closures, with slots, are partially inserted into the neck of the vial. These closures are made from an elastomeric material and are referred to as lyostoppers. This term indicates that it is a stopper specifically to be used for freeze-drying, or lyophilization, as this process is also known. Thus placed, when the vapor is formed within the vial, it can escape through the slots in the closure. These bottles are packed onto shelves in a freeze-drying chamber without the use of trays, or with trays with removable bottoms, so that heat transfer from the shelf is not impeded by another layer of material.

The freeze-dryer for industrial production of injections consists of a large chamber containing heated shelves onto which are placed the vials of injection. A vacuum pump is connected to the interior of the chamber and a moisture trap is placed between the chamber and the vacuum pump. Since the operation of the chamber is at a low temperature (eg, −30°C to −40°C), both the moisture trap as well as the vacuum pump must be capable of working under these conditions. The entire system must be capable of achieving specified temperatures and

pressures and, for this purpose, gauges are placed in multiple spots within the chamber (to ensure uniform conditions in the chamber) as well as in the condenser. A simplified diagram of a freeze-dryer is shown in Figure 12-2. With systems that do not use terminal sterilization, it is imperative to understand that the entire interior of the chamber and condenser must be sterilized. This is done, without dismantling the entire system, using techniques referred to as clean-in-place and sterilize-in-place. A description of these techniques is beyond the scope of this chapter.

The product is first frozen to a sufficiently low temperature so that complete solidification of the product occurs. The chamber is then evacuated to a pressure lower than the vapor pressure of ice. After this pressure is reached and the condenser is cooled, heat is applied to the shelves in sufficient quantity to provide the heat of sublimation of ice. It is extremely important that the temperature of the product does not rise appreciably. If it does, the system would not be at the required conditions, and some of the ice will melt. At the correct pressure and temperature conditions, the ice sublimes directly to water vapor. This is referred to as the primary drying step. It should be noted that the ice sublimes from surface layers and, as the water vapor rises, it leaves behind a porous material. Further drying causes moisture depletion of deeper levels of ice and the vapor must pass through the porous material created earlier. The material is porous because only the solid particles that were found in the interstices between the ice particles remain.

For most products, not every trace of water freezes and, after primary drying, secondary drying is needed to remove the residual water. Since there is no longer any ice to consume the latent heat of vaporization, the temperature of the product rises and, towards the end of the secondary drying cycle, the temperature of the product is close to that of the heating shelf. It is common practice to close the vials while they are still within the drying chamber and under partial vacuum. This prevents entry of any foreign matter that may have been in the external environment, outside the chamber, and enables the stoppers to be seated more tightly because of the negative pressure within

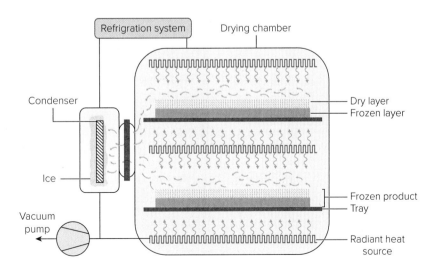

FIGURE 12-2 A simplified diagram of a freeze-dryer. (Reproduced, with permission, from Garcia-Amezquita L, Welti-Chanes J, Vergara-Balderas F, Bermúdez-Aguirre D. Freeze-drying: the basic process. In: *Encyclopedia of Food and Health*. Academic Press; 2016: 104-109.)

the vial. This factor also makes it easier to add solvent to the vial, in the clinic, prior to injection. It is fairly common practice to fill the vials with nitrogen before the stoppers are fully seated, thus ensuring an inert atmosphere. Freeze-drying is a long process, typically taking 2 to 3 days for an industrial batch. Therefore, the process is expensive to conduct, in addition to the large capital outlay for the purchase of equipment.

Recap Questions

1. Name two reasons for using injectable suspensions.
2. What do you understand by the term, "syringeable"?
3. Why is the globule size of an injectable emulsion important?
4. Why is it necessary to provide an emulsion intravenously to a patient who cannot consume food orally for an extended period?
5. What is a freeze-dried powder?
6. Distinguish between primary and secondary drying during freeze-drying.

EXTENDED-RELEASE INJECTIONS

In many instances, it is therapeutically desirable to have a longer duration of action for an administered medication. The reasons for this are described in detail in Chapter 11, Modified-Release Oral Dosage Forms, in the context of oral delivery systems. A similar rationale applies with respect to injectables. One of these reasons, the inconvenience of taking multiple dosage forms in a day, is much more relevant with respect to injections because of the fear of the needle and the actual pain to be endured. It is also possible, with injectables, to have a much longer duration of action measured in weeks and longer in some instances. For many drugs of biological origin, the injectables route is the only viable route at the present time but it is also the most patient-averse route. For such products, extended-release injections have made a significant impact on therapy.

While there are many advantages to extended-release injections, there are also some disadvantages. One major disadvantage is the inability to stop drug effects when medically required. Another is the fact that individualization of release rates is generally not possible. Some products are now offered in multiple versions, each with a slightly different extended-release rate. Some of the first extended-release injections, from the 1950s, were suspensions of drugs in aqueous and oily vehicles. This was followed by poorly soluble drug derivatives in the form of esters of long-chain fatty alcohols or acids. These became available in the 1960s and 1970s. The longer duration of action is due to the fact that the process of de-esterification, to release the parent drug, is slow with the long-chain esters. Haloperidol decanoate is a long-acting anti-schizophrenic drug administered once a month as an oily injection. In comparison, haloperidol lactate is a short-acting injection. Lactic acid has three carbon atoms

whereas the chain length of decanoic acid is 10. Extended-release injections are particularly useful for psychiatric drugs because of the difficulty in administering such drugs repeatedly to patients, especially in psychiatric institutions. Fluphenazine is an example of such a drug, esters of which are administered as injections in sesame oil. Haloperidol, mentioned above, is another example. The use of polymers for extended-release injections began in the 1970s and their historical development is briefly outlined in the section, "Microparticulate Injections."

The choice of drug for an extended-release injection is driven by the following factors:

1. The drugs should be potent enough that a relatively small quantity is sufficient for dosing for the extended time.
2. The drug should not be degraded or metabolized rapidly after injection.
3. The drug must be stable not only during the typical shelf life of a product but also for the extended duration of activity within the body which is related to factor 2 above.
4. Injection site irritation is a major concern for the entire formulation, not only the active.

Extended-release injections can take the form of a solution or suspension in oil, an aqueous suspension, and a gel that, after injection, forms a solid in situ. Extended-release injections are also referred to as depot delivery systems.

Oily Injections

When a drug is water-insoluble but soluble in oil, the extended-release injection can be formulated as a solution in oil. This formulation may be considered as the simplest form of an extended-release injection since it consists simply of the oil and the API dissolved in it (together with required excipients such as antioxidants). Benzoyl benzoate may be used to enhance the solubility of some drugs, such as steroids in oils, when necessary. In addition, the need for strict particle size control, as required for a suspension, is eliminated and the sterilization step is made easier due to the ability to use sterilization by filtration. However, even this type of preparation is not necessarily easy to formulate since there are many parameters to consider including the stability of the oil and its viscosity. The latter affects the filtration rate. If heat is required to dissolve the drug, what is the effect of elevated temperature on the stability of the drug? Upon injection, the oily solution should disperse within the muscle, to some extent, in order to spread the solution. In the subsequent step, the dissolved drug partitions into the water phase of the tissues. The oil/water partition coefficient of the drug is important for this step as well as for absorption into tissues, and into blood vessels for generalized circulation.

The oily suspension is somewhat more complex since the drug must first dissolve from the solid suspended particle, to form an oily solution, before diffusion can occur into the surrounding aqueous fluids. Drug release from an oily solution is first order: as the drug content of the oil decreases, so does the absorption rate. Drug release from oily suspensions is zero order since the suspended particles will dissolve to replace the drug absorbed. Initial absorption takes place from the small amount of dissolved drug in the administered dose.

Technically, the oily suspension should, therefore, be considered a separate class of long-acting injection. However, the Food and Drug Administration (FDA) considers oily solutions and oily suspensions together as one category, namely, oily injections. In this writing, therefore, both categories will be considered "oily injections." Some oily injections available in the US are mentioned in Table 12-3.

These injections are administered intramuscularly usually, but may also be injected subcutaneously. The oil itself is usually one of the vegetable oils such as peanut, corn, olive, cottonseed, and sesame oils. The latter is the most preferred oil for injections since it is the most stable vegetable oil except for its ability to be oxidized, as explained below. Exposure to light and/or heat promotes oxidation. Therefore, the injections are usually presented in amber-colored containers and should not be stored at high temperatures. Several synthetic, or semi-synthetic oils are also available for injection formulation. Examples include isopropyl myristate, ethyl oleate, polyethylene glycols (PEGs). The low viscosity grades of ethyl oleate and sesame oil are preferred. The major instability of all oils is their ability to be oxidized. Sesame oil contains natural antioxidants, especially sesamol, and ought not to be sensitive to oxidation. However, this low-molecular-weight compound is driven off during the deodorizing step of production. Hence, this oil needs protection from oxidation.

The oils should be non-irritating and not react chemically with the drug. All oils used in injections must be able to be slowly eliminated from the injection site so that no oil residue remains for a significant time after the drug has diffused out of the oil. Generally, the oil slowly dissolves in body fluids, especially after conversion to a soluble species. It may also be eliminated by the shedding of microdroplets from the depot surface, and subsequent transport of the droplets from the injection site. The type of oil used must be stated in the labeling since some individuals are allergic to certain vegetable oils.

Injection site irritation is a concern with all injections. Excessive unsaturation of the oil may result in tissue irritation upon injection. The use of oily injections has somewhat diminished in recent years in preference to aqueous suspensions which may be less irritating, less sensitizing, and cause less pain

upon injection. Table 12-3 lists some oily injections for extended release. Extended-release injections are particularly useful for psychiatric drugs because of the difficulty in administering such drugs repeatedly to patients, especially in psychiatric institutions, and for the consistent blood levels that are achieved. Fluphenazine is an example of such a drug; esters of this drug are administered as injections in sesame oil. As previously mentioned the esters formed from long-chain fatty acids or alcohols confer a longer duration of action since de-esterification, to release the parent drug, is slow. Haloperidol decanoate is a long-acting anti-schizophrenic drug administered once a month as an oily injection. In comparison, haloperidol lactate is a short-acting injection. Lactic acid has three carbon atoms whereas the chain length of decanoic acid is 10. An oily injection may appear slightly cloudy upon standing. Usually, this will disappear with slight warming of the injection and shaking of the vial. If it does not, it may be a sign of a more serious stability problem and the vial should not be used.

Aqueous Suspensions

Aqueous suspensions of insoluble drug particles were amongst the first extended-release or depot injections to be marketed. While some of the older products have been taken off the market, examples of injections containing aqueous suspensions that continue to be commercially available, at the time of writing, are listed in Table 12-2. It should be noted that there are many suspensions for once-a-day administration that may be considered "long acting" since their duration of action is longer than an injectable solution of the same drug. Some insulin formulations fall into this category. However, these injections are not considered to be depot formulations (and are not mentioned in this section) since depot formulations typically give durations of action measured in weeks.

After standing for long, a parenteral suspension formulation should not cake and it should be easily resuspended with mild agitation. It should be easy to administer through a 20- to 25-gauge needle. After IM administration, the vehicle is rapidly absorbed and the particles form fine agglomerates within the fibrous muscle tissue. In this respect, it is different from an oily injection in which the vehicle is retained at the site of injection

TABLE 12-3	Some Oily Injections Available in the US			
TRADE NAME	**ACTIVE**	**COMPANY**	**OIL**	**INDICATION/ FREQUENCY**
Delestrogen	Estradiol valerate	Par Sterile Products LLC	Lowest strength: sesame oil; higher strengths: castor oil	• Vasomotor symptoms of menopause—every 4 weeks • Palliative treatment of prostate cancer—every 1-2 weeks
Depot-Testosterone	Testosterone cypionate	Pfizer	Cotton seed oil	Hypogonadism—every 2 to 4 weeks
Depot-Estradiol	Estradiol cypionate	Pharmacia and Upjohn Co. (Pfizer)	Cotton seed oil	• Vasomotor symptoms of menopause—every 3-4 weeks • Female hypogonadism: Monthly
Haldol	Haloperidol decanoate	Janssen Pharmaceuticals Inc.	Sesame oil	Antipsychotic—every 4 weeks

for some time. Many of the formulation characteristics are similar to those for quick-acting injectable suspensions and, in this section, only differences will be highlighted. Viscosity enhancement may be used to improve stability from settling during storage. After injection, viscosity may also influence the diffusion of dissolved drug, through the surrounding medium. However, a balance must be attained between increased viscosity and syringeability. An example of this kind of formulation is penicillin G procaine. The thixotropic behavior of some viscosity enhancers may be useful in this regard. Thixotropy is a phenomenon in which a liquid may be viscous on standing but becomes thinner under a shearing stress such as mixing. Typically, the thin liquid, on standing, becomes thicker again. In the present context, a polymer-containing liquid may be viscous in the vial and, hence, retard settling of dispersed particles. However, withdrawal of the liquid into a syringe represents a shearing strain causing the liquid to be less viscous. Similarly, the act of depressing the plunger to empty the syringe is also a shearing strain which reduces viscosity. This thixotropic behavior of the liquid assists syringeability and therefore delivery of the injection is easier.

Microparticulate Injections

Historical Development

Microparticulate materials may also be used to provide extended release of the drug. The history of their development can be traced to the use, starting in the 1930s, of implanted (larger) pellets to produce sustained release of hydrophobic drugs. Drugs administered in this way included estradiol for prostate cancer and testosterone for deficiency of this hormone. Implant development continues with the synthesis of new polymers and block copolymers. The latter are long-chain polymers made up of two, or more, different polymeric materials. Within a polymer chain, a length of pure polymer of the one type is adjacent to a length of pure polymer of the second type, with these blocks repeating at intervals. For example, poly (ethylene-co-vinyl acetate) consists of blocks of alternating ethylene, and vinyl acetate, polymers. The success of many of these devices led to the concept of using similar polymers as drug-loaded microparticles that could be injected.

Ideally, the microparticle, or "bead" as they are also known, should consist of a polymer that is slowly biodegradable. Degradation of the polymer should occur from the surface of the particle or bead, going inward. If the drug slowly diffused out of the bead and the biodegradation of the bead material occurred at a somewhat slower rate, it would result in the following situation. The outermost layer of the bead would deliver its drug content and then the drug-depleted portion of the bead would degrade, exposing a fresh surface of the bead, containing its drug load. This could be repeated numerous times to give a nearly zero-order release rate. If this did not occur, diffusion would take place through an increasing thickness of drug-depleted bead polymer, and the diffusion rate would become progressively slower.

Poly-hydroxy acids are used for sutures that dissolve slowly. These polymers were utilized for drug delivery, beginning from the 1960s and 1970s, and continue up to the present time.

For example, poly (glycolic acid) (PGA) was used as a suture and was one of the polymers used initially for drug delivery from beads. Subsequently, lactic acid was used in the degradable suture composition, that is, the suture material consisted of poly (lactic-co-glycolic acid) (PLGA). As a result, this material was considered for the manufacture of microparticles. The material is available in different viscosity grades, with higher viscosity grades consisting of longer polymer chains. The major advantage of these materials is the fact that they degrade to glycolic acid and lactic acid, both normal constituents of the body.

In the late 1960s, drugs were added to PLA and microparticles and pellets were formed from this material, for use as depot delivery systems. In the 1970s, steroid-loaded PLGA microparticles for contraceptive use were developed and clinically tested. Around this time, important studies were also carried out to investigate the properties and in vitro degradation of PLGA copolymers. While much of the early work was on small molecule drugs, subsequently PLGA systems were developed with molecules of biological origin, for long-acting effects. The 1986 introduction, in Europe, of a PLGA microparticle system of triptorelin, for the treatment of prostate cancer, was the first injectable, degradable microparticle depot drug delivery system in the world. Lupron Depot was introduced in the United States in 1989 after being developed earlier in Japan by the Takeda Pharmaceutical Company. It is a PLGA microsphere product containing leuprolide, a luteinizing-hormone-releasing hormone analog.

Polymer Selection

Once an ideal dissolution profile has been proposed for the microparticulate product, the next step is the selection of the polymer. For a single constituent polymer (eg, PLA), the length of the polymer chain affects viscosity. Higher viscosity grades correspond to slower drug release (usually, different viscosity grades are available from the supplier.) Drug release rate is mainly dependent on the rate of chain cleavage of the polymer, to form progressively shorter chains. Cleavage occurs throughout the polymer that has become wet, so that cleavage can occur some distance from the surface.

With block copolymers, each constituent has a different hydrophobicity. For example, in PLGA, the lactic acid component is more hydrophobic than the glycolic acid component. Thus, if there is more lactic acid in a particular block copolymer, the release rate would be slower than one with less lactic acid, other factors being the same. The slower release rate occurs since water penetration into the hydrophobic portions of the material is slower and, hence, hydrolysis of the ester links would be slower. PLGA is by far the most commonly used polymer for the manufacture of injectable microspheres. This polymer has become very popular due to its biocompatibility, the fact that it can encapsulate many drugs, and that release profiles of several weeks are attainable. The release profile can be tuned by adjusting the relative proportion of the two components. Whatever the manufacturing method, the microcapsules should be smaller than 250 μm, preferably less than 125 μm, and they should not aggregate after production.

Manufacturing Methods

Techniques that may be used in the manufacture microparticles for injectables are, first, emulsion/solvent evaporation, spray drying, spray congealing, phase separation/coacervation, and extrusion. The first technique, in its simplest form, involves the formation of an O/W emulsion where the oil phase is an organic volatile solvent, such as methylene chloride or ethyl acetate, and the drug is hydrophobic and insoluble in water. The drug and polymer are dissolved in this organic phase and the emulsifying agent is dissolved in the aqueous phase. The emulsion formation process is similar to that described in Chapter 7, Emulsions. While the emulsion is being stirred, the solvent is evaporated, in the next step, frequently using the application of a vacuum to facilitate the process. The result of this process is the formation of coated particles suspended in the aqueous phase, with no discernible internal phase remaining. The particles are coated with the polymer from the organic phase. The aqueous phase is then decanted, and the resulting microcapsules are washed and dried.

Many adaptations of the basic method have evolved, including the formation of complex emulsions such as a water-in-oil-in-water emulsion (W/O/W) that is used for water-soluble drugs). A water-soluble drug is dissolved in the first water phase which is emulsified with an organic solvent such as dichloromethane, containing PLGA. This emulsion is then introduced, with stirring, into the second water phase containing an emulsifier to form the W/O/W emulsion. The organic phase is removed under vacuum and further processing is done as described above. In another application, solid particles (S) are dispersed, but not dissolved, in the organic phase, resulting in a solid-in-oil-in-water emulsion (S/O/W). The emulsion process is now commonplace to produce fine particles for injection.

Spray dried, and spray congealed, particles for extended-release injections may be prepared as described in Chapters 9 and 11, respectively, with the essential difference that the particle size for injections must be much smaller than in the applications described in these chapters. Typically, a size of <250 μm is required, with <125 μm being the preferred particle size. The process of phase separation/coacervation has been used to coat particles suspended in a liquid medium. Commonly, this process has been used to make coated particles for taste-masking or controlled release where the coated particles are compressed into tablets, for example. A similar process can be utilized to make injectable particles with the major difference being the size of the final particles.

Starting with a solution of a polymer or a colloidal dispersion, a polymer- or colloid-rich dispersion can be created in several ways. One of the simplest methods is the slow addition of a non-solvent for the polymer or colloid. In the remaining explanation only a polymer will be referenced but these methods apply equally to colloids. If a large amount of non-solvent is added, a precipitate will be formed. If the non-solvent is added very slowly, and in a limited amount, a point is reached where a polymer-rich phase separates within the body of liquid, the rest of the liquid being polymer deficient. With continued stirring and the addition of drug or other insoluble particles, the polymer will wrap around the particles. This coating is in the liquid state. By a further change of conditions such as the addition of more non-solvent the coating can be made to solidify. The coated particles are then filtered and dried in air. Ethylcellulose dissolved in chloroform with the addition of a non-solvent, such as an ether, is an example of this process. This is a simple coacervation process consisting of a single polymer. In a complex coacervation, two polymers make up the coacervate. An example of the latter is alginate and chitosan which are attracted to each other by their respective, negative and positive, charges. For coacervated injection microparticles, the proviso is that a much smaller particle size and a narrow size distribution must be maintained in addition to sterility requirements.

The extrusion technique involves melting a polymer and dispersing the drug in this melt. The material is then transferred to an extruder. The molten material in this apparatus is maintained at the correct temperature, by a heating jacket or electric coils, to avoid solidification within the apparatus. The maintenance of the material at the correct temperature is imperative. Within the apparatus, the molten material, at slightly above the solidification temperature, is forced through openings in a rigid metal plate, or screen, by the application of force. This may be done, for example, by an elongated, horizontal screw (Figure 12-3). As the screw turns, it forces the semisolid material forward. An alternate to a rigid metal plate with holes, is a die at the end of the cylinder (as shown in Figure 12-3). The force exerted by the

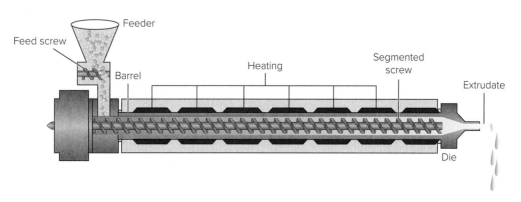

FIGURE 12-3 Diagram illustrating extrusion. Drug Development & Delivery.

screw finally squeezes the material through the die. The general process of squeezing material through apertures to form strands is referred to as extrusion; since the material is heated to melt, in this case, the process is referred to as hot-melt extrusion. The strands of the drug-containing polymeric material that are extruded may be referred to as the extrudate. The extrudate breaks up into smaller, ovoid particles as it falls from the extruder into a collection vessel. The polymer must have sufficient plasticity for this technique to work.

Whatever the method of manufacture, the resulting microparticles are formulated into an injection. Upon administration, a depot is formed for the long-lasting effect of the medication. Over time the constituents of the microparticles break down in the biological system and are removed, by biological processes, from the injection site. Table 12-4 provides information on some injectable microparticle formulations. Where the microparticles are unstable in the intended liquid vehicle, they may be supplied as a dry powder for reconstitution immediately before injection.

Just as microparticles (particles with individual diameters in the micrometer size range) are formed, new technology produces particles in the nanometer size range, frequently a few hundred nanometers in diameter. These particles could take several forms such as drug complexes, micelles, solid lipid nanoparticles. The latter are complex in that they are attached to moieties for targeting specific active sites. Nanotechnology has developed at a rapid pace, so an entire chapter, Chapter 13, is devoted to its description.

Recap Questions

1. Why is an extended-release injection necessary?
2. Name three types of extended-release injections.
3. Name one factor to take into consideration when selecting a drug candidate for extended-release injections.
4. Name three oils that can be used in an oily injection for extended release.

5. What is the most common polymer in microcapsule-containing-extended-release injections?
6. What is the difference between spray-dried and spray-congealed formulations?

STERILIZATION METHODS

Introduction

Sterilization refers to the inactivation of microorganisms or spores, or their removal from the product. Any method used for sterilization must not change the sterilized product in such a way that it is no longer suitable for its intended use. It is important to understand the kinetics of microbial inactivation. There is an exponential relationship between the extent of treatment with a sterilizing mechanism and the number of microorganisms that are killed. The decimal reduction value, or D Value, is the time of exposure, or the radiation dose, to kill microorganisms so that only 10% remain viable at the end of the exposure. For example, suppose there are 10,000 viable microorganisms on a specific surface area of a device to be sterilized and, after the sterilization process, only 1000 viable microorganisms survive. The dose of radiation used in this example is the D value.

As a second example, assume that 10,000 viable microorganisms are in a specific volume of a liquid. The number of minutes of steam sterilization that achieves an inactivation of 9000 microorganisms, leaving 1000 viable organisms, is the D Value. The next treatment of the same dose of radiation would leave 100 viable organisms, that is, 1/10th of the original number, and so on. When planning a sterilization procedure, there is, obviously, no intention to leave any viable organisms remaining on, or within, the sample. Rather, it is empirically known that a particular set of sterilizing conditions, in a specific apparatus, leads to the probability of a specific number of viable organisms remaining. This theoretical method is useful to determine the sterilizing conditions that will attain sterility, that is, the number of cycles to be used.

Sterilization methods that are commonly used in industry are moist steam under pressure or autoclaving, dry heat, ionizing

TABLE 12-4	Some Injectable Microparticle Formulations Available in the US			
TRADE NAME	**ACTIVE**	**COMPANY**	**INDICATION**	**FREQUENCY OF INJECTION**
Lupron Depot	Leuprolide acetate	AbbVie Inc.	Endometriosis	1 month or 3 months*
Vivitrol	Naltrexone	Alkermes Inc.	Alcohol & opioid dependence	1 month
Risperdal Consta	Risperidone	Janssen Pharmaceutica	Schizophrenia Bipolar disorder	Every 2 weeks
Sandostatin†	Octreotide acetate	Novartis	Acromegaly Carcinoid tumors & VIPomas	Every 4 weeks

*Two doses available for different durations.
†Microspheres consist of PLGA.

radiation, and ethylene oxide (EO). Sterilization by filtration can only be used practically for small volumes of liquid and, for this reason, this technique is not used much in the pharmaceutical industry. It is used extensively in compounding pharmacies to produce sterile preparations in relatively small volumes.

Moist Heat Sterilization (Autoclaving)

Moist heat kills organisms by coagulating and denaturing their proteins, both structural and enzymatic. The former causes the loss of physical integrity of the microorganism, while the latter alters its physiology. Moist heat is useful for the sterilization of culture media and other materials that allow steam to penetrate into the material. Typically, sterilization can be done at lower temperatures for the same time of exposure, as compared to dry heat sterilization, since moist heat is more effective. If higher temperatures are used for moist heat sterilization, a shorter duration of exposure is possible. For some drugs, a short exposure at a high temperature does not adversely affect their stability whereas, other drugs are unstable at a high temperature, even for a short duration. Spores are usually more resistant than the microorganisms themselves. Exposure to moist heat at 121°C for 15 minutes is sufficient to kill many spores, while the most resistant spores may require 30 minutes of exposure at this temperature. Many sterilization processes involving moist heat have been developed and some of these methods are briefly described below.

Gravity Air Displacement

Steam is introduced from the top into the sterilizing chamber which contains the materials to be sterilized (Figure 12-4). The steam remains as a layer above the air. As more steam is let into the chamber, the steam layer increases and pushes the air down. Eventually, air is pushed out through a drain at the bottom of the unit. Once the air is removed, the steam pressure builds and, simultaneously, the temperature rises. Once the sterilizing temperature has been reached, a few minutes are allowed for the temperature equilibration of the contents of the chamber. Thereafter, the exposure time begins. Gravity sterilizers are used for surgical instruments, liquids, and linen.

Dynamic Air Removal (Prevac)

This system uses a vacuum pump to remove air from the product chamber before steam is introduced. It is typically used to sterilize porous materials, or in situations where the item to be sterilized has cavities from which air is difficult to remove. Since the vacuum is efficient at removing air, this system is more efficient than gravity air displacement systems because the steam readily penetrates the material or the item (container or package) from which the air has been removed. Figure 12-5 shows a system in which multiple cycles of partial evacuation and steam introduction are used. This system is more efficient than a single evacuation followed by steam introduction.

Whatever steam sterilization process is used, there are four critical parameters: the quality of the steam, temperature, pressure, and time. Steam of high quality should be used: this contains no more than 3% liquid water (and 97% water vapor). This condition is described by stating that the relative humidity is 97%. The appropriate temperature depends on the type of sterilizer in use. For example, sterilizers that operate on the principle of gravity air displacement require a temperature of 121°C, whereas, sterilizers operating on the principle of dynamic air removal require a temperature of 132°C to 135°C, with an exposure time of approximately 4 minutes. Thus, dynamic air removal sterilizers are very efficient, in spite of the higher temperature needed. The pressure should be 15 psi and 27 psi, to achieve 121°C and 135°C, respectively.

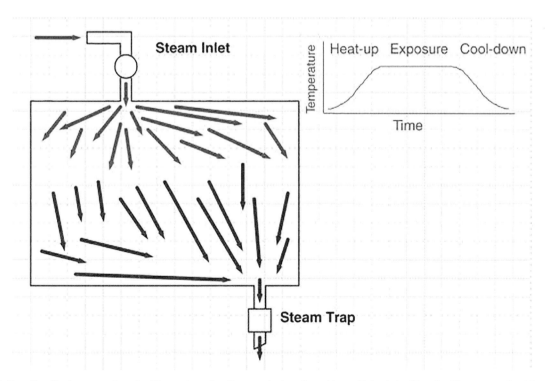

FIGURE 12-4 Gravity displacement cycle. (Reproduced, with permission, from Nema S, Ludwig JD, eds. *Pharmaceutical Dosage Forms - Parenteral Medications*. 3rd ed. Volume 2: Facility Design, Sterilization and Processing. New York, NY: Informa Healthcare; 2010.)

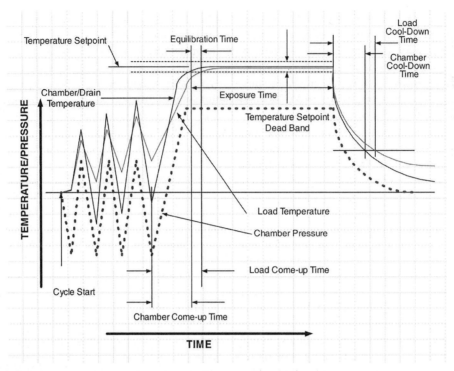

FIGURE 12-5 Multiple prevacuum cycle. (Reproduced, with permission, from Nema S, Ludwig JD, eds. *Pharmaceutical Dosage Forms - Parenteral Medications*. 3rd ed. Volume 2: Facility Design, Sterilization and Processing. New York, NY: Informa Healthcare; 2010.)

Dry Heat Sterilization

Dry heat kills organisms by destructive oxidation of cell constituents. As essential constituents are destroyed, the cell dies. Inactivation of the most resistant spores, using dry heat, requires a temperature of about 160°C for 60 minutes. For this reason, dry heat may not be considered as effective as moist heat. Dry heat is employed for glassware, syringes, some surgical instruments, and items that are wrapped in paper. One must ensure that the latter are not spoiled by the high temperatures involved. An alternative for the sterilization of syringes and other small instruments is the use of ionizing radiation.

Sterilization Using Ethylene Oxide

An epoxide is a cyclic ether and ethylene oxide is the simplest epoxide, having the structural formula C_2H_4O. Its shape is similar to an equilateral triangle (Figure 12-6). The three-membered ring is composed of two carbon and one oxygen atoms. The approximately 60° angle makes the molecule strained and, therefore, more reactive than other ethers. Ethylene oxide is an alkylating agent and its use in sterilization is dependent on its ability to disrupt the DNA of microorganisms. Ethylene oxide

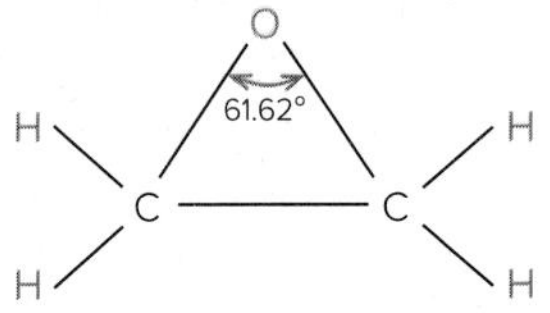

FIGURE 12-6 Ethylene oxide structure. Note that the approximately 60-degree bond angles lead to stress within the molecule.

is compatible with a large range of materials requiring sterilization but the material must allow penetration of the gas, and of humidity, into the interior spaces. Likewise, the product package must be permeable to gases. The latter quality will also allow air to pass through during the aeration step, after sterilization has been completed. This is required to remove the ethylene oxide from within the packages. Four variables control the efficacy of ethylene oxide sterilization processes. These are gas concentration, humidity, temperature, and the time of exposure. While a continuous process, ethylene oxide sterilization may be divided into the following four phases for ease of visualization: preconditioning, conditioning, addition of ethylene oxide, and aeration.

Preconditioning

As the name implies, this is the preliminary portion of the process and it involves the introduction of humidity into the sterilization chamber (Figure 12-7). The purpose of the prehumidification step is to enable moisture to penetrate into the materials to be sterilized. The humidification starts prior to loading the material to be sterilized and continues thereafter as well. This affords the best chance for proper penetration of moisture. It is important to realize that gas cannot be introduced first, with moisture introduction thereafter, for the following reason: ethylene oxide being a light molecule will pervade rapidly. In so doing, it will expel the air found in spaces in the material and will reside in such locations. When moisture is subsequently introduced, it will have difficulty expelling ethylene oxide in order to inhabit the spaces. The introduction of moisture first ensures proper penetration and the fast diffusion of ethylene oxide. The latter does not displace the moisture significantly.

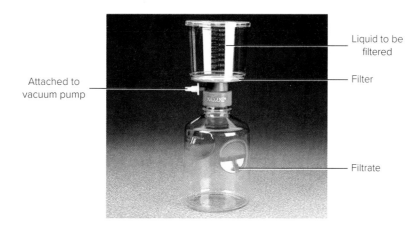

FIGURE 12-7 Sterilizing filtration apparatus (small scale).

Conditioning

In this step, the heat within the chamber is turned on and the "conditioning" is the fact that the humidified chamber is brought up to a certain temperature that has been determined to be effective for ethylene oxide sterilization. The temperature that is generally used is 50°C to 60°C.

The rate at which microorganisms are killed due to exposure to ethylene oxide is dependent on the temperature of the material to be sterilized. The factor that takes into account temperature, during the ethylene oxide sterilization, is the Q_{10} value. It describes how the death rate changes with every 10°C change in temperature. This value is typically between 1.8 and 2.7, depending on the material being sterilized. Consider a Q_{10} value of 2. If the temperatures increased by 10°C, the kill rate would be doubled. It also means that a drop in temperature of 10°C, from the set value, would reduce the kill rate to half. In other words, the exposure time (D) would have to be doubled. For this reason, precautions are taken to minimize fluctuations in temperature during ethylene oxide sterilization. The apparatus must be able to maintain the set temperature within a range of less than 10°C.

Addition of Ethylene Oxide

Ethylene oxide is then let into the system until a predetermined pressure is attained. Since the product and packaging materials will absorb some ethylene oxide the pressure within the chamber will drop. As this occurs more ethylene oxide needs to be pumped in to the system. Generally, ethylene oxide is recirculated throughout the sterilizing chamber to maintain an effective concentration in different areas of the chamber. As the pressure in the chamber is primarily due to the ethylene oxide, pressure readings give an indication of the concentration of the sterilizing gas.

The ethylene oxide concentration, in the range of 50 to 500 mg/L, has a dramatic effect on microbial kill rate. Concentrations between 400 and 650 mg/L are generally considered effective. The reasons for not using much higher concentrations are two-fold. First, above 800 mg/L the rate of kill does not increase significantly. Second, the residual ethylene oxide must be removed from the product before it can be used and it cannot easily be removed at higher concentrations.

At the end of the sterilization time, the recirculation of ethylene oxide is stopped. Forced air is circulated through the chamber and, by this means, ethylene oxide is pumped out. There must be optimal spacing between product containers, so that air can circulate efficiently. Optionally, nitrogen may be introduced to remove ethylene oxide faster from the chamber and from within the product.

Aeration

At the end of the sterilization cycle, the product is removed from the chamber and it is aerated in large chambers or rooms. This is done because residual ethylene oxide in the product, after forced air circulation, may be hazardous. Forced, HEPA-filtered air is circulated through the chamber or room. There must be optimal spacing between product containers so that air can circulate efficiently.

Ionizing Radiation Technologies

Two types of irradiation processes are used in industrial sterilization of medical products, namely, gamma rays and the electron beam. Gamma radiation is the more common type. It is used for the sterilization of small medical equipment since this process must be carried out in a non-aqueous environment.

Gamma rays are a form of electromagnetic radiation, frequently referred to as photons. They are emitted from a radioactive isotope, the most common being cobalt 60 (60 Co). Photons have no electric charge or mass. They transfer energy to the material being sterilized by Compton scattering collisions with electrons within the material being sterilized. The photon strikes free electrons in the material and, in so doing, passes a part of its energy to the electron as kinetic energy. The increased kinetic energy causes the electron to be displaced and such electrons continue moving, deflected from their original path.

The scattered gamma ray carries the balance of its energy (original energy minus that lost to the electrons) as it moves deeper into the material. It interacts again with electrons in its path, becoming slightly less energetic with each collision. The incident photon is replaced, at this point, with a number of energetic electrons and a photon of reduced energy (which is capable of going on to excite other electrons). As the gamma ray passes through the material, however, the probability of Compton scattering is low. Therefore, the primary beam of gamma rays will penetrate deep into the material before a large extent of scattering occurs. This means that the gamma rays deposit energy deeply (up to 50 cm), but the dose at each depth level is low due to the low Compton scattering. The absorbed dose is the quantity of ionizing radiation energy imparted per unit mass of a specific material. It is expressed as the gray (GY). The dose decreases exponentially with depth, that is, the gamma rays lose energy in an exponential fashion as they penetrate the material.

In contrast to gamma rays, electrons focused into a beam by a linear accelerator have both mass and charge. They interact easily with other charged particles. In so doing, they transfer their kinetic energy by means of elastic and inelastic collisions. As soon as charged particles penetrate solid materials, they are subject to the Coulomb force exerted by atomic nuclei. Therefore, they are in constant interaction with the material. These interactions result in many directional changes of the electrons which are slowed down. In the material, ionizations and radioactive processes occur. Because of the large amount of interactions, the penetration of an electron beam is small, relative to gamma radiation in the same type of material. The material density affects penetration extent. In fact, the penetration is inversely proportional to product density. Thus the nature of the material must be specified when making comparisons.

Microorganisms are killed by both gamma rays and electron beams primarily by ionization. Electrons are direct ionizing radiation whereas photons are indirect in their action, that is, they activate electrons in the substrate which act as the ionizing agent. The energy transferred by these radiations brings about chemical and/or physical changes at the molecular level which results in the death of the microorganism. (This may be due to DNA strand rupture or through chemical reaction in the cytoplasm, or in the environment of the microorganism.) Energy can be taken up in a bond of a DNA or RNA strand, causing a disruption of its structure. Alternately, free radicals can be generated in the water contained in the cytoplasm of the cell. The free radicals can react with, for example, an enzyme (protein) to alter its normal cellular metabolism.

Sterilization by Filtration

Filtration is a method to sterilize solutions by the use of a sterilizing grade filter to remove microorganisms from the liquid, producing a sterile effluent. This technique is commonly used for small volumes of liquids in compounding pharmacies. It is also used for the sterilization of freeze-dried liquids. Most filters at the current time have a pore size of 0.22 µm or less. Each filter is discarded after the filtration of a single lot. It is important to realize that the entire filter assembly and the container into which the filtrate flows must be sterile for the solution to be sterile. For compounding pharmacies, small volume units (eg, 500 mL) can be purchased, complete with the filter, as a sterilized assembly in a sealed package (Figure 12-7). The unit is discarded after one use.

Industrial filters, in addition to being much larger, must also be able to withstand the higher pressures involved with the sterilization of large volumes. The apertures in the filter, while individually small, are numerous and occupy a large proportion of the surface area of the filter. Thus, they are able to filter rapidly in spite of the small aperture size. Filter integrity is an important aspect to ensure efficacy. With a larger surface area for filtration (ie, more spaces), relative to the total surface area, the filter material must be strong and not tear easily. Some filter materials are not suitable for aqueous solutions because of their hydrophobic nature but they will be more suitable for organic, hydrophobic solutions.

Sterility Testing

The compendia (such as the USP) as well as the FDA, in a guidance document, describe methods for sterility testing. While there are small differences in these methods, the basic principles are the same. Therefore, in this chapter, a general description of test procedures is given which will be applicable to any of the methods referred to. For this reason, specifics (such as the volumes of liquids or incubation temperatures) are not mentioned.

There are two procedures by which these tests are conducted: the membrane filtration and the direct transfer methods. In the first method, a specified volume of liquid is filtered through a filter having a nominal pore size of 0.22 µm. For injection testing, the fill volume of the individual units of the injection and the batch size determine the volume to be filtered. The filter is then submerged in a defined recovery medium (one that supports microbial growth) and incubated at a specified temperature for 14 days. The entire test is repeated using a second microbial growth medium that is specified in the method.

The second test method omits filtration. Instead, the product is directly immersed into a suitable volume of each of the two media to allow growth. The media are selected to support growth, respectively, of aerobic organisms, and those that thrive in an environment having limited oxygen. Both types of tests require a positive control, that is, a demonstration of growth in samples that had been intentionally inoculated with microorganisms. The test, obviously, evaluates representative samples only. One of the criticisms of the test has been the fact that it can only prove the sterility of those samples tested—samples which are destroyed by the test process. For this reason, some writers have expressed the opinion that the sterility test is simply a quality control test, and that it cannot prove the sterility of the batch.

Endotoxin Testing

The toxic effects of endotoxins include fever which is a pyrogenic response, hypotension, tachycardia, shock, and lethal toxicity. A local sensitivity reaction that is seen is referred to as the Schwartzman reactivity. It is visible after a second non-toxic dose of an endotoxin is injected intravenously, as bleeding at the first injection site. Since fever is usually the first reaction seen with a low dose of endotoxin, the latter is also referred to as a pyrogen. However, endotoxins are not the only pyrogens; many other substances may also cause a fever upon injection and are, hence, pyrogens. Endotoxins are the most potent pyrogen and techniques to get rid of endotoxins would eliminate other pyrogens. Sterilization techniques, if continued for long enough, usually eliminate or reduce endotoxins to a safe level. Dry heat sterilization is the most effective at eliminating endotoxins. Extensive washing especially with acids or bases or other effective chemical agents can reduce the endotoxin load prior to sterilization. Treatment with hydrogen peroxide similarly reduces the endotoxin load. The effect of an endotoxin is, essentially, an inflammatory response brought about by secretion of cytokines mainly by macrophages.

Endotoxins are only produced by gram-negative bacteria. The endotoxin is a structural component of the cell envelope of this bacterium. The inner membrane is a typical biological membrane similar in structure to that of a gram-positive cell. It consists of a phospholipid bilayer with embedded proteins. It is the outer membrane that results in the endotoxin reactivity. This membrane consists of two layers: an inner phospholipid layer and an outer layer which consists mainly of lipopolysaccharides (LPS), and not phospholipid. It is the LPS that acts as the endotoxin.

A pyrogen test was previously used and it detected pyrogens from any source. The Limulus amebocyte lysate (LAL) test is specific for endotoxins and has replaced the pyrogen test since endotoxin is the most potent pyrogen and the most likely pyrogen to be found in an injectable. The name of this test is derived from the systematic name for the horseshoe crab, *Limulus polyphemus*. The blood of this organism, unlike that of mammals, does not contain all of the factors required for clotting: an endotoxin is required to complete the clotting mechanism. The clotting proteins that Limulus does have are contained in granules in the amebocytes (blood cells) of this crab.

For producing the test reagent, these proteins are extracted in the form of a lysate obtained from the disrupted amebocytes. This material is formulated into the LAL reagent. A primary standard has been prepared and is maintained in official standards laboratories while secondary standards, for use in everyday laboratory work, have been prepared at equivalent potency.

The two methods of conducting the test are, first, one in which the injection to be tested is reacted with the LAL reagent (the "pre-gel"). If an endotoxin is present in the injectable liquid, the reagent is converted into a gel-clot. A photometric method is also available. The LAL reagent is mixed with the injectable material and studied spectrophotometrically at specified wavelengths. In the presence of endotoxins, the solution becomes turbid and the turbidity can be measured. The reaction can be detected far sooner by this method than by the gel clot method. This method is actually a turbidimetric measurement since the extent to which light passes through the turbid material is measured.

Recap Questions

1. Name three methods of sterilization.
2. Name two sterilization methods that require the use of steam.
3. What is the D-value, a term used with regard to sterilization?
4. How does ethylene oxide kill microorganisms?
5. Which has better penetrating power: gamma rays or the electron-beam?
6. What is an endotoxin?

SUMMARY POINTS

- Injections are complex formulations that must be well understood by pharmacists involved with their use.
- Injections are prepared as solutions, suspensions, and powders for reconstitution. Very long-acting, or depot, formulations are increasing in number and provide controlled drug delivery with consistent blood levels over an extended period.
- Depot injections are extremely useful in institutional settings where it may be difficult to administer short-acting injections repeatedly to many uncooperative patients.
- Sterility and quality control of injections is vital.

BIBLIOGRAPHY

Nema S, Ludwig JD. *Pharmaceutical Dosage Forms – Parenteral Medications.* 3rd ed. Vol 1: Formulation and Packaging. New York, NY: Informa Healthcare; 2010.

Nema S, Ludwig JD. *Pharmaceutical Dosage Forms – Parenteral Medications.* 3rd ed. Vol 2: Facility Design, Sterilization and Processing. New York, NY: Informa Healthcare; 2010.

Wright JC, Hoffman AS. Historical overview of long acting injections and implants. In: Wright JC, Burgess DJ, eds. *Long Acting Injections and Implants.* Series: Advances in Delivery Science and Technology. doi:10.1007/978-1-4614-0554-2.

What do you think?

1. List all the points, from manufacturing up to administration of an injection, which could contribute to dose variation? Can one error cancel out another?
2. In terms of crystal growth in a suspension, which is worse: an elevated temperature or a reduced temperature, of short duration, during storage?
3. How can a formulation be sterilized without killing, or inactivating, microorganisms?
4. It has been said that one of the major difficulties in producing sterile injections is the fact that people are involved in their manufacture. Explain this statement.
5. Why do you think the development of injectable polymer microparticles mirrored the development of subcutaneous implantable beads?

Nanotechnology

13

PREVIEW

- Why nanotechnology is a new paradigm, not just a new technology
- Small size and large surface area
- Thinking about solubility in contrast to the rate of solution
  - Is solubility an intrinsic property or can it be changed by processing?
- Different types of nanoparticles and their basic function
  - Nanocrystals
  - Metallic nanoparticles
  - Micellar nanoparticles
  - Solid nanoparticles with drug embedded in or on them
  - Nanoparticles consisting of a shell encasing a liquid
- Marketed pharmaceutical products based on nanotechnology
- A perspective on the future of pharmaceutical nanotechnology

INTRODUCTION

As the name implies, nanotechnology refers to the science and technology of very small particles. In the pharmaceutical context, nanotechnology refers to very small particles used for drug delivery, for diagnostic purposes, and for other-related functions that will be outlined in this chapter. While much more will be said, in a later section, about particle size for pharmaceutical nanotechnology, it is a good idea to obtain a perspective on size at the outset. Figure 13-1 is a step diagram showing units used for measuring linear dimensions where each step is a factor of $1000\times$. As can be seen from this diagram, a micrometer is 1 thousandth of a millimeter. The latter, itself, is a very small dimension in terms of sizes familiar in daily life. The diagram depicts other familiar linear dimensions, for comparison. Some perspective on the size of nanoparticles is also obtained by considering that a human hair is 80 to 120 μm in diameter. If we consider the "average" human hair to be 100 μm in thickness, then a 100-nm particle is one thousandth the thickness of a human hair. Such a nanoparticle would be a reasonable size for consideration in pharmaceutical nanotechnology, and not an extreme example. Protein molecules are very large in comparison to inorganic molecules, and some protein molecules are in the nanometer size range. For example, the diameter of the hemoglobin molecule is 5 nm. The C_{60} molecule (also known as the Buckyball) has a diameter of 0.7 nm. The smallness of a nanometer may also be gauged from the fact that the ratio of a nanometer to a meter is approximately the same as the ratio of the diameter of a toy marble to that of the earth.

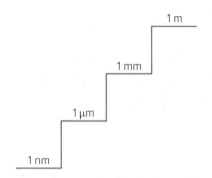

FIGURE 13-1 Step diagram of units for linear dimensions.

RATE OF SOLUTION AND SOLUBILITY

It is a common practice in the laboratory to grind a solid material before dissolving it. Why, exactly, is this done? The small size of the particles increases the rate of solution, that is, a fixed weight of the powder will take less time to dissolve under the same conditions (such as stirring rate).

Why should drug particles or crystals be made progressively smaller? Consider a poorly soluble substance that is available as large crystals, in the millimeter size range. Now consider the effect of reducing these particles into even smaller sizes. Particles of a few millimeters diameter are converted to particles of hundreds of micrometers, then to tens of micrometers, and to single-digit micrometer dimensions. The rate of solution of an equal weight of each of these differently sized particles increases with decreasing particle size. The reason for this is the fact that the total surface area of a given weight of powder increases dramatically with decrease in particle size. The relationship between particle size and dissolution rate is given by the Noyes-Whitney Equation, Eq. (4-10). One factor in the equation is the total surface area of unit mass of the powder particles (S). The dissolution rate is proportional to S.

The effect of size can be visualized by considering a cube measuring 2 × 2 × 2 cm. Suppose this cube is subdivided by cutting each side into half, as illustrated in Figure 13-2. The total surface area of the resulting eight small cubes increases as illustrated in this figure. It is assumed, for this illustration, that no material is lost in the cutting process. If each side of the eight small cubes is again divided into two, the resulting 64 tiny cubes have a greater total surface area than the eight small cubes, and a much greater total surface area than the original cube. By decreasing the size, as illustrated, until one side of the cube is one-fourth of its original dimension, the surface area is increased four times. If the process of subdivision were to continue for a few more orders of

magnitude, the total surface area would be increased to an even greater extent.

Hence, a coarse powder ground to progressively finer particles has a progressively greater dissolution rate. Suppose a coarse powder was progressively ground, as described above, and the final product was in the 1 to 20 μm range, that is, not in the nanometer category. The total surface area of a given weight of this material has increased greatly compared to the original particles. An even greater increase in the surface area can be expected when size reduction is continued into the nanometer range and, correspondingly, a greater rate of solution can also be expected. However, the actual rate of solution obtained from nanoparticles is significantly greater than that predicted from surface area comparisons.

In the above discussion, only the rate of solution increases with decrease in particle size, that is, if the solubility of the material was 0.2 g per 100 mL, subdivision of the particles decreases the time it takes to dissolve a fixed quantity of substance, under standardized conditions, but the solubility is not affected and is fixed at 0.2 g per 100 mL. Historically, the solubility of the material was considered an intrinsic property of the material, that is, it does not change with changes in other parameters such as particle size. However, this is only true when dealing with materials of larger-than-nanometer dimensions. The concept of the sanctity of solubility only prevailed when material could not be converted into nanoparticles and the properties of the latter were not fully understood. Nanoparticles display increased solubility which is partly responsible for the apparent increase in dissolution rate that is observed. The reason for the increase in solubility is a complex subject which requires mathematical treatment for a full understanding. However, for the purpose of this chapter, a very brief explanation is offered below.

Consider a single-component liquid, such as water, in a beaker with air above the surface of the liquid. All the molecules of the liquid, in this case water, have the same chemical composition (H_2O). However, the surface molecules of the water, in contact with the air, behave very differently from the molecules in the interior of the water. Interior molecules experience attractive forces from nearby molecules, in all directions. The surface molecules, on the other hand, experience strong attractive molecular forces, from the water molecules within the body of the water, which tends to pull the surface molecules inward. The surface molecules also experience an upward force which is far weaker than the downward pull. The nature of the material above the liquid, which exerts the upward force, is responsible for this difference. Air has fewer molecules (largely N_2) compared to an equal volume of water, and each molecule of air also exerts a smaller attractive force. The fact that the surface

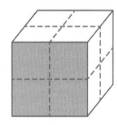

Cut no.	Side (cm)	Total area (cm²)		Increase over original
0.	2	2 × 2 × 6	= 24 cm²	–
1.	1	1 × 1 × 6 × 8	= 48 cm²	2 ×
2.	0.5	0.5 × 0.5 × 6 × 8 × 8 × 8	= 96 cm²	4 ×

FIGURE 13-2 Subdivision of a cube.

molecules of water are being pulled inward is not obvious in a beaker of water due to the interaction of the water molecules with the glass of the beaker. However, if the surface of liquid is free to contract, the effect of the larger inward forces will be observed. Dispersed droplets, for example, assume a spherical shape due to this inward pulling force. Having established that the molecules on the surface of a liquid behave differently from those in the interior, how does the behavior of the atoms on the surface of a crystal differ from that of atoms in its interior?

Consider a crystal such as one of sodium chloride. It consists of positively charged sodium ions and negatively charged chloride ions packed together as a cube (Figure 13-3). The atoms within the interior of the crystal, referred to as the bulk atoms, experience strong attractive forces from neighboring atoms of the opposite charge. Such attractive forces are exerted in all directions in the three-dimensional cubic structure. The attractive forces from more distant atoms, of the opposite charge, are lower than those that are closer, this force decreasing rapidly with distance. For this reason, significant attractive forces are only experienced from the first few (closest) atoms of opposite charge in all directions. The attractive forces from the more distant atoms are insignificant. Surface atoms do not experience attractive forces from oppositely charged atoms above the plane of the surface of the crystal. As mentioned, air molecules exert little attractive force on the surface molecules of a substance, in this case the crystal.

The net effect of the above considerations is that surface molecules are not as tightly held to the crystal as are interior molecules. As can be seen from Figure 13-3, the corner atoms are least tightly held to the crystal. A common imperfection in a crystal is the absence of atoms from the corners.

Since the surface atoms are more loosely held to the crystal, these atoms will detach from the crystal most easily in a solvent in which the substance is soluble. When sodium chloride is placed into water, the attractive forces of water for the surface atoms of the crystal will cause these atoms to leave the surface, that is, they dissolve in water. Hence, dissolution is said to be a surface phenomenon. In all crystals, then, dissolution occurs from the surface, and the crystal becomes progressively smaller. Atoms within the depth of the crystal, as mentioned, are tightly bound and do not experience these surface effects.

As surface layers dissolve, the next layer is exposed. Eventually, the tightly bound atoms in the interior become surface atoms and they, too, will dissolve. Now, the ratio of bulk atoms to surface atoms in a nanocrystal is greatly decreased relative to larger crystals. This results in insufficient nearest atoms to strongly attract the surface atoms. Thus, the surface atoms are able to leave the surface more easily, that is, the surface is said to be "fluidized," leading to a greatly increased dissolution rate. A crystal of nanometer dimensions is so small that the difference between surface atoms and interior atoms becomes less distinct. Practically all atoms behave as surface atoms, that is, they leave the crystal easily to become solvated. In effect, it means that the solubility of the substance is increased.

Now consider the situation from the perspective of the solvent, water, in the examples discussed. First, consider the general case, that is, that of large crystals. The solvent must have the ability to attract the atoms of the crystal. As the solvent becomes saturated, this ability decreases. It is for this reason that dissolution, of conventional solids, is rapid initially and becomes increasingly slower. As the saturation point is reached, the dissolution rate becomes very slow because the near-saturated liquid has little power to attract solute from the crystal. In a nanocrystal, less attractive force is required from the solvent to dissolve the substance with the result that the solvent can continue to dissolve more substance. This continues even as concentrations are reached that would be considered close to saturation for large crystals. As the solvent continues to dissolve the crystal, it exceeds the traditionally established solubility of the substance. Consequently, the solubility, and not only the dissolution rate, of a nanocrystal is greater than that of larger-sized crystals.

Because the attractive force between oppositely charged atoms drops off rapidly with distance, it is only a few nearest atoms (in each direction) that can exert significant attractive force, as stated. Therefore, the solubility is not a continuum from a high value for very small particles (of nanometer dimensions) and gradually decreasing to a low value for large particles. Instead, there is a sudden drop to a lower solubility value for particles larger than a few hundred nanometers.

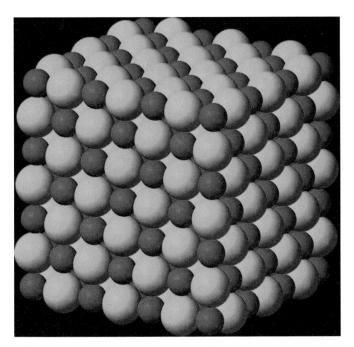

FIGURE 13-3 Diagram of a sodium chloride crystal.

Recap Questions

1. Distinguish between the terms, "dissolution rate" and "solubility."

2. What are surface atoms and how do they differ from atoms in the interior?

3. Why do the corners of cubic crystals tend to break off?

4. What are "nearest atoms," in terms of dissolution theory?

DEFINITION AND SIZE

The reader may think it is obvious that the term, "nanoparticles," refers to particles of nano dimensions, with no room for ambiguity. However, the reality is more complex: the definition is not simply a literal definition determined by units but depends also on function. For this reason, the definition has changed as nanotechnology developed. Initial work on nanomaterials was done by physicists and the definition depended on the optical and electronic properties of materials. Such properties change dramatically below 100 nm and, therefore, this becomes the size limitation embodied in original definitions of nanoparticles. Since almost any particulate material is a heterogeneous mixture of different-sized particles, newer definitions embodied language to describe a particular fraction of the population of particles such as "50% or more" (have a particular size dimension). As described in Chapter 5, Pharmaceutical Powders, in assigning a percentage, the analyst must also mention the basis on which the value was determined: a weight basis or a number basis.

An additional factor that relates to the irregular shape of the particles is the question of which dimension to consider. Most standards require the diameter, or one dimension, to be between specified size limits. The definitions of some official compendiums were being revised at the time of writing. A practical definition for pharmaceutical nanoparticles is the following: particles in which the diameter, or one dimension, of the majority of particles, is up to 200 nm.

TYPES OF NANOPARTICLES

Numerous types of nanoparticles have been developed over the last few decades. Not only is their complexity increasing due to innovation, but combinations or hybrid forms of the traditional nanoparticle types have also been produced and are described in the literature. Hybrids may require new terminology, and sometimes it is difficult to describe the "type" or class to which a particular complex nanoparticle belongs.

The following description starts from elementary nanoparticles to the more complex, with a few commercial examples given. The intention is not to provide a comprehensive listing of all nanoparticle types since they are numerous and the description would be confusing. Many of the nanomaterials presently in the research phase are unlikely to see commercialization. This is the nature of the research enterprise: many ideas are tested and several may be abandoned, some may even reach an advanced stage of clinical testing, only to be abandoned for the lack of significant efficacy, or due to toxicity. Few actually reach the market. Included in the descriptions in this chapter are some that are in commercial production, or show this potential.

The approach to the categorization of the different types of nanoparticles is simple: nanoparticles may be small drug particles; small inorganic particles which constitute the active pharmaceutical ingredient (API) or have the API embedded in or on them; small solid matrix particles, consisting of polymers or solid lipids, with drug embedded in or on them; or small volumes of drug-containing liquids that are bounded by a shell or some type of containment material, where it is understood that the term "small" refers to nano dimensions (Mind Map 13-1). Several of these categories have subcategories, or other complexities, and the reader is advised to keep this diagrammatical summary in mind while reading the rest of this chapter.

This chapter will not provide detailed methods by which nanoparticles are made: that is beyond the scope of the book and, probably, the interest of the intended reader. Instead, an introduction is given to the types of nanoparticulate dosage forms that are likely to be encountered in pharmacy practice. Some theoretical introduction is also provided in the hope that it will allow the pharmacist to read and understand information

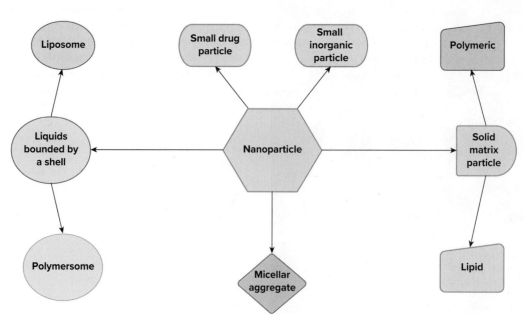

MIND MAP 13-1 Major classes of nanoparticles.

about novel nanoparticulate dosage forms that are presently on the market but not mentioned in this chapter, or that come to market in the future.

NANOSIZED DRUG PARTICLES

The nanoparticle, in this case, consists entirely of the drug, whereas other types of nanoparticles, as will be described later, have additional chemicals combined with the drug. A formulation consisting of the drug only enables maximal drug load. The particle is usually crystalline and, therefore, the term "nanocrystal" is used. The nanocrystals may be formed in two ways: the top-down and the bottom-up techniques. In the first technique, large particles are subdivided into progressively smaller units until particles in the nanosize range are achieved. This is the more common technique for producing nanocrystals. The NanoCrystal® technology was developed by NanoSystems, an American company, which was acquired by the Irish company, Elan Corporation. This technology is probably the best known of the top-down techniques and has yielded several marketed pharmaceutical products.

The bottom-up technology starts with a solution of the drug. By manipulating the physico-chemical conditions, the drug is precipitated from this solution. Highly controlled processes, such as the addition of nonsolvent at a precise rate, with continuous stirring, are used to induce the precipitation of very small drug particles. Some of these particles are in the nanosize range. It is emphasized that it is the very tightly controlled conditions that enable particles in the nanosize range, to be formed; under conditions that are not well-controlled, macroscopic crystals form or a wide range of particles sizes result. This process is less frequently used than particle size reduction or grinding (a top-down process).

It is also possible to use a combination of the two processes. For example, the Nanoedge™ technology of Baxter Pharmaceutical Company utilizes micro precipitation (a bottom-up technique) to form microparticles. These are ground by high-pressure homogenization (a top-down process) to form particles of nano dimensions. The nanocrystals may then be incorporated into other dosage forms, most frequently into injections which may be formulated for extended release (ER). For example, Invega Sustenna is an ER injection of the antipsychotic, paliperidone palmitate. The injection is administered once a month and offers far better control of the psychoses than previous antipsychotics. Table 13-1 lists some products on the US market that utilize nanocrystals.

Inorganic Nanoparticles

A variety of inorganic materials have been used as drug carriers, APIs, or diagnostic agents. These materials may further be divided into metallic and nonmetallic nanostructures. With respect to metallic nanostructures, gold, palladium, copper, iron, silver, platinum, selenium, and lanthanides have been used in research studies. Up to the time of writing, only iron, zinc (as zinc oxide), and titanium (as titanium dioxide) have been used to a significant extent in medications and cosmetics

that have reached the marketplace. Metals have been used to synthesize a range of novel nanostructural shapes for research studies but, as yet, none has reached the marketplace. Apart from noting that some of these interesting shapes, such as nanoprisms and nanopyramids, could possibly become medications in the future, these novel metallic nanoparticles will not be described further.

Metallic nanostructures can, generally, be synthesized by top-down or bottom-up approaches similar to those described for nanocrystals. The bottom-up method involves the construction of the nanostructure by the addition of individual molecules or atoms, to gradually form the required shape. In the top-down approach, the bulk material is reduced in size using physical or chemical methods. Top-down approaches often result in structural units with surface imperfections which can have a critical impact on surface chemistry. Since nanoparticles have a high aspect ratio (the ratio of surface area to volume), surface chemistry may have a large influence on their properties. Carbon and silica are the most common nonmetals used in nanoparticle development. Carbon has been utilized to create interesting structures. Carbon, as well as many metal, nanostructures are not biodegradable and may accumulate in the body to cause long-term toxicity. This is a possibility even when short-term toxicity is not obvious. Due to these toxicity concerns, they have not been used in marketed nanoparticle products and will not be considered further in this chapter.

Because organic nanoparticles are biodegradable they are used far more than inorganic nanoparticles. A notable exception is iron oxide nanoparticles which have been used internally. As is well known, iron is a constituent of hemoglobin and iron-containing formulations have been used for the treatment of anemia long before the advent of nanomedicines. In recent times, nanoparticulate iron has been found to be more effective in the treatment of iron deficiency, especially in certain special classes such as iron deficiency with kidney failure. An example is Feraheme which is an iron compound coated with a carbohydrate material. The ultra-small particles are trapped by the reticulo-endothelial system (RES) in the liver, spleen, and bone marrow. Within the macrophages of these organs, the carbohydrate coating dissolves to release the iron component into vesicles. The iron, thereafter, either gets incorporated into the intracellular iron pool (for storage) or enters the plasma as a transferrin complex. Iron is slowly released and less frequent injections are needed (one treatment consists of two injections 3 to 8 days apart).

An interesting class of compounds is the super paramagnetic iron oxide nanoparticles (SPIONs) which are used as contrast agents in magnetic resonance imaging (MRI). They consist of ferric iron (Fe^{3+}) and ferrous iron (Fe^{2+}) in the particle core. The latter is surrounded by a polymer such as polyethylene glycol (PEG). Since SPIONs are captured by the RES, they are suitable for imaging the liver, spleen, and lymph nodes. The SPIONs appear dark on the MRI image, improving the sharpness and sensitivity of tissue images. In addition, an agent may be attached to the polymer coating for targeting a particular cell type, possessing a specific receptor, and located in organ(s) of interest. It should be noted that the iron in Feraheme is in the form of a SPION, but it is not intended for imaging. In fact,

TABLE 13-1 Some Marketed Nanocrystal Products

TRADE NAME (MANUFACTURER) YEAR INTRODUCED*	DRUG NAME (PHARMACOLOGICAL ACTION)	COMMENTS
Rapamune® (Wyeth) 2000	Sirolimus (Immunosuppressant)	Tablet and oral solution. First nanopharmaceutical product to be marketed (1990).
Emend® (Merck) 2003	Aprepitant (Anti-emetic)	Capsule and powder for oral suspension. Very poorly soluble drug. Small particle size/large surface area allows enhanced dissolution and absorption.
Tricor® (Lupin Atlantis) 2004	Fenofibrate (Hyperlipidemia)	Tablet. Increased bioavailability and decreased dose
Triglide® 2005 DISCONTINUED	Fenofibrate (Hypolipidemic)	Tablet. Decreased dose
Megace® ES (Par Pharmaceuticals) 2005	Megestrol acetate (Anti-anorexic)	Oral suspension. Reduced dosing
NanOss® (Rti Surgical) (Pre-market)	Hydroxyapatite (Bone substitute)	Prefilled syringe. Nano-structured hydroxyapatite—extremely high surface area, for more cell attachment sites for osteoclasts and osteoblasts. Improved mineralization and bone formation.
EquivaBone® (Zimmer Biomet) (Pre-market)	Hydroxyapatite (Bone substitute)	Kit for reconstitution of semi-solid. Nanocrystalline and amorphous calcium phosphate, comparable to mineral composition of human bone. Scaffold for new bone growth mimics bone structure.
Invega® Sustenna® (Janssen Pharma) 2009/2014	Paliperidone palmitate (Schizophrenia/schizoaffective disorder)	ER suspension of poorly water-soluble drug (racemic mixture)
Abraxane (Abraxis Bioscience LLC) 2005	nab-paclitaxel (Advanced breast/pancreatic/non-small cell lung cancer)	nab = nanoparticle albumin bound. Improved bioavailability without use of solvent. Replaces Cremophor EL–containing formulation which caused toxicity and hypersensitivity reactions.

*According to Orange book, which may reflect the most recent reformulation, or update of information, not the date of first marketing.

the product literature states that imaging studies should not be done shortly after Feraheme administration, because it may affect the image.

Many mesoporous silicon nanostructures are able to host "guest" molecules in the numerous small cavities and pores on the particle surface. Such guest molecules may consist of drugs (including macromolecules), and imaging or contrast agents. Nanoparticulate titanium dioxide has been used as a sun screening agent, usually in combination with other such agents. While effective as a sunscreen, these particles have come under criticism for potential undesirable effects. Such reactions are thought to occur in two ways: first, the nanoparticles may penetrate the skin, causing toxic reactions; and, second, because of the way titanium dioxide dissipates the UV light energy that it absorbs. After absorption of potentially skin-damaging UV light (a protective mechanism), titanium dioxide releases superoxides which are known to cause damage to the skin, including damage to the DNA of cells. The net protective effect of titanium dioxide is questioned.

Recap Questions

1. Why is the definition of nanoparticles not simply "particles of nanometer dimensions"?
2. Which form of nanoparticle has the highest drug content?
3. Distinguish between top-down and bottom-up nanoparticle formation processes.
4. Why are organic nanoparticles more popular than inorganic types?

MICELLES

Micelles may consist of surfactant molecules, that is, molecules which have relatively well-balanced hydrophobic and hydrophilic groups. The hydrophilic group usually consists of a small polar group whereas the hydrophobic group is a long hydrocarbon chain or "tail." The amphiphilic nature of these molecules contributes to the formation of micelles, as described below. At low surfactant concentrations, individual surfactant molecules are present in solution (in an un-aggregated form). However, their distribution in the aqueous phase is not uniform: there is a tendency for some of the molecules to be located at the surface of the medium, with their hydrophobic tails protruding into the air. This arrangement reduces the contact of the hydrophobic tails with water, with which they have no affinity.

As surfactant concentration is gradually increased; however, another phenomenon is observed. Initially, the concentration of surfactant in solution simply increases. At a particular concentration, referred to as the critical micelle concentration (CMC), the molecules aggregate to form a sphere with a special configuration and purpose (Figure 13-4). The hydrophobic tails reduce contact with water by pointing inward, toward the interior of the sphere, and the hydrophilic groups are on the external spherical surface, where they are in contact with the aqueous medium. The CMC is dependent upon the temperature of the medium. While other micellar shapes are possible, a sphere is formed most often and is the only shape considered in this chapter.

By forming this arrangement, the surfactant molecules reduce exposure of the hydrophobic tails to the aqueous environment. (This is analogous to pointing the tails into the air at lower concentrations of the surfactant.) The hydrophilic groups point toward the aqueous environment, to which they are favorably disposed. By this aggregation mechanism, the hydrophobic tails could be viewed as creating their own hydrophobic environment in the interior of the sphere. For drug delivery, hydrophobic drugs can be captured in the hydrophobic interior of the micelle, while the micelle, itself, is within an aqueous environment. Thus, the hydrophobic drug is in an ideal environment, surrounded by the hydrophobic tails of the surfactant molecules, while being transported within an aqueous

environment throughout the body. A hydrophobic drug moving freely through a hydrophilic medium, such as blood, would otherwise be a contradiction.

While micelles were traditionally formed from surfactants, as described above, in the realm of pharmaceutical nanotechnology it is more useful to form micelles from specially-developed block copolymers. These have somewhat longer hydrophilic, than hydrophobic, blocks in the polymer chain. When the micelle forms, the hydrophilic ring, surrounding the hydrophobic core, is much larger than in traditional micelles in which the ring is formed from small hydrophilic groups (Figure 13-5). These larger groups are involved in compact packing, referred to as Palisade packing, within the micelle. The hydrophilic ring is consequently much tougher. As a result, these micelles are more stable than traditional micelles. Their circulation time is also longer and they display improved biodistribution. In addition, PEG, or similar compounds, used as the hydrophilic portion, have OH groups which can be used for linking targeting moieties. An additional type of micellar component consists of polymers conjugated with lipid molecules. In aqueous solution, they form micelles which have found utility in drug delivery.

Reversed micelles have also been described in the literature. These have the hydrophobic tails on the outside and the hydrophilic groups on the interior. These micelles could usefully be employed to carry hydrophilic drugs in an oily environment, for example, in a cosmetically-acceptable oil for topical administration.

The only micellar formulation on the US market, as judged from Orange Book listings, was Estrasorb, an ethinyl estradiol formulation. The micellar nanoparticles are presented as an emulsion, packaged in foil pouches. Each pouch contains 1.74 g of emulsion equivalent to 0.025 mg of estradiol. The patient applies the contents of one pouch to each of her legs (thigh and calf). Thus, two pouches were needed to supply the required amount of estradiol to treat the vasomotor symptoms of menopause. From the foregoing, it will be realized that this is

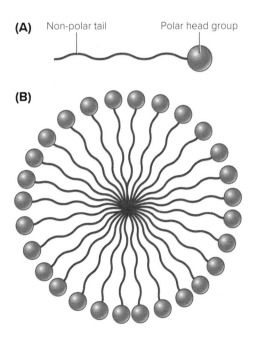

FIGURE 13-4 Structure of a typical micelle.

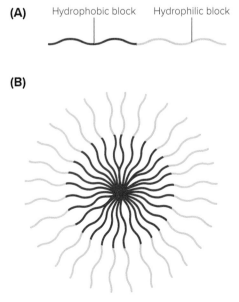

FIGURE 13-5 A block copolymer and a micelle formed from it.

an example of a nanotechnology product presented as a topical dosage form. Estrasorb was discontinued in 2021.

LIPID MATRIX NANOPARTICLES

This class of nanoparticles is further divided into solid lipid nanoparticles (SLN) and nanostructured lipid carriers (NLC). The former are well-known and have been described in the research literature for long, whereas the latter are newer and may be considered an improved version.

SLNs are composed of a lipid (or a blend of lipids) that is solid at room temperature (Figure 13-6). They are frequently stabilized by a surfactant layer over the surface of the particles. These nanoparticles show improved physical stability in comparison to "nanocapsules" which, as the name suggests, have a shell with a liquid lipid core (described in a later section of this chapter). SLNs are relatively easily produced and are of low cytotoxicity due to the fact that they are produced from physiological lipids, or common lipid excipients which are known to be non-toxic.

SLNs can only be loaded with relatively low amounts of drugs. When the lipids are mixed with the drug, during production, the drug molecules become located between the fatty acid chains of the matrix. During further processing, as well as during storage, the crystallinity of the fatty material increases. This leads to expulsion of the drug molecules from their location between the fatty acid chains, and to their presence on the surface of the nanoparticle after processing, or after storage. The surface drug dissolves rapidly when the particles are placed in an aqueous medium. This phenomenon

may be observed as a burst drug release from SLNs. A burst release refers to the rapid, initial release of a portion of the drug load. It is the highly crystalline nature of the lipid matrix that is responsible for this rapid drug release. In addition, the drug exhibits agglomeration within the crystal lattices of the lipid material, resulting in the formation of drug crystals. Consequently, when the drug is pushed out to the surface of the nanoparticles, it is in the crystalline form, a form which exacerbates the rapid drug release.

NLCs were especially developed to reduce some of the undesirable properties of SLNs and may be considered the second generation of lipid nanoparticles. They consist of a mixture of lipids which, at room temperature, contain both solid and liquid components. This mixture of lipid materials results in the crystal structure of the matrix being less organized, that is, it is less crystalline and more amorphous than the SLN. The loaded drug can be in both the molecular form and in clustered aggregates at lattice imperfections of the crystalline lipid. Due to this structure, NLCs exhibit better drug loading and reduced drug leakage or burst effect. Lipid nanoparticles are more efficient for hydrophobic drug loading than they are for hydrophilic drugs.

For SLN and NLC production, the molten lipid is allowed to slowly drip into a cold aqueous medium that is being rapidly stirred. The hot lipid solidifies as droplets due to the cooling effect of the aqueous medium. The incorporation of hydrophilic drugs can be challenging in this method of nanoparticle formation since these drugs may partition toward the aqueous phase during the formation process. A major problem observed with lipid nanoparticles in vivo is the fact that they are rapidly cleared from the circulatory system by entrapment in the RES. This major disadvantage has been overcome by the application of surfactants to the surface of the nanoparticles or by PEGylation. The latter is the process by which the surface (lipid) molecules are treated with hydrophilic PEG.

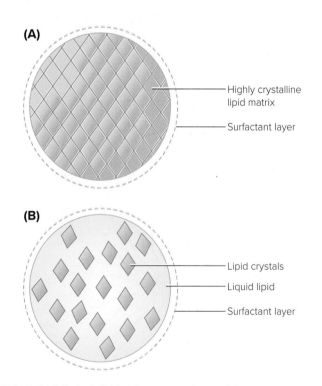

(A)

— Highly crystalline lipid matrix

— Surfactant layer

(B)

— Lipid crystals

— Liquid lipid

— Surfactant layer

FIGURE 13-6 A. Solid lipid nanoparticles and **B.** nanostructured lipid carriers.

Recap Questions

1. What is meant by the CMC with respect to micelle formation?
2. What is a reverse micelle? Name one application of reversed micelles.
3. Why are nanostructured lipid carriers better than solid lipid nanoparticles for drug delivery?
4. Why is it easier to produce lipid matrix nanoparticles with hydrophobic drugs, rather than hydrophilic ones?

POLYMERIC MATRIX NANOPARTICLES

As the name suggests, these nanoparticles consist of solid polymers which, to be useful, must be biocompatible and biodegradable. When water enters the matrix, it will dissolve the drug contained in the superficial portion of the nanoparticle. The drug, which is now in solution, will diffuse out of the nanoparticle to mix with the external fluid. In the presence of water, the biodegradable polymer chains will also be hydrolyzed, creating shorter polymer segments. These segments are more hydrophilic because of the polar end groups created by the hydrolysis reaction. Due to their greater affinity for water, as a consequence, they will leave the matrix. In this way, the nanoparticle erodes and exposes deeper layers containing additional drug. This process slowly releases the nanoparticle's drug content as erosion proceeds to progressively deeper layers.

The shortened fragments of biodegradable polymer that are released from the nanoparticle are then metabolized. Biocompatibility is not synonymous with biodegradation. The former means that the polymer is not toxic nor does it have untoward effects on biological systems. However, it may not be hydrolyzed to smaller fractions, as described above, due to the lack of hydrolyzable groups. The absence of such functional groups in a long polymer chain results in it remaining intact. There are two types of polymer matrix: hydrophobic and hydrophilic which are described below.

Hydrophobic Polymers

For matrix nanoparticle formulation, hydrophobic polymers are more common than the hydrophilic type. Common hydrophobic polymers include poly lactic acid (PLA), poly glycolic acid (PGA), and the copolymer made from these polymers, poly (lactide-co-glycolic acid) (PLGA). These polymers are biodegradable and, for this reason, are very popular for the fabrication of nanoparticles. Eudragit and ethylcellulose are examples of non-biodegradable polymers that have also been used for polymeric nanoparticles. The nanoparticles are usually administered by IV injection and are trapped by the RES. The inclusion of even small amounts of toxic, irritating, or sensitizing materials as formulation excipients is a concern in terms of both systemic and injection site reactions. An example of such an excipient is a surfactant that may be required for manufacturing, or to solubilize the drug. The Cremophor range of surfactants has been used extensively to aid in the solubilization of drugs. In several instances they have been found to cause injection site reactions and, in some cases, systemic toxicity. The polymers for nanoparticles can be formed *in situ* as the nanoparticle is being formed, that is, smaller subunits combine to form a larger polymer during nanoparticle formation. On the other hand, preformed polymers could be used for nanoparticle manufacture. The latter technique is described below.

The most common method of forming nanoparticles from preformed hydrophobic polymers is by emulsion techniques. The polymer and, usually, a hydrophobic drug are dissolved in an organic halogenated solvent. Such a solvent is very toxic but is required for adequate solubilization of the polymer. This solution is next emulsified in an aqueous medium containing a surfactant. This forms an oil-in-water (O/W) emulsion, where the organic solvent is the "oil." As the solvent is subsequently evaporated from the internal phase, it causes solid polymer to form at the solvent–water interface. Continued loss of solvent increases the extent of solid polymer precipitation at the

boundary of the internal phase droplet. Precipitation occurs because there is insufficient solvent, within the droplet, to keep the polymer in solution. Initially, precipitation occurs at the boundary because there is water, a non-solvent for the polymer, on the other side of the boundary. As precipitation continues, the volume of the internal phase droplet also decreases and, ultimately, a solid nanoparticle is formed. The nanoparticle consists of a hydrophobic polymer in which the hydrophobic drug is embedded. The external liquid phase is filtered off and the nanosized particles are washed and then dried. Many variations of this technique are possible and are used for various applications in nanoparticle fabrication. All of these techniques are, unfortunately, not suitable for protein and nucleic acid drugs due to denaturation of the drug in the organic solvents. Low encapsulation efficiency may also be observed for larger molecules, such as proteins. While high encapsulation efficiencies, that is, high drug loading capabilities, are possible with these techniques using small molecule hydrophobic drugs, they are unsuitable for water-soluble drugs. Additional problems are the facts that the surfactant may be toxic, and that the residual organic solvent may not be totally removed from the nanoparticles. Small quantities of solvent, embedded deeply, frequently resist removal even with extended drying. The FDA takes particular note of residual solvents, remaining after the manufacture of drug products. Even relatively small amounts of some solvents are unacceptable. The FDA places solvents into different classes, depending on their potential danger. For the most toxic solvents (class I), the limits are the most stringent. Each of these solvents has a different limit, measured in parts per million.

As opposed to the emulsion techniques, polymer precipitation has good entrapment efficiency. The drug and polymer are dissolved in a solvent. When this polymer solution is slowly added to a nonsolvent, with stirring, polymer precipitation occurs due to the fact that the solvent rapidly diffuses into the external medium. The precipitating polymer traps the drug. While, superficially, this process may resemble the emulsification process, there is no surfactant in the external medium and, therefore, an emulsion does not form. Because of the rapid transfer of the solvent to the external phase, the process is rapid. Since there is no surfactant added to the formulation, toxic effects from the latter are also absent. Some drugs, such as proteins, may be sensitive to the solvents used during processing. In addition, the presence of trace amounts of solvent, after the manufacturing process is over, is a problem.

Hydrophilic Polymers

Commonly used examples of hydrophilic polymers are chitosans, alginates, and gelatin. These polymers are incorporated into water to form hydrogels which contain more than 50% w/w water. Although they appear as solids macroscopically, at the molecular level they behave like liquids. The hydrogels are formed into nanoparticles and, to form a more rigid mass, the polymer is then cross-linked. Covalent and ionic cross-linking are both possible. The latter is referred to as ionotropic gelation and involves the use of low-molecular-weight poly-anions such as tripolyphosphate (TPP).

In the case of chitosan, an acidic solution of the polymer (pH = 4-6) is first prepared. Next, an alkaline TPP solution (pH = 7-9) is slowly added while stirring the bulk solution. The anionic phosphate groups of TPP react with the cationic amine groups of chitosan, forming inter- and intra-molecular linkages. Alginates, on the other hand, are anionic and will react with cationic groups. For example, calcium chloride has been used to cross-link alginates.

Recap Questions

1. Distinguish between biocompatibility and biodegradation.
2. Name two types of matrix nanoparticles.
3. With reference to polymeric nanoparticles, what is meant by the term "erosion"?
4. Why are proteins particularly difficult to formulate as polymeric nanoparticles?
5. Name two hydrophilic polymers used to form nanoparticles.

VESICULAR SYSTEMS

A vesicle, in biology, is a small structure containing a liquid which is bound by a membrane. Analogously, in pharmaceutics, a vesicular structure refers to one containing a liquid and bound by some type of film or membrane, or other structural material which contains the liquid. In contrast to matrix systems, which are solid, vesicular systems consist of an outer shell and an inner core of liquid. Four basic types of vesicular systems can be identified on the basis of the shell material and the nature of the liquid in the core. For purposes of classification and simplicity, the different vesicular systems could be considered to have two major classes:

1. Vesicles with aqueous cores
   a. Liposomes have a phospholipid bilayer which forms the shell surrounding the aqueous core.
   b. Polymersomes have a polymer which forms the shell surrounding the aqueous core.
2. Vesicles with oily cores
   a. Polymeric nanocapsules have a polymer shell surrounding the oily core.
   b. Lipid nanocapsules have a surfactant shell surrounding the oily core.

Vesicles with Aqueous Cores

Liposomes

Liposomes consist of a lipid shell encasing an aqueous core. The lipids are phospholipids which have a hydrophilic head group and two long hydrophobic tails. Phospholipids are poorly soluble in water and, therefore, spontaneously self-assemble into flat bilayers or sheets, with the lipid tails facing each other, to reduce contact with water. Further, the bilayer closes on itself to form a sphere to further reduce contact with water (Figure 13-7). Thus, phospholipids placed into water will spontaneously form spherical vesicles, or liposomes.

Liposomes may consist of a single bi-layer of lipid material, in which case they are referred to as unilamellar, or they may consist of several bi-layers of lipid material in which case they are referred to as multi-lamellar (Figure 13-7). Liposomes may also be small or large (while being, generally, of small dimensions). These options for liposome production give rise to several liposome types, the most important of which are small unilamellar vesicles (SUV), small multilayer vesicles (SMV), large unilamellar vesicles (LUV), and large multi-lamellar vesicles (LMV). SUVs can be made sufficiently small that they are of nano dimensions.

When placed into water, phospholipid materials will spontaneously organize themselves into one or more spherical bilayers, as mentioned. Therefore, if the phospholipids are dissolved in a drug solution, some of this solution will be encapsulated in the formed liposome. In this way, drug-containing liposomes can be formed. In addition, hydrophobic drugs may be trapped between the lipophilic tails of the bilayer. The latter may be achieved by the incubation of preformed liposomes with a solution of the hydrophobic drug. Therefore, hydrophilic or hydrophobic drugs may be encapsulated within liposomes and, in some cases, it may be possible to encapsulate both drug types into one liposome. This could be a major advantage when multiple drugs are needed to adequately treat a disease condition.

Potentially, a drug and a diagnostic agent could be co-located in a liposome, resulting in a so-called "theranostic" (therapeutic plus diagnostic). The fact that the drug, or other agent, is entrapped within the vesicle and not on its surface is an advantage. With surface drug loading, which occurs to an extent with some solid nanoparticles, the drug will be rapidly released when the nanoparticles are exposed to water. In such cases, in addition, extensive drug degradation is possible. Liposomes can be rapidly eliminated by the RES but they are usually coated with PEG (they are said to be PEGylated), to form so-called "stealth-liposomes" which avoid capture by the RES.

Most liposomal products are required to be injected, although they may also be used for oral, inhalation, or topical application. While there are several liposome products on the market at the present time (Table 13-3), it must be remembered that basic research on liposomes has been going on since the 1960s. In many cases, the liposome presentation took very long to reach the marketplace, from initial conception. Some of the reasons for the long development time are burst drug release, low drug loading potential, and poor stability. An additional disadvantage with liposomes is the poor control of triggered release. Triggered release refers to the release of the drug upon encountering a particular stimulus or trigger, for example, when the liposome is in a particular environmental pH, or in the presence of specific enzymes. Triggered release is a feature utilized with several novel drug delivery systems, in particular nanoparticulate systems. In the case of liposomes, it was found that utilization of a trigger (presence of an enzyme or a particular pH) did not cause release of the drug in as controlled or predictable a manner as is the case with other nanoparticulate dosage forms. It should be noted that it may also be possible to have drug

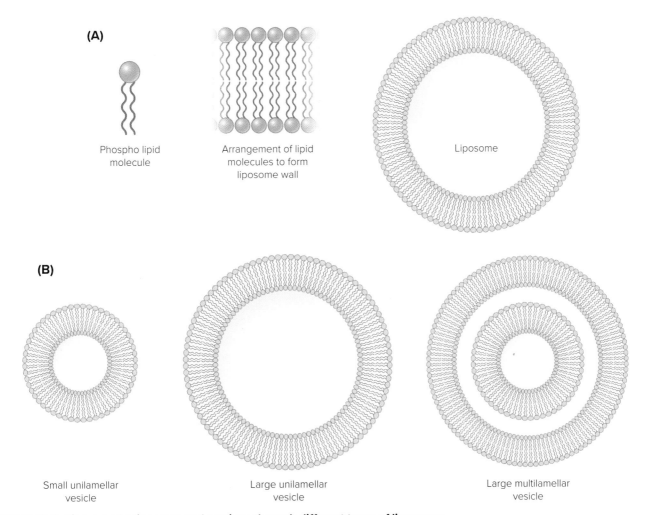

(A)

Phospho lipid
molecule

Arrangement of lipid
molecules to form
liposome wall

Liposome

(B)

Small unilamellar
vesicle

Large unilamellar
vesicle

Large multilamellar
vesicle

FIGURE 13-7 Diagram of a liposome and sections through different types of liposomes.

released from a liposome (or another dosage form) due to an intentional stimulus exerted externally to the body. Examples of such stimuli include heat or low-frequency ultrasound.

Premature drug release, or leakage, in vivo is particularly noticeable when the liposomes are constructed of natural phospholipids. These include phosphatidylcholine which is obtained from soybeans or eggs. These first-generation materials form more permeable, and less stable, bilayers. Liposomes formed from saturated phospholipids which have long acyl chains form more rigid, less permeable bilayers and they are more stable. Dipalmitoylphosphatidyl choline is an example of such a phospholipid. Similarly, liposomes containing cholesterol and sphingomyelin, as additives, show improved properties. These substances also confer rigidity and impermeability to the bilayers. Liposomes can be functionalized for active drug targeting. This is done by adding, to their surfaces, functional groups capable of reacting with the desired receptor. In addition, liposomes can be made into sustained-release formulations, and formulations for vaccine delivery.

While a great deal of information regarding the structure of liposomes, and methods of formation, were developed from active research since the 1970s, no product appeared on the market for many years. More recently, however, products have become available to the public. Some liposome formulations on

the US market are listed in Table 13-2, which also shows products that have been withdrawn from the market.

Polymersomes

A polymersome is similar to a liposome but is synthesized from block copolymers in place of the phospholipid surfactants used in liposomes. Several hydrophobic monomers joined together to form the hydrophobic block. This is linked to a block of several hydrophilic monomers to form the block copolymer (Figure 13-8). This is a di-block copolymer, that is, a block copolymer consisting of two blocks, one of which is hydrophobic while the other is hydrophilic. When the di-block copolymer units are placed into water, they will self-assemble to form polymersomes which are also illustrated in Figure 13-8. From the figure, it can be seen that the polymeric material, as a double layer, forms the shell.

The above description of a polymersome uses the example of a di-block copolymer. This is the simplest form of block copolymer, and it is used for illustrative purposes. More complex block copolymers, consisting of multiple blocks, can also be used for the development of polymersomes, but will not be discussed in this chapter. The fact that polymersomes are constituted from copolymers leads to the major functional differences between them and liposomes.

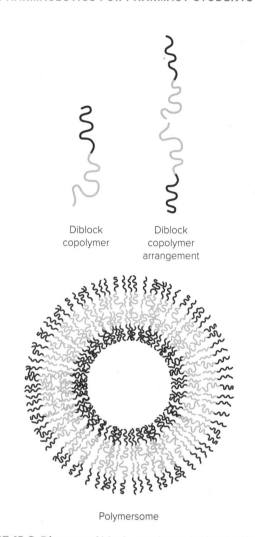

Diblock
copolymer

Diblock
copolymer
arrangement

Polymersome

FIGURE 13-8 Diagram of block copolymer and polymersome.

The diameter of a polymersome is similar to that of a liposome. However, liposomes have thin walls of approximately 5 nm with little variation in wall thickness. On the other hand, polymersomes can have a wide range of wall thicknesses. On the low end, the thickness of a polymersome wall may be similar to that of a liposome and, on the high-end, they can be significantly thicker. The reason for this is the fact that a wide range of monomers can be used to make up each block of the copolymer, resulting in great variability in the length of a copolymer unit. In addition, the copolymer may be constituted of multiple blocks, instead of two in the diblock copolymer described above. If three different blocks are used to form the polymer, it is a triblock copolymer, and so on. This leads to greater variation in the wall thickness of the polymersome. Conversely, liposomes are made from phosphatidylcholine or similar lipid compounds, which have approximately the same length. Consequently, the wall thicknesses of the liposomes do not show a great variation.

The thicker shells lead to greater strength of polymersomes and, more importantly, the tight packing of the block copolymer units leads to slower diffusion of drug from polymersomes. Polymersomes are also more stable than liposomes. The term, "stability of vesicles" refers to both the potential for the vesicle

to disassemble, and also to the chemical stability of the components. The latter is more important with vesicles. The lipid components of liposomes, in the presence of reactive oxygen species (ROS), undergo oxidation to form lipid peroxides, whereas the non-lipid components of polymersomes do not undergo this reaction. In addition, polymersome components are less subject to hydroxylation than are the lipid components of liposomes. Overall, the greater chemical stability of polymersomes leads to less changes in their physical structure and less "leaking" of the contained drug. In addition, due to the vast range of components that could be used to form polymersomes, their properties can be adjusted, or tuned, as necessary. For example, if the drug release rate is too slow, it can be adjusted by choosing a different block copolymer system. If PEG is a constituent of the block copolymers, long circulation times can be anticipated since the polymersome escapes entrapment by the RES.

Vesicles with Oily Cores

Lipid Nanocapsules

Lipid nanocapsules are composed of an oily core and a surfactant shell. They are used for delivery of hydrophobic drugs which are dissolved in the oil phase. The surfactants comprising the shell are lipophilic, with some hydrophilic component. Lipid nanocapsules are formed in situ by an emulsification process which results in lipid nanocapsules dispersed in an aqueous phase. The Cremophor® range of surfactants, in combination with other surfactants, has been used extensively in the formulation of lipid nanocapsules. The distinction between a lipid nanocapsule and an o/w nanoemulsion (an emulsion with the dispersed oil phase globules having diameters in the nanometer range) is not very clear. The former has a more rigid surfactant shell which may, in part, be responsible for the ability to produce nanocapsules as sustained-release formulations. Lipid nanocapsules also, naturally, avoid capture by the RES due to the fact that the surfactant blend usually contains PEG or a similar hydrophilic material. Thus, there is no need to chemically add a hydrophilic component, as is done with PEGylation. Avoidance of the RES capture is also assisted by the fact that lipid nanocapsules are generally quite small, 100 nm or less.

Polymeric Nanocapsules

As mentioned above, polymeric nanocapsules contain an oil surrounded by a solid shell of polymeric material. Hydrophobic drugs are dissolved in the oily core material. As a result of the fact that nanocapsules contain a drug solution (as do liposomes), premature drug release is an issue. Compared to lipid nanocapsules, polymeric nanocapsules show reduced premature drug leakage, and increased stability due to the solid shell. In addition, the polymer shell disrupts less easily because it is stronger. Less water permeation occurs through intact polymer shells than through intact lipid membranes and, hence, polymeric nanocapsules show reduced burst release compared to lipid nanocapsules.

When compared to liposomes (which contain aqueous drug solutions), polymeric nanocapsules display significantly greater stability and protection against premature drug loss. Compared to polymeric nanospheres (which are solid), polymeric nanocapsules allow a higher drug loading and have a lower polymer

TABLE 13-2	Some Marketed Metallic Nanoparticle Injectable Products		
TRADE NAME (MANUFACTURER) YEAR INTRODUCED	**DRUG NAME (PHARMACOLOGICAL ACTION)**	**COMMENTS**
INFeD® (Sanofi Aventis) 1957	Iron dextran (low MW) (Chronic kidney failure with iron deficiency)	Increased dose capacity
DexIron®/Dexferrum® (SanofAventis) 1957	Iron dextran (high MW) (Chronic kidney failure with iron deficiency)	Increased dose capacity
Ferrlecit® (Sanofi Aventis) 1999	Sodium ferric gluconate (Chronic kidney failure with iron deficiency)	Increased dose capacity
Venofer® (Luitpold Pharmaceuticals) 2000	Iron sucrose (Chronic kidney failure with iron deficiency)	Increased dose capacity
Nanotherm® (MagForce®) 2010	Aminosilane-coated Iron (Brain tumor thermotherapy)	Destroy tumor cells or sensitize for additional therapies
Feridex®/Endorem® (AMAG pharmaceuticals) 1996/2008	SPION* coated with dextran	Imaging material
GastroMARK; Umirem® (AMAG Pharmaceuticals) 2001/2009	SPION coated with silicone	Imaging material
Feraheme™ (AMAG Pharmaceuticals) 2009	Ferumoxytol (ultrasmall SPION) with polyglucose sorbitol carboxymethylether (Chronic kidney failure with iron deficiency)	Prolonged steady release and decreased number of doses

*Superparamagnetic iron oxide nanoparticles

content. Therefore, if a non-biodegradable polymer (which is the less desirable type) must be used, it would be better to formulate polymeric nanocapsules, rather than polymeric nanospheres, due to their far lower polymer content. The lower polymer content is advantageous when considering the biological elimination of the polymer.

Drug release from polymeric nanocapsules is by diffusion of the drug molecules through the capsule shell. This process is governed largely by the partition between the oily core material and the external aqueous medium. The thickness of the shell and the molecular weight of the polymer comprising the wall also control diffusion through the shell material. Shells with thicknesses of 1.5 to 20 nm have been reported. Higher molecular weight polymers retard drug release to a greater extent than lower molecular weight polymers when used in the same amounts.

A brief note to distinguish some of the nanoparticulate types may be useful at this stage. A micelle, at first sight, appears very similar to a liposome. However, the micelle does not have a double layer of phospholipid material. Although micelles may be formulated to contain a hydrophobic drug, they can be distinguished from oily nanocapsules by the fact that they lack the oily core of the latter. In fact, there is no liquid core in a micelle since the hydrophobic tails repel the water molecules of the aqueous environment. Furthermore, the micelle can be distinguished from a polymeric nanoparticle in that the latter is a solid particle consisting of polymer(s).

FUTURE DEVELOPMENTS

While intense activity in the nanopharmaceutical arena has been ongoing for the last 30 years and several products have been marketed since 1995, this scientific discipline has yet to achieve its full potential. However, the existing pharmaceutical nanotechnology products have already established the value of this group of technologies. Bioavailability has been increased and toxicity and side effects due to the drug have been reduced. By the ability to eliminate certain excipients used in conventional formulations, the toxicity and side effects of these excipients have also been eliminated. In addition, dosing compliance has been greatly increased. For example, Invega Sustenna offers significantly better control of schizophrenic patients than has been possible with previously-available drug products. One injection provides relief of symptoms for one month. The company literature states that the cycle of incarceration and hospitalization, frequently experienced by such patients, can be broken with the use of this product.

Considering advantages of this magnitude, and commercial feasibility demonstrated by dozens of products, the stage is set for the rapid expansion of nanopharmaceuticals in the near future. Pharmaceutical research and development, production, and marketing are extremely expensive and risky. The risk is greatly compounded where novel technologies are concerned. Products that come to market, and are successful, provide a

TABLE 13-3	Some Marketed Liposome Products	
TRADE NAME (MANUFACTURER) YEAR INTRODUCED	**DRUG NAME (PHARMACOLOGICAL ACTION)**	**COMMENTS**
Doxil® (Caelyx®) (Baxter Healthcare Corporation) 1995	Doxorubicin (Karposi's sarcoma; Ovarian cancer; multiple myeloma)	First approved nanopharmaceutical; first nano-product to have a generic. SUV stabilized with PEG.
Abelcet® (Lediant Biosciences Inc.) 1995	Amphotericin B lipid complex (Fungal infections)	Decreased toxicity
AmBisome® (Astellas Pharma US Inc.) 1997	Amphotericin B (Fungal and/or protozoal infections)	Drug is intercalated into membrane. Reduced nephrotoxicity.
DaunoXome® (Galen Ltd) 1996 *DISCONTINUED*	Daunorubicin (Karposi's sarcoma)	Increase delivery to tumor and decrease toxicity
DepoCyt© (Sigma-Tau) 1996 *DISCONTINUED*	Cytarabine (Lymphomatous meningitis)	Intrathecal treatment of lymphomatous meningitis. Increase delivery to tumor and decrease toxicity.
Curosurf® (Chiesei Farmaceutici) 1999	Porcine lung surfactants (Rescue treatment of Respiratory Distress Syndrome [RDS] in premature infants)	Suspension for intratracheal administration. Surfactant consists of 99% polar lipid (phospholipids) and 1% surfactant-associated proteins. Decreased toxicity and increased delivery for smaller volume.
Visudyne® (Valeant Pharmaceuticals) 2000	Verteporfin (Ocular histoplasmosis, myopia, decreased vision)	Increase delivery to lesion vessels—photosensitive release
DepoDur® (Pacira Pharmaceuticals Inc.) 2004 *DISCONTINUED*	Morphine sulfate (Reduction in postoperative pain)	Prolonged release
Marqibo® (Acrotech Biopharma LLC) 2012	Vincristine sulfate (Acute lymphoblastic leukemia)	Liposomal injection has different dosage than vincristine injection. Increased tumor delivery with decreased toxicity
Onivyde® (Ipsen Biopharmaceuticals Inc.) 2015	Irinotecan (Pancreatic cancer)	Increased tumor delivery and decreased toxicity
Exparel® (Pacira Pharmaceuticals Inc.) 2011	Bupivacaine (anesthetic)	Multivesicular liposomes—sustained release. Postsurgical local analgesia and brachial plexus nerve block (rotator cuff repair)

huge impetus to other companies to develop their own products in the same technological area. Indeed, several innovative nanotechnology products are in late-stage development and/or in clinical testing at present.

Several nanocrystalline drug formulations are currently commercially available. Although these are the least complex type of formulation, in terms of product design, they are not necessarily easy to produce at a level that accords with reproducibility and safety for public consumption. The latter requires the development and implementation of adequate quality control and quality assurance measures. Publications and presentations on methods to produce nanocrystalline products preceded the availability of such a product by several years, illustrating the difficulty of achieving a well-designed product

having a well-controlled production process. The latter involves good quality control procedures.

While several liposomal products have reached the market, there are still some issues with this type of dosage form, including stability concerns. A few products have been withdrawn from the market as indicated in the table of liposome products (Table 13-3). Polymersomes display improved stability and can be tuned for slower release of the contained drug. The possibilities for developing polymersome products with different characteristics depend, largely, on the ability to synthesize varied block copolymers that are suitable for this application. The latter is limited only by the ingenuity of the chemist. The description of polymersomes, in this chapter, takes into account the use of only one block copolymer type, with several of these units forming the polymersome, and this is also reflected in Figure 13-8. However, polymersomes having more than one type (or mixed) block copolymers, within the same unit, are possible and increase the range of properties that may be attained. This is another avenue for growth.

Most nanopharmaceutical research has been directed to cancer therapy and, in the future, it is anticipated that many more products will become available for this condition. In addition, products for other major diseases such as Alzheimer's, diabetes, and hypertension will also be developed in the future. The development of a single product with both diagnostic and therapeutic functions is an exciting prospect, especially if they are also self-regulating with respect to drug release rate. The latter is theoretically possible with the use of feedback mechanisms which provide information on the amount of drug available in the medium, such as the blood or tissue fluid. The rate of further drug release is then regulated using this information.

Future nanopharmaceutical development will be greatly aided by developments in other scientific areas, in particular material science (development of new polymeric materials), improved microscopic and imaging methodologies (to pinpoint drug location and extent of pathology such as tumor size), and improved technologies for identifying and quantifying disease markers. The latter two groups of technologies (imaging and disease markers) will allow earlier detection of diseases, or the pre-disease state, for earlier treatment. It is also possible that these technologies will spur the development of different modalities for early-stage treatment of disease conditions.

While most nanotechnology products at the current time are administered by intravenous injection, nanoparticulate materials may also be administered by inhalation, topically, or by subcutaneous injection. Thus, the development of alternative means of administration will provide another direction for expansion, over and above newer and improved nanotechnologies. Green chemistry and the utilization of GRAS ingredients in the development of nanotechnology products will be another direction of improvement. Possibly, the biggest impetus to increase the output of nanotechnology products will come from the intersection of this technology and personalized medicine. The complexities of formulation development and, especially, the ability to define the optimal formulation from limited experimental data will be greatly assisted by artificial intelligence.

Recap Questions

1. How do vesicular systems differ from matrix nanotechnology systems?
2. What do liposomes and polymersomes have in common, and in which ways are they different?
3. What term is used to denote a vehicle with an oily core?
4. What causes liposomes and polymersomes to spontaneously form when placed in water?

SUMMARY POINTS

- The introduction to nanotechnology emphasizes that it is not only about size; functionality is also important.
- The major types of nanotechnologies for drug delivery, that are currently marketed, or which have a potential to be marketed, are described.
- Some of the shortcomings and limitations were mentioned, where appropriate. For example, several liposomal formulations were withdrawn from the market.
- Examples of marketed nanotechnology products, available in the US, are listed in several tables.
- Finally, some thoughts are provided about the direction in which pharmaceutical nanotechnology is anticipated to be heading, and the types of products that the pharmacist may encounter in the years to come.

What do you think?

1. In which way are the interior molecules, or atoms, of a nanocrystal different from those of a large crystal?
2. Can one substance have a slower dissolution rate, but a greater solubility, than a second substance?
3. If enhanced solubility depends on the nanometer dimensions of a solid substance, why is it necessary to think of solubility in terms of the solvent as well?
4. Many diabetic patients currently take 750 mg of metformin daily. If the dose could be reduced to half (375 mg) by the use of nanotechnology, which specific technology would you recommend using considering that the dose is still relatively large?
5. If it were desired to convert a low-dose (5 mg) hydrophobic drug to a nanomedicine, which technology would you recommend and why?
6. A low-dose hydrophilic drug is presently administered in a liposome formulation. The manufacturers have found that premature drug release is an issue with this formulation. Suggest an alternative nanotechnology to improve the performance of the product.
7. If nanopharmaceuticals are so advantageous, why are all medications not converted to nanoparticulate form?

BIBLIOGRAPHY

Cornier J, Kwade A, Owen A, Van de Voorde M, eds. *Pharmaceutical Nanotechnology: Innovation and Production.* 1st ed. Wiley-VCH Verlag GmbH & Co. KGaA; 2017.

Patra JK, Das G, Fraceto LF, et al. Nano based drug delivery systems: recent developments and future prospects. *J Nanobiotechnol.* 2018;16:71.

Rideau E, Domova R, Schwille P, Wurm FR, Landfester K. Liposomes and polymersomes: a comparative review towards cell mimicking. *Chem Soc Rev.* 2018;47:8572.

Packaging 14

PREVIEW

- The container—not simply a vessel to contain the medication
- Protection of the product—and other functions
- With modern drugs, the bar has often to be set higher
- Moisture protection and desiccants
- Child-resistant, tamper-evident, and compliance packaging—the new paradigm
- Safety and diversion
- The FDA's view of the package

THE CONTAINER

How important is the container that stores a medication?

Consider what goes into the development of a new medication. An array of scientific disciplines must be considered in the development of one new product. This includes medicinal chemistry to synthesize the drug, formulation science and analytical chemistry to ensure that an adequate formulation has been prepared, and pharmacology and therapeutics to understand the effect of the dosage form. When considering these various aspects, the student may be apt to place less emphasis on the container. However, the choice of the container that is used to store a medication is of vital importance. Apart from serving as the utensil to contain the medication, the container must protect the stored medication from the physical damage

that may occur due to the rigors of shipping over long distances. These include not only bumping, shaking, and vibration but also changes in the environment or air quality. The container must keep out oxygen and moisture and, in many cases, also light which may degrade components of the medication, including the drug. The container, thus, plays a vital role in ensuring the stability of the product. For this reason, the Food and Drug Administration (FDA) gives consideration to the stability of a particular medication *in its final container*. Stability data that is generated in any other container (apart from the container that will be used for marketing the product) will only be considered as "supporting data." This emphasizes the fact that the product and its container are one integral unit and the stability of the product must be defined in terms of its container. This indicates that the container is of vital importance.

The importance of the container can also be gauged by consideration of the following question: can the improper choice of container cause an otherwise good product to be rejected at the FDA? It definitely can. The FDA is concerned with the safety of the public which includes the provision of stable medications to consumers. If the FDA feels that the container does not adequately protect the drug product from harmful environmental factors and that the resultant instability is sufficiently serious that it is undesirable for the product to be supplied to the general public, it will not approve the product for marketing. The case study at the end of this chapter provides an interesting example of the FDA not approving a product due to the packaging, where the problem was not related to stability of the product. Upon making changes to the packaging to comply with FDA requests, the product was subsequently approved. The more important functions of the container are summarized graphically in Mind Map 14-1.

In recent years, a relatively new function of packaging has come to the forefront, especially with regulatory bodies such as the FDA. This function is referred to as compliance packaging. This term refers to the ability of the packaging to help a patient comply with the dosage regimen, that is, assist the patient to take the medication regularly, as prescribed. Among the earliest examples of compliance packaging are contraceptive tablets which may be packaged in a blister with the days of the month printed on the packaging material.

Another specialized form of packaging, tamper-evident packaging, has been in use for many years and is the type of packaging that, when the product is tampered with, reveals evidence of intentional interference. The importance of having evidence of tampering is important in the case where there is intentional interference with the medication in some way, including the willful creation of a toxic product by the addition of chemicals. To get to the medication, the package has first to be opened. Thus, evidence of interference with the packaging is a warning that the product, itself, may have been tampered with and is unfit for consumption. A modern application of packaging is the ability of the package to help reduce pilfering and theft of potent drugs by people close to the patient, for example, the

theft of individual opioid tablets by family members for the purpose of recreational use.

MOISTURE PERMEABILITY

Generally, most containers keep out significant amounts of moisture. However, special attention has to be given to moisture permeability for many pharmaceutical products. Why is the relative impermeability of the container so important? Some pharmaceutical products are extremely sensitive to moisture and the penetration of even a small amount can be deleterious to the product. The ability, of the different materials used in packaging, to keep out moisture can be very different. Generally, the best materials are in the given order:

$$\text{aluminum foil} \gg \text{glass} \gg \text{plastic}$$

If the packaging material cannot keep out all the moisture, and the product is very sensitive to moisture, what else can be done in order to have a stable product? A material that absorbs moisture can be added within the container (alongside the product). If a small amount of moisture permeates the wall of the container, the added material takes up this moisture. The result is that only very small amounts of moisture reach the product. In this way, the stability of the product is ensured. Materials, which behave in this fashion, are termed desiccants.

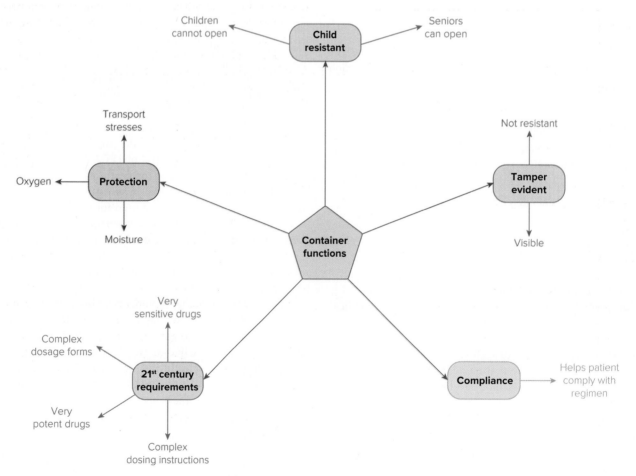

MIND MAP 14-1 Functions of a pharmaceutical container.

There are different types of desiccants including silica gel, molecular sieve, and calcium sulfate. These materials have different moisture absorbing capacities. Some materials, absorb moisture poorly at low relative humidity values but may absorb much more moisture at high relative humidity values. Figure 14-1 shows that molecular sieve has a high moisture-absorbing capacity at relatively low relative humidity values up to about 40%. At high relative humidity values, it soon reaches a plateau. On the other hand, silica gel has a low moisture absorbing capacity for relative humidity values up to about 40% but its uptake is rapid at high relative humidity values. Silica gel and molecular sieve are used more frequently than the other desiccants mentioned, especially for very moisture-sensitive products.

Apart from the rates at which moisture is taken up, the total amount of moisture that a desiccant can hold is also important. For example, calcium oxide has a rapid rate of moisture uptake but its utility is limited by the fact that it cannot hold a large amount of water. It becomes saturated fairly quickly. Sorbents Systems, a company that specializes in desiccants, has extensively studied moisture uptake rate and the extent to which different sorbents can absorb moisture. A desiccant may contain a combination of two materials for best overall moisture absorptive capacity. For example, a combination of molecular sieve and silica gel provides good moisture absorbing capacity at both low and high relative humidity values. If the product is moisture as well as oxygen sensitive, a pouch that contains desiccants in one half, and an oxygen-absorbing material in the other half, may be purchased.

What route do gases, such as oxygen or water vapor, take as they enter a container of tablets or capsules? In a screw-cap glass or plastic container for solid oral dosage forms, one source of entry is the rim of the bottle which is invariably not perfectly smooth but has imperfections. This leads to some space between the rim of the bottle and the cap. However, the closure normally has a soft liner which deforms to take up some of the space created by imperfections of the rim. Therefore, the volume of the spaces available for gaseous penetration is small and this route is not a large source of gaseous contamination.

On the other hand, gases may permeate through the wall of the container. While the rate of penetration may be slow, the large surface area makes this a source of significant contamination. Glass is better than plastics in preventing gaseous permeation but glass is expensive and, also, heavy for transport, leading to additional costs. In any event, the permeation of gases through glass is not zero. How can one prevent the gas from permeating through the large surface area of a bottle of tablets? A solution that some companies have developed is to use a double-walled plastic container with desiccants between the walls. This effectively inhibits the permeation of moisture vapor all the way through the wall into the container. Moisture will, however, penetrate the first wall layer and will then be taken up by the desiccant.

Glyceryl trinitrate is sensitive to moisture and is, therefore, dispensed in glass bottles which are significantly less permeable to moisture vapor than plastic bottles. By limiting moisture penetration, greater stability of the drug can be assured. In addition, glyceryl trinitrate is volatile and can escape one tablet to permeate the wall of a plastic container. Subsequently, the drug may leave the wall to occupy the airspace of the bottle. From here, the drug may migrate to a different tablet. This results in differences in potency of the tablets. Since this drug does not permeate glass, the problem of tablet-to-tablet migration is reduced with the use of glass bottles. The use of stabilized glyceryl trinitrate limits the volatilization of the drug in the first place.

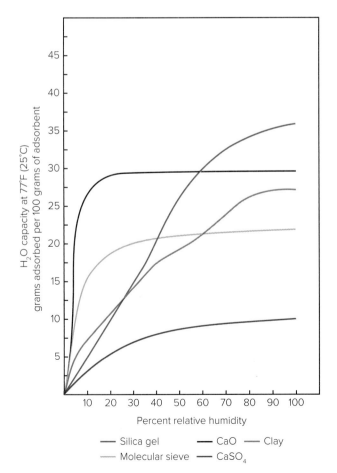

FIGURE 14-1 Different moisture adsorbents and relative potency. (Sorbent Systems website.)

Recap Questions

1. "The sole function of the container is to keep the product stable." Do you agree or disagree with this statement? Give reasons for your answer.

2. What is the most likely way that moisture can penetrate into a plastic container of tablets: through the side walls or under the cap? Knowing how the moisture penetrates, what is an example of innovative packaging to protect medication that is extremely moisture sensitive?

3. What is the rationale to combine different absorbent materials to capture moisture that penetrates a container of medication?

CHILD-RESISTANT PACKAGING

The poison prevention act (1970) provides for packaging designed and constructed to be:

1. Significantly difficult for children under 5 years to open and retrieve all of the items in a package, or a toxic or harmful amount of the substance contained, within a reasonable time, and

2. That is not difficult for senior adults to use properly.

Many medications are now packaged in child-resistant packaging. As more potent medications were developed, the use of child-resistant packaging became more prominent. An important principle to keep in mind is the fact that there are two requirements for child-resistant packaging. First, as the name implies, children should not be able to easily open the package. Second, senior citizens should be able to open the package relatively easily. The second requirement makes it difficult to prepare child-resistant packaging since the manufacturer must walk a fine line. If the only requirement was to prevent children from opening the package, this type of packaging may have been easily achieved. However, if the package is made very resistant to opening by children, then some seniors would, likely, also not be able to open the package. Special testing procedures are prescribed by law to test both facets of these requirements.

Child Test Procedures

The following procedures are utilized in testing the product with children:

1. The children must be under 5 years of age, 50% male and 50% female.

2. Two children together attempt to open one package.

3. The instructor says "please try and open this for me."

4. After 5 minutes the children are asked to stop working on the package.

5. The instructor demonstrates the opening of the package but offers no verbal instructions.

6. The children are again asked to try to open the package and are told that they could use their teeth if they want to.

7. The children are given 5 more minutes.

8. The number of children that succeed in the first 5 minutes, and the number that succeed in the second 5 minutes as well as the panel size are used in conjunction with statistical tables to determine whether the product failed the test.

The Senior Adult Panel

1. The senior adult panel consists of people between the ages of 50 and 70, 70% of whom are female.

2. If a tool, for example, scissors must be used according to the manufacturer's instructions, this is supplied to the adults (but not to the children).

3. Two packages are supplied to each panelist. The panelist must be able to open the first package within 5 minutes, and must be able to open and close the second package in 1 minute.

4. If the senior adult accomplishes both tasks mentioned in 3 above, it counts as one success.

5. The number of successes divided by the total number of participants, expressed as a percentage, is the senior adult user effectiveness (SAUE).

6. The SAUE is calculated separately for men and women and a formula is used to determine the overall SAUE score.

7. Overall, the SAUE should be greater than 90%.

Examples of Child-Resistant Packaging

A good example of child-resistant packaging for an opioid drug is the packaging used for Actiq. This product contains fentanyl in a base placed on the end of an applicator. The earliest versions of this medication had a candy base but the nature of the base has been modified subsequently. The medication is intended to be held by the handle and rubbed onto the inside cheek, using alternate sides of the mouth and also rotating the applicator.

Actiq Packaging

Since fentanyl is a very potent drug, the manufacturers of Actiq took special precautions to make the product child resistant. Each unit is individually contained in a child-resistant pouch with the pouches packaged within a carton. This pouch is made of a heavy grade of laminated foil. The material is multilayered and is heat sealed. It requires scissors to open the package and, partly for this reason, is very effective as a child-resistant package. Children had difficulty opening the package since it requires coordination. Seniors were able to open the package with only a little difficulty. In child-resistance testing, it obtained a 99% effectiveness rating. Upon opening the package, only one Actiq unit is exposed. This is a safety measure since multiple units have the potential to cause greater harm.

Since the pouch is opaque, the child cannot see the unit which, possibly, could have been mistaken for candy or a lollipop. The earliest version of this product did look a lot like a lollipop and the company changed the appearance to avoid children mistaking the product for candy. Furthermore, the front of each pouch has a symbol which warns about child safety and opioid tolerance. The back of the pouch has the same symbol and warnings, in plain language, about child safety and proper storage. There is also a reminder that the patient or caregiver should read the Actiq patient leaflet. The Actiq shelf carton contains several messages explaining the risks involved and provides warnings about accidental ingestion by children. Each carton contains eight strips of three pouches each, giving a total of 24 pouches or a 10- to 14-day supply.

TAMPER-EVIDENT PACKAGING

Tamper-evident packaging is not the same as child-resistant packaging. In the former type of package, the only requirement is that any tampering that has occurred should be self-evident, that is, the nature of the package must be such that any attempt to tamper with the product should be clearly visible; there is no requirement that it should be difficult for anyone to open the package. This distinction is critical.

Tamper-evident packaging came to the fore in 1982 because of the drug-related deaths of seven people. This occurred at various locations in the Chicago area and was due to tampering with Tylenol capsules which were intentionally laced with potassium cyanide. There are many interesting stories as to why this was done, but no proof of the exact nature, or sequence, of events. It would appear that this tragedy was perpetrated for industrial espionage purposes. Whatever the background to these events, the nation was shocked and industry got into high gear to find ways to make tampering evident, the idea being that the customer would not take off a pharmacy or supermarket shelf, and pay for, a package that had obviously been interfered with. The major focus was on over-the-counter medications since these could easily be accessed by members of the public. By contrast, prescription medications are under the control of the pharmacist and pharmacy staff at all times.

The Johnson & Johnson Company was quick to initiate a product recall and compensated customers. It also recalled all acetaminophen-containing products from the market. The company received praise for its prompt action under these tragic circumstances. While the company's image was initially hurt and business decreased considerably, the actions that they took led to them regaining public confidence and market share within a relatively short time.

The Johnson & Johnson Company also developed the caplet, a capsule-shaped tablet, as a response to this unfortunate event. While in the form of a capsule, it is a solid tablet which is much more difficult to intentionally contaminate without leaving visible signs of tampering. Subsequently, Johnson & Johnson also developed a gelatin-coated capsule-shaped tablet (the so-called "gel tab"). This was intended to have the elongated shape of a capsule and also the slipperiness of gelatin, when wet, for easier swallowing.

After the Tylenol scare, new requirements for over-the-counter (OTC) products for human consumption were put into place. These requirements are contained in the code of federal regulations (21 CFR 211.132). These regulations define a tamper-evident package as follows:

> "A tamper-evident package is one having one or more indicators or barriers to entry which, if breached or missing, can reliably be expected to provide visible evidence to consumers that tampering has occurred."

All over-the-counter (OTC) products are now required to be marketed in tamper-evident packaging. This type of packaging may take several forms. One of the simplest is a piece of tape with printing on it, used to seal a container, such as a cardboard carton, containing medicines (Figure 14-2). When peeled off the package, it removes some of the printing from the carton. The removal of printing, or other damage to the carton, makes it very obvious that tampering has occurred. Also, in some instances, the removal of the tape leaves printing that states that the package has been tampered with. This is a double layer of tape in which only one layer can be peeled off, leaving the mentioned printing on the second layer.

Further, the regulations require a labeling statement on the container to indicate to the consumer the specific tamper-resistant features that have been used. The labeling statement

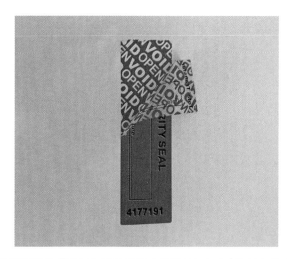

FIGURE 14-2 **Tape to seal carton for tamper evidence.** Note: if removal of the seal is attempted, evidence of interference with the package becomes visible instantly.

will also mention that the product should not be used if a seal is broken. The labeling statement is required to be placed in such a way that it will not be affected by the unauthorized opening of the package, that is, the statement can still be read after the package has been opened. Some examples of relatively simple tamper-evident features will now be mentioned with the suggested labeling to instruct the consumer when they should not use the product.

An entire package, such as a carton, may have a film wrapped around it (Figure 14-3). The labeling statement will indicate that the product should not be used if the film wrapper is damaged or missing. Tablets or capsules, or other products, may be sealed in a blister with the statement that the product should not be used if the blister seal is broken (Figure 14-4). The container may have a heat shrink band, that is, a piece of plastic that is tightly bound due to shrinkage, around and under the cap. This

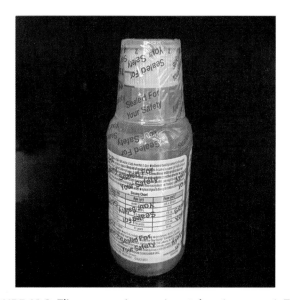

FIGURE 14-3 **Film wrapped around container (overwrap).** The bottle is wrapped with a heat-sealed material or cellophane which is glued or taped at the edges.

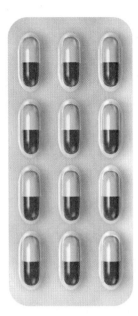

FIGURE 14-4 **Blister strip.** (Used with permission from Artpartner-images/The Image Bank/Getty Images.)

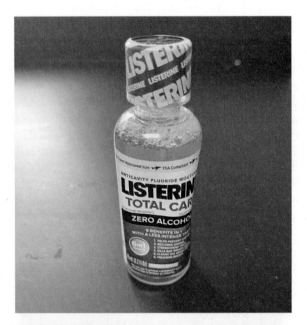

FIGURE 14-5 **Heat shrink band.** A loose band is placed over the cap; it extends below the cap as well. When heat is applied, the material shrinks to form a tight seal. To remove the medication, the seal must be broken.

is typically used for liquids (Figure 14-5). The labeling statement states that the product should not be used if the seal around the cap is broken or missing.

Other forms of tamper-evident packaging are more complex. Tablet packages, for example, may contain several mechanisms to identify tampering. All of the following methods may be found on the same container, thus affording multiple layers of evidence. A tablet container may consist of an inner container (plastic tablet vial) and an outer container (cardboard carton). One flap of the closure of the latter may be glued to the cap of the vial to create a tamper-evident container (Figure 14-6). In order to open the package to remove tablets, the cardboard has to be

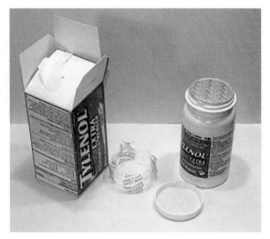

FIGURE 14-6 **Pharmaceutical tablet product with multiple tamper-evident protections.** Note that the product has the following protective measures: (1) Flap of carton is glued to rest of carton and is damaged during opening (or it may be glued to the cap of the immediate container); (2) there is a heat-sealed band under and over cap which must be torn to open immediate container; (3) the container is sealed under the cap with a foil which must be torn to retrieve contents. (Used with permission from Katerina Primula/Shutterstock.)

torn off the vial. This results in obvious evidence that the package was opened. The screw-on lid of the tablet vial may have a plastic banding seal around, and under, the lid. This seal is similar to that described above for liquids and it has to be broken to remove the tablets. The broken seal is very obvious evidence of the fact that an attempt was made to open the package. Once the screw-on lid has been removed, a thin inner foil or polymer film may cover the open mouth of the container and is glued in place. This seal helps, first, to keep the product within the container. Second, if the product is oxygen sensitive, the oxygen can be replaced by nitrogen before sealing. Most importantly, in the context of this chapter, the seal provides further evidence of tampering since the seal has to be broken before the tablets can be removed.

Recap Questions

1. Child-resistant packaging, as the name implies, is intended to prevent children from accessing medications. Why, then, should the product be tested using both children and seniors as subjects?

2. Why do you think children under 5 years old are tested? Are older children, for example, 8 years old not at risk?

3. Name three mechanisms by which the manufacturers of Actiq attempt to prevent the consumption of this medication by children.

4. What incident led to a greater consciousness in the pharmaceutical industry about the potential for medication packages to be tampered with?

5. Name three tamper-evident mechanisms that are used for pharmaceutical products.

COMPLIANCE PACKAGING

As previously mentioned, a novel utility of packaging is "compliance" packaging. The basic idea is that the package must be so designed as to assist the patient or caregiver to be compliant with a dosing regimen. It is critical for contraceptive tablets to be taken daily as prescribed. The consequences of forgetting to take a tablet may be serious. Therefore, it is highly desirable that the package provide a reminder, or assistance, to the patient to be compliant, that is, to take one contraceptive tablet each day. Thus, this form of packaging assists the patient in a vitally important aspect of her medication. This function is brought about not just by the printing on the container but also by other factors such as the blister packaging which allows easy removal of a single tablet each time, without access to the rest of the container of tablets (Figure 14-7). The broken blister and empty cavity also indicate that the tablet has been removed (and likely taken) which helps avoid double dosing. The printed day of the week on the blister encourages compliance.

Some asthmatics take steroid medications by inhalation. A typical instruction for such an inhalation may be, "take two puffs twice daily." Ideally, the two puffs constituting a single dose should be taken at least 1 minute apart. It may be difficult for a busy person who is multitasking while taking the medication, to recall whether they have taken one or two puffs. Several of the steroid medications provided for inhalation have counters, which decrease by one unit, each time a puff is taken. Figure 14-8 shows an Incruse inhaler used for chronic obstructive pulmonary disease which also has a counter to guide the patient in using the medication optimally. The patient may note the number of doses remaining before taking the medication at any time point. Hence, they have a reference to whether they have taken one dose or two. On the other end of the spectrum of patients who use this medication are very ill patients who may not be totally focused on the number of puffs that they have taken. Again, the counter assists patients to determine whether they have taken one puff or two, or none at all.

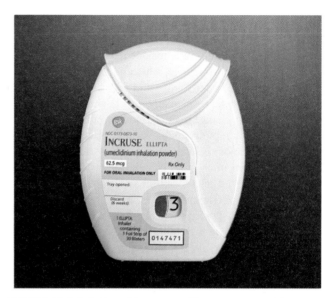

FIGURE 14-8 Inhaler with counter. The patient should not use the inhaler if the count is not 30 since this may indicate tampering. In addition, the counter helps with compliance. (mims.co.uk)

Ventolin is a rescue inhaler, which contains albuterol, for the symptomatic treatment of asthma and other conditions in which bronchoconstriction is a characteristic. This medication also has a counter to assist the patient in knowing how many puffs they have taken at any point in time. It also helps them to know how much medication is left and when to re-order. Ventolin is used on an as-needed basis and, unlike regularly-taken medications, the supply of medication will not necessarily be exhausted on the same day each month. It should be noted that Ventolin, the original product, has the counter while many of the generics do not.

An interesting example involving compliance packaging is provided as a case study in the last section of this chapter.

PACKAGING IN THE TWENTY-FIRST CENTURY

The packaging of modern drugs is far more complex than the packaging of medications even 20 years ago. Some of the reasons for this are the following:

Sensitive Drugs

Many drugs are far more sensitive to environmental conditions than drugs were previously. Therefore, better packaging is required to keep out even small amounts of moisture, oxygen, or light. This places a great deal of emphasis on packaging materials and containers, and on the work of packaging engineers. The double-walled container with desiccant between the walls, which was previously mentioned, is an example of the development of novel packaging by packaging engineers.

Complex Dosage Forms

Apart from the fact that many newer drugs are sensitive to environmental conditions, many newer dosage forms (as distinct

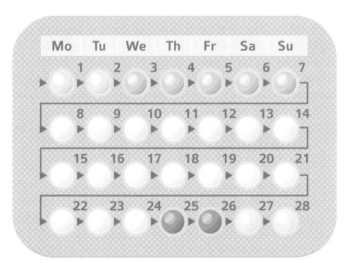

FIGURE 14-7 Compliance packaging (contraceptives). The packaging is marked with the days of the week and shows the consumer which tablet to start with. The packaging supports compliance with the dosing regimen. (Used with permission from Katerina Primula/Shutterstock.)

from the drug) are also very sensitive to environmental conditions and require special packaging. The hardness of the tablet, and hence its dissolution rate, may be altered by the moisture content of the atmosphere in which the product is stored. Some polymers are water soluble and ingress of moisture into the container may cause small amounts of the polymer to dissolve and this may change the functionality of the dosage form. Methylcellulose is rapidly soluble in cold water and hydroxypropylmethylcellulose is hygroscopic. When the moisture content of a container of capsules is high, the capsules can soften and deform since the gelatin capsule shells are very sensitive to the level of atmospheric moisture. Conversely, when the moisture content is very low, the capsule shells can become brittle. These effects influence the ability of the patient to handle the capsules, and may also affect the functionality of the unit.

Very Potent Drugs

Many modern drugs are extremely potent and their potency dictates that special precautions should be taken to avoid diversion of drugs, as well as unintentional consumption of a dangerous medication. Many of the opioid products are subject to abuse, and pilfering of such products is a major problem. This can occur when a teenager takes one or two tablets of a relative's potent pain medication for recreational use but it can also occur when large quantities of this type of product are stolen during shipping. While there are many methods that medical professionals and law enforcement use to limit such misuse, the role that the container plays is tremendously important. The container should also limit mistaken consumption of the drug. Large shipping containers of potent drugs may contain tracking devices which inform the shipping company when the product has been diverted. For home use, potent drugs may be individually packed so that one unit can be taken out at a time, with the rest of the medication securely stored. Actiq provides a pouch that the patient may wear around the waist to contain a few doses for the patient's needs for a specific period, for example, for a day trip to the hospital. In this way, the medication is under the direct control of the patient or the caregiver. Additionally, this is a limited quantity, not the entire pack, that is carried on the trip.

Complex Dosing Instructions

Many of the modern dosage forms have very complex dosing instructions. One of the roles of packaging is to encourage the correct use of the medication and to limit inappropriate use, or overuse. One example is the dosing instructions for Actiq, which involve moving the applicator from side to side (as mentioned) and also the fact that the patient is instructed to stop using the medication as soon as relief from pain is felt. What happens to the remainder of the dosing unit? There were some accidental consumption incidents by children who probably thought that the medication was a lollipop. The manufacturers later provided detailed instructions on the disposal of partially consumed Actiq units, possibly in response to such incidents. Another interesting example is given in the case study described below which also deals with oral mucosal drug delivery.

CASE STUDY IN PACKAGING: INTERMEZZO

Insomnia is a problem that affects many Americans. What most laypeople regard as insomnia, an inability to fall off to sleep at bedtime, is but one form of insomnia, referred to as sleep onset insomnia. Roughly one-third of insomniacs are able to fall off to sleep at bedtime but awaken in the middle of the night (MOTN) and cannot fall off to sleep again. Such patients cannot take a sleeping tablet when they awaken during the night, since the product would put them off to sleep for a long period and they may not be able to get up at the appointed time in the morning. All marketed sleep preparations, up to the time of this case study, would induce sleep for 6 to 8 hours. There were no effective treatments that could be used in the MOTN and which would reliably provide a short period of sleep, such as 3 to 4 hours. Since MOTN insomnia does not occur every night, the patient would have to guess whether they would have an MOTN event on a particular night. Then, they would take regular sleep medication at bedtime. This could result in overuse of the medication since the patient may not have had an event on that night.

Transept Pharmaceuticals produced a sublingual, low-dose formulation of zolpidem tartrate for MOTN insomnia. The product was specially formulated for quick absorption of the drug and fast onset of action and was to be taken when the patient could not get back to sleep due to an MOTN awakening. The formulation was shown to be effective in sleep studies where awakening in the MOTN was followed by an inability to fall asleep again. In response to the company's new drug application, the FDA stated, in its complete response letter (CRL), that it thought that the company showed evidence of effectiveness of its product, Intermezzo, intended to treat MOTN insomnia. The FDA also conceded that the company had produced a treatment for a unique insomnia indication, with a unique dosing strategy. In addition, there were no next-day effects when taken as directed.

Among other comments made by the FDA, in deciding not to approve the formulation, it stated two concerns which related to the packaging of the product. One of these was that dosing in the MOTN could lead to next-day residual effects if the medication was taken in an inappropriate manner. A particular concern of the FDA was the patient's ability to drive the next morning. With reference to the packaging of the product, the FDA specifically asked Transept to address methods:

1. To avoid inadvertent dosing with less than 4 hours of bedtime remaining.

2. To avoid inadvertent re-dosing in a single night.

An example of the first point could be the situation where a patient cannot fall off to sleep after an awakening but cannot, or does not, calculate how much sleep time he has left and consumes a tablet. An example of the second case would be the patient who could not fall off to sleep and takes a tablet. Thereafter, she gets a little drowsy but does not fall off to sleep quickly, and decides to take the MOTN medication, forgetting that she had already taken a tablet.

The company addressed the FDA concerns as follows. Whereas the tablets that were the subject of the NDA application were strip packed in cards of 10, Transept proposed, after receiving the CRL, to package the tablets in a new bedside unit dose pack. Essentially this was an envelope containing one tablet. Ten of these envelopes were packaged in a box. The intention was that the patient would place one of the tablets, in its envelope, on the nightstand. Upon awakening, in the MOTN, and being unable to fall off to sleep again, the patient would consume the tablet and return the empty envelope to the nightstand. Upon awakening again, the patient would pick up the envelope. If it was torn open, it meant the patient had already taken a dose and, therefore, should not take another dose. In any event, another dose would not be easily available, since only one envelope is kept on the nightstand. If the envelope was intact, it meant that the patient had not taken a dose and was at liberty to do so at that point.

The question of taking a tablet with less than 4 hours of bedtime remaining was addressed by the company as follows. Printed on the envelope was a table with two columns: one contained various times at which the patient had to arise in the morning, while the other had the latest time at which a tablet could be consumed, considering the time of arising. For example, if the patient's wake-up time was 6 AM, the alternate column indicated that the sublingual tablet should not be consumed after 2 AM.

In the ways described, the packaging assisted the patient not to overdose by taking a second tablet, or by taking a tablet too late at night, when there was insufficient bedtime remaining. In other words, the packaging assisted patients to be compliant. With these changes to the packaging, the FDA approved the product which was then a marketed product for the treatment of middle-of-the-night insomnia. At the time of approval, it was the only product in the US market for this indication. Due to poor sales, which were probably due to poor marketing, the product was later withdrawn from the market. Nevertheless, the changes requested by the FDA for approval (and the innovative packaging design responses presented by the company and approved by the FDA) are worthy of consideration when contemplating compliance packaging.

SUMMARY POINTS

- The container is important for ensuring the stability of the product.
- Moisture, light, and oxygen are the major contributors to instability.
- Different types of desiccants may have complementary roles to ensure that the product is not deleteriously affected by moisture.
- Ensuring stability is not the only function of the container; in the modern period, the container should also aid in patient compliance, child resistance, and be tamper evident.

What do you think?

1. Would it be better to prevent people from tampering with medications instead of simply making products tamper evident?
2. Why does the package have to ensure compliance, is that not the role of the pharmacist during patient counseling?
3. How does the packaging of single doses (eg, in a blister) contribute to safety?
4. What function does the FDA have with respect to the packaging of a product that is the subject of a New Drug Application?

Dosage Form Stability

PREVIEW

- Different ways a dosage form can become unstable
- Tests to **estimate** how long a product will remain stable
- Assignment of product shelf life and continued testing after marketing
- Stability problems: advise patients, speak knowledgeably to pharmaceutical companies

It is important for manufacturers to produce, and for pharmacists to dispense, elegant, patient-acceptable dosage forms that contain the correct amount of the drug. It is obvious that the product should also be able to withstand normal handling, such as transport from home to office, and removal from the container. The drug should be released at the desired rate upon consumption of the dosage form by the patient. However, there is little point in having a dosage form that meets all quality criteria when it leaves the manufacturing plant, only to deteriorate rapidly over 3 or 6 months, making it unfit for consumption by the time the patient is ready to consume it. With the exception of a few specialized products, such as injections produced using biotechnology, a longer shelf life is needed.

CHANGES DUE TO INSTABILITY

What changes make a dosage form unacceptable for use? Contrary to popular belief, dosage forms do not "go bad" or putrefy in most instances. While the development of toxic breakdown products is possible, it is not frequently encountered. A more frequent problem is that of sub-therapeutic drug levels, due to the aging of the product, where drug deterioration is not accompanied by toxic breakdown products. In general, dosage forms may show many types of instability, as mentioned in the following sections.

Chemical Degradation of the Drug Contained in the Dosage Form

This is the primary, but by no means the only, concern regarding dosage form stability. It is obvious that decreases in the content of drug from the labeled amounts are not in the best interests of the patient.

Generally, drug content decreases over time but the decrease is usually not large enough over the shelf life of the product to change the therapeutic efficacy. For example, the drug content of a tablet formulation may decrease from 99% of the labeled amount (at the time of manufacture) to 96% over 2 years. Usually, this change is too small to cause any noticeable alteration in a therapeutic outcome. However, with narrow therapeutic range drugs (such as theophylline or digoxin), it may be difficult to maintain blood drug levels in the therapeutic range even with 100% of the labeled drug content. This is due to biological variability. Hence, it gets increasingly more difficult to do so with a product that displays decreasing drug content as it ages, even when the percent decrease in drug content is generally regarded as reasonable with other products.

Formation of Toxic Products from Low Levels of Drug Degradation

The drug content of a product may not change appreciably over time but the degradation of even a small percentage of the drug leads to the formation of toxic degradation products. Examples of this phenomenon include:

1. The conversion of tetracycline to epianhydrotetracycline
2. The conversion of p-aminosalicylic acid to m-amino phenol
3. Photolytic reactions of chlordiazepoxide and nitrazepam

Sensitization from Degradation Products

A good example is the infusion of degraded penicillin G which can lead to the sensitization of lymphocytes and the production of antibodies.

Physical Changes *in Dosage Forms* Leading to Sub-Optimal In Vivo Performance

Physical changes in dosage forms, such as a decrease in dissolution rate, could decrease bioavailability even when the dosage form is tested to reveal acceptable amounts of the drug, that is, the assay is acceptable. The product may have a normal appearance in such cases. The observed physical changes, such as hardening of the tablets, decrease in dissolution rate, etc., may be mediated via a chemical change in an excipient, such as the disintegrant. (Exposure of the tablet to high humidity can lead to a decrease in disintegrant efficiency which, if sufficiently pronounced, can lead to reduced biological efficacy of the product.)

Changes in the Physical Form of the *Drug*

The assay may reveal that the dosage form contains the correct amount of the drug but changes in the polymorphic form may lead to a change in the dissolution rate, leading to a decrease in bioavailability. Such transitions may occur during processing, for example, during the drying of granules, and the change in this instance would be regarded as a processing problem.

These changes can also occur during the storage of pharmaceuticals, especially under non-ideal conditions, for example, when large changes in the temperature, pressure, or relative humidity (RH) occur. Steroids, sulphonamides, and barbiturates are examples of drugs that may change polymorphic form. Of great importance is the fact that the physico-chemical properties of a polymorph, such as solubility and dissolution rate, may be significantly different from that of the starting material and could affect the bioavailability of the drug.

Degradation of Excipients

The integrity of the dosage form may be compromised by the degradation of excipients, including antimicrobials, solubilizers, emulsifiers, or suspending agents. Depending on the nature of the change, the drug product may have decreased bioavailability, or could be unfit for human use for other reasons. The latter could include situations when the bioavailability is acceptable.

Appearance

Physical changes may occur that affect the appearance of the product without influencing the efficiency of the dosage form. Mottling of tablets is an example of this type of effect. Although such changes may not directly change the effectiveness of the dosage form, they may cause a decrease in compliance which, indirectly, influences effectiveness.

From the above description, it can be seen that the drug product may undergo changes that make it physically, chemically, toxicologically, and therapeutically unstable. It may be surprising to the reader that not all instabilities are linked to chemical changes; several issues involve physical changes in the dosage form. An interesting phenomenon is seen with nitroglycerin tablets. Nitroglycerin vaporizes and may redistribute into other tablets within the bottle. Hence, if one determines the average content of the drug in the tablets, this value may remain fairly consistent with the value at the time of manufacture. However, the standard deviation of the average content of nitroglycerin per tablet may increase with storage time. Stabilized nitroglycerin products contain macromolecules that decrease volatilization of the nitroglycerin and so minimize this problem.

From the initial considerations of the nature of changes that may occur, attention is now focused on methods to determine the extent of change. These methods emphasize the chemical content of the drug in consideration of the fact that decrease in drug content is by far the most common form of instability. For this, some theoretical concepts must be introduced.

THE RATE AND ORDER OF A CHEMICAL REACTION

For every chemical reaction, a reaction rate can be determined. Generally, when a chemical reaction is thought of, a reaction of the following type is considered:

$$[A] + [B] \rightarrow [C]$$

However, in the present context, degradation reactions are of greater interest. In this context, a drug of known concentration

TABLE 15-1	Characteristics of Common Reaction Orders		
ORDER	**RATE IS PROPORTIONAL TO …**	**EQUATION**	**EQUATION NO.**
Zero	$[Conc]^0$	$C_t = C_o - k \cdot t$	15-2
First	$[Conc]^1$	$C_t = C_o \cdot 10^{-kt/2.303}$ Or, in Log form: $Log\ C_t = Log\ C_0 - kt/2.303$	15-3
Second	$[Conc]^2$	$\dfrac{1}{Ct} = \dfrac{1}{Co} + kt$	15-4

is denoted as [D]. As the drug degrades, its concentration decreases and byproducts are also created. In terms of the present interest, only the reduction in the concentration of the drug will be considered. However, it should be noted, in those instances where toxic byproducts result from drug degradation, there may be a great interest in the concentration of these toxic products. The rate of degradation, or the rate at which drug concentration is reduced, may be expressed as follows:

$$-\frac{d[D]}{dt} = k \qquad (15\text{-}1)$$

Reactions follow an "order" which indicates whether the reaction continues at a consistent rate, or the rate changes over time. If the rate is of the latter type, how does the rate change? Is it somewhat fast in the beginning and decreases slowly over time? Is it very fast in the beginning with rapid decrease in the rate? The order is also dependent on the extent to which the reaction rate is in proportion to the concentration of the drug remaining at any time point.

A zero-order reaction continues at a consistent rate throughout the period of observation, that is, in the beginning, when there is a large amount of drug, and at the end of the period, when the amount of drug is significantly less, the reaction rate is the same. This may be expressed by saying that the rate of degradation is proportional to $[Conc]^0$. Since any number raised to the power 0 is equal to 1, it means that the reaction rate is independent of concentration. The first-order reaction is proportional to $[Conc]^1$ and, therefore, as concentration decreases, the rate of degradation is reduced. The characteristics of the three major types of reaction order are summarized in Table 15-1.

GRAPHICAL REPRESENTATION

Observation of Eq. (15-2), given in Table 15-1, reveals the equation has the form of the general equation of a straight line:

$$y = a - mx\ (\text{or } y = -mx + a) \qquad (15\text{-}5)$$

The latter is the more general expression. Thus, if concentration (at various time points during the storage of the drug) is plotted against time, with the latter on the X-axis, the plot shown in Figure 15-1 results. The plot has a slope of $-k$, and the point at which it intersects the Y-axis is C_o, the original drug concentration.

Similarly, Eq. (15-3) also has the form of a straight line:

$$y = a - mx\ (\text{or } y = -mx + a) \qquad (15\text{-}6)$$

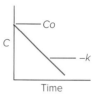

FIGURE 15-1 **Plot of concentration vs time (zero-order reaction).**

Considering the log form of this equation, if log C is plotted against time, the plot shown in Figure 15-2 results. The plot has a slope of $-k/2.303$ and it intercepts the Y-axis at log C_o, the log of the original drug concentration. Similarly, a plot can be drawn for a second-order reaction, using Eq. (15-4) ($1/C$ would be plotted against time). This plot is not shown but analogous conclusions could be drawn from such a plot.

Thus, we can state in the general case: to determine k, the reaction rate constant, some factor of C (concentration) is plotted against time and the value of k is determined from the slope of the resulting plot.

Conversely, when dealing with a set of degradation data in which the order of the reaction is unknown, the concentrations can be plotted versus time (ie, in the format of the zero-order equation). If a straight-line results, as shown in Figure 15-3A, the data represents a zero-order reaction. If plotting the data results in a curve, it means the reaction is not zero order (Figure 15-3B). If the same data is plotted as log concentration versus time, and

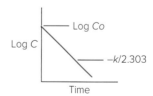

FIGURE 15-2 **Plot of Log C versus time (first-order reaction).**

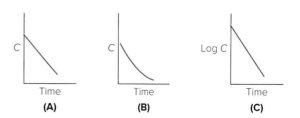

FIGURE 15-3 **Plots of degradation data of unknown order to different profiles. A.** Zero order (data fits); **B.** Zero order (data does not fit); **C.** First order (data fits).

a straight-line results (Figure 15-3C), it is a first-order reaction. Similar reasoning can be applied to a second-order reaction.

In this example, there was no reason to start with a zero-order reaction and the first choice could have been a first-order reaction. In practice, the investigator (through experience, for example) may have reason to choose one or the other equation type.

STABILITY TESTING

It is self-evident that any product that contains chemical compounds will deteriorate over time. The following questions then arise:

How long is the product stable?

When is the product no longer fit for human consumption?

Both questions may be reframed as: what is the maximum storage time, under specified conditions, after which the product will still be acceptable? The answer to this question can be determined experimentally by finding the changes in the dosage form and comparing it to its original condition or initial test results, conducted soon after manufacture. With this information, an expiry date can then be assigned. The consumer refers to the expiry date printed on the package to know how long the product is fit for human use.

Stability testing may be conducted by storing packages of the medication at room temperature (or at the recommended storage temperature specified by the manufacturer). Then, testing could be undertaken monthly, for example, to ascertain when any test parameter falls below an acceptable limit. This is when the product fails the test. The shelf life is then assigned as one test cycle less. For example, if the product fails at 37 months (with monthly testing), the acceptable shelf life is 36 months. Such a study would take too long to conduct and, although it may not be appreciated at first, involves a great deal of work. This includes labeling the products appropriately before storing, removing samples at the appropriate time, testing, recording, and evaluating the results. Hence, so-called "accelerated" stability testing is usually conducted and gives results in a shorter period.

The basic premise of such testing is that by stressing the product, using harsh storage conditions, any change that would have occurred over a long time will now occur over a significantly shorter period. If a convenient method were available to connect the time of product failure under stress conditions with the time of failure under normal conditions, it would be much quicker to determine the shelf life of the product. An example of product failure during stability testing is a drop in drug concentration to less than 90%. This is the essence of accelerated stability testing.

Early research studies showed that temperature influenced degradation of chemicals. Hence, it seemed reasonable to store materials at elevated temperature conditions to assess changes that would occur. The Arrhenius equation was developed as a mathematical model to understand the effects of temperature on the degradation of chemicals. Using this equation, chemical degradation was studied extensively. This equation and the methods developed from it allow one to study degradation at 50°C, 60°C, and 70°C, for example, and use the information

obtained to predict degradation at 25°C or room temperature. This method involves rigorous mathematical application, using equations and graphical methods. However, only chemical degradation can be assessed using this method.

Since it is known that pharmaceutical products undergo degradation which may be both chemical and physical, application of the Arrhenius equation alone does not give a complete picture of the deterioration of the product. For example, the softening, or the hardening, of tablets will affect the rate at which the drug is released which, in turn, influences bioavailability. However, there is no room for testing these parameters with the use of the Arrhenius method only. The FDA described accelerated test methods for evaluating all aspects of a pharmaceutical dosage form's quality in a guidance document for the use of pharmaceutical companies when conducting stability testing. This is the basic method used in industry today and it assesses both chemical and physical changes in dosage forms.

The Arrhenius method will be briefly described, for the development and appreciation of a theoretical background. More attention will be paid to the method described by the FDA in its guidance document. This method uses the Arrhenius equation as background information, without applying the mathematical rigor implicit in this method. It also goes beyond the Arrhenius method by utilizing other test methodologies. Elevated temperature as well as humidity are used as simultaneous stress conditions to obtain an indication of stability relatively quickly. However, room temperature data are also required for final acceptance by the FDA of the product's stability.

Recap Questions

1. Name three changes that may occur in a dosage form due to aging.
2. Which is the most common type of change occurring in dosage forms as they age?
3. Which order of chemical reaction represents change at a constant rate?
4. Why are elevated temperature and humidity conditions used to test the stability of a drug product?

ARRHENIUS METHOD

As mentioned, the Arrhenius equation was developed to study the effects of temperature on the degradation of chemical compounds. It provides a theoretical basis for such a study. Some theoretical considerations that were taken into account in the development of this equation will be briefly considered. One theory for chemical reactivity is the collision theory. All molecules are in random motion and this theory holds that the collision of two reactant molecules, under the correct circumstances, will lead to a reaction between the two molecules. Two factors control the rate of reaction: the activation energy (Ea) and the collision frequency.

Ea is the energy in excess of the average molecular energy of all molecules of the type under consideration. An energy level, in excess of the average energy level, is required for a reaction to occur. Collisions between molecules of lower energy do not result in a reaction. As the temperature is increased, the number of molecules at or above the activation energy level is increased, resulting in a greater number of effective collisions.

The collision frequency is the number of collisions per unit of time. The more collisions that occur, the greater the number of effective collisions (those between molecules above the activation energy level) and, hence, also the greater the number of molecular reactions. A higher concentration of the chemicals, for example, leads to more collisions and, therefore, a faster reaction rate. A later modification to the theory included an orientation factor. Since many molecules have the reactive group surrounded by large atoms, steric hindrance may be a factor and only collisions which occur between molecules at the correct orientation are effective and result in a reaction. The Arrhenius equation is provided below:

$$k = A \cdot e^{-\frac{Ea}{RT}} \qquad (15\text{-}5)$$

where k = reaction rate constant
A = Arrhenius factor or frequency factor
Ea = Energy of activation
R = gas constant
T = temperature (°K)

The natural log form of this equation is:

$$\text{Log } k = \text{Log } A - \frac{Ea}{2.303R} \cdot \frac{1}{T} \qquad (15\text{-}6)$$

The reaction rate constant (k) is specific for a particular set of experimental conditions, especially the reaction temperature. From the form of Eq. (15-6), it can be seen that the plot of log k versus 1/T will yield a straight line with a slope of − Ea/2.303R and a Y-axis intercept of Log A (Figure 15-4). The utility of the equation is as follows. The reaction is conducted at several elevated temperature values and k is obtained for each temperature. Then, the obtained values of k are plotted against the inverse of T (which is stated in degrees K). This results in a straight line which can be extrapolated to obtain k at 298°K (or 25°C) (Figure 15-4). Inserting this value for k into the appropriate rate equation (eg, Eq. (15-7) for a zero-order reaction), the time taken to reach a given level of degradation, such as 10%, can be obtained. This duration of time is the period during which the product has the required potency, assuming that 90% is the lowest drug concentration that is acceptable.

Steps to Determine Expiry Date

The above explanation provides the major steps for determining the expiry date using the Arrhenius equation. The detailed method is provided below as a list of steps to take:

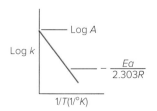

FIGURE 15-4 Arrhenius plot.

1. Obtain k, the reaction rate constant, for different temperature values (eg, k_{50}, k_{60}, k_{70}, where the subscript indicates the temperature in degrees centigrade):
   a. Store the sample in stability ovens (described in a later section) at three different elevated temperature values (eg, T_{50}, T_{60}, T_{70}).
   b. Withdraw samples from each oven at predetermined time intervals, for example, 1 month, 2 months, 3 months and determine the concentration of drug remaining in each sample.
   c. Determine the order of the reaction, as previously discussed (Figure 15-3).
   d. Plot concentration (remaining) versus time for **each** elevated experimental T, assuming step c determined that it is a zero-order reaction (for a different order, a function of C, such as Log C, is plotted, as previously described).
   e. Obtain three k-values from the slopes of the three plots, that is, one for each temperature.

2. Obtain k_{25} from Arrhenius plot of three k values:
   a. Convert the three temperature values (50°C, 60°C, and 70°C in example above) to °K.
   b. Find the inverse of the °K temperature values.
   c. Plot log k versus the inverse values of T obtained in step b above (Figure 15-5).
   d. Extrapolate the plot to the inverse of 298°K (25°C) (or 3.36×10^{-3}).
   e. Assuming a zero-order reaction and 90% as the lowest acceptable drug concentration, insert the percentage values into the rate equation.
   $$C_t = C_o - k \cdot t$$
   $$90\% = 100\% - k_o \cdot t \qquad (15\text{-}7)$$
   f. Insert the value of the slope from the Arrhenius plot and solve for t, which is the time to reach 90 % concentration
   g. The shelf life is typically one test cycle less than the value obtained in step f, for example, if 25 months is the answer obtained from step f, the shelf life is 24 months.

FDA-REQUIRED STABILITY STUDIES

Historically, the stability of a drug in a dosage form was considered in terms of the Arrhenius equation, as described above. Pharmaceutical stability studies have their historic origin in the application of the Arrhenius equation. However, modern studies are quite far removed from the strict application of the Arrhenius equation, as described above. Nevertheless, the Arrhenius equation is the theoretical underpinning for much of modern drug product stability studies.

Somewhat empirically, it can be tentatively deduced, after 6 months of study at elevated temperature and humidity, that the drug in the product will be stable for 24 months at room temperature. Obviously, changes that are not directly related to chemical degradation, including physical changes such as softening or hardening of tablets, are not related to the Arrhenius equation. Nevertheless, demonstration of the stability of these

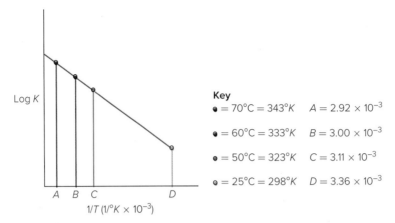

Key
● = 70°C = 343°K $A = 2.92 \times 10^{-3}$
● = 60°C = 333°K $B = 3.00 \times 10^{-3}$
● = 50°C = 323°K $C = 3.11 \times 10^{-3}$
● = 25°C = 298°K $D = 3.36 \times 10^{-3}$

FIGURE 15-5 Calculation of room temperature rate constant using the Arrhenius plot.

parameters over 6 months at elevated temperature and humidity is also considered evidence of stability for 24 months at room temperature. The use of elevated storage conditions to assess physical changes in the dosage form is not totally rigorous from a theoretical perspective. Over time, however, this application has been shown to be reasonably accurate and provides results from which sound conclusions may be drawn. Consequently, it has become widely accepted, especially by the FDA.

To assess the changes that occur in a dosage form over time, and to determine the length of time during which deterioration is low enough to consider the product acceptable for human use, a stability program is initiated by the pharmaceutical company. The FDA has published a guidance document on how stability studies are to be conducted for drug products overseen by them. This document is the framework for stability testing of all products to be sold in the United States and can be used in the assessment of chemical, as well as physical, changes. A description of the major elements of this document is provided in a later section of this chapter.

The results of stability studies conducted on products intended to be marketed in the United States are reviewed by the FDA. The details of the stability program and the results are an important part of the data that a company provides to the FDA in the application for marketing approval of the drug product. The FDA requires testing be done under accelerated conditions for 6 months as well as testing at room temperature for 2 years. The latter period is the usually assigned shelf life for the majority of new drug products. A summary of the major aspects of the FDA-required stability testing is shown in Mind Map 15-1.

With the submission of a new drug application (NDA), the FDA requires the inclusion of 6 months' stability data under accelerated conditions as well as 12 months' long-term ("room temperature") data. The FDA, additionally, stipulates that the long-term testing continue and that data be provided by the company as it becomes available. This dispensation saves the company a great deal of time since the full long-term testing results will not be available at the time of application submission, and often not even at the time of approval of the application. Testing continues during the period of review by the FDA and after the granting of marketing approval.

The FDA will assign 2 years shelf life based on acceptable 6 months' data at elevated temperature and humidity, and acceptable data with each submission of continuing stability test results. In this way, accelerated stability testing is advantageous since long-term testing is continued while other activities are ongoing. The FDA allows this dispensation on the basis of acceptable accelerated test results and this saves the pharmaceutical company a great deal of time.

STABILITY CHAMBER

From the above description, it is clear that products must be stored under specific elevated conditions (including elevated temperature) for extended periods to force rapid product deterioration. From the rates of deterioration at elevated conditions, product deterioration under normal conditions of use can be estimated. This data allows the deduction of the period during which the product will be stable. The combination of elevated temperature and humidity is used since it is also known that this combination can accelerate changes in products. Certain fixed combinations of temperature and humidity have been used and are standardized. Given this information, how can one conveniently store products under these elevated conditions (eg, 40°C/ 75% RH) for extended periods, such as 6 or 12 months?

It is important, naturally, that the selected conditions must be maintained consistently during the test period. If large fluctuations in conditions occur, results will not be reproducible from lab to lab and, also, will not give confidence in the results obtained within a lab. Even if conditions dip below the critical values only briefly, but repeatedly, it may result in the product receiving less stress than stated. The product may appear to be stable over the period of study when, in fact, it would not be stable if test parameters were held consistently. More importantly, deductions made from such results about stability under normal conditions of use may be unreliable in that they may overestimate shelf life.

The requirements for the physical test environment can, therefore, be summarized as follows:

1. Simultaneous provision of the temperature and humidity conditions as required for the test.

2. Ability to easily set and attain the required conditions.

3. Maintenance of the desired test conditions within narrow limits over the duration of the study.

4. Ability to know, retroactively, if the test conditions were not met, and the period during which they were not met.

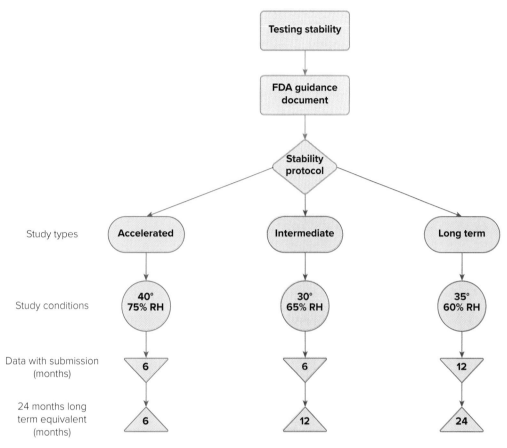

MIND MAP 15-1 Overview of FDA-Required Stability Testing Studies

These requirements can be achieved with the use of stability chambers, an oven-like device used to maintain the desired temperature and humidity conditions. Typically, they are specially developed for stability testing. The test conditions are dialed in using the instrument panel which also shows the actual temperature and humidity conditions prevailing at any point in time. Modern stability chambers have efficient systems for heating the interior of the chamber and insulated walls to prevent loss of heat, thus maintaining consistent temperature. Stability chambers may vary in size from bench top models, the size of a small refrigerator, up to walk-in types, capable of storing thousands of samples for multiple stability studies.

Sensitive temperature sensors turn on the heating elements as the temperature drops and turn them off as the temperature rises marginally beyond the set point. The chamber has a water line to continuously supply water, as needed, in order to establish and maintain elevated humidity at the set point. Condensed water vapor is removed via a drainage system. The system is capable of holding the conditions at the set points consistently. Obviously, any mechanical system cannot hold conditions perfectly but the fluctuations are generally small and acceptable.

The temperature and humidity are recorded on circular graph paper. The line drawn is a continuous spiral and, thus, a record of the actual temperature and humidity prevalent within the chamber is maintained for every minute of the day and night of the study. The circular graph paper with spiraled information means that information for an extended period is stored on one

sheet of circular paper. These can easily be stored as a record of the prevalent conditions during the study.

In use, temperature and humidity changes can be observed when the operator opens the door to remove samples for testing. Minimal changes of this type are acceptable. These systems are usually linked to backup power generators so that power supply is maintained even during short power outages. Additional to alarms giving an audible signal, in modern pharmaceutical companies, the stability chambers are also linked to computer systems which generate a message to a designated company employee, informing this person that there was a power outage and the times during which the backup power supply went into operation. Other important functions of the computer system, in relation to stability testing, are mentioned later in this chapter.

Recap Questions

1. Why does the FDA ask for testing under multiple conditions?

2. In which ways does the FDA make it easier for companies to do stability testing?

3. What is the purpose of subjecting a drug product to high temperature and humidity as part of a stability study?

4. Which components of the chamber allow temperature to be accurately maintained?

5. Which component of the chamber prevents heat loss?

6. Which components of the chamber facilitate humidity being consistently maintained?

7. Suppose the temperature and humidity within a stability chamber were recorded manually three times per day at 8-hour intervals. Besides the inconvenience to operators, what potential problem in relation to fluctuations of storage conditions could occur?

STABILITY PROTOCOL

The stability program is governed by a **stability protocol** which is a formal document prepared by the scientist conducting the stability study and which must be approved by certain company officials, including the manager of the Research and Development group that is conducting the study. This document sets out precisely how the stability study will be conducted and specifies several parameters, for example:

1. The number of containers that will be stored in the stability chamber.

2. The conditions under which they will be stored, that is, the specific temperature and humidity conditions to which the chamber is set.

3. The time intervals at which containers of the product will be withdrawn from the stability chamber for testing, for example, 1, 2, and 3 months.

4. The tests that will be conducted on the product at each pull point.

5. What constitutes a passing result for each test (acceptance criteria).

6. How the data will be analyzed (statistical methods).

The setting out of the study details in a protocol, which must be rigorously followed, prevents operators from making arbitrary decisions during the conduct of the study.

FDA GUIDANCE DOCUMENT

Since the stability of pharmaceuticals is so important, the FDA has published the previously-mentioned guidance document on stability testing. As the name implies, a guidance document is not the law but it is there to guide companies. Generally, companies follow the guidance document closely. If, for certain aspects, a company does not, there should be good reasons.

The International Conference on Harmonization (ICH) prepared guidelines for the performance of stability studies that are acceptable to Japan, the United States, and Europe. The guidance document mentioned above reflects the findings of this conference. Prior to the ICH, each country had its own standards. Hence, international companies, marketing a product multi-nationally had to do different stability tests, in accordance with the requirements of each country, for the same product. Sometimes, the two countries had minor differences in their requirements. However, the company had to perform two stability tests to satisfy each country's requirement. For example, if one country wanted a study to be done at 30°C/60% RH and another country needed the study done at 30°C/65% RH, the company had to perform studies under both conditions to obtain results that accord with each country's requirements. To conduct a stability study for each product in many iterations is an enormous amount of work and is expensive, ultimately making the product expensive. In an attempt to avoid duplication and reduce costs of internationally marketed drugs, the United States, Europe, and Japan established this mechanism to find common procedures that would be acceptable to the three regions. These regions consume the major percentage of world pharmaceutical production.

The guidance document describes the testing of active pharmaceutical ingredients (ie, the drug itself, usually available in powder form), and of dosage forms incorporating the drug. The main concepts pertaining to the latter will be discussed in this chapter since this is of greater interest within the discipline of Pharmaceutics and, also, may be of greater interest to the practicing pharmacist. Some drugs are intended to be stored in the refrigerator or freezer and the guidance document has a special section dealing with these. This topic will not be covered in this chapter. This FDA guidance document (and this chapter) do not discuss the testing of biological products, which is a separate subject with its own issues. In addition, the referenced guidance document specifically describes the testing of new drugs and new drug products, while the testing of generic products is described in a separate guidance document which was published in 2014. This document follows the same general principles as used in the testing of new drugs, with some changes to procedure. These changes do not alter the conceptual framework of stability testing which this chapter attempts to convey. However, no further reference to generic drug testing with regard to stability will be mentioned.

Stability test procedures will now be briefly discussed to provide an overview of the process. The pharmacist will, usually, not be expected to conduct stability trials. In the event, however, that a stability issue is encountered, or is suspected, the pharmacist should be able to conduct an informed discussion with the patient or, if necessary, a representative of the manufacturing company. This chapter provides the basic framework of information for such discussions. The chemical analysis tests and statistical methods utilized in stability testing are beyond the scope of this book.

CONTAINERS USED FOR STABILITY TESTING

Since the container is an integral part of the unit that is tested to demonstrate stability, it is important to understand that the FDA-assigned shelf life is for the product **stored in**

a particular container. The package that contains the drug product units (eg, tablets or capsules) used for the stability test should, ideally, be the actual container to be used for the marketed product. Sometimes, this container is not available for a variety of reasons. For example, a company may want to use custom-made containers for the commercial product. It is possible that these containers were not produced at the time the stability tests are to be started. Then, the container used for the stability studies must resemble the commercial package as closely as possible. It should consist of the immediate container and outer container that are of the same dimensions and made from the same material as the intended commercial containers. The above provision allows the company to use a container that is similar (but not identical) to the one to be used for commercial sales. If cotton wool (or other material for stuffing) or a desiccant pack is to be used in the final commercial package, these should be incorporated into the stability test package as well.

Recap Questions

1. If a company has well-trained people, why is it necessary to have a stability protocol?

2. Why is it important to have the manager sign off on a stability protocol?

3. What are the reasons for potentially faster product deterioration in an alternate container?

STABILITY TEST CONDITIONS

Elevated temperature and humidity are not the only "stress" conditions mentioned in the guidance, but they are important ones that affect almost all drug products. The ultimate test of stability involves storage of the product for its intended shelf life, with testing for various quality attributes. The storage would occur under the manufacturer-recommended storage conditions which are usually room temperature and ambient humidity for most products. Since at least 24 months' shelf life is desired for most consumer products, this test process would take long. In an effort to obtain faster results, accelerated testing procedures are resorted to, as described in the introductory remarks. These conditions are usually elevated temperature and humidity, but may also involve exposure to intense, but controlled, light; or to freezing and thawing the product. These procedures and test methods are described in the FDA guidance document but the document leaves room for manufacturers to vary the process, or to use other methods, where scientifically justified. This chapter focuses on the use of elevated temperature and humidity as the accelerated conditions since these are the most commonly used conditions.

As the name implies, guidance documents are not legally binding but they do represent the thinking of a legal authority which has made a concerted effort to provide sound guidelines. Typically, a draft document is circulated, and industry is offered the opportunity to comment. The typical guidance document takes years to prepare, including the time for comment and amendment of the document in the light of the opinions of industry scientists and academia.

The following are the three test conditions mentioned in the guidance document that utilize temperature and humidity as the major factors that affect product quality:

Long-Term Testing

Commonly referred to as "room temperature" testing, this test utilizes a temperature that is typical of room temperature, and humidity that is similar to the ambient condition. However, the study is performed in a stability chamber with significantly smaller fluctuations of either parameter than in a typical room. Products are stored for 24 months with testing at selected times during this period as indicated in Table 15-2. It is intended to reflect conditions of storage generally used by consumers. The intention is to show 24 months' stability to obtain a shelf life of 24 months, which is the most common initial shelf life approved by the FDA.

Accelerated Testing

Accelerated testing is conducted to give a quicker indication of the stability of the product without waiting for 24 months. The tests are conducted at 40°C and 75% RH. As mentioned previously, these conditions are intended to accelerate any changes that would occur at a slower rate at room temperature. The test conditions and times at which samples should be taken (pull points) are summarized in Table 15-2.

Intermediate Testing

Accelerated conditions may be too harsh for certain drugs or for certain types of dosage forms. This is reflected in very rapid deterioration of the drug or in rapid changes in the dosage form which make the test conditions unsuitable for continued testing for 6 months. It is important to realize that very harsh conditions, which do not represent normal use conditions, were used to test the drug to get quick results, with the intention of extrapolating these results to a longer term, under normal conditions of use. Hence, the product does not "fail" at this point. The only conclusion that can reasonably be drawn is that testing under

TABLE 15-2	Summary of Stability Study Conditions		
STUDY	SIMPLIFIED* STORAGE CONDITION	PULL POINTS GIVEN IN GUIDANCE (MONTHS)
Long Term	25°C/60% RH	0, 6, 12†, 18, 24
Intermediate	30°C/65% RH	0, 6†, 9, 12
Accelerated	40°C/75% RH	0, 3, 6†

Notes:
*The acceptable deviations from temperature and humidity, and the alternate storage conditions mentioned in the guidance document are not given in the table.

†The minimum time period covered by the data at the time of submission for each stability condition is given in red font (stability testing continues thereafter).

less harsh, or "intermediate," conditions has to be used in this instance. These conditions still allow a shorter testing program than long-term testing, and an assessment can also be made of the stability of the formulation under normal conditions of use. Since the testing conditions are less harsh, testing will go on for longer than under accelerated conditions. Table 15-2 provides the test conditions and pull points.

In order to assign a shelf life, the FDA considers both the data collected under accelerated conditions, as well as the long-term data. If the company found that accelerated conditions were too harsh for the delivery system in question, the FDA will review intermediate and long-term data.

It is important to realize that the product may be approved for marketing before all long-term data are available, that is, before 24 months have elapsed since the stability tests were begun. The approval is based on the available long-term data and the accelerated data. The use of accelerated data in this way allows for a quicker decision by the FDA. Consequently, products are marketed earlier than would be the case if all stability data were required for FDA review prior to approval. The earlier approval may be of great significance to patients waiting for the approval of a novel treatment. The company may have invested hundreds of millions of dollars (or more), up to that point, for product development. The earlier approval allows the company to begin recouping some of its investment at an earlier point.

CONDUCT OF THE STUDY

It may not be immediately apparent, but one study could involve:

1. Hundreds of containers of the drug.

2. A great deal of data, graphs, tabular summaries, and reports.

The large number of containers is due to the fact that they must be stored at different temperature and humidity conditions, and for several "pull points" (the dates on which the containers must be removed from the stability chamber for testing). As mentioned, a computer program is usually used to track all of these activities. The computer system is programmed to send an email to the responsible person, shortly before a pull point, instructing them to withdraw a stability sample on the appropriate date. Typically, a protocol statement allows the sample to be pulled up to 3 days before, or after, a specified date. This proviso makes it possible that the scientist or technician does not have to come in on a Sunday or holiday to withdraw a sample. The protocol also specifies the period during which the sample must be tested, after removal from the stability chamber. Since this period is written into the protocol before the start of the study, an operator cannot decide "on the fly" that he will take additional time to complete the task. If the testing is not completed within the period allowed, a deviation from the protocol has occurred. The test period incorporated into the protocol must, therefore, be a reasonable period to complete the work and must, also, take into account probable delays. A typical test period may be 2 weeks but could be longer.

After the samples are analyzed, the results are stored within the computer program. Reports can be generated using the stability report templates stored within the computer program.

These reports are formatted in a manner that is acceptable to the FDA. It is not essential or mandated that a computer program be used but such programs greatly facilitate stability testing and reporting.

Recap Questions

1. How can we rapidly test whether a drug is sensitive to light and will degrade, apart from storing it for 2 years under normal light conditions and then testing for drug potency?

2. If it is not intended that patients store drugs in extreme conditions, why are such conditions used for testing? Does it not make sense to test pharmaceutical products under the conditions in which they will be stored and used?

3. In your own words, explain the use of intermediate test conditions.

4. Name two benefits of using a computer program to assist with stability testing.

ADDITIONAL TESTING

If the company desires a longer shelf life, it would have to test, and prove product stability, for a longer period. Typically, companies obtain 24 months of stability with their initial application and, after marketing the product, start new stability studies and continue these studies for the intended, longer shelf life. If the data supports the extended shelf life and are found to be acceptable to the FDA, the longer shelf life will be assigned. It is important to remember that companies cannot assign a shelf life, only the FDA can do this (for products that are approved for sale in the United States). This is done after evaluating the data supplied by the company and considering the company's assessment of the data.

It should be noted that the guidance document mentions a "minimum" number of time points at which samples should be removed from the stability chamber for testing. These time points are captured in Table 15-2. The company is free to withdraw, and test, additional samples. These have to be decided before the study is commenced and incorporated into the protocol since changes cannot be made "on the fly." In any event, a larger number of samples must be placed into the stability chamber and accounted for in the protocol. The additional testing may be done to get a clearer understanding of the changes occurring in the product and to discern trends. For example, additional samples may be pulled at 3 months in a long-term study. Sometimes, additional samples are tested to give the company a level of assurance, at an earlier point in time, that the product's stability will be acceptable. Conversely, if the test results are less good than anticipated, the company may choose to begin work on an alternate formulation while continuing to test until a failure is seen. The additional test time point, in this case, allows the company to start work on the alternate formulation earlier.

The guidance states that the company that began an accelerated study and observed significant change in the product should then begin an intermediate study. A significant change is defined in the guidance. In each of the following scenarios, consider the implications for the company:

1. A company starts an accelerated study and, after 3 months, a significant change is observed; the company then starts an intermediate study.

2. The company starts the accelerated and intermediate studies simultaneously.

In the first scenario, they would be 3 months late with the start of the intermediate study in comparison to the second scenario. For this reason, it is customary in the industry to follow the latter method. Time is very valuable to the company. In contrast, only a minimal cost would be incurred by starting an intermediate study that may not be needed. Since one cannot buy time, this is the typical practice within the pharmaceutical industry.

SELECTION OF BATCHES FOR TESTING

The guidance states that at least three primary batches of the product must be tested. A primary batch is one that is produced from scratch. Using the example of tablets, the batch is begun from the blending of the primary powdered ingredients. It cannot, for example, be two batches derived by splitting one large batch at any stage of the process, for example, after powder blending or after granulation. Two of the primary batches must be of pilot scale. The pilot scale is defined as 100,000 tablets or 1/10th the intended commercial batch size (as defined in the NDA), whichever is the larger. The third batch may be smaller. Tablets are used as an example in the above description. Obviously, these requirements apply to other dosage forms as well where appropriate batch sizes are also mentioned.

While these test batches are typically smaller than a commercial batch, the method of manufacture must be the same. To stay with the tablets example, the powders used to make the tablets may be blended in equipment that is smaller than the commercial blending equipment but the blending action must be similar. The company should not, for example, use a high-intensity mixer for the pilot batch and a low-intensity mixer for the commercial batch. The tablet compression should either be done on the same machine, or on another machine that is smaller but has very similar operating mechanisms.

The three batches of product should be manufactured using at least two different batches of the drug substance, where possible. This requirement is intended to show that any minor differences in the drug substance (typical batch-to-batch variation) do not result in major differences in the resulting product. The reason that some leeway is allowed by the use of the statement "if possible" is that refinement of synthetic chemical techniques and scale-up of the drug substance production may be going on simultaneously with tablet scale up and pilot batch manufacture. Hence, multiple batches of the drug, in sufficient quantities for a pilot batch of product, may not be available.

STABILITY COMMITMENTS

If all the product information and test results contained in the NDA, including the stability information, appear satisfactory to the FDA, they will approve the product. Commercial production, and sales, may begin as a result of the approval. Since the FDA, in several ways, has afforded the company some leniency in the stability testing program, the company must now commit to completing a full and rigorous stability program after product approval. The instances of leniency are summarized below:

1. Stability studies are, most often, not complete at the time of NDA submission and, additionally, may not be complete by the time the product is approved. The company commits to completing the stability studies already begun.

2. Stability studies are usually conducted with two batches of pilot scale size and with one batch that may be even smaller. The company commits to repeating the entire stability exercise using the first three production batches (which are usually 10 times larger). For example, the pilot batch may consist of 100,000 capsules while the production batch consists of 1 million capsules. Although the pilot batch is manufactured in a way that resembles the full-scale production batch, this requirement is in place to ensure that a usual production batch is tested and will be demonstrated to provide the required stability. Only a small portion of the production batches are used in stability testing and the remainder of the batches can be sold, whereas the pilot batches manufactured for stability testing cannot be sold. In this context, it is helpful to remember that the pilot batches were manufactured before FDA approval, while the production batches were made after product approval.

These commitments are a condition of approval, that is, the company does not have an option as to whether they will complete these tasks or not. It is important to understand that a company may choose to complete stability studies based on pilot batches before submission of the NDA. In addition, they may choose to use full production batches for the stability study. In such cases, the above commitments may only apply partially, or not at all.

Recap Questions

1. Which provision of the stability protocol makes it unnecessary for operators to come to work on a Sunday to pull samples?

2. Which provision of the stability protocol attempts to prevent an operator from taking a very long time to complete the testing of containers that were pulled?

3. Suppose one point on an accelerated stability test shows degradation values that are slightly higher than expected. Does this mean that the stability study has failed and that further stability testing is not needed?

4. If the product is removed on the correct day but cannot be tested the same day, would this constitute a deviation?

SUMMARY POINTS

The Arrhenius equation is used to assess chemical degradation. By studying degradation at three higher temperatures, an extrapolation to room temperature can be made and the stability of a compound is assessed in a shorter time. The method used in the FDA guidance document relies on the Arrhenius equation as background theoretical information. All aspects of the stability of a dosage form are considered, not just chemical (drug) degradation. Stability testing methods are standardized in the major global markets.

FDA testing is required on two pilot (1/10 scale) batches and one smaller batch. Stability testing is conducted according to a guidance document. A stability protocol must be developed by the company. Computerized systems facilitate control and data handling. The fact that the FDA permits companies some leeway in stability testing should not be viewed as the FDA having a poor sense of the stability of the product it is approving. During the period in which the application is under consideration at the FDA, companies must continue to submit stability data to the FDA as the results become available. Hence, the submission of incomplete data at the time of application is not overly lenient. Even when approval occurs before all data have been submitted, it is only done when the stability data, up to that point, leaves little question about the continued stability of the product. Even the use of pilot batches, in place of full-scale production batches, is acceptable considering that batch production must be on the same, or similar, equipment as the production batches. Then, full-scale batches have to be tested after marketing approval. In addition, if the results submitted prior to approval leave any doubt, the FDA has every right to allocate a shortened expiry date or even, in extreme cases, may not approve the product for marketing. As a consequence of all these activities and reviews, the FDA is assured that the product has adequate stability by the time it is ready to make a decision on the application.

When the three full-scale batches are tested, after approval, the drug is in production and being sold, and the cost implications for the company are less severe. The three production batches which are subjected to stability testing are referred to in the industry as "commitment batches" and the remaining product, not used in the stability tests, may be sold commercially.

What is the significance of "adequate stability"? It reflects that the product has sufficient shelf life for normal use by patients, when stored under the manufacturer-specified conditions. If room temperature is the specified storage condition, there may be minor excursions out of the temperature range contemplated, and these are permitted. The company cannot guarantee stability if the product is not stored as required. For example, if the product is stored in the patient's car which is parked in the sun during a large part of the day, summer temperatures may cause excessive deterioration of the drug. Likewise, products are not intended to be stored in the bathroom where temperature and humidity levels may be excessive.

The primary aim of the formal stability study is to obtain evidence of such stability. The results of earlier, informal stability studies may have been used to find the causes of instability and to develop methods to control the deterioration of the product, in efforts to improve stability. The shelf life is assigned by the FDA after consideration of all the data supplied by the company. This is the expiry date that is noted on the label. Usually, this will be 2 years from manufacture. A company may not assign a longer shelf life than the one determined by the FDA. After marketing of the product has begun, the company may conduct another stability study for a period longer than 2 years, for example, 3 years. Upon submission of the data to the FDA, and if the FDA concurs that the data reveals stability for a longer period than 2 years at room temperature, the FDA will assign a longer shelf life, such as 3 years. A company may not extend the shelf life on its own.

What do you think?

1. What information does one need in order to calculate the order of a reaction?

2. A student is working in a pharmaceutical production company during the summer. He is assisting with the manufacture of a pilot batch of tablets for a stability study. The commercial product consists of 1/2-in tablets but the punches and dies that should be used are not available. The student suggests using a 9/16-in set of punches and dies, arguing that this is only 11% larger in diameter than the set that should have been used. Comment on his suggestion.

3. Mrs. Jones informs you that the tablets she purchased from your pharmacy were a pale blue color when purchased a month ago and now are a lighter blue color, with darker blue in patches. She shows you the tablets and you confirm her description. She does not want to continue taking the medication since she feels that the drug has gone "bad." She wonders how much harm has been caused by the three doses that she took before coming to discuss this with you. Upon checking the pharmacy's prescription records, inquiring from Mrs. Jones, and looking up the active ingredient's stability you discover the following:

   a. The tablets were purchased 6 months ago and have an expiration date 1 year ahead of the present time

   b. Mrs. Jones stores all her medications in a bathroom cabinet

   c. The API is very stable at room temperature, and under elevated temperature and humidity conditions

   How would you advise Mrs. Jones?

4. A patient shows you, the pharmacist, a container of sustained-release tablets that she purchased from you approximately 3 months ago. The tablets appear to be

soft and the coating is peeling. The patient thinks it is okay to use the tablets since it is "only the color coming off." How would you advise the patient?

5. From a scientific perspective, why is it important to complete the testing of pulled samples within the prescribed time?

6. How should the company react, with respect to an ongoing stability study, if the stability chamber, a mechanical device, goes out of the set range, for example, 30°C/65% RH?

7. How would the company know if a stability chamber had gone out of its set range for, say, 6 hours and then come back into the correct range?

8. Would a stability study, generally, have to be terminated if there is an electrical outage in the area of the company and the company has products stored under test conditions within a stability chamber?

9. If exposure to moisture is thought to be the cause of a particular chemical transition, what test could be performed to illustrate that moisture absorption has been high?*

10. Which tests tell us that the product has undergone polymorphic transitions?**

Notes:
*Answer not given in this chapter.
**Answer not given in this book.

BIBLIOGRAPHY

Guidance for Industry Q1A(R2): Stability Testing of New Drug Substances and Products. FDA, November 2003.

Guidance for Industry ANDAs: Stability Testing of Drug Substances and Products. FDA, June 2013.

Good Manufacturing Practices 16

PREVIEW

- Why are good manufacturing practices important?
- Overview of current good manufacturing practices and regulatory status
- How quality is built into a product
- Good manufacturing practices at various stages of processing

INTRODUCTION

A complex pharmaceutical dosage form has many steps in its production and every step has to be done correctly, with appropriate testing after each step, to ensure the quality of the final product. In this way, **quality is built into the product** at every step. It is important to understand this principle in the overall process of creating a pharmaceutical product. Quality cannot be developed, after the fact, by rigorous post-production testing. The latter can only confirm the fact that a quality product has been produced or, alternately, that the batch should be rejected because it does not meet quality standards.

Some of the steps involved may not be readily recognized as steps toward the production of a quality product. For example, the testing of raw materials is considered an integral part of this process; without such testing, products produced in a manufacturing plant *may* be defective and unsuitable for human use, even though the methods employed in its production were correct, that is, a good product cannot be manufactured from poor ingredients even though the manufacturing steps were conducted appropriately. Hence, scientists working in the pharmaceutical industry are careful to pay attention to the quality of the drug substance and excipients that go into pharmaceutical products, and the testing of ingredients is regarded as an integral part of the overall manufacturing process. Mind Map 16-1 provides an overview of GMP manufacturing and the control measures used to maintain quality.

Quality Assurance and Quality Control

Since there is a quality control (QC) group as well as a quality assurance (QA) group in pharmaceutical companies, it will be useful to explain the difference between these two similarly-named groups before a more detailed discussion of their respective activities.

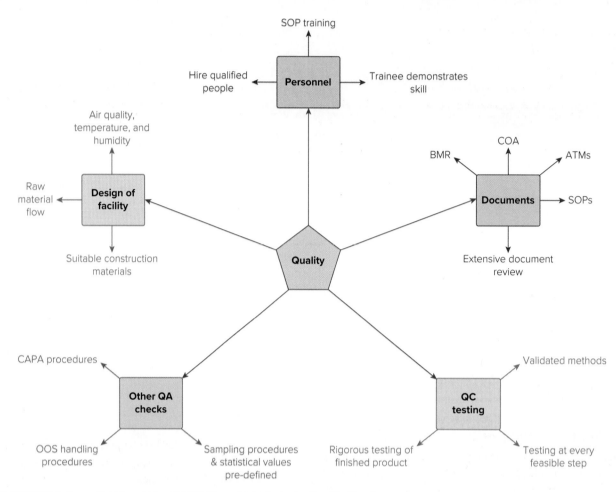

MIND MAP 16-1 Essential Elements of GMP Manufacturing of a Quality Product

Quality Control Department

The QC group conducts all laboratory testing within the company, apart from a few, relatively simple in-process tests. The latter are done in the manufacturing suite during the production process. The test results may dictate an adjustment to a parameter on a production machine. For example, in-process tablet hardness testing may show that the tablets produced in the initial few minutes of a batch are too soft. Consequently, the hardness setting on the machine would be increased. Tablets produced up to that point would be trashed. Apart from such tests, the QC group does the vast majority of laboratory testing required in a pharmaceutical company.

Quality Assurance Department

Distinct from the QC department, the QA Department has responsibility for the overall quality of the products produced by the company. In this role, the department has oversight over many other departments with respect to quality issues. Generally, it exerts this oversight function through the development of appropriate documents and minute oversight of these documents. Some of these documents are complete when written (and resemble policy documents) whereas others are in the nature of forms with blank spaces that require the filling out of important information. QA reviews the completed documents for the information entered by the operator each time the document is used. For this purpose, it usually has a checklist.

DOCUMENTS USED IN GMP

Numerous documents are used in the course of GMP manufacturing and a reasonable understanding of GMP necessitates at least a cursory examination of the main documents types, and an understanding of their use to control various activities within GMP plants. While there are many document types used for control purposes, only the most important of these will be briefly discussed here. Each of these types has a standardized format within a particular company. It is important to realize that a significant part of the control of GMP production is achieved through the use of these standardized documents, and by an insistence that they be correctly, and completely, filled out and checked by multiple people before release of the batch of product to consumers. Also, these documents reference abundant test results and other information pertaining to the batch which are stored on company computers (or as paper copies in company files). In this way, a massive amount of original information can be located, even years later. Thus, there are numerous opportunities to find, and potentially to correct, errors.

Standard Operating Procedure

Standard operating procedures (SOPs) are documents in which general methods of conducting a particular operation within a company are detailed. Examples of SOPs are:

1. Procedure for disassembling and cleaning a capsule-filling machine
2. Method for operating a Korsch Model 123 tablet press
3. Method for using a propeller mixer

All operators in the company are expected to be trained on each SOP that they will be using and are required to follow the instructions contained in the SOP strictly. SOPs are also written for equipment used for chemical analysis, such as high-pressure liquid chromatography (HPLC) equipment. In addition, there are SOPs that are not equipment related but may be procedural, for example, an SOP for reviewing a batch manufacturing record (see next section). This gives direction to managers, for example, when they review the records of a batch manufactured by personnel in their group. Another example of an SOP is one for the gowning procedure to be used before operators enter a GMP area. An abbreviated version of a typical gowning SOP is shown in Appendix 1 as an example of such a document while Table 16-1 provides a more extensive list of SOPs, categorized by type.

Batch Manufacturing Record

The standard operating procedure is a general method for using a piece of equipment, for example, a tablet press. For very specific details related to the manufacture of a particular product, the company uses batch manufacturing records (BMR) or "batch records", for example, batch record for the manufacture of cetirizine tablets. This document is used each time a batch of the specified product is manufactured. The printed batch record has spaces for the operator to fill in significant information when preparing the batch of medication, for example, the reference number of the balance that was used to weigh the drug. Other examples of information to be filled in include the humidity and temperature in the room at the time of production, and the actual weight of drug used in the batch, as compared to the theoretical weight. This is done since there may be a difference between the actual weight that was measured and the (theoretical) weight printed in the batch record. It is clear from the above that the BMR details the specifics of the batch rather than the operation of a machine. The SOP deals with the latter.

Analytical Test Method

For analytical methods related to a specific product, an analytical test method (ATM) is used, for example, HPLC analysis of cetirizine hydrochloride in tablets. Instructions in ATMs provide detailed steps to be taken in the analysis of the drug, as performed in a specific company. The instructions are also very specific, for example, they will usually not state that the operator should mix two liquids until well blended (if liquid blending were a step in the analytical procedure). It is more likely to say "shake for 2 minutes on a Heidolph vibrating test tube shaker using speed setting 2."

The above are some examples of the documents used in GMP and they are described to provide a flavor of the types of documentation used. There are many more documents that

TABLE 16-1	Examples of Standard Operating Procedures Used in the Pharmaceutical Industry
SOP TYPE	NAME OF STANDARD OPERATING PROCEDURES
Manufacturing	Housekeeping in the manufacturing area
	Maintaining the equipment log
	Calibration of balances
	Weighing
	Line clearance in the manufacturing area
	Cleaning of Manesty 16-station Tablet Press
	Operation of Manesty Tablet Press
	Tablet inspection
	Packaging of tablets and capsules in primary and secondary packaging
Quality Control	Password policy, and data backup for computer systems
	Technology transfer
	Sampling and testing schedule for purified water
	Calibration of tablet hardness tester
	Handling and testing of in-process samples
	Rounding of analytical test results
	Disposal of expired chemicals and reagents
	Sampling procedure for raw materials
	Method of preparation of volumetric solutions
Quality Assurance	Qualification of vendors
	Release of raw materials
	Corrective and preventative action (CAPA) implementation
	Preparation of batch manufacturing record
	Handling of out-of-specification results
	Review of batch manufacturing records

are generally used, the details of which are not necessary for an introductory description of this topic.

QUALITY CONTROL FUNCTIONS

The testing done at the QC labs may be divided into four types:

1. Testing of raw materials and drug substances that go into the manufacturing of pharmaceutical products.

2. Testing of all containers and closures, etc., that are used for the packaging of pharmaceuticals. One aspect of such testing is the dimensions of the packaging supplies, for example, the diameter of bottlenecks.

3. Testing of samples of partially processed material at different stages of manufacture. For example, testing is done after granulation (before tablet compression).

4. All finished products that the company manufactures are also subjected to extensive testing before the product can be released for sale or for clinical trial use.

The testing of all materials and drug substances is usually done before products are manufactured. In addition, the water and all solvents that are used in drug manufacture are tested and released for use in manufacture. Some solvents do not form a part of the final product, for example, solvents used to dissolve tablet coating material. Once the tablets are coated, the solvent is evaporated. Nevertheless, these solvents are tested and must be suitable for the manufacture of medications to be consumed by humans.

All materials must comply with previously established criteria to ensure, first, that the ingredients are always of suitable quality for incorporation into pharmaceutical products and, second, that the products made from these ingredients are suitable for consumption. The criteria are stipulated in a document referred to as a "specification." The specification for the drug substance, for example, may state that the drug should be not less than 99% pure. Since the drug substance may contain very small, or trace, amounts of impurities, it would also state the maximum amounts of each impurity that may be present. The level of many impurities is stated in parts per million (ppm) or parts per billion (ppb). For example, lead is a naturally occurring substance that may be present in trace amounts in chemicals that are used in pharmaceutical products. If a purchased chemical, or drug, does not meet the requirements, as stated in the specification, that chemical cannot be used for the production of drug products for human consumption.

The specification is the pharmaceutical manufacturing company's standard for the chemical. A related document, one that is supplied by the chemical manufacturer, is a certificate of analysis (COA). The COA lists all the tests conducted by the chemical manufacturer on that chemical, as well as the final results of such tests for the batch of chemical supplied. The pharmaceutical manufacturer may quote some COA values and also do some of its own testing, in the assessment of the acceptability of the ingredient. The extent of reliance on each depends on the nature of the chemical and its use within the pharmaceutical product. The drug is usually assayed by the pharmaceutical company in addition to reviewing the COA. Each company also has its own policy on what should be tested in-house.

Testing is done at the completion of several major steps in the manufacturing process. For example, in the manufacture of tablets, sampling, and testing are done at the following stages: after blending of the excipients and drug to ensure that the blend contains the correct amount of drug, as well as to ensure that the powder is uniformly blended; and after granulation, to ensure that the drug content has been maintained and is still uniform throughout the mass of granules. The testing of powder blend uniformity and granule uniformity requires the removal of multiple samples from statistically chosen locations within the bulk material. Variation in active ingredient content is assessed by examining the standard deviation between the samples which should not exceed a certain preset value. In addition, there are other tests of granule properties, such as density determination, which are conducted.

Analogously, the QC department also tests finished products that the company produces. For example, consider a capsule product that has just been manufactured by a particular pharmaceutical company. The capsule, according to the specification for the product, should contain 20 mg of drug in each capsule. Since all mechanical processes have some inherent variability, the specification would also indicate the acceptable extent of variability for drug content and for other test values mentioned in the specification. For example, it may state that it is acceptable to have between 95% and 102% of the stated amount (20 mg) of drug in each capsule. The QC department would test the capsule by appropriate chemical analytical procedures. If the drug product does not comply with this requirement, that is, if its drug content is less than 19 mg or more than 20.4 mg, the product would fail. Similarly for the many other test values mentioned in the product specification. All of the tests alluded to are conducted by the QC department.

QUALITY ASSURANCE FUNCTIONS

SOPs, BMRs, and ATMs have been described in the section, Documents Used in GMP. While research and development (R&D) scientists usually write SOPs and BMRs since they are well-versed in the scientific procedures involved and are the people that develop new formulations, QA reviews these documents for completeness, formatting, and other aspects, usually with the aid of a checklist. QA also stores all important documents. QA may suggest updates to SOPs and other documents from time to time, as necessary due to changes in pharmacy law and regulations, or to current GMP requirements.

The referenced section of this chapter also mentions the fact that the BMR and the COA require information to be filled in. In the former case, information is entered by the operators in the course of the production of a batch of product. Such information includes the temperature and relative humidity (RH) of the manufacturing suite, the exact weights of ingredients measured out, the total weight of all ingredients, the yield of product, etc. The COA requires that the measured values relating to the batch of product (such as its drug content) and the variability in the values be recorded. It is emphasized that no material facts can be changed in this review process. The final review of a BMR and of the COA is by QA.

QA is the department that sees to it that quality is built into the product. This begins with the correct construction of buildings and provision of ancillary services such as air conditioning. The QA department has input into construction and works with architects and engineers to ensure that appropriate design and construction are carried out and that the final building complies with GMP specifications. The QA department also ensures that appropriate procedures are developed and documented for functions that need to be performed routinely. An example of such a function is the review of a BMR for which there is an SOP detailing the critical information that the QA reviewer must identify in the BMR and the quality checks to be undertaken. Manufacturing processes, such as the operation of a tablet press, are done in accordance with SOPs and it is a QA function to ensure that there are SOPs for all processes, that all people carrying out these functions are appropriately trained on these SOPs, and that they are updated as needed. After an update, all users must be re-trained on the SOP. Sometimes the training may be as simple as reading the SOP and demonstrating that the person has understood the document. In some instances, it is necessary to demonstrate competence. This can be done, for example, by the operator demonstrating his ability to operate a tablet press, or by her ability to correctly operate a capsule filling machine. A batch can be failed solely on the fact that the operator, responsible for the production of the batch, was not appropriately trained. The failing designation would usually be made by the QA department.

In addition to SOPs for manufacturing processes, there are also documents that govern analytical procedures, cleaning of equipment, and calibration of instruments. Nothing is left to chance, and no assumptions are made that personnel will conduct procedures appropriately. Instead, all personnel are trained and have to follow step-by-step, written procedures that are documented. Tablets, and the tableting process, are used as examples several times in this chapter in order to explain GMP processes or concepts. Tablets are the most popular solid oral dosage form and it is reasonable to use this example. However, GMP applies to the manufacture of all pharmaceuticals. If any terms relating to tableting technology are unfamiliar, Chapter 9, Tablets, should be referred to for an explanation.

SOPs for manufacturing procedures are usually written by a scientist, frequently an R&D scientist, familiar with the operation of the equipment. This scientist may have been trained by the manufacturer of the equipment. For large-scale equipment, used exclusively for commercial manufacturing, the document may be written by a manufacturing scientist. The BMRs are written by scientists who develop new formulations. The QA department maintains these documents, and ensures that they are formatted to company specifications, contain the required information, that they are updated as needed, and that all persons who use the relevant equipment are properly trained on the relevant SOP. QA is also the repository for the final, "official" versions of documents. For example, QA is the only department that has the master BMR for a specific product. When a batch is to be produced, QA supplies an "official" copy of the BMR to the person responsible for manufacturing the batch. This may be the person who wrote the BMR in the first instance. This person may not simply print a copy from their own computer but must use the copy provided by QA, appropriately coded to confirm its origin from the QA department. In this way, the company ensures that no changes can be made on the fly and that only the QA-released documents may be used. These reflect approval of the document by QA in the form of the signature of a QA representative. It also has oversight over training of personnel in terms of training protocols and maintains a training log for each piece of equipment or process.

The QA department also ensures that the warehouse is correctly situated and that it functions appropriately with raw materials and finished products being stored in a very well-controlled manner. Figure 16-1 shows the relationship between the warehouse and the manufacturing suite in a simplified format. The diagram is also annotated to reflect the movement of materials between the warehouse and the manufacturing suite, as well as the packaging area.

Recap Questions

1. Name three types of document used in a GMP facility in connection with drug product manufacture.

2. If, according to the specification, a product must contain 30 mg of drug and the specification also states that the drug content may vary between 95% and 102%, calculate the highest, and the lowest, amounts of drug that the product might contain, and yet be acceptable.

3. If the drug substance is tested and found to be 99% pure (within specification), why is it necessary to conduct further tests on individual impurities found with the drug?

FACILITIES

The company must ensure that the building is suitable for the production of pharmaceuticals, that manufacturing suites are correctly built and laid out, and that suitable equipment is installed. The building should be built to appropriate standards, and consideration must be given to proper facilities for waste removal. This includes wastewater, smoke, solid chemical, and solvent disposal. The flow of materials must be such that quarantined and approved manufactured products do not cross paths as they are respectively brought into, or taken out of, the warehouse. Quarantined products are those that have been manufactured but not tested. This is done to ensure that quarantined products are not shipped out before they are tested and released for shipment. In a properly designed building, the path through the building for trash removal does not cross the path used for taking finished products to the warehouse, prior to transportation to wholesalers/agents or pharmacies.

The building must be designed so that cross-contamination between batches is prevented. If there were a common air conditioning system for many production suites within the building, there is the possibility of transferring small amounts of drug from one suite to the next via the air conditioning system. Even minute amounts of drug, transferred in this way, may end up in unrelated products. Because some people are extremely sensitive to penicillin, they may have a serious allergic reaction even to trace amounts in an unrelated product. The FDA, for this reason, requires separate buildings for the manufacture of penicillin and cephalosporin products, in comparison to those used for the manufacture of other medications. A log of repairs to the building should be maintained because this may be important

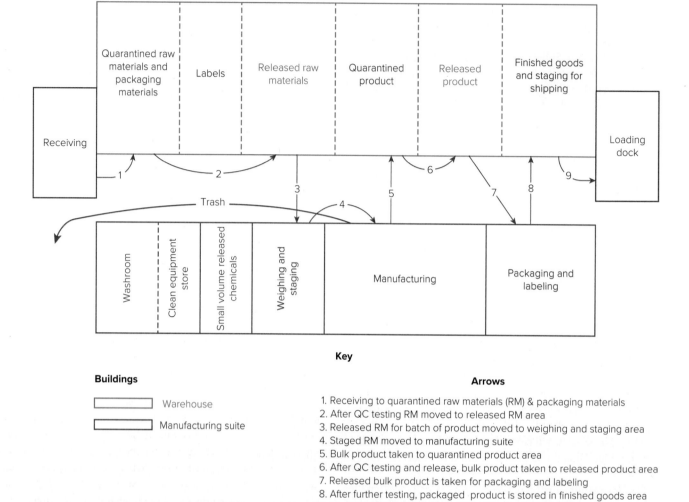

FIGURE 16-1 Simplified diagram of a pharmaceutical manufacturing suite and warehouse.

in the context of the correct manufacturing of the pharmaceutical product. For example: was a failing batch made just before a problem with the air conditioning in the room was discovered and repaired?

Manufacturing suites are built such that they can easily be cleaned. For example, the room has no window ledges that may attract dust, including drug particles. Floors and walls are made of materials that can be wet-mopped for thorough cleaning. Each manufacturing suite must have individual temperature and humidity controls. Control of humidity usually needs to be better than it is in a regular office building. This requirement is necessary because some pharmaceutical products are extremely susceptible to humidity. Regular air conditioning cannot maintain the lower levels required, while effervescent products are especially sensitive to humidity.

Each manufacturing room has a chart recorder which continuously records both the temperature and humidity prevalent within the room. During batch manufacture, these values are also noted in the BMR at intervals, as specified in this document. When the product is known to be sensitive to either of these parameters, it may become necessary to note these values more frequently. Everything within the manufacturing suite is labeled. It may appear amusing to note that the trash can is

labeled as such. However, considering that a trash can in a manufacturing suite may contain broken tablets or tablets that are otherwise defective, the effort to unmistakably distinguish this container is done to prevent the sale of rejected tablets.

Manufacturing equipment must be correctly chosen based on the following GMP attributes (among others):

1. They should be able to operate consistently, for example, if a component of the machine is set to rotate at 500 rpm, the actual rotation speed must not be much less than, or much greater than, this speed for the entire duration of product manufacture.

2. They are able to be cleaned thoroughly: if the product contact surface of the machine has small apertures and narrow angles, it may be difficult to remove every trace of the drug during cleaning.

3. Components of the machine should not absorb chemicals from the processed drug product, nor should the machine shed contaminants into the product.

While temperature and humidity conditions may be relatively easily maintained in a small room, this is much more difficult to achieve in a large warehouse. Large fluctuations in different parts of the warehouse may be observed even when the air conditioning system is apparently working well and its monitors reflect that the parameters are controlled at the set values. For this reason, "mapping" of the warehouse is necessary. This involves taking the temperature and humidity in different locations of the warehouse including at different heights. Areas close to the ceiling of a multi-story warehouse may be several degrees higher in temperature than areas close to the floor, due to hot air rising and remaining at the top of a confined space.

PRIOR TO BATCH MANUFACTURE

A logbook is maintained for each room in which product is manufactured. Each cleaning of the room, and each repair of the room itself will also be noted in this log. Repairs to the lighting or air conditioning in the room are examples of such repairs, distinct from repairs to manufacturing equipment which are described below. Every batch of product that is manufactured in the room is noted in the log in addition to the cleaning of the room done after manufacture. Since different products may be manufactured in the same production suite, it is essential that cleaning be done between batches, and the logbook is an easy way to verify the completion of this task.

A separate equipment logbook is maintained for each piece of equipment, that is, a tablet press will have its own logbook as will a capsule machine or a blender used to mix liquids. Consider one piece of equipment and its logbook. Each use of that equipment (for different batches of the same product, or for different products) will require a separate entry to reflect the production of that batch. Each time the equipment is cleaned, it is also noted. Equipment repairs and servicing will also be noted in the equipment log. It is important to realize that in several companies, production equipment may be used in different rooms, or production suites. Hence, the equipment logbook remains with the equipment.

A separate log is maintained for the calibration of all equipment. The calibration of a balance, for example, may involve checking the reading when a certified weight is placed on the balance. If a 20-g weight, for example, gives a reading of 18.2 g, the balance will be adjusted by the calibration department to produce a reading that is closer to 20 g and which is within the limits of acceptability. In this logbook, the date of the calibration as well as that of the next required calibration of the equipment is noted. A sticker is placed on the equipment, noting the latter date. Operators should not use a piece of equipment if it is out of date in terms of calibration.

Before manufacturing can commence, components have to be received by the warehouse personnel. "Components" includes the drug, excipients, containers, labels, and packaging materials. These items are stored in one section of the warehouse that is designated as "quarantined" (Figure 16-1). Brightly colored stickers, for example, red or orange, with the word "Quarantined" are placed onto the containers of these components. The use of this label indicates to operators that they should not use these materials in production, since the materials have not been released for this purpose. In due course, QC will take a sample of the product for testing.

Each component receives a component number and a control number. The component number is a unique number, within the company, for each component. For example, the component number for lactose may be "L 4000." Each time lactose is purchased, it will have the same component number. The control number is a unique number for the particular batch of lactose purchased and received on a particular day. (The same grade of lactose purchased on 18th August and 28th September will have different control numbers.) This number stays with the component throughout its history within the company and is always mentioned in any documents relating to batches produced with that particular lot of lactose. For example, if a sample of lactose is taken for analysis in the QC laboratory, it will be labeled with this component number (in addition to other information). Once the component has been tested by QC and found to be suitable, a member of the QA group will place another brightly colored sticker (eg, green) over the first sticker. This sticker bears the word "Released" to indicate that the component has been tested and has passed. The container will now be moved out of the quarantined area into the released products section of the warehouse. Both the sticker and the location of the container within the warehouse indicate to personnel that the lactose may be used for the production of pharmaceutical products.

If a problem is suspected with a pharmaceutical product, it is possible to trace back to the lot of lactose that was used in the manufacture of the product, and also to determine the date on which it was received. This information could be used to investigate and to assess if there was an issue with the lactose that was used in the batch in question which, in turn, caused the particular problem that is observed, or suspected, with the pharmaceutical product. This is an example of traceability mentioned earlier. Obviously, each ingredient used in the production of a batch of product may, similarly, be traced.

All components, and not only the drug, are tested for suitability for use in the manufacture of pharmaceuticals. This includes bottles that are used as containers for the product; even closures used to seal the product from the elements are subject to testing. For critical components, such as the drug, testing may go as far as auditing the manufacturer of the drug substance. Auditing involves a team of scientists and QA personnel visiting the drug manufacturer to tour the factory and to review their SOPs, batch records, and other paperwork with the purpose of assessing whether the drug substance is manufactured in a controlled fashion and to the highest standards in compliance with GMP requirements. If any deficiencies are found, the pharmaceutical manufacturing company will inform the drug manufacturer who may be able to make improvements to the satisfaction of the pharmaceutical manufacturing company. On the other hand, the pharmaceutical company may decide to use an alternate drug manufacturer.

EQUIPMENT CLEANING

Just as it is important for finished products to be tested and the drug content analyzed, it is also important to use thoroughly clean equipment. If the equipment had been used for manufacturing a different product, it must be thoroughly cleaned before the next product can be made. If it is not, there may be small amounts of the drug from the previous product remaining on the equipment which can contaminate the next batch, of a different product. The whole question of residual traces of drug from the previous batch came to the fore with the manufacturing of penicillin products.

It is well known that some patients are allergic to penicillin and, therefore, cannot be given a normal dose of penicillin, for example, 250 mg. What was surprising when it was first observed, however, was the fact that some patients displayed an allergic reaction when consuming a non-penicillin product that they had previously taken with no adverse reaction. Upon investigation, it was discovered that the allergic reaction was not a reaction to the product consumed but to traces of penicillin from the previous batch of penicillin product which was manufactured on the same machine. It came as a surprise when the first instances of this reaction occurred because the production equipment was considered to have been thoroughly cleaned before manufacture of the non-penicillin product that caused the problem.

The equipment had certainly been cleaned sufficiently well that no trace of powder could be seen on the machine. It is interesting to note that drugs, and drug blends with excipients, are often white or off-white, unless colored by the use of a dye. Hence, the presence of such a powder is easily visible against stainless steel machinery (the most common material used in manufacturing equipment). Any material remaining after cleaning, which was responsible for the allergic reaction, would probably have been so small in quantity that it was not easily visible to the human eye. Yet this caused patients to experience an extreme reaction. It should be mentioned, in this context, that some interior surfaces of the equipment may be obscured from full view and could, potentially, be a source of contamination.

As a consequence of the above, a very careful reconsideration had to be given to what constitutes "clean." Is it clean when the operator's visual inspection determines that it is clean? Will one operator's perception differ from that of another, even when operators are trained to make such observations? It may be surprising to learn that there are now very detailed procedures for the cleaning of equipment in pharmaceutical plants. The instructions include detailed information about breaking down the machine into its constituent parts and about cleaning the various components. After cleaning is complete, the equipment must not only pass visual inspection by the operator conducting the cleaning and then by a supervisor but, in addition, the equipment is also swabbed at various critical locations using a solvent for the drug in question. Next, the swabs are tested for the presence of the drug. If traces of drug are found, it means that cleaning was not efficient in terms of pharmaceutical production standards that ensure no "carryover." In such a situation, cleaning will be repeated until tests reveal that the equipment is clean (free of any trace of the drug).

As mentioned, cleaning usually involves the breakdown of the machine into as many components as can easily be removed, and which is necessary for proper cleaning. These small components are then thoroughly cleaned using the specific method mentioned in the cleaning protocol. For example, a Perspex cover may need a different cleaning liquid from stainless steel components. Since it is cleaned after removal from the machine, instructions for the removal of the cover will also be given in the cleaning protocol.

The remaining "core" machine is also cleaned according to the protocol. This typically involves brushing to remove all loose powder. Next, the equipment is dry wiped with a cloth that does not shed fibers. Then, the equipment is wiped down with 70% isopropanol, typically. This solvent is chosen because it is not toxic, dissolves many drugs, and is noncorrosive to the equipment. When the operators are satisfied that the equipment appears to be clean, a QA manager also inspects the equipment. If the manager is satisfied that the equipment is visually clean, a request is made to QC to swab parts of the equipment and to test the swab for the presence of drug. The portion of the equipment that is swabbed is typically a hard-to-reach area for cleaning purposes. If testing by a sensitive analytical method, such as HPLC, reveals the presence of drug, the equipment will be re-cleaned and tested once more, as mentioned. If necessary, this will be repeated until testing reveals that the equipment is clean. The test procedure, whereby the equipment is swabbed and the swab tested to display absence of drug is referred to as "cleaning verification."

From the above description, it will easily be understood that the cleaning process is long and consumes resources. It is not unreasonable for a batch of tablets to take 3 or 4 days to manufacture, and for the cleaning, including all testing, to take more than 1 week to complete. This long, expensive procedure is justified since products produced by a pharmaceutical company should be pure and un-contaminated, including by elements of the previous batch.

Now, suppose that the company has manufactured a particular product several times and has cleaned the equipment according to a standard cleaning protocol (contained in a Cleaning SOP) after manufacture of each batch. This cleaning method was used repeatedly over the course of 1 year with several batches produced and with different operators performing the cleaning, and the same results were obtained each time, that is, after the first cleaning of the equipment, the test swab contained no trace of drug. This gives confidence about the appropriateness of the *cleaning procedure* that was developed (embodied in the "Cleaning SOP") and followed by operators. This result also indicates that the training of the operators conducting the cleaning was adequate. Under such circumstances, and in accordance with detailed FDA requirements (which are beyond the scope of this book), the company may decide that their cleaning procedure works well, and had been demonstrated to work well, that is, the cleaning procedure had been "validated." Subsequently, the company need not conduct cleaning verification each time the machine is cleaned, except as described below.

After such proof of efficient cleaning has been established, the FDA permits the company to conduct cleaning verification periodically (eg, once a year) to confirm the previous results. This is an enormous saving in time for the company. However, it should not be construed as a shortcut, since the company has had to expend significant effort to first prove that the method of cleaning is efficient and leaves no trace of the drug. This involved several batches of product that were manufactured over a significant period of time. Only with such justification is the company allowed to continue manufacturing the product in question without performing cleaning verification after each batch. Nevertheless, cleaning verification is still conducted once a year, for example.

Recap Questions

1. Name three aspects of the design of a manufacturing suite that are important with respect to GMP.
2. Name two features of the layout of a pharmaceutical plant that are conducive to GMP.
3. If a machine has been thoroughly cleaned and there is no visual evidence of drug or product on it, is this sufficient?
4. B.J. is an 80-year-old male who has obtained all his medications from your pharmacy for several years. He explains that he felt a little unwell after taking the last supply of pain medication. He has heard of people getting allergic reactions to peanuts, from food that did not contain peanuts, just because the food processing machine had been used to manufacture a peanut-containing product previously. He wonders if the same thing might have happened to his medication since he is allergic to penicillin. He reminds you that your pharmacy does have his patient profile on record. How would you respond to B.J.?

BATCH MANUFACTURE

The manufacturing of a batch of product will now be discussed in terms of the GMP requirements. For convenience, this will be discussed under different headings although the different topics are interrelated.

Overview of Manufacturing

Every step of the manufacturing procedure for the pharmaceutical is verified during the course of production. Two operators must always be present in the manufacturing suite: one person performs a manufacturing step (eg, weighing an ingredient) while the other person observes. In the example given, the weighing of an ingredient, the person who performed the weighing step will note, on the batch record, the amount weighed. For example, a batch may call for 20 kg of an inactive ingredient. If 19.9999 kg of the drug were actually weighed, this figure will be noted on the batch record by the person performing the weighing operation. This person will initial the batch record in the space provided ("Performed by"). The second operator will observe the procedure and will add his or her initials as the observer ("Observed by" column). All work procedures are documented in this way. The operators generally interchange functions, that is, the person weighing the drug, in the above example, may be the observer for the weighing of the second ingredient.

The procedures, as outlined in the batch record, are intended to be conducted exactly as mentioned. Any minor variation has to be recorded. For example, most procedures are intended to be continuous processes. If, due to some unforeseen event, work actually stops for a short time, for example, 30 minutes, and is then resumed, this change will be noted and signed by both operators. Changes such as this will be considered when managers and QA consider whether the batch should be approved. A 30-minute unintended pause in an 8-hour production run for a batch of tablets will usually not be considered negatively but the nature of the product, and the processing step that was interrupted, must be taken into account. A lunch break may be taken at a convenient point in production, but should not interrupt a step such as mixing.

Major changes to the formula or the process cannot be made in the course of manufacturing a batch. If the operator thinks that he or she has discovered an improved procedure, this change cannot be made during the production of the batch. Such a potential change would have to be discussed at a meeting of the appropriate people. If the change is agreed upon, the batch record will be amended accordingly. This procedure then becomes the "official" procedure. Thereafter, every time a batch of the product is manufactured, the new procedure, or amended formula, will be used.

Personnel

The people who are responsible for the manufacturing of pharmaceuticals are usually scientists who have had training in the pharmaceutical sciences, typically at the Masters or doctoral level. Other workers, especially in the manufacturing area are operators. The term "operators" is probably derived from the fact that these employees control or operate the machinery that manufactures pharmaceutical products. Typically, they do not have higher degrees but many, with years of experience, are very knowledgeable about pharmaceutical manufacturing and their opinion may be sought by scientists especially where the appearance or the "feel" of the material at a specific stage in the manufacturing process is critical. The operators are trained on the equipment they will use. For the manufacture of GMP batches, documentary evidence of this training is important for both operators and scientists who work on a batch.

Efforts are made to limit contamination of the product. In this respect, the personal hygiene of the operator is very important. In addition, the operator is not allowed to wear cosmetics or jewelry. Any person who has been convicted of fraud with regard to the production of pharmaceuticals (most commonly presenting fictitious test data) may not be employed in the manufacture of products for human consumption. The FDA maintains a list of such persons who have been debarred. Manufacturers are expected to check this list and not to employ any person whose name is listed.

Preliminary Steps

No batch manufacture can begin before QA inspects the manufacturing suite which has to be clear of all materials such as the previously manufactured batch, additional equipment and raw materials, and labels pertaining to the previous batch. This is done, obviously, to ensure that there are no mix-ups, for example, using a material from a previous batch. Once QA has certified the room to be clear, it provides a blank BMR to the operators who will be manufacturing the new batch. This document has printed instructions for manufacturing the batch with spaces for the operator to note certain information. Examples of information to note on the batch record are given in the next section.

Manufacturing Procedure

First, the temperature and RH in the room are noted on the batch record. This is done by the operator at the start of the batch. This is repeated at the end of the batch, and also at predetermined intervals throughout the duration of batch manufacture. Thus, the temperature and RH are recorded at predetermined intervals during the course of the operation. This may be critical for some formulations. For example, tight limits on RH values are required for the manufacturing of effervescent products and hygroscopic drugs.

Next, ingredients are weighed and the actual weights are recorded on the BMR. For small R&D batches (typically made for clinical studies), the ingredients are weighed as they are needed for incorporation into the product. For large batches, the ingredients are more likely to be pre-weighed and staged in a separate weighing room which has a large capacity balance. One operator weighs and notes the weight in the appropriate spaces in the batch record. The second operator observes the operation. The document contains designated spaces for the operator, and observer, to initial and date after each step to signify, respectively, that they have performed the function or observed and can verify the performance of the function. For example, if 10.001 kg of drug were weighed, the observer's initials signify that he observed this number on the balance, and also verified that the name and tracking numbers of the drug as it appears on the container are the same as that entered in the BMR. Initialing of the document occurs at every major manufacturing step. It is not uncommon for the observer and operator to switch roles during the manufacture of the batch. In addition, when samples are removed for analytical testing, the weight and the times at which the samples are removed are noted. Samples could be taken during powder blending, or samples of granules may be taken during the process of granulation.

Start and stop times of important steps, such as mixing, are noted. The batch record also has spaces for calculations that need to be made. In this way, the calculations form a part of the BMR and are available for review, shortly after batch manufacture, by the manager of the group and also by QA. In the future, should an error be suspected, the calculation shown in the batch record may be checked again for correctness.

An example of such a calculation is the percent yield of the batch. If the starting materials weighed 200 kg, and 190 kg of product is produced, the yield is 95%. The 5% of material that did not go into the finished product, in this example, is a "loss." Losses can be divided into "accountable losses" and "unaccountable losses." Accountable losses in tablet production may consist of broken tablets, tablets that are underweight or overweight, or otherwise defective. Initially, while the tablet press is being set up and adjusted for tablet weight and hardness, tablets that do not meet specifications are produced and must be discarded. Powder that remains on the tablet press at the end of the tableting run is another source of accountable loss. The defective tablets and the powder remaining on the die table and in the hopper of the press are collected, weighed, and the weight noted in the batch record. Unaccountable losses are those losses that cannot be accounted for in production. This includes some powder that remains on the press after reasonable attempts at collection, and powder that may fly off the press as fine dust. Naturally, it is desirable to keep unaccountable losses as small as possible.

During processing, the batch record instructions must be adhered to rigidly. However, a few minor deviations are usual, and generally acceptable. Any minor deviation from the written procedures are noted. Sometimes, these variations trigger a deviation investigation which might be conducted by the manager of the manufacturing group and/or the QA group. A deviation investigation report is prepared and, depending on its nature, deviations may be found to be acceptable. If this is the case, the batch is considered suitable for use, provided it passes all QC tests. If the deviations are deemed unacceptable, the batch must be rejected.

Reconciliation of quantity is conducted at all important steps, for example, after powder mixing, granulation, tableting, and packaging. This is one of the measures taken to ensure that the product includes all required ingredients in the correct quantities (and no additional ingredients, or required ingredients in excess). This is a standard step in pharmaceutical production. If there is no significant deviation from the required quantity (and there is conformance to other tests), the processing of the material will continue to the next stage. If there is a significant deviation, an investigation must be launched to determine the reason for the loss of material, or for the excess weight. In the packaging department, for example, excess weight might mean that tablets from another batch (potentially of a different product) might inadvertently have been mixed with the batch intended to be packaged and now being reconciled. An alternative explanation is that the containers may have been under-filled, leaving an excess weight of tablets remaining after packaging the required number of containers.

After the Batch

After the completion of a batch, the two operators review the BMR, in detail, check for accuracy and completeness. The BMR may easily be 20 pages long and often longer. Simple errors can be corrected and omissions can be filled in. A common calculation error may be in rounding of numerical values where the error does not affect the quality of the batch. Corrections are annotated with the reason for the correction, for example, "rounding error" and are initialed and dated. A typical omission consists of the operator initialing a processing step but omitting the date. When all such corrections have been made, the operators sign and date the document as opposed to initialing which is done for each processing step. Next, a manager checks every detail on the batch record, including calculations, and signs off that he or she has checked the document.

Common elements that may be missing include one of the two dates for a certain step adjacent to the initials of the operator or observer.

The manager may ask the operators about anything that is unclear in their notations, prior to signing the BMR. QA is the last to sign off after completing a detailed review. If QA has any questions, they would generally consult with the manager of the group responsible for that batch. If the questions are satisfactorily resolved, QA will sign off on the batch record. When analytical test results have been received by QA, sometime after the batch has been manufactured, they are also reviewed and, finally, the batch is released by QA.

Recap Questions

1. If pharmaceutical production follows step-by-step written procedures, how is it possible that errors still occur?

2. During GMP manufacture the operator is required to record the reference numbers of the balances that were used for that batch.

    a. Why is it important to know the reference number of the balance that was used to weigh the drug?

    b. Why is it important to know the reference number of the balance that was used to weigh the excipients?

3. If a drug has been verified as being ibuprofen, for example, why is it necessary to check the following?

    a. The component no.

    b. The lot no.

4. Why is it necessary for two people to initial every step of the manufacturing process? Why not simply have them sign off on the entire batch record?

5. In a mixing process, if the operators comply with an instruction to mix for 30 minutes, for example, why is it necessary to note the start and stop times?

6. What are some of the important steps taken by the operators after the batch is manufactured?

7. Why does QA review analytical test results sometime after the manufacture of the batch, and not right after the batch has been made?

CLINICAL TRIAL MATERIAL

Clinical trial materials, which are generally smaller batches of product, may be manufactured as described above. At this stage of development, the chemical analytical and other quality control measures, while adequate, may still be undergoing further refinement and development. Controls get stricter from phase 1 to phase 3 of clinical testing since the clinical population becomes larger through the phases. However, it should be kept in mind that at no stage is there lax control over the quality of the product given to any subject or patient.

Often, in the production of clinical trial material, there is a need for double-blind packaging. A double-blind study is one in which neither the patient nor the clinical staff, know which patients are getting the drug product and which the placebo. Therefore, comparative products suitable for such a clinical trial (eg, drug formulation and placebo) look identical and may only be distinguished by the batch number. In a double-blind study, the latter is not shared with clinicians or patients. Only the pharmacist handling the clinical supplies, at the clinic or hospital, has the key to the identity of the batches. Thus, patients and clinical staff can be expected to provide unbiased assessments of the clinical efficacy of the product.

There is a good rationale for double-blinding products. However, there has to be strict control of supplies to prevent mix-ups. This control must be maintained on all the batches (placebo and drug-containing), labels, and of the process of labeling the products. In some studies, multiple doses of the product may be involved, with each dose indistinguishable from the other. Where the pharmaceutical dosage forms and the packages are identical to each other and to the placebo product and package, this control is difficult. It is therefore best to leave double-blind packaging to specialists who handle this type of packaging routinely.

FDA AUDITS

The FDA can conduct an audit of the pharmaceutical plant at any time and for various reasons. There are regularly-scheduled inspections of pharmaceutical plants, in which case the company knows in advance and can prepare for the inspection. There are also inspections prior to the approval of new products, termed "pre-approval inspections." In this case, the FDA does not announce its arrival to companies. However, companies can deduce the approximate time at which the FDA will arrive, after submission of their NDA, and they should be inspection-ready close to this time. The above is not a comprehensive list of FDA inspections but merely a few examples.

As a result of any visit, the FDA can issue Form 483 observations. Observations noted after visits may range from mild to very serious. The FDA can also issue warning letters to the company for more serious defaults. In addition, a consent decree can be issued. The latter means that no production or distribution of drug products can occur until an approved third party (consultant) certifies that the company has met the required standards. Obviously, this is an even more serious action by the FDA and very expensive to the company, especially since it is usually accompanied by a hefty fine. The FDA can take other actions, including the closing down of a pharmaceutical plant. By these mechanisms, the FDA offers monitoring of pharmaceutical companies and ensures that pharmaceutical products are manufactured to the highest standards and in compliance with GMPs. The FDA audits all companies that supply products to the USA, including companies located overseas. The examples of FDA actions mentioned above, and others not discussed, apply to overseas companies with respect to products that the company supplies to the US.

In addition, the FDA regularly inspects overseas companies that provide drug products to the US. Obviously, the FDA has no jurisdiction over products that an overseas company manufactures for its home market.

ACHIEVING AND MAINTAINING QUALITY

Every step of the manufacturing process is conducted according to written procedures and all actions are documented so that detailed information about the production of a specific batch can be retrieved, even years later. Since the manufacturing process usually consists of several steps, it is possible to take samples at the end of each major step along the way. The testing of the partially manufactured product gives assurance that the product is acceptable, up to that point, in the manufacturing process. Alternately, it may reveal deficiencies that may be corrected. For example, the addition of more drug to a powder blend, if the blended material was found to be sub-potent and records reveal that an insufficient amount of drug was weighed initially. (If the correct amount was added initially and the blend is subpotent, it would trigger an investigation, not simply the addition of more drug.) It is possible that the testing may result in the rejection of the partially manufactured batch if the deficiency cannot be easily corrected.

The following is an example of correcting a processing deficiency: when powders (such as drug and excipients) are blended, samples of the blended powders are taken from various points within the mixing vessel and are tested for drug content. If the content is not uniform, blending would be continued with repeat testing to ensure an acceptable level of content uniformity. This ensures that the tablets subsequently made from these powders will also be uniform in drug content. The BMR will reflect the additional time of blending as a deviation.

The results of the laboratory testing conducted at this stage may also be taken into consideration in determining the overall quality of the product when the finished product is tested and the results of such testing are evaluated. For example, the content uniformity of the tablets (variability in the content of individual tablets) is determined after the batch has been produced. Suppose the content uniformity of a particular batch is found to be acceptable, but borderline. The results of the prior powder blending test may be examined to see if they offer supporting evidence of the acceptability of the batch of tablets with regard to content uniformity.

Every step in the manufacturing process must be traceable, that is, there must be a paper trail which may prove to be very useful at a later point. In the event that a product is found to be defective after marketing, it can be traced back by its batch number and every manufacturing step can be scrutinized. In this way, the reason for the defect may be determined. It would also be possible to determine which operators manufactured the batch, and which managers from the production department reviewed the batch records. It would also be possible to review analytical results and to determine the names of the analyst who tested the batch and the analytical supervisor, from

the quality control department, who checked and signed off. Furthermore, since all documentation is reviewed once more by the Quality Assurance Department (QA) after manufacture and before release of the batch, it would also be possible to trace the individual from the QA department who signed off on the documents. Depending on the time that has elapsed, it may be possible to interview these individuals and such discussions may throw light on the problem at hand.

It is also possible, in the case of a defective product, to obtain (from the BMR) the batch numbers of the ingredients that were used in its production. From this, two sets of testing data may be referenced: first, the in-house test results and, second, the COA, both of which are stored by the pharmaceutical company. From the batch number of the ingredient, stated on the COA, detailed information about the tests conducted, and the results, may be obtained from the ingredient manufacturer. In this way, it may be possible to resolve a problem, or find its source. For example, the source of a trace contaminant, found in a pharmaceutical product, may be found to have come from the particular batch of lactose that was used.

The steps described above help with the resolution of ingredient-related issues. The error may also relate to incorrect processing (eg, inappropriate mixing). Ineffective mixing may relate to the use of less than optimal equipment, or the use of the correct equipment under inappropriate machine settings, for example, the speed and run time settings. An example of the latter is mixing at 100 rpm for 20 minutes when mixing at 200 rpm for 10 minutes was intended.

Electronic trails are rapidly replacing paper trails in modern manufacturing concerns for several reasons, such as the obvious saving of space for storage of information and the easier searching of old records. Depending on the nature of the error, a product recall may be necessary. This is very expensive for the pharmaceutical company and, hence, they make every effort to avoid a product recall by manufacturing high-quality products which are rigorously tested and documented to establish evidence of product quality. Some examples of pharmaceutical product recalls that occurred at the time of writing this chapter are listed in Table 16-2. Since limited information as to the nature of the problem is provided to the public with the recall announcement, the author has provided probable explanations for, and background to, the problem. It is emphasized that the reasons provided are "probable." Since the author does not have direct access to the actual circumstances under which the error occurred, a definitive explanation cannot be offered.

Product recalls are a fact of life in the pharmaceutical manufacturing industry and the pharmacist may be called upon to offer a brief explanation to patients who must return their medications. Furthermore, if the drug is unavailable for a time after the recall, they may be required to explain the situation to the patient and, possibly, also to the physician. In addition, the pharmacist may be requested to suggest an alternative medication to the physician and must be able to justify his choice. A basic understanding of manufacturing and quality control dynamics will help the pharmacist to explain the situation to the patient in somewhat brief, but factually correct, lay terms so that she does not think the drug supply, and occasional substitution, are shrouded in mystery.

TABLE 16-2	Some Recent Drug Product Recalls in the United States*			
DATE	BRAND NAME	DESCRIPTION	REASON FOR RECALL	COMMENTS
2/03/2021	Apotex (Generic)	Enoxaparin Sodium Injection, USP	Packaging error resulting in incorrect dosage listed	Syringe barrel had 150 mg/mL markings (used for a different strength of the product) instead of 100 mg/mL markings
01/27/2021	Meitheal (Generic)	Cisatracurium Besylate Injection, USP 10mg per 5mL	Mislabeling	A portion of 1 lot was mislabeled as Phenylephrine Hydrochloride Injection, USP.
01/25/2021	Nostrum (Generic)	Metformin HCl Extended-Release Tablets, USP 750 mg	Levels of nitrosamine impurities above the ADI* limit of 96 ng/day	Nitrosamines are potentially carcinogenic byproducts in certain drugs. The acceptable daily intake is limited.
01/08/2021	Fresenius Kabi (Generic)	Ketorolac Tromethamine Injection, USP, 30 mg/mL	Presence of particulate matter	Injections containing particulate matter could cause injection site reactions and obstruction of blood vessels and cause blood clots to form.
1/04.21	Soho Fresh	70% Rubbing Alcohol	Contaminated with methanol	Ethanol is useful while methanol is toxic and can be absorbed through the skin.
01/04/2021	Nostrum Laboratories	Metformin HCl Extended-Release Tablets, USP 750	NDMA exceeds acceptable daily intake limit	N-nitrosodimethylamine is a nitrosamine, a potential carcinogen
12/31/2020	GUM Paroex	Paroex Chlorhexidine Gluconate Oral Rinse, 15 mL unit dose cups	Potential contamination with Burkholderia lata	Contamination with this bacterium could cause oral and, potentially, systemic infection.
12/28/2020	Paroex	Paroex Chlorhexidine Gluconate Oral Rinse, 4 oz and 16 oz	Potential contamination with Burkholderia lata	Contamination with this bacterium could cause oral and, potentially, systemic infection.
12/23/2020	IMC	Wash-Free Hand Sanitizer	Undeclared Methanol	Ethanol is useful while methanol is toxic and can be absorbed through the skin.
2/09/2020	AvKare	Sildenafil 100 mg tablets and Trazodone 100mg tablets	Due to product mix-up	The two tablet products mentioned were inadvertently mixed while packaging. Each labeled pack contained some of the other product.
12/09/2020	Torrent Pharmaceuticals Limited	Anagrelide Capsule USP 1 mg	Due to dissolution test failure	Slower dissolution could mean slower release of the medication to the body, a potentially slower absorption, and inadequate blood levels.
12/02/2020	MPM Medical	Regenecare HA Topical Anesthetic Hydrogel	Burkholderia cepecia contamination	Applied to the skin, the gel could cause skin infections. For immunocompromised patients, the skin infection could spread into the bloodstream causing sepsis.
11/19/2020	Fresenius Kabi USA	Dexmedetomidine HCL in 0.9% Sodium Chloride Injection	Cross Contamination with Lidocaine	A trace amount of lidocaine was found in this lot. If the patient is allergic to lidocaine, an allergic reaction could be precipitated.

(Continued)

TABLE 16-2	Some Recent Drug Product Recalls in the United States* (*Continued*)			
DATE	BRAND NAME	DESCRIPTION	REASON FOR RECALL	COMMENTS
11/09/2020	Lohxa	Chlorhexidine Gluconate Oral Rinse USP, 0.12% Alcohol-free	May be contaminated with Burkholderia lata	Contamination with this bacterium could cause oral and, potentially, systemic infection.
11/03/2020	Nostrum Laboratories	Metformin HCl Extended-Release Tablets, USP 500 mg	NDMA exceeds acceptable daily intake limit	N-nitrosodimethylamine is a nitrosamine, a potential carcinogen.

*Summarized from https://www.fda.gov/safety/recalls-market-withdrawals-safety okay-alerts (accessed February 2021). Full details can be found on this website. Comments are from the author.

SUMMARY POINTS

- Quality must be built into a product, it cannot be "created" by repeated testing.
- The QC department is largely involved with testing, including raw materials and drug products, utilizing various methods of chemical analysis, and other test procedures.
- The QA group is concerned with overall quality which includes proper planning and layout of facilities, and the development and control of appropriate documentation.
- The layout of pharmaceutical production units is intelligently designed to facilitate the movement of materials, to prevent mix-ups and to reduce the potential for cross-contamination.
- Every manufacturing step is conducted according to written procedures and witnessed by a second operator; both operators initial and date the BMR as a record of the completion of the step.
- Wherever feasible, testing is done at the completion of each step of a manufacturing process.
- Traceability is important: the paper trail is now largely replaced by an electronic trail.
- Traces of penicillin contamination from an unrelated product led to emphasis on thorough cleaning after the previous batch produced on the same equipment and also led to a focus on cleaning verification.
- Control is accomplished, to some extent, by the use of extensive documentation and a thorough review of completed processes.
- Documents used in the pharmaceutical industry include SOPs, BMRs, ATMs; and calibration, room, and equipment logbooks.
- Some other important GMP features are meticulous calibration; labeling and separation of quarantined and released raw materials, and of quarantined and released manufactured products; use of components numbers for all raw materials; and proper design of facilities.

What do you think?

1. Why are many samples removed for testing from one powder mixing container? Would one sample not suffice considering that this sample may be subdivided into smaller amounts and each tested individually? In this way, the original sample will, effectively, be tested multiple times to ensure accuracy of the test procedure.

2. If a pharmaceutical product is intended to be extensively tested once all manufacturing steps are completed, and only released for sale to the public if all test results are acceptable, why is it necessary to conduct tests during the course of processing, that is, so-called "in process testing"?

3. List three advantages of using electronic trails instead of paper trails in the pharmaceutical manufacturing industry.

4. If the weight of every ingredient in a batch is recorded and verified by two people, why is the batch of completed product (mixture of all ingredients, each of known weight) reweighed at the end of production?

5. Why does the FDA need to visit overseas companies? Would retesting the product in the US not suffice and be cheaper?

6. Can recalls be eliminated by the use of very high standards in GMP?

BIBLIOGRAPHY

https://www.fda.gov/safety/recalls-market-withdrawals-safety-alerts

21 CFR-Subpart B — 211.28-(a)-(d)

Appendix 1
Facility Dress & Conduct Code

1.0 PURPOSE:

1.1 This SOP defines the dress, hygiene, and conduct of Jasmine Pharmaceuticals, Inc., personnel.

2.0 APPLICABLE DEPARTMENTS:

2.1 All Jasmine, Inc., personnel involved with GMP manufacture of products, whether for R&D purposes or commercial production, and all visitors to the GMP areas.

3.0 SAFETY:

3.1 This SOP addresses standard safety apparel. Specific safety issues are addressed in other SOPs, where they are relevant, and in the Chemical Hygiene Plan.

4.0 REFERENCES:

4.1 21 CFR-Subpart B — 211.28-(a)-(d)

5.0 DEFINITIONS:

5.1 **Laboratory Personnel** – Employees of Quality Control and Research and Development departments who have duties in the GMP areas.

5.2 **Uniforms**—Types of uniforms provided by the company as defined below

   5.2.1 *Production Uniforms* – Long-sleeved white shirt with navy blue pants.

   5.2.2 *Maintenance Uniforms* – Long-sleeved grey shirt and grey pants.

   5.2.3 *White lab coats* – For use in laboratories and GMP areas.

   5.2.4 *Blue lab coats* – For use by contractors and Maintenance/Engineering personnel in the GMP areas.

   5.2.5 *White lab coats with "Visitor" embroidered across front panel* – For use by all visitors to the company (who are not maintenance/service people).

6.0 RESPONSIBLE PERSONS:

6.1 Supervisors, Managers, and Directors are responsible for the training of their employees and their compliance with this SOP. Supervisors and Managers are responsible for issuing uniforms and other apparel listed in this SOP.

6.2 All employees are responsible for compliance with this SOP.

7.0 PROCEDURES:

7.1 General:

   7.1.1 No food, beverage, chewing gum, tobacco, or makeup products may be carried, consumed, or used in any Production, Laboratory, or R&D area.

   7.1.2 Hands must be washed after using the lavatory, before and after eating, or whenever they are dirty.

7.2 Personnel working in the GMP areas must prevent contamination caused by dandruff, hair, scalp, skin particles, or other particulates, by adhering to the following:

   • Sleeves must be rolled down and buttoned.

   • Shirts must be completely buttoned.

   • Shirts must be tucked inside trousers.

   • No make-up, including facial, fingernail, etc. may be worn in the GMP areas.

   • No jewelry may be worn in the GMP areas.

   • Hairnets must be worn, covering ears and with all loose hair tucked in.

   • Facial hair must be completely covered with dust mask or facial hair cover.

   • Gloves must be worn when working over or with exposed product and on clean machinery.

   • Shirt pockets contain no loose items (white production shirts have no pockets). When wearing a lab coat, the lab coat must be buttoned.

   • Eye protection must be worn in production areas.

Introduction to Bioavailability

17

INTRODUCTION

Drug therapy may range from a single dose taken for relief of an acute condition, such as a headache, to drugs taken for life-long treatment of chronic conditions, such as diabetes, hypertension, asthma, or epilepsy. The dosage and frequency of administration of a drug is referred to as the **dosage regimen**. The duration of therapy and the regimen depend upon the therapeutic objective.

When a drug is administered orally, a sequence of events takes place before a therapeutic response is elicited and these events can be summarized as shown in Figure 17-1. The therapeutic, as well as the toxic, effects of drug therapy depend upon the concentration of the drug at the site of action. With respect to an orally-consumed medication, the drug is released from the dosage form, absorbed into the bloodstream, and distributed to other tissues (such as muscles, connective tissue, and the brain). The drug is also excreted from the gastrointestinal tract (GIT) via the feces, and may be partially metabolized in the GIT as well. Excretion and metabolism are collectively known as elimination. The drug may also be metabolized in the blood, or from the tissues into which the drug has been distributed. In addition, the drug is also distributed from such tissues back into the blood (or central) compartment. For each of these kinetic processes (absorption, elimination, distribution, etc.), mathematical equations can be written to define the rates at which they occur which, in turn, affects the amount of drug that is present

in the systemic circulation or the "availability of the drug." For example, if absorption is rapid, then the drug concentration in the blood will rise rapidly, if other factors are constant. On the other hand, if elimination of the drug is very fast, then the observed blood levels will decrease rapidly. Bioavailability is the rate and extent at which a drug reaches the systemic circulation in active form after administration of a pharmacological dose. The reader should take particular note that it is the drug

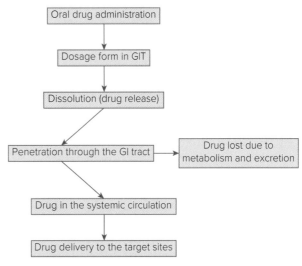

FIGURE 17-1 Sequence of events leading to a drug reaching the target sites.

reaching the systemic circulation and not the absorbed drug that is referenced. What is the difference in the amount of drug absorbed and the amount of drug reaching the systemic circulation? This difference is the amount of drug that is metabolized during the first passage of the blood through the liver. Briefly, any absorbed material that is not a nutrient will be metabolized by the liver. By having blood pass from the small intestines, after absorption, to the liver means that the liver can de-toxify any compounds that may have been consumed. In this way, hepatic first-pass metabolism (as the process is termed) is protective. This process has been described in detail in Chapter 3, Oral Route of Drug Delivery.

The study of these kinetic processes and their impact on the body, fall into the study area of pharmacokinetics. The techniques to study the bioavailability of a drug and its mathematical treatment, as well as the graphical methods that are utilized, are also a part of pharmacokinetics. Generally, pharmacokinetics is taught as a separate subject area from pharmaceutics. However, in describing several topics in pharmaceutics, such as novel delivery systems and sustained-release medication, some reference to the topic of bioavailability is required. It was, therefore, considered prudent to include some very basic concepts of bioavailability in order to facilitate an understanding of several later chapters in this book.

Since the site of action may be in deep tissues, such as the muscles or even the brain, the level of drug at the site of action is difficult to measure. On the other hand, the blood compartment can easily be accessed and blood withdrawn. Blood, or plasma, concentrations of the drug can readily be measured with accuracy and these drug levels can be correlated with the efficacy of the drug, for example, one may be able to say that 20 µg of the drug per 100 mL of blood correlates with significant reduction of headache.

While the drug acts on the brain to relieve pain, it is possible to correlate blood drug levels with the relief of pain. The central assumption of this type of testing is that the level of the drug in the blood or plasma correlates with the level of the drug at the site of action (the brain in the example of pain). With certain drugs, there may be ways to substantiate that this relationship is true. In other instances, we assume it to be true, in order to be able to make certain deductions. The accuracy of conclusions, thus drawn, are dependent on the extent to which this assumption is true. With the use of non-steroidal anti-inflammatory drugs (NSAIDs) in the treatment of arthritis, for example, the level of the drug in the synovial fluid (ie, the fluid in the space between the bones at the joint) is significant for the action of the drug, and this drug level does not correlate well with blood levels. This is an example of a situation where it is inaccurate to assume that the blood, or plasma, level represents the drug level at the receptors. In most other instances, as understood up to the present time, however, this assumption leads to useful results.

After oral consumption, the dosage form enters the GIT, the drug is released and is absorbed through the gastrointestinal (GI) membranes (usually those of the small intestine) into the portal vein and, ultimately, into the systemic circulation. As the drug gets absorbed, there will be a rise in the level of the drug in the plasma (blood). As long as the drug concentration is below a certain level, called the **minimum effective concentration** (MEC),

there will be no therapeutic response (and vice versa). When the drug concentration is above a certain level, called the **maximum safe concentration** (MSC), an adverse reaction may be observed. The MSC is also known as the **minimum toxic level** (MTL) or the **minimum toxic concentration** (MTC). The plasma, or blood, drug concentration between these two limits is the **therapeutic concentration range** or the **therapeutic window**. The ratio of the maximum safe concentration to the minimum effective concentration of the drug is called the **therapeutic index**. In order to achieve therapeutic success, plasma concentrations of the drug should be maintained within the therapeutic window.

Recap Questions

1. Distinguish between the terms: dosage, regimen, and duration of therapy.
2. Explain the difference between metabolism and elimination.
3. Why is blood tested for drug content when, in fact, the important drug level is at the receptors in the affected tissue?
4. The minimum effective concentration of theophylline is 10 µg/mL and the maximum safe concentration is 20 µg/mL. What is the therapeutic index of theophylline?

PLASMA DRUG CONCENTRATION-TIME PROFILE

Consider a dosage form, such as a tablet, which is administered orally. In the GIT, it disintegrates into particles and then releases the drug, which is absorbed into the systemic circulation. The drug concentration in the plasma is low initially and increases steadily, as the drug is absorbed, until a peak is reached, after which the plasma levels tend to fall off. In general, a direct relationship exists between the concentration of the drug at the site of action and the therapeutic response (the effect of the drug). The concentration of the drug at the site of action is significantly lower than the plasma concentration but usually correlates well with the concentration of the drug in the plasma, for a large part of the plasma concentration-time profile. Thus, the concentration at the site of action goes up when the plasma concentration goes up, and vice versa. A plasma drug concentration-time profile may be obtained from animals that have been dosed with the drug, or from humans (volunteers or patients) to whom the drug has also been administered. Such human studies are conducted in clinical settings. The basic steps involved with obtaining this profile in a human study will be briefly explained.

The subjects are normally admitted to the clinic the day before the study. By means of a questionnaire regarding their medical history, and also by physical examination and discussion between the patient and physician, it would have been previously established that the volunteer is a normal, healthy individual. It is confirmed on the evening before the start of the study that the patient's condition has not changed. It is important to exclude those individuals with any disease condition or other abnormalities which would affect the rate and extent of drug absorption and elimination, or who may be adversely affected by the drug to be administered to them. Typically, the patients' or subjects' food intake would be controlled by providing all subjects with a set meal at a fixed time. In this way, the effect of food on the absorption of the drug is controlled.

On the morning after admission, a blood sample is taken from a vein, typically a vein on the forearm. This is the time-zero blood sample. The drug is then administered, often by the oral route. If an indwelling catheter is inserted into the patient's vein, samples of blood can be withdrawn at predetermined intervals via this catheter. This avoids having to puncture a vein each time a blood sample is withdrawn. Blood samples continue to be taken according to a predetermined schedule, as specified in the clinical protocol for the study, for example, every 2 hours for 24 hours. The blood samples are typically centrifuged to separate cellular components (white blood cells, platelets and red blood cells). The plasma is then frozen until analyzed. At the time of analysis, the plasma samples are first allowed to thaw. Since plasma contains proteins and other materials which may interfere with chemical analysis of the drug contained in the plasma, the drug is typically extracted from the plasma using an organic solvent. The solvent may be evaporated and the residue dissolved in an aqueous buffer and this solution serves as the analytical sample. By an appropriate analytical method, the drug content of a fixed volume of the sample is determined. A very common method for analyzing plasma samples is high-pressure liquid chromatography (HPLC).

The results of the analytical study are a list of plasma concentrations, at various time points, for each subject in the study. The time points are the times after drug administration at which a particular plasma sample was drawn from the patient. Next, the concentration of the drug in the plasma samples is plotted against the time, with drug concentration on the Y-axis and time on the X-axis. This results in a typical **plasma drug concentration-time curve (profile),** an example of which is presented in Figure 17-2. We can calculate various parameters from the curve which are helpful in understanding drug action.

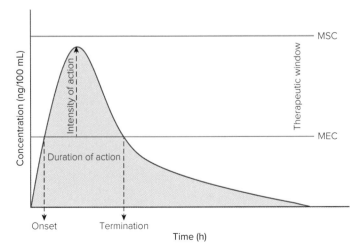

FIGURE 17-2 Concentration-time profile for an orally administered drug.

The portion of the curve to the left of the peak represents the absorption phase, that is, when the rate of absorption is greater than the rate of elimination. The section of the curve to the right of the peak generally represents the elimination phase, that is, when the rate of elimination exceeds the rate of absorption. One should always remember that elimination starts as soon as the drug enters the body and, hence, during the absorption phase there is also elimination. However, the rate of absorption exceeds the rate of elimination and, therefore, the concentration increases. To the right of the peak, elimination is faster than absorption and, therefore, the plasma levels decrease. The peak concentration is often related to the intensity of the pharmacologic response and it should, ideally, be above the minimum effective concentration (MEC) and below the maximum safe concentration (MSC).

Three important pharmacokinetic parameters describe the plasma level-time curve and are useful in describing the bioavailability of a drug from its formulation. These are C_{max}, T_{max}, and AUC and these terms are described briefly below.

Peak Plasma Concentration (C_{max})

The highest point of the curve is called the peak, and the concentration of the drug at the peak is known as the peak plasma concentration. At this point, the rate of absorption is equal to the rate of elimination. The C_{max} gives an indication of the intensity of the action of the drug from that formulation. In other words, if formulation A gives a higher peak concentration than formulation B of the same drug, the intensity of drug effect can be expected to be higher from formulation A. Side effects from formulation A may also be higher.

The C_{max} indicates whether the drug is sufficiently absorbed into the systemic circulation to provide a therapeutic response. The C_{max} differs with the route of administration, dose, and also with formulation factors within the same type of dosage form. For example, in a tablet formulation, the ingredients used, and the method of manufacture of the tablets (such as the compression force used) may all have an impact on the C_{max}. Two tablet formulations that appear to be identical may differ with respect to C_{max} due to variations in the parameters mentioned. The C_{max} by the IV route is always higher than the C_{max} obtained from any other route because IV administration places the drug directly into the systemic circulation. There is no absorption phase, and no loss of drug due to binding with the constituents of food, or loss due to first-pass metabolism, for example. These factors can be significant with oral medication. The C_{max} is an important parameter to consider when determining if two products are bioequivalent. Research studies may also place importance on the T_{max} (ie, the time at which the maximum concentration occurs) but the FDA places less reliance on it because of the observed variability in this factor.

Time of Peak Concentration (T_{max})

The time it takes for the drug to reach peak concentration in the plasma, after extravascular administration, is called the time of peak concentration or, simply, the peak time. The peak time (T_{max}) gives an indication of the rate of absorption of a drug. Its value is dependent on the rate of absorption and, to a lesser extent, on the rate of elimination of the drug. The T_{max} varies with the formulation factors applied in the design of the dosage form, for example, the type and age of capsule shells used in an encapsulated dosage form. Obviously, the type of dosage form is important in the consideration of T_{max}. Is the formulation a conventional tablet, a sustained-release dosage form, or an enteric-coated dosage form? The route of administration is also important. For example, the T_{max} for the oral route is later than that for the IV route.

Area under the Curve

The area under the curve (AUC) is the total area that the plasma level time profile encompasses (shaded area in Figure 17-2). The size of this area is a measure of the total amount of drug that reaches the systemic circulation following administration of the drug. It is an important parameter in evaluating the bioavailability of a drug from its dosage form. It represents the amount absorbed minus the amount metabolized by the liver during the first passage of blood from the intestine to the liver. All substances (nutrients as well as other substances) pass first to the liver before entering the general circulation. In the liver, substances that are perceived to be foreign, or harmful, are metabolized to detoxify them or to promote easier excretion. This is a defense mechanism that protects the body against toxic substances.

The AUC is of particular use in estimating the bioavailability of drugs. To assess a drug's oral bioavailability, for example, the ratio of the AUC after oral administration to that after intravenous injection is calculated when the same dose is administered by each route to the same subject. Since an intravenous injection is considered to be 100% bioavailable, if a capsule dosage form reflects half the area under the curve compared to the IV injection, the extent of the capsule's bioavailability is said to be 50%. While the AUC serves as the characteristic for the extent of absorption, the C_{max} and T_{max} characterize the rate of absorption. If two formulations of the same drug have the same bioavailability, it means that the rate and the extent of drug reaching the systemic circulation from these two dosage forms are the same and that they will exhibit similar therapeutic benefits.

Often, one cannot give an IV injection at the same dose as the oral formulation. This is due to the fact that the entire dose is instantly absorbed via IV and may result in toxic effects, whereas with the oral formulation only a fraction of the dose is absorbed, and this amount is absorbed over a period of time. In such a case, the theoretical area that would have been obtained with the higher IV dose (a dose that is equivalent to the oral dose) is determined from the area for the lower dose, by ratio and proportion.

During drug product development, the AUC measured after administration of a new drug formulation is an important parameter. Often, it is compared to the AUC obtained with an existing formulation of the same drug. Studies may be performed where one drug formulation is given to a panel of subjects, and a different drug formulation, of the same drug at the same dose, is given to another panel of subjects. The data from the two panels are compared using various parameters, including AUC values. Such tests could show that one product, or formulation, is superior to the other product because it gives a greater bioavailability. On the other hand, bioequivalency testing involves testing of two products, containing the same dose of the drug, to see if they give substantially the same AUC values when they would be considered bioequivalent (provided the C_{max} and T_{max} are similar).

MINIMUM EFFECTIVE CONCENTRATION

The minimum effective concentration (MEC) is defined as the minimum concentration of a drug in the plasma that is required in order to produce the desired therapeutic effect. It reflects the minimum concentration of the drug at the receptor sites which will elicit the desired pharmacologic response. Because we cannot easily measure drug levels at the receptors, we use the plasma level as an indirect estimate. Concentrations of the drug below the MEC are referred to as sub-therapeutic levels. In the case of antibiotics, the term minimum inhibitory concentration (MIC) is used. It describes the minimum concentration of antibiotic in plasma required to kill or inhibit the growth of microorganisms.

The MEC gives an idea about the dose required and the dosage regimen to be maintained. The dose should be selected so that the plasma drug concentrations will be above the MEC for a reasonable length of time, without exceeding the maximum safe concentration. When the concentration falls below the MEC, another dose is needed for continuation of therapy. The next dose is actually administered before the drug level falls below the MEC, to minimize or eliminate the period when no pharmacological action is observed. In the case of antibiotics, the plasma drug concentration is usually maintained above the MEC to avoid the risk of the microorganisms developing resistance. Therefore, skipping a dose or early termination of therapy is generally discouraged.

In general, at plasma drug concentrations below the MEC, the drug concentrations at the receptor may not be adequate to elicit a pharmacological response. There are many factors that complicate the relationship between plasma drug levels and drug levels at the receptor but these will not be dealt with in this chapter.

MAXIMUM SAFE CONCENTRATION (MSC)

The maximum safe concentration (MSC) is also called the minimum toxic concentration (MTC). It is the concentration of the drug in the plasma above which adverse or unwanted effects will usually occur. Concentrations of drug above the MSC are referred to as toxic levels. As plasma drug concentrations reach or pass the MSC, side effects become more predominant. The unwanted effects may be elicited on a different organ than the one which experiences the beneficial or expected effects.

ONSET OF ACTION

The onset of action is the beginning of the pharmacologic response and occurs when the plasma drug concentration becomes higher than the MEC. A rapid onset of action is desired in acute conditions such as pain, allergic reactions, etc. However, there may be conditions where a delayed onset of action is preferred. For example, most heart attacks occur in the morning and a specially-formulated delayed-release medication may be taken at night to prevent heart attacks in the so-called morning risk zone (6 AM to 12 noon). Without a special dosage form (eg, Innopran®), the patient would have to be awakened very early in the morning, for example, at 4 AM, to take a dose of conventional medication in order to obtain sufficiently high blood levels to prevent a heart attack during the morning risk zone. Clearly, it is not an ideal situation to wake the patient at that time in order to take medication.

A second example is the formulation of drugs that irritate the stomach, such as NSAIDs. They may be formulated as enteric-coated products which only release the drug in the small intestines where the drug is absorbed. By avoiding release in the stomach, irritation of the stomach is avoided. However, the onset of action is delayed. This effect, though not desirable in terms of efficacy, is acceptable for this type of medication. Other formulation factors may also, unintentionally, delay the onset of action of a dosage form. A prime example of this is the use of magnesium stearate as a tablet lubricant. Magnesium stearate is an excellent lubricant but, in certain instances, it may delay the dissolution and release of the drug. In turn, this delays the onset of action.

Onset of action is also dependent on the route of administration. The IV route, in general, has the quickest onset of action since the drug is placed directly into the blood compartment and no absorption phase can be identified. When the same drug is administered orally, the onset of action is much slower because there is an absorption phase and some time elapses before the drug level reaches the MEC. A higher dose of oral medication will provide quicker onset of action than a lower dose, if the drug follows first-order absorption. First-order absorption is the most common type of absorption and occurs when the absorption rate is proportional to the amount of drug raised to the first power. Therefore, the presence of more drug leads to faster absorption.

Recap Questions

1. Why are subjects in a bioavailability study not given any choice with regard to the meals they consume before drug administration?
2. Name three parameters, apart from those appearing in question 3, that are obtained from a plasma concentration versus time curve?
3. Distinguish between C_{max} and T_{max}.
4. Why is the onset of action from an enteric-coated product delayed?
5. From an observation of Figure 17-2, why does a larger dose result in a faster onset of action?

DURATION OF ACTION

The period of time during which the drug plasma concentration remains above the MEC is called the duration of drug action. The duration of action indicates the length of time that a drug produces an effect. Most drug products produce effects over a relatively constant period, for example, a particular pain medication is intended to provide relief for 4 to 6 hours and this period is fairly consistent. The drug response will continue as long as there is a sufficiently high concentration, that is, one that is above the MEC. As the drug is metabolized and excreted, the response decreases because the plasma level of drug decreases. Termination of action means the response is no longer observed. This is because the drug level is now less than the MEC. The duration of action depends on the half-life of the drug (time taken for the plasma concentration to reach half its value) and on the dosage form formulation factors. The longer the half-life, the higher will be the duration of action. Controlled-release dosage forms are designed to have a prolonged time during which the drug is released from the dosage form and, consequently, they have a long duration of action compared to conventional dosage forms.

INTENSITY OF ACTION

The difference between the peak plasma concentration and the minimum effective plasma concentration provides a relative measure of the intensity of the therapeutic response to the drug.

THERAPEUTIC RANGE

The drug concentration between the MEC and MSC represents the therapeutic range or the therapeutic window. This indicates the range of concentrations at which a drug or other therapeutic agent is effective with minimal toxicity. Medication may be said to have a narrow or wide *therapeutic index* or *therapeutic window*. (As mentioned previously, the therapeutic index is calculated as the ratio of MSC to MEC.) A compound with a narrow therapeutic index (value close to 1) exerts its desired effect at a dose close to its toxic dose. Conversely, a compound with a wide therapeutic index (greater than five) exerts its desired effect at a dose substantially below its toxic dose.

Those drugs with a narrow therapeutic index are more difficult to dose and may require therapeutic drug monitoring. This process involves the routine determination of blood levels of the drug at a selected time point(s) after dosing in patients taking the medication (as opposed to clinical trials). This may be at the point when the blood level is expected to peak, or at the expected trough (low) blood level. The peak is the highest point in the curve (C_{max}) and the trough is the lowest point that is reached before the next dose causes a rise in the concentration once more.

It should be emphasized that therapeutic drug monitoring is different from a plasma concentration-time profile. The latter involves the taking of several blood samples, often with a clinic stay. Here one or perhaps two blood levels are taken with the aim of estimating whether the dosing is adequate (in patients who are taking the medication). Subsequently, there may be a modification of the dose, depending on the results observed. If the dose change did not result in optimal therapy, the blood sampling and dosage adjustment may be repeated. Examples of drugs with a narrow therapeutic index are warfarin, some anti-epileptics such as phenytoin, aminoglycoside antibiotics, vancomycin, and theophylline. Most anti-cancer drugs have a narrow therapeutic index: toxic side effects are almost always encountered at doses used to kill tumors.

HALF-LIFE ($T_{1/2}$)

The duration of action of a drug can be estimated by its half-life. This is the period of time required for the concentration or amount of drug in the body to be reduced by one-half. We usually consider the half-life of a drug in relation to the amount of the drug in the plasma. A drug's plasma half-life depends on how quickly the drug is eliminated from the plasma. A drug molecule that leaves the plasma may have any of several fates. It can be eliminated from the body (eg, in the urine), or it can be transferred to another body fluid compartment, such as the intracellular fluid, or it can be metabolized in the blood. The removal of a drug from the plasma is known as clearance.

BIOAVAILABILITY

Bioavailability was previously defined, in this chapter, as the rate and extent at which a drug reaches the systemic circulation in active form after administration of a pharmacological dose. It is an important parameter in comparing different dosage forms of the same drug (eg, tablets vs capsules). For example,

one may state that the bioavailability of drug X from a suppository is 75% of that from an oral dosage form. It is also possible to compare different formulations (or brands) of the same dosage form, for example, generic tablets versus the innovator tablets. (The term "innovative product" is the first product of this type to be produced and marketed, that is, the product that was an "innovation".) It is very important to understand that AUC, C_{max}, and T_{max} are important parameters to measure bioavailability and thus govern the efficacy of a dosage form. Mind Map 17-1 summarizes the more important bioavailability concepts.

The bioavailability or systemic availability of an orally administered drug depends largely on the extent of its absorption and the extent of first-pass metabolism (metabolism in the gut wall and the liver). In practice, the most common method of assessing the bioavailability of a drug from a dosage form is by measuring the area under the plasma drug concentration-time profile. Blood samples are obtained at various times after administration of the dosage form to a subject, and the plasma is separated and analyzed for drug content. The plasma concentration (Y-axis) is plotted against time (X-axis). A curve similar to that shown in Figure 17-2 is obtained. The area under this curve is a measure of the bioavailability of the drug. Instead of plasma, the drug concentration in whole blood, or in serum, may also be determined. This type of study is used a great deal in the generic industry when the generic product is compared to the innovator's product. If the described curve is plotted for an innovator product, and for a generic, and the areas under the respective curves are approximately equal, it can be said that the two products have the same bioavailability if there is also a similarity in C_{max} and T_{max}.

The described study is used to assess bioavailability, and such studies are called "bioavailability studies" and are commonly used in the drug approval process. Bioavailability studies may be conducted in animals or in humans and are called, respectively,

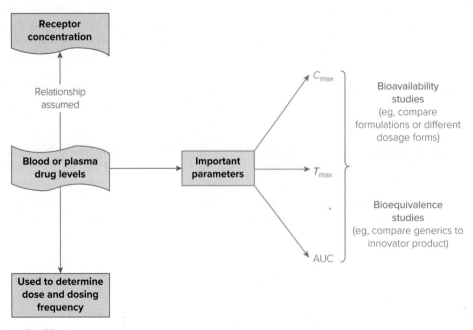

MIND MAP 17-1 Bioavailability Concepts

animal bioavailability studies or human bioavailability studies. For new drug products, such studies are conducted in animals first and later in humans. For generic drugs, typically, only human studies are conducted since the drug would be well characterized and understood by the time a generic is being developed. These methods needed to perform bioavailability studies and the calculations required are usually studied in detail in a pharmacokinetics course and will not be described further in this chapter. This introduction is provided, at this stage, since the concept of bioavailability will be used in discussing different dosage forms.

As mentioned, the formulation of the dosage form and the route of administration affect the bioavailability of a drug and these factors may, therefore, influence the intensity and duration of the pharmacological effect. An indication of the rate of drug absorption can be obtained from the peak plasma concentration and the time to reach the peak plasma concentration. The absorption rate constant (Ka) can also be calculated and this parameter provides a convenient way to compare different drugs, or formulations.

Bioavailability can be determined after a single dose of drug is administered or after multiple dosing at regular intervals when a steady state in plasma concentration is reached. The steady state denotes minimal fluctuation in drug plasma levels after regular dosing at predetermined intervals (eg, daily, twice, or thrice daily). When dosing is initiated, the peaks and troughs in the plasma concentration-time profile are large, but these become smaller as regular dosing continues. For controlled-release formulations, it is usually necessary to determine additional parameters in order to be able to state that two products have the same bioavailability. For example, not only will the total AUC be compared, but the AUC during different time intervals is also important, for example, AUC from 0 to 4 hours, and AUC from 4 to 8 hours. These are usually denoted as $AUC_{0-4\,H}$, etc. Each of these areas denotes the availability of the drug during that time period. If two sustained-release formulations display similar areas under the curve from 0 to 12 hours but one formulation displays a very small area from 0 to 4 hours, it would signify that very little of the drug is available from this formulation during this early period and that drug therapy would not be optimal during this time. It may also indicate that blood levels will be excessively high at some later point, if the total area from 0 to 12 hours is similar for the two formulations. In general, the bioavailability may also be assessed from the amount of drug excreted in the urine, or in saliva. It is also possible to determine bioavailability from the levels of a drug metabolite.

To recap, the following parameters should be assessed for comparing the bioavailability of a drug from two conventional, or immediate-release, formulations: Peak plasma concentration (C_{max}), time to reach peak plasma concentration (T_{max}), and the area under the plasma concentration-time curve (AUC). Minor changes in bioavailability may not be of clinical significance for the majority of drug products but for narrow therapeutic range drugs, minor differences in bioavailability could result in clinically significant effects. For this reason, brand substitution of narrow therapeutic range drugs, such as warfarin, is not encouraged.

It is important to differentiate the terms absolute bioavailability and relative bioavailability.

Absolute Bioavailability

Consider two situations: in one a drug is administered intravenously by a bolus injection, that is, an injection administered all at once in contrast to a slow drip; in the second, the same drug is administered orally at the same dose. The entire dose (100%) of the intravenously administered drug is rapidly placed directly into the systemic circulation. In contrast, orally administered drugs have an absorption phase. The speed of their absorption will vary with the properties of the drug in question but it will be slower, in all cases, that an IV bolus injection. In addition, the orally administered drug will probably not be completely absorbed. The proportionate amount that reaches the systemic circulation is obtained by comparing the AUC after oral administration to the AUC after IV administration and is usually expressed as a percentage, that is,

$$\text{Absolute bioavailability} = \frac{AUC(oral)}{AUC(IV)} \times \frac{100}{1} \qquad (17\text{-}1)$$

The absolute bioavailability is the ratio of the AUC after oral administration to the AUC after intravenous administration. The amount reaching the systemic circulation is not the same as the amount absorbed since the absorbed drug passes directly to the liver where a portion is metabolized. The drug that is not metabolized during this first passage through the liver and reaches the systemic circulation is the bioavailable drug. The following extreme example may help to clarify this concept. Resveratrol is 98% absorbed but only 2% bioavailable, that is, most of the absorbed drug is metabolized during the first passage through the liver. For most other drugs, the difference is not as pronounced but this example illustrates the difference between the absorbed drug and the drug reaching the systemic circulation.

It should be recognized that the principle embodied in this type of study and in Eq. (17-1) is that the amount of drug reaching the systemic circulation from an IV injection is the total, or "true," or absolute amount. Every other route of administration provides less systemic availability and, therefore, every other dosage form may be compared to this "gold standard." For a new drug, this comparison may be between the first oral formulation and an IV injection. This will provide the absolute bioavailability of the formulation and is studied in addition to the other parameters such as the safety and efficacy of the new drug. It should also be noted that this assumes a rapid, or bolus, injection. During the course of a slow injection (eg, an intravenous drip), there is sufficient opportunity for the elimination of the drug to begin and, hence, the area under the curve does not represent the "absolute" amount of drug administered.

Equation (17-1) holds true if the same dose of drug is administered by each of the two routes that are being compared. When a different dose is administered orally, the formula has to be adjusted for dose:

$$\text{Absolute bioavailability} = \frac{\dfrac{AUC(oral)}{Dose(oral)}}{\dfrac{AUC(IV)}{Dose(IV)}} \times \frac{100}{1} \qquad (17\text{-}2)$$

$$\text{Absolute bioavailability} = \frac{AUC(oral) * Dose(IV)}{AUC(IV) * Dose(oral)} \times \frac{100}{1}$$

(17-3)

Relative Bioavailability

The relative bioavailability is a measure of the fraction of the dose that is absorbed into the systemic circulation from a test dosage form compared to the fraction that is absorbed from a standard dosage form of the same drug. This is obtained by determining the ratio of the AUC of the test formulation to that of the standard formulation. This is used when comparing a new formulation to the original formulation, or when a generic formulation is compared to the innovator's formulation. How well does the new formulation compare to the old formulation? In this case, comparison of the new formulation test data to IV data may be less significant.

$$\text{Relative bioavailability} = \frac{AUC(test)}{AUC(standard)} \times \frac{100}{1}$$

(17-4)

If different doses are used under similar conditions, the relative bioavailability is calculated from the following equation (derivation is analogous to Eq. [17-3]):

$$\text{Relative bioavailability} = \frac{AUC(test) * Dose(standard)}{AUC(standard) * Dose(test)} \times \frac{100}{1}$$

(17-5)

Bioavailability Studies

Most bioavailability studies are conducted to compare two formulations and, hence, have a common theme. If an injection formulation is not available, or for some other reason, the bioavailability of a new formulation may be compared to the

bioavailability after an oral solution, which is a relative bioavailability determination. For a reformulated product (by the same manufacturer), the comparison is intended to show that the new formulation has an improved bioavailability compared to that of the old formulation. On the other hand, if the old product contained an excipient that research showed to be undesirable, the purpose of the bioavailability test is to show that the reformulated product, which does not contain this ingredient, has a similar bioavailability to the old formulation.

In the case of generics, the purpose of the bioavailability study is to show that the generic formulation has the same bioavailability as the innovator's formulation. In testing the performance of a modified-release formulation, the innovator may want to show that the absorption is slower than the immediate-release product, as desired, but that the bioavailability of the drug from the sustained-release formulation is similar to that of the immediate-release formulation, such as a conventional capsule, after accounting for the different strengths of the two formulations.

Figure 17-3 presents serum time profiles of three low-dose oral mucosal fentanyl formulations for breakthrough cancer pain. Treatment A was a newly developed tablet formulation with a mechanism to enhance absorption. Treatment C represents the marketed product (Actiq by Anesta Corporation), used as a comparator, and treatment B was a tablet formulated in a similar manner to Tablet A, except that the mechanism to enhance absorption was excluded. The profiles show that the experimental tablet formulation resulted in greatly enhanced drug absorption compared to the commercial formulation, especially in the critical first 30 minutes, providing rapid relief from breakthrough cancer pain. The curve for formulation A rises much more steeply than the curves for formulations B and C. In addition, the AUC (0–30 minutes) is much larger for formulation A compared to formulations B and C. In this example, the experimental formulation was compared to both a formulation without the enhancing mechanism and the commercial formulation. This is an example of a comparison of 3 formulations in one study.

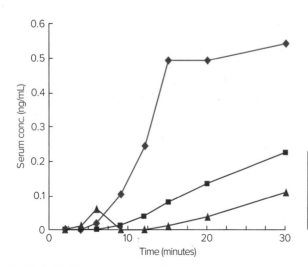

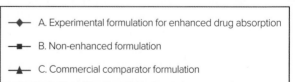

FIGURE 17-3 Initial fentanyl absorption.

Recap Questions

1. Show the derivation of Eq. (17-5) from Eq. (17-4).

2. After administering a dose of a new oral formulation of a drug to a patient, the AUC obtained was 55 µg.h/mL. The AUC obtained after administering the same oral dose of the old formulation was 83 µg.h/mL. What is the percent relative bioavailability of the new formulation?

3. Based on the information given in question 2, should the new formulation replace the old formulation?

4. In your own words, explain the difference between relative bioavailability and absolute bioavailability.

SUMMARY POINTS

- Bioavailability gives an indication of the rate and extent at which a drug reaches the systemic circulation.

- An IV bolus injection places the drug directly into the systemic circulation and the area under the IV curve represents the full dose (or absolute amount, with no loss) within the systemic circulation.

- Bioavailability can be absolute or relative.

- Various parameters can be identified from a plasma concentration-time curve, including C_{max}, T_{max}, and AUC.

- MEC and MSC give an indication of the therapeutic window.

- Superimposition of the MEC and MSC over a plasma concentration-time curve will allow an estimation of the onset time and termination time and the duration during which the plasma concentration is within the therapeutic window.

- Bioavailability studies are important for new product development including novel dosage forms and generics.

What do you think?

1. If the concentration at the site of action is the important factor, why do we not test for drug levels at this site?

2. Can two formulations of the same type, with the same amount of drug, display different C_{max}, T_{max}, and AUC values? Explain your answer.

3. List the formulations in Figure 17-3 in order of decreasing C_{max}.

4. Which formulation in Figure 17-3 has the greatest AUC?

5. How could the unenhanced formulation (TRT B) display improved bioavailability over the commercial formulation?

Introduction to the Drug Regulatory Process

18

PREVIEW

- Highlights of the legislative steps that helped to develop control of the drug supply, promoting safety, efficacy, and quality

- The steps required to gain marketing approval for a new drug product: identification and development of a new drug substance, preclinical (animal) testing, obtaining approval to conduct clinical studies, details of the clinical studies, and the submission and approval of the new drug application (NDA)

- Alternate marketing approvals: the abbreviated new drug application (ANDA) and the 505(b)2 application

- Inspections by the FDA, and actions that the FDA might take to ensure compliance with laws and regulations

OVERVIEW AND HISTORICAL HIGHLIGHTS

The manufacture and sale of drug products is a highly regulated industry. There are over 200 laws and myriad regulations that cover drugs and drug products that are commercially available in the US. The subject is vast and complex, and this chapter provides an introduction, so that the pharmacist may have insight into the regulatory process, especially the approval of drugs for sale in the US. The chapter starts with some historical highlights to give the reader an impression of how the present regulatory status was arrived at. Table 18-1 summarizes the evolution of drug laws in the US, mentioning some of the more important legislation that was promulgated, and the impact of these laws.

The Pure Food and Drugs Act was promulgated in 1906. This act prohibited misbranded and adulterated food, drinks, and drugs in interstate commerce. A misbranded drug product is one that is falsely labeled as to quality or ingredients (eg, a herbal remedy that contains added drugs not mentioned on the label). An adulterated product is one that has putrified and is unfit for human use, or has been diluted or otherwise changed by the addition of substances to it (eg, a 20% solution that has been diluted to 10% but continues to be labeled 20%). Prior to this act, even this basic, common sense requirement was not in the law, and products of dubious effectiveness, as well as of questionable safety, were openly sold in the US. This law was enforced by the Bureau of Chemistry in the Department of Agriculture. This Bureau became the Food and Drug Administration (FDA) in 1930. Apart from the fact that there was no approval process, there was not even the requirement that product information be submitted, prior to marketing a new product, to the Bureau of Chemistry or, later, to the FDA. The burden of proof was on

TABLE 18-1	Evolution of Drug Laws and Impact on Drug Utility	
PREVALENT SITUATION OR PROMPT TO PASS NEW LAW	**NEW LAW OR AMENDMENT**	**EFFECT OF NEW LAW**
Misbranded and adulterated drugs openly sold (questionable safety)	1906 Pure Food and Drugs Act	Prohibited misbranded and adulterated drugs in interstate commerce
Johnson's Mild Combination Treatment for Cancer seized SCOTUS*: challenge of false claims not within scope of 1906 Act	1912 Sherley Amendment	Prohibited labeling with false claims with intent to defraud
"Intent"—difficult to prove. In 1937 sulfanilimide elixir contained ethylene glycol, 100 people died.	1938 Federal Food, Drug and Cosmetic Act (FDCA)	Evidence of safety before distribution required. Application required for new drug product—approved if no negative comments from FDA
	1945 Amendment to FDCA	Certification of safety and efficacy of penicillin (later all antibiotics)
	1951 Durham-Humphrey Amendment	Defined drugs that required a prescription
	1962 Kefauver-Harris Amendment	Evidence of efficacy from adequate and well-controlled trials, greater safety, written approval from FDA. Advertisements must be accurate
Manufacturers could not research ANDAs during patent of the innovator. Development of generics delayed.	1984 Hatch-Waxman Amendments	Research and even submit application to FDA, but not sell product until approval and expiry of patent
	2007 Food and Drug Administration Amendments Act	FDA: Ensure that clinical trials info to CliicalTrials.gov; and pre- and post-marketing drug safety (trials, labeling changes, and REMS)
	2012 Food and Drug Administration Safety Innovation Act	Fee for ANDA (shorter review period); mid- and late-cycle communications from FDA; and breakthrough therapy designation for faster review and product availability

*SCOTUS, Supreme Court of the United States

the government to show that a drug's labeling was false and misleading before it could be taken off the market. A test of the validity of the 1906 act came about when, in 1910, the government seized a large quantity of Johnson's Mild Combination Treatment for Cancer, a worthless product. In the legal battle that ensued, the Supreme Court ruled against the government stating that, in terms of the then-current law, the government could not challenge the false claims of this product since this was not within the scope of the 1906 act.

In an attempt to overcome this deficiency, the Sherley Amendment was passed in 1912. This amendment prohibited the labeling of medicines with false claims, with the *intention* to defraud the purchaser. While the purpose of this amendment was good, in practice it was difficult to prove "intent." To establish such a proof, the government was required to demonstrate that the seller knew that the product was deficient or, often, worthless. Several cases were lost because the *intent to defraud* could not be proved. A bill was introduced in the US Senate in 1933 to make good the deficiencies of the 1906 act. The bill stalled in Congress and, as often happens, the desired revision only came about after an unfortunate drug-related problem. In 1937, sulfanilamide was developed as a new wonder drug. It was

formulated into an elixir that contained ethylene glycol, which is toxic, rather than propylene glycol, which is a good, non-toxic solvent. More than 100 people died and this forced the rethinking of drug product quality.

The Federal Food, Drug, and Cosmetic Act (FDCA) was approved in 1938. This act required, for the first time, that manufacturers show evidence of safety for new drug products before they were distributed to the public. It also extended regulatory oversight to cosmetics and devices, and required that an application be made to the FDA for every new drug product that a manufacturer wished to sell in the US. Prior to 1938, there was no such requirement. The 1938 act stipulated that the manufacturer wait for a statutory period before marketing the product. If the company did not receive a (negative) response from the FDA within this period, the product was automatically approved for sale. The 1938 act also eliminated the Sherley Amendment.

In 1945, the FDCA was amended to require the certification of the safety and efficacy of penicillin. Subsequent amendments included all antibiotic products. The Durham-Humphrey Amendment in 1951 defined those drugs that cannot safely be used without medical supervision, and required such drugs to bear a label, indicating that they may only be sold upon presentation of a prescription from a licensed medical practitioner. The Kefauver-Harris Amendment to the FDCA in 1962 required evidence of efficacy for the first time. The amendment stated that such evidence must be obtained from adequate and well-controlled studies, a revolutionary requirement at the time since the typical drug study had been conducted in a sloppy manner.

It also required that greater drug safety be demonstrated and that the manufacturer should receive a written approval notice from the FDA before marketing the product (instead of the absence of a negative comment in a specified period signaling approval). In addition, advertisements were required to be accurate regarding adverse reactions and efficacy. No longer could manufacturers claim that a product was a "breakthrough" treatment without appropriate evidence. This amendment also required informed consent for study participants. This amendment was a major advance in that the efficacy of the product had to be *demonstrated* and no longer could manufacturers, or sellers, offer for sale products of dubious value to human health.

In 2007, the Food and Drug Administration Amendments Act (FDAAA) was promulgated. It greatly increased the responsibilities of the FDA and re-authorized several critical programs such as the Prescription Drug User Fee Amendment Act (PDUFA). The latter continued to allow the FDA to charge a fee for the review of each New Drug Application (NDA), in exchange for reduced review times. One of the responsibilities given to the FDA was greater involvement in ensuring that clinical trial information is provided to ClinicalTrials.gov, a website that is run by the National Institutes of Health (NIH). The FDAAA also requires the FDA to play a larger role in pre- and post-market drug safety. In terms of this act, the FDA has the authority to require post-market studies, including clinical trials, safety labeling changes, and risk evaluation and mitigation strategies (REMS). An example of the latter is an evaluation of the risk involved with marketing a new opioid drug for oral delivery, that is, how great is the risk that abusers will extract the drug from the oral delivery product to use intravenously? In terms of this act, the FDA can ask companies to actively identify and analyze such risks.

In 2012, the Food and Drug Administration Safety Innovation Act (FDASIA) was passed. It added a fee for abbreviated new drug application (ANDA) review, providing for a shorter review period, similar to shorter reviews for NDAs upon payment of a fee. (The difference between NDAs and ANDAs is described later in this chapter.) FDASIA also provides for greater transparency with respect to the review process since it includes mid- and late-cycle communications from the FDA to the applicant. FDASIA also provides for innovation by allowing faster access to safe and effective products by patients with serious illnesses. This is done in terms of FDA assigning a "breakthrough therapy" designation to certain drug products which allows a faster review. FDA may do this when there is preliminary clinical evidence suggesting that there might be substantial improvements over available therapies. In terms of FDASIA, the FDA is also working to ensure that interested parties have the ability to provide input to the FDA. Enhanced information technology will be used to increase stakeholder involvement in FDA processes. This may take the form of patients providing information on how the disease impacts their daily lives.

It may be surprising to learn that 40% of finished drug products and nearly 80% of active ingredients are supplied to the US from overseas countries. In light of this fact, it is important that the FDA protect the global supply chain and FDASIA provides the authority to the FDA to do so. An FDA requirement, in terms of this law, is that all drug establishment facilities must be registered. The FDA also advocated higher penalties for adulterated and counterfeit drugs, a suggestion that was accepted by the US Sentencing Commission.

For many years, the major pathways for drug approval in the US were as follows:

1. The 505(b)1 pathway covers pharmaceutical products that contain new drug substances (API) that have not been used in man before and for which an NDA was required to be submitted to the FDA.

2. The 505j pathway for generic drugs, that is, a drug product that is identical with respect to dosage form and strength, etc., to the original product of this drug. The original product would have been approved after an NDA submission. This product is also referred to as the "reference listed drug" (RLD), indicating that all proposed generics, containing the same active ingredient, would have to be compared to this product.

3. Manufacturing in compliance with drug monographs that are listed in the United States Pharmacopeia (USP) or the National Formulary (NF) for over-the-counter (OTC) drugs. The drug monograph describes in detail the properties of the product and also describes test methods, and acceptable standards, for each test. Products must be manufactured according to the standards, and must meet the test specifications, contained in each monograph but do not need FDA approval, although some companies will submit data to the FDA, for review, to ensure that they are in compliance. If an OTC product cannot be made in compliance with every aspect of a monograph, and the company wishes to market the product, then an IND and an NDA would have to be completed, as described in a later section of this chapter.

4. Submission of an NDA for a non-monograph OTC product which is either a prescription to OTC switch, or a new non-monograph OTC product.

The first person or company to develop a new pharmaceutical product usually has patent protection for a period of time, approximately 20 years at present. The patent offers the developer protection so that others may not imitate the product during the stated period. The original developer of the product is referred to as the innovator, and this term will be used in the remainder of this chapter. The patent protection allows the innovator time to recoup research and development costs without the concern that competition would inhibit sales. This was the legal situation up to early 1984. In terms of prevailing legislation, manufacturers could not research generic equivalent formulations, during the lifetime of the patent, without infringing the innovator's patent(s). In practice, this meant that development of generic products would only begin after the expiry of the patents. Only after appropriate research and testing, thereafter, could an application to the FDA be made. While it was accepted that the innovator should get protection during the lifetime of the patent, this arrangement delayed public access to more affordable generics for an additional period of several years. The 1984 Hatch-Waxman Amendments to the FDCA allowed companies to research their products and even to submit an application to the FDA, but they could not sell the product until the expiration of the patent period (and the approval of the application by the FDA).

More recently, a new drug approval pathway has been utilized in the US. This is a 505(b)2 pathway. This pathway covers the use of an existing drug substance in a new manner, such as in a new dosage form or a new route of administration, or for a new indication, etc. For example, consider a drug that had previously been offered as a swallowed tablet. When this drug is reformulated as an orally disintegrating tablet, that is, a new dosage form, the 505(b)2 application can be utilized to obtain marketing approval. This application is faster and cheaper to develop because many studies that are required for an NDA, such as several safety studies, do not have to be performed by the applicant. However, such *information* is still needed but may be supplied from literature sources. There is some evidence that the 505(b)2 pathway is becoming more popular than the NDA pathway.

Recap Questions

1. The 1906 Pure Food and Drugs Act is an example of early legislation to control drugs. What type of problem with marketed drug products did it attempt to control?

2. How did the Sherley Amendment try to improve the Pure Food and Drugs Act and why did it fail to do so?

3. The FDCA, approved in 1938, required manufacturers to show evidence of the —————— of drug products. (Fill in the blank.)

4. What major improvement to the FDCA did the Kefauver-Harris Amendment (1962) make?

5. Which amendment allowed quicker access to generic drugs?

NEW DRUG APPLICATION

For every new drug product that a developer wishes to market in the US, a new drug application (NDA) must be submitted to the FDA to obtain *marketing authorization*. The latter terminology is used by the FDA to define what most laypeople refer to as "registration" of the drug product with the FDA. The "drug product," in FDA terminology, is the dosage form, that is, the form in which the patient takes the medication. The "drug substance" is the chemical entity that has a pharmacological effect. The application is a complex process and requires the submission of a great deal of data concerning the new drug substance and the drug product. This includes the test results obtained by the pharmaceutical company wishing to market the product (or by other companies or individuals contracted to it). The company wishing to obtain marketing approval for the product is referred to as the "applicant" or the "sponsor." The FDA will approve a marketing application if, after careful consideration of the submitted data, and any other available information (eg, published information), it is of the opinion that the drug product meets the standards for safety and effectiveness, manufacturing and controls, and labeling. It will also have the company inspected prior to approval. In reaching its conclusion, the FDA may also consult with outside experts and seek public opinion.

The work of the FDA is divided across the four main "offices." The Office of Medical Products and Tobacco has the Center for Drug Evaluation and Research (CDER) which deals with small molecule drug substances and drug products, and a Center for Biologics Evaluation and Research (CBER) which deals with most, but not all, Biologics Licensing Applications (BLA). The latter are products of biological origin, for example, proteins and peptides. The marketing applications for such products, as well as for devices, are not covered in this chapter. This chapter describes the regulatory landscape regarding small molecule drug substances and drug products, which represent the majority of new medical product applications. These applications are submitted to CDER which provides regulatory oversight with regard to the development and marketing of new drug products, generic drugs, and over-the-counter drugs. It is worth considering a brief description of the overall drug development process, at a basic level, in order to place the NDA, and activities connected with it in context, before going into more detail with regard to each aspect of the regulatory process.

Synopsis of the Drug Development Process

The drug development process starts with the discovery of a chemical substance that appears to have drug properties (Mind Map 18-1). Such a chemical may be developed from natural products such as the roots, leaves, barks or other parts of plants, or from crude extracts of plants. Such natural products may have been used in folk remedies with claims of beneficial effects. Pharmaceutical scientists extract the active ingredient from such natural products and test them in laboratory and animal models. If the results appear to be promising, development of the drug product may be pursued. Drugs may also be developed as synthetic analogs of existing drugs. Medicinal chemists study chemical structures and may predict that small changes to an existing molecule will bring about an improved therapeutic response, or a reduction in adverse reactions. The altered molecule may be obtained by synthetic or semisynthetic means, and is then tested in the laboratory, or in test animals, to determine if the desired effect is produced. Importantly, they will also assess if the changes introduce new adverse reactions. If the molecule is significantly improved, it may be developed into a drug product.

Biologists and pharmacologists may also review normal and abnormal chemical processes in the body. They may hypothesize that a particular molecular structure, or change to an existing compound, is likely to interact with biological molecules to correct abnormal chemistry or function that is observed in specific disease conditions. These molecules, prepared by synthetic

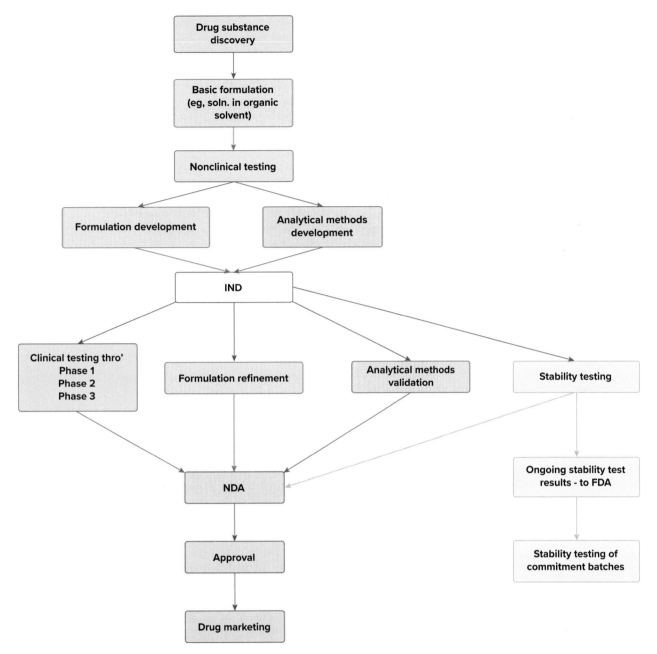

MIND MAP 18-1 The Drug Development Process

chemists, will then be tested in the laboratory, and in animals, to ascertain whether the expected effect occurs.

Substances with drug potential, discovered by any of the methods in this simplified description require more detailed animal testing to fully describe their effects, adverse reactions, and toxicology. For this purpose, simple injection formulations may be utilized, frequently in organic solvents. Many newer drugs are not water soluble, necessitating the use of nonaqueous solvents. At a later point in animal testing, somewhat more sophisticated formulations may be needed and some formulation work may be performed at this stage of development. Even the formulation of a "simple" injection may not be straightforward. The use of a mixture of multiple solvents (a solvent system), or a solvent and a cosolvent, with or without the addition of surfactants, may be needed.

If the animal testing proves to be successful, the decision may be taken to proceed with the development of a drug product for human consumption. For this purpose, a formulation has to be developed and clinical testing performed. To test drugs in humans, there are two requirements from a regulatory perspective: first, the approval of an institutional review board (IRB) needs to be obtained and, second, an investigational new drug application (IND) has to be submitted to the FDA. For testing in humans, there must be a formulation to administer to the human subjects or patients and this formulation has to be developed by the company. For quality control testing of this formulation, analytical test methods must be developed with sufficient reliability for initial human testing. (Subsequent testing in larger numbers of subjects, or marketing to the general population requires even more stringent test methods.)

Details of the formulation, the test methods used, and the test results obtained are a part of the IND.

The IRB is a non-governmental body. It is a board that may be associated with a university or even a private company. The members of the board review the research proposal and other documents to determine if the research can be expected to be conducted ethically and without undue harm to the patients or subjects. If IRB approval has been obtained and the FDA has no concerns with the proposed human testing, as gleaned from the IND, such testing may be carried out by the company. During the clinical testing phase, the formulation may be refined, and the analytical test methods will be further refined and more extensively validated.

The methods and results of the clinical testing, formulation development, analytical methods development and validation, and product stability will be combined with other information about the drug (such as its chemistry and pharmacology) into an NDA. This is a voluminous document that has to be prepared according to FDA guidelines using an FDA template. Upon review of this application, if the FDA determines that the drug is suitable for the intended purpose, is safe for human consumption, is sufficiently stable, is manufactured reproducibly and tested appropriately, it will approve the NDA after a satisfactory inspection of the facilities and equipment. Upon such approval, the drug may be marketed in the US.

The above synopsis provides a very brief overview of the whole process to keep in mind as the details are discussed in the following pages of this chapter. If drug discovery (as described above) is considered a prerequisite step, then the regulatory process involves chemistry, manufacturing, and controls (CMC); preclinical; clinical; and marketing phases.

Pre-IND Meeting

The submission of an IND notifies the FDA that the company intends to conduct clinical studies. It is also noteworthy that the FDCA states that a product may not be the subject of interstate commerce unless the FDA approves a marketing application for that drug, that is, it is approved to be marketed. Therefore, if the company were to send the test product across state lines for clinical testing, without any further legal provision, it could be accused of illegal interstate commerce. The IND provides an exemption from this requirement of the FDCA.

Prior to the submission of the IND, the company may send representatives to meet with the FDA for a pre-IND meeting to discuss questions pertaining to the IND document that will be submitted. The delegation that visits the FDA will probably be led by a senior member of the regulatory affairs group within the company. The group will also consist, very likely, of a representative from clinical affairs who was involved with the design of the clinical studies, and a representative from the formulations group who understands the development of the formulation, and has knowledge of the analytical work and of the stability testing of the product that has been done up to that point.

As with other FDA meetings, the names of the delegates, as well as the questions that are to be discussed, must be submitted ahead of the meeting. Only questions provided in writing may be discussed further at the meeting. Clarification questions pertaining to the written questions may be asked but no new questions can be introduced at such a meeting. Data that the company usually has at this point includes the results of preclinical studies, stability study data representing testing for a short duration, and the formulation and quality control data. Such data will be presented in summary form and submitted with the questions. This allows the FDA to be familiar with the available data and to relate such data to the questions being asked. Major questions that the company poses may relate to the design of the clinical studies and the statistical procedures that will be used to evaluate the data obtained. It is acceptable to ask the FDA if the proposed investigation (clinical study) is likely to lead to the data required for eventual NDA submission. Additional questions may relate to the formatting of the IND.

The basic intention of the pre-IND meeting is to minimize the potential for a clinical hold (described below) by gaining FDA support for a proposed clinical strategy, and specific agreement that the design of the proposed studies is likely to provide useful information, supporting the company's hypothesis regarding the utility of the drug. This meeting, however, also provides the opportunity for a good exchange of ideas between company scientists and FDA regulators, on aspects of product development, which could result in a more creative development strategy. For example, detailed dissolution testing parameters may be discussed (if the broad topic of dissolution was mentioned in the meeting documentation). While the obvious objective of company scientists would be to gauge whether the designed studies appear to be sufficient for regulatory approval, an unexpected benefit of the meeting may be the advice from the FDA that certain contemplated studies are unnecessary. In this way, the meeting may be time and cost saving.

Investigational New Drug Application

After the pre-IND meeting, the team who met with FDA representatives will report back to the relevant parties within the company. In the light of FDA suggestions and advice, the development of documents for incorporation into the IND will continue with appropriate modification, as needed. Once the IND paperwork is complete, it is submitted to the FDA. A summary of the more important components of the IND is given below:

- An introductory statement.
- The general investigational plan.
- The investigators brochure: *this document provides pertinent information regarding the drug product to multiple clinical investigators who may be conducting clinical studies at different locations.*
- The clinical study protocols: *for each clinical study, a document is provided describing the precise steps to be undertaken, including dosing, blood sample collection, patient evaluation, clinical endpoints, and statistical methods for evaluating the results.*
- The chemistry, manufacturing, and controls information: *information regarding how the drug substance is tested and deemed acceptable, that is, drug substance specifications; how the drug product is manufactured and tested, and the specifications for the product.*
- Pharmacology and toxicology information.

- The results of preclinical testing.
- A summary of previous human experience, if any: *for a new drug, there may be no previous human experience; if the drug has been used in other countries (whether marketed or for clinical studies), there may be information to provide.*
- Any additional information that may be of value to the FDA in assessing the safety of the drug.

The FDA reviews the application and, per the regulations, the FDA is obligated to inform the company of a negative response within 30 days of receipt of the application. In terms of the regulations, if there is no response by the 30th day, the company may continue with the clinical studies. However, if the FDA has a favorable response, there will, usually, be a letter from them stating that the company may proceed with the study. A "negative" response from the FDA is referred to as a "clinical hold," meaning that the study may not continue. A clinical hold may arise if the application documents are incomplete, if the FDA has concerns about the clinical plan or the drug product, or safety concerns with any aspect of the study. The latter may arise from observations that the FDA makes during the review of the preclinical data.

New clinical protocols may be submitted to the FDA at any time under an "open" IND. This, typically, occurs as the clinical program matures and new needs are discovered. The fact that later submissions will be accepted means that a clinical hold can occur at any time, for example, a clinical hold may be placed in response to a recently submitted protocol or to information that has recently become available.

Institutional Review Board

An institutional review board (IRB) may be set up by a hospital, university, or other institution to ensure that human subject research carried out at that institution is done in an ethical manner, and in accordance with relevant laws. The US Department of Health and Human Services (HHS) promulgated regulations for human subjects research based on the Belmont report. The Belmont report was written by the National Commission for the Protection of Human Subjects of Biomedical and Behavioral Research. The report was commissioned partly due to problems arising from the Tuskegee syphilis study in which the subjects were treated unethically. The full title of the report is: "Ethical Principles and Guidelines for the Protection of Human Subjects of Research." The report's recommendations were expanded into the current regulations which cover all research involving human subjects. The three fundamental principles for human subjects' research embodied in the Belmont report are mentioned below since these principles direct an IRB's review of proposed research.

1. Respect for persons: protecting the autonomy of all people and treating them with courtesy and respect.
2. Beneficence: The concept of "do no harm" which embodies maximizing benefits for the research project while minimizing risks to the research subjects.
3. Justice: ensuring that reasonable, non-exploitative, and well-considered procedures are administered fairly and equally.

Human research may involve biomedical research, such as the testing of a new drug product, but it may also consist of psychological research or educational research. The task of the IRB is to ensure that no harm is done to the subjects or patients and that any pain or suffering, endured in the course of the research, is minimal and justified in terms of the expected research outcomes. For example, drawing blood samples may be considered minimally invasive and does not cause a great deal of pain to the subjects (when professionally done) but the IRB may object if many blood samples are drawn without justification for the large number. Greater invasiveness may be acceptable if the anticipated outcome is expected to have a huge impact on human health, for example, if it is expected to be lifesaving.

The harm done to the patient may not only be physical but there may be psychological trauma as well. If the questions asked in the course of psychological research require the subject to analyze intense feelings or to recount negative experiences, the nature of such questions can cause psychological injury. The IRB will be cognizant of this type of potential harm to the subjects as well. In educational research that is conducted at a University, do students feel obligated to participate in the study because their professor is the lead investigator? Are students uncomfortable in answering the questions that are asked about their study habits but feel obliged to participate because they think their grades may be affected if they do not? These are some of the questions that IRB members will be asking as they review applications. As some of these examples indicate, injury to the subject may not only be physical, such as the adverse reactions of drugs, although the latter will certainly be taken into account in a drug study. While psychological and educational research is not involved in drug registrations, these examples were mentioned to provide a fuller understanding of the function of the IRB and also to reveal the extent to which IRB members are concerned about the welfare of study participants.

The IRB consists of five or more persons who are scientifically qualified and familiar with the type of study generally undertaken at that institution. In large institutions, the IRB may consist of many more members, all of whom do not participate in the review of every application that the IRB receives. From the large membership, selected persons would be asked to serve as reviewers for specific applications, based on their experience and knowledge of the type of study being reviewed. One member of the IRB is a layperson, that is, a person who does not have a scientific qualification or background. This person is typically a member of a community organization and serves on the IRB to represent the layperson's perspective of the research being reviewed. Before undertaking any review of study materials, the IRB members must, in terms of legal requirements, undertake a course of study covering the ethics of research and obtain a passing grade. The course materials usually contain case studies which enable the participants to practice decision-making regarding approval or non-approval of an application.

The IRB reviews the major documents pertaining to a clinical study. These include the protocol, informed consent, and the investigator's brochure. These documents are usually prepared by the clinical department of the sponsoring company, or by consultants. The IRB should be fully satisfied with these documents before approving the study. The IRB may address questions, via its chair, to the sponsoring company. Only when the IRB is satisfied that questions have been fully and satisfactorily answered and that the documentation is complete, will the study be approved. Since the IRB meets at specific times (eg, once a month), companies must send the documentation in good time not to delay the start of a study. In certain instances, it may not be necessary for the entire IRB to reconvene to consider the answers to questions that were sent to the company by the IRB. Depending on the nature of the questions, the chair may approve a previously reviewed study upon receipt of satisfactory answers.

Protocol

The protocol provides a detailed description of the study including its purpose, the number and type of subjects or patients to be included, the test procedures, and the methods of analyzing the results, including statistical methods. The protocol usually includes a description of what constitutes a positive result. As an example, consider a medication that is intended to reduce blood pressure. The protocol may state that a successful treatment is a reduction in the systolic blood pressure of at least 20 mm Hg. In a placebo-controlled trial, the results may be stated as the number of patients in the treatment group who achieved this level of blood pressure reduction versus the number in the control group. These parameters are stated in the protocol before the study begins to eliminate the possibility of "softening" the parameters for success once the data are available.

In describing the study, it will be stated whether the study is double-blind or open-label, for example. A double-blind study is a comparative study involving two or more products in which neither the subject (patient) nor the clinic staff can identity which product option was taken by a specific patient. Such blinding is done to preserve the objectivity of the results which includes an assessment of the improvement in the patient's condition, and the prevalence of adverse reactions. The study materials, commonly a test drug and a comparator, are fully described to clinic staff but they are unaware which product each patient takes since the products are visually identical.

The study subjects are fully described in terms of the number of subjects, age group, gender, etc. The inclusion criteria are also stated; some examples (that may each be used in a different type of study) are the following: healthy males between the ages of 20 and 40 years; males and females between the ages of 40 and 60 years who are experiencing moderate pain; and post-menopausal women with a diagnosis of osteopenia. The protocol may also contain exclusion criteria, a common example of which is women who are pregnant.

The procedures to be used in the study are described in detail. Examples of procedural factors that may be included are: the fact that patients are required to fast overnight, the medication to be taken and the dosage, and the fact that the medication has to be taken after a standard breakfast. The time of dose administration, as well as of blood draws, is specified. These parameters are typical for a pharmacokinetic (PK) study. How the blood samples are to be drawn, that is, the equipment to be used, the vein from which the blood is drawn, and the volume of blood, are specified. The processing of the blood samples will also be described fully in the protocol. This includes, for example, the fact that the blood must be centrifuged, and plasma removed and frozen. The chemical methods of analysis are also mentioned, as are the ways in which the results will be calculated and presented. The fact that adverse reactions must be noted and the method of reporting will also be specified in the protocol.

The standard breakfast is described by the FDA and includes items that contain some fat. The idea of fasting overnight and then taking medication after a standard breakfast ensures that all subjects are taking the medication under similar fed states. The standard breakfast also allows the impact of food to be taken into account. The procedure for drug administration is identical whether the test product or the comparator (placebo or another drug product) is administered. In many instances, a great deal of data may be recorded electronically at the time of data collection. Included in this category may be blood pressure readings and other clinical data, and the protocol will specify the systems for data collection and storage.

Informed Consent

Ethical conduct of human research requires that the patient or subject give their consent to participate in the study. This consent must be informed, meaning that the patient should understand the fact that he or she is participating in a clinical study for the purpose of obtaining data that may, or may not, be useful in the treatment of other patients. The patient should also understand the procedures that will be carried out on him or her and, most importantly, that participation is voluntary and that the patient may only be included in this study with the patient's consent. The need for informed consent arises out of the concept of "respect for persons" which is one of the principles of the Belmont report.

The informed consent document must be written in lay language and the content of the document must also be explained to patients before the commencement of the study. Patients should have an opportunity to ask questions, and to have their questions answered satisfactorily in lay terms. This document must explain the potential risks involved in being a participant in the study, and the potential benefits (if any). Also, it must clearly state that a patient may withdraw from the study at any time, and for any reason, without penalty. If a patient withdraws from the study, the withdrawal does not preclude continued use of the services of the physician conducting the study, or of the clinic at which the study is being conducted, for any medical issues that the patient may have (that are unrelated to the study). This document will be signed by both the patient and an employee of the clinic who has oversight responsibility. By signing, the patient is giving consent to the clinic to perform the procedures outlined in the informed consent document, that is, he or she agrees to be a participant in the study. The patient must be given a copy of the signed informed consent document.

All of the above requirements must be appropriately embodied in the informed consent document. Members of the IRB will review this document carefully as part of the process to consider approval of the study. It is not uncommon for an IRB not to approve a study until some aspect of the informed consent document is amended.

Investigator's Brochure

The investigator's brochure contains information about the drug product under test to familiarize clinic staff. For a new drug, the brochure may contain a synopsis of preclinical testing of the drug. It will also contain some information on the dosage form and how it is expected to work, especially for a novel drug delivery system. If the drug has been used in humans previously, for example, in other countries, the brochure will contain a summary of previous human experience with the drug. If the drug is well known but is now presented in a different formulation or dosage form, the summary of previous human experience would describe the existing presentations of the drug.

The investigator's brochure also describes the effects of the drug, the adverse reactions (as known at the time of the study), and the frequency of each adverse reaction mentioned. Obviously, if the study is "first in man," that is, the drug has not been administered to humans before, such information would not be available. The study under consideration may, in fact, have been designed to obtain such information. In such a case, information from in vitro and preclinical studies may be offered as an indication of the effects to be expected. The personnel at the clinic are expected to be familiar with the information in the investigator's brochure. For example, if respiratory depression is an expected adverse reaction determined from previous human use of the drug, or gleaned from preclinical studies, the test facility must be prepared to handle such an event. They may do this by having drugs to counteract respiratory depression, as well as oxygen, on hand.

Phase 1 Studies

A phase 1 study is also referred to as a "first in man" study. The number of subjects is low, frequently 10s of subjects. This study utilizes normal, healthy volunteers. Since patients are not involved, participants are referred to as "subjects." These studies are primarily performed to observe the safety and adverse reactions of the drug. The study may be a dose-escalating study. This means that a very low dose is given to a few subjects, typically three, initially. If no adverse reactions are noted, dosing is repeated at an incrementally higher level using the next small cohort of subjects. This may be continued, using the same number of subjects (three in this example), for a few dosing levels. When some adverse reactions are observed, the escalation of doses, and the study, is stopped. The entire study may be at lower drug levels than the eventual dose of a commercial drug product, assuming it is approved.

A dose-escalating study may be a single-dose, or a multiple-dose, study. The latter differs from the former in that the first dose is given multiple times, at fixed dosing intervals, to the first cohort of subjects. If no adverse reactions are observed, the next dose level is administered, using the same dosing regimen, to a different cohort of subjects, and so on. The primary goal, as stated, is to observe the safety and tolerability of the drug in this first exposure of the drug to man. If, however, some idea of the effectiveness of the drug is obtained from a pharmacodynamic (PD) response (such as a reduction in blood pressure), this is a bonus. Some pharmacokinetic data may also be obtained from the study.

Phase 2 Studies

Phase 1 study provides information on safety and tolerability and gives an indication of the dose, or the dose range.

The purpose of phase 2 study is to test this preliminary idea of the dose in a larger group of patients, to continue safety observations and to observe the pharmacological effects of the drug. PK parameters such as absorption, distribution, metabolism, and excretion are determined in phase 2a studies. These include single-dose and multiple-dose PK and PD studies, dose proportionality, and absolute and relative bioavailability determinations. Additional studies may be undertaken to clarify the effects of food. Additionally, the company may conduct subpopulation studies, for example, to determine any differences due to gender, ethnicity, or pediatric populations.

In phase 2b studies, referred to as dose-ranging studies, a series of doses may be tested to determine the optimum dose. These range from slightly less than, to somewhat higher than, the anticipated therapeutic dose, as estimated from phase 2a studies. From an observation of beneficial effects, as well as of adverse reactions, an optimum dose is chosen for use in phase 3 studies, assuming other drug parameters are acceptable.

Phase 2 studies may involve numbers of patients in the low 100s, or even a few hundred. Because of the larger number of patients, some adverse reactions not seen in phase 1 may be seen in these studies. Adverse reactions may also result from the larger doses used, especially in phase 2b studies. In addition, some adverse events may only be seen in patients, not in healthy volunteers. The formulation used in phase 2 studies may not be the final formulation. In addition, stability studies may not have been completed at the time of these studies but may be ongoing. However, the company should be able to demonstrate, to the satisfaction of the FDA, that the test product has stability for a little longer than the time from production to the end of dosing to patients. Formulation development will likely be ongoing during phase 2 studies but should, ideally, be finalized by the time of the late phase 2 studies because this formulation will be used for phase 3 studies. Formulation details and available test results will also have to be submitted to the FDA in preparation for a meeting with the FDA, described in the next subsection.

End of Phase 2 Meeting

While an IND holder may request a meeting with the FDA at any time, certain meetings are recommended at critical points of the product development timeline. These meetings are described in this chapter under the commonly used name for the meeting. The end of phase 2 meeting (EOP2) is one such meeting that the sponsor company may request with the FDA. The primary purpose of this meeting is to obtain the FDA's concurrence that it is safe to begin phase 3 testing (in which there will be a much larger number of participants than in phase 2) and to obtain agreement from the FDA on the overall plan for phase 3. At this meeting, therefore, the plans for phase 3 clinical testing of the product, as well as topics such as the specifications for the product may be discussed. The concept of specifications for a product was discussed in Chapter 15, Dosage Form Stability. Prior to attending the EOP2, specifications should have been developed internally at the company. If the company has questions relating to specifications, these may be discussed with the FDA at this meeting.

The company should also have limited stability data collected up to this point and may wish to discuss this with the FDA. The company may not have stability data for the intended shelf life of the product, at this stage of development. However, it should be able to demonstrate, using the available stability data, that the product will be stable during the clinical testing period.

As described for the pre-IND meeting, the names of the delegates to the meeting, as well as the questions to be discussed, must be sent to the FDA in advance of the meeting. Again, the meeting will only discuss the questions stipulated in writing, prior to the meeting. The purpose of this meeting is to obtain FDA buy-in before a great deal of resources and time are spent on clinical studies. At the end of a long and expensive study, it would be undesirable for the company to hear that the study design does not permit determination of the effectiveness of the drug. Therefore, prior to study commencement, company officials can explain the reasons for designing the studies the way they did. It is also an opportunity for the FDA to comment and, perhaps, to state why they felt the study, as designed, would not allow one to draw the anticipated conclusions. This meeting is also an opportunity for the FDA to comment on the overall clinical program and to state whether it felt certain studies were unnecessary, which would save the company time and money.

It also gives the company the opportunity to discuss gray areas with regard to the testing of the product. For example, dissolution testing may not fit textbook examples and the company can explain nonstandard methods used, or unusual results obtained. This would be an opportunity for the FDA to state whether the test methods are appropriate and if the results, obtained up to this point, appear to be reasonable. Again, a question pertaining to dissolution testing methods should have been provided in the written documentation, prior to the meeting, for this question to be discussed at all. This would give the company confidence to continue using the described dissolution test methods, for example, in the assessment of dissolution changes during stability testing, if these were previously observed. The FDA may give an indication of its views toward the product at this stage of development but will not state that the product is acceptable for marketing approval until all study results are available and the NDA is submitted and reviewed. Nevertheless, it would be useful to obtain an indication of the FDA's thinking, at this stage.

Phase 3 Studies

Phase 3 studies determine the efficacy of the drug for the stated indication while also analyzing the adverse reaction profile in a larger group. Phase 3a studies are completed before the submission of the NDA to the FDA while phase 3b studies are not complete at this time. They may be in progress and will be completed before the marketing of the drug begins. While the NDA is under consideration, the FDA will be given updates on the progress of these studies.

The study may be "placebo-controlled," meaning that the therapeutic effect of the drug and the adverse reaction profile are compared to these effects in patients who take a placebo. Whenever two products are compared, the study may be performed as a crossover study. For this study, two groups of subjects (Group A and Group B) are formed. Subjects are randomly placed into each of these groups which have approximately equal numbers. Group A receives the test product, whereas Group B receives the placebo. All the subjects take the medication (test product or placebo) on the same day. After a wash out period (a period in which no drug is taken), the group that took the test product will receive the control and vice versa. The washout period is used to ensure that the drug is cleared from the body before the second dosage form is taken. This ensures that no residual effects from the first administration will be observed after the second administration and mistaken for an effect of the second product.

In a parallel design, the subjects are also divided into two groups (Group A and Group B), with one group taking the drug and the other group taking the placebo on the same day. In contrast to a crossover design, all of the dosing occurs on one day; there is no second dosing and no crossover. To achieve the same power (same statistical significance of the study), twice the number of subjects are used, as compared to the crossover design. The difference between the two designs is illustrated in Table 18-1 which shows that a total of 50 subjects were used in the crossover design, whereas a total of 100 subjects were required in the parallel design, in order to achieve the same study size. The parallel design may present more difficulty with recruiting. In the parallel design, all dosing and blood collection are over in one day. This is in contrast to the crossover design where there is a washout period after which the clinic is utilized again for a second dosing, blood collection, and other activities required for the study. In the crossover design, each subject takes both the test medication and the placebo (on different days). In the averaged data, this may be viewed as the patient being his or her own control. This individualized control is lacking in the parallel design. While the parallel design study has controls, such control is afforded by a different group of subjects. The validity of a parallel design study's results may depend on how well the two groups are balanced. The main characteristics of cross-over and parallel designs are compared in Table 18-2.

TABLE 18-2	**Crossover and Parallel Clinical Study Designs**			
Design (Type/Total No. of Subjects)	**Dosing Period**	**Group A (No. of Subjects / Medication)**	**Group B (No. of Subjects / medication)**
Crossover 50	1	25 Test drug	25 Placebo
	2	25 Placebo	25 Test drug
Parallel 100	Single dosing	50 Test drug	50 Placebo

In the above description of crossover and parallel designs, the test drug and placebo were mentioned. However, these study designs may also be used for other controlled studies as described in the regulations:

1. Dose-comparison concurrent control: *a study in which two different doses of the drug are compared.*

2. No treatment control: *the test drug is compared to no treatment but there are objective measurements of effectiveness. This is used where the placebo effect is known to be negligible.*

3. Active treatment control: *the control is an established drug that is known to be effective.*

4. Historical control: *the collected data for the test drug is compared with the well-documented progression of the disease using historical treatments (eg, a new treatment for an aggressive cancer compared to the previous standard of treatment).*

The third controlled study mentioned above includes several types of studies, examples of which are:

1. A new formulation of the drug against the old formulation of the same drug

2. A new generic formulation of the drug against the innovator's formulation

3. Two different dosage forms of the same drug, such as a capsule compared to a tablet

4. Two routes of drug administration for the same drug, such as the oral route compared to the rectal route

5. One drug against another drug in the same therapeutic category, for example, chlorpheniramine maleate (a well-known antihistamine) compared to a newer, "non-drowsy" antihistamine

The crossover and parallel study designs are commonly used but they are by no means the only types. They are among the simplest designs. There are many other designs of increasing complexity which will not be described in this introductory chapter. Since phase 3 studies may continue for a relatively long time, usually more than one year, it is conceivable that some minor changes may be made to the formulation during this time. Such changes may arise from ongoing testing, or from new information that comes to light. Assuming that the clinical studies show the desired results, the final formulation would have to be subjected to a pharmacokinetic study once again to demonstrate that the bioavailability of the drug in the new formulation is, for practical purposes, the same as that of the earlier formulation that produced good therapeutic outcomes.

Special Protocol Assessment

The regulations provide a mechanism for the FDA to assess and subsequently to discuss with the sponsor any special protocol that will be used to obtain data for an NDA. As the name implies, these protocols are "special" in that some aspect of the study is different from, or unusual, compared to conventional studies. The basic philosophy is that the company should get FDA input before undertaking a study that may be complex, time-consuming, and costly. When there is agreement with the FDA on the design of the study and the required endpoints, then the company may be more comfortable expending human and financial resources on the study. Each special protocol assessment (SPA) is intended to cover one protocol only. For example, if there are four studies that constitute phase 3, two of these may be straightforward and the company may only request an SPA for each of the other two studies.

The type of clinical protocol that qualifies for SPA review includes phase 3 protocols for clinical trials that demonstrate efficacy of the drug. The latter may be new protocols, developed after the EOP2, or they may be modifications of the protocols discussed at the EOP2. Such modifications, increasing the complexity of the protocol, may become necessary in the light of initial clinical data or new information. Certain applications receive accelerated review if the sponsor can demonstrate that there is an urgent need for the drug. An example is the case where there is no other drug in that therapeutic category, and the disease condition has serious effects on human health. For applications that are submitted for accelerated review, the efficacy protocol may be done earlier in the development program (not as a phase 3 study). The efficacy protocol for such a study will be reviewed under SPA, no matter in what phase it is done.

The SPA is only available if the sponsor has had an EOP2. In the case of an accelerated review, the efficacy study may be a phase 2 study, as mentioned above. In such a case, the sponsor should request an end of phase 1 meeting. Prior to requesting an SPA, the sponsor should hold a pre-meeting with the FDA to discuss the proposed trial and the regulatory issues. This is done so that the FDA will be familiar with the study when the formal request and documentation are received. Since the FDA would like notice of an SPA request, for planning purposes, this notification may be given verbally at the pre-meeting or the company may send an email after the meeting, giving notice that they intend to file a request for an SPA.

The next step is the formal request for the SPA which is submitted referencing the company's IND, so that the study protocol becomes part of the IND. The request, together with the submission of materials for FDA review, must be made at least 90 days before the proposed start of the trial. The protocol and statistical analysis plan must be complete. Apart from clinical studies, animal carcinogenicity protocols and stability protocols may be submitted for review. Typically, the latter are significantly different from standard stability protocols, or raises specific questions not ordinarily encountered or not addressed in the FDA's guidance for conducting stability studies.

The sponsor should submit specific questions, for FDA response, regarding unusual features of the protocol. These may include how efficacy and safety are determined, the data analysis plan, and the potential limitations of the proposed study. The FDA will undertake a summary review to decide if the protocol meets the requirements for FDA review. If the FDA agrees to review the protocol, the review will be focused on the aspects of the protocol that are related to the questions posed by the company. It will not be a line-by-line review of the entire protocol.

The outcome of this review is the issuance of an SPA letter which will be sent to the sponsor within 45 days of receipt of the submission. This letter includes the areas of agreement, and those of non-agreement, with the company's contentions and will also contain comments from the review team. Since it is the FDA's intention not to delay studies, they will attempt to resolve issues, prior to the end of the 45-day period, by communicating with the sponsor regarding problems that they see. If the sponsor responds in a timely manner, their comments may be incorporated into the final decision. However, no additional questions or data may be added during this correspondence. If the company receives SPA agreement, it means that the FDA agrees with the opinions and the views presented by the company in their document concerning aspects of the study. It does not mean that the FDA has thoroughly reviewed the protocol and agrees with every element of it.

If a company receives a non-agreement letter, the company could request a meeting to discuss the non-agreement when any remaining issues will be discussed. If the issues are resolved, there could be SPA agreement resulting from such a meeting. The company may also decide not to initiate the trial and to respond in writing to address the FDA's concerns. The FDA will consider this documentation to be a resubmission. The company may, alternatively, decide to initiate the trial without SPA agreement. In this case, the company risks possible rejection when the final application (NDA) is submitted. However, it is also possible that the outcome will be favorable, that is, upon reviewing the completed study data, the FDA is in agreement with the company's contentions.

It is not a requirement that a sponsor participate in an SPA. The company may decide that they are comfortable undertaking the study, even if it is complex. However, an SPA is advised (in cases where there are complex protocols) to provide a better chance that the FDA would agree with the company's design and general approach. An SPA cannot be requested for clinical trials that have already started.

Pre-NDA Meeting

The pre-NDA meeting is held before the submission of the NDA. Questions that may be asked are those pertaining to the submission of the NDA, such as the presentation of the data and details of the formatting of the document. In addition, questions regarding the acceptability of studies already completed may be asked. The results of partially completed clinical studies (phase 3b) may also be discussed, as well as how the remaining data should be presented to the FDA after NDA submission. Usually, stability studies are incomplete at the time of NDA submission and the submission of the remaining data may also be discussed.

The pre-NDA meeting is also intended to help with unresolved problems and to identify the pivotal studies relied upon to establish the effectiveness of the drug. It also helps regulators to become acquainted with the study and the nature of the data to be submitted for review in the NDA. A written request for the pre-NDA meeting must be sent with documentation which includes test results and supporting published literature. These have to be sent ahead of the meeting, together with the names of attendees and the specific questions that are to be addressed at the meeting.

NDA Submission

The NDA is submitted to the FDA at the conclusion of the clinical trials, although phase 3b studies may be ongoing. Sufficient information should be provided to give regulators a good idea of the history of the development of the drug product in question. Most often, by the time the company reaches this development stage, it would have a massive amount of data, including some studies that led to a dead end. While inclusion of all this data would be overwhelming and impractical, the applicant, nevertheless, must provide a succinct development history for the product including a synopsis of work performed that is not relied upon for NDA approval.

An NDA must be in a standard format referred to as the common technical document (CTD), a format that is also used by other regulatory agencies, such as the European agency. A new drug application, including all appendices (several of which contain extensive data), would usually consist of many volumes in printed format. When such a format was the norm and considering the number of copies that was required to be submitted, a paper submission could easily have run into more than a hundred volumes in total. An electronic format is, therefore, much easier to handle, and the FDA requires all NDAs (and several other submissions) to be electronic submissions. The Electronic Common Technical Document (eCTD) is the standard, accepted electronic format. Some of the more pertinent information to be submitted in this document includes:

- Chemistry, manufacturing, and controls.
- Non-clinical pharmacology and toxicology.
- Human pharmacokinetics and bioavailability.
- Microbiology (for anti-infective drugs).
- Clinical study design and data.
- Statistical evaluation of clinical data.
- Pediatric investigations, if any.
- Proposed labeling.
- Exclusivity request: *under certain circumstances the FDA gives the applicant the exclusive right to market the product without competition from other companies.*
- Certification that the required information pertaining to clinical trials, undertaken as part of the NDA, has been submitted to the National Clinical Trials Database maintained by the NIH.

Recap Questions

1. What is the purpose of an IND and why is it filed?
2. What is the purpose of a phase 1 study?
3. Name three of the important documents that are submitted to an IRB.
4. What are some of the topics discussed at an EOP2?
5. Name two types of study designs that can be used when a product is compared with a placebo.
6. What is a special protocol assessment?

FDA REVIEW AND APPROVAL

Upon receipt of an NDA, the FDA initially determines if the application is complete and acceptable for a full review. During this initial review period of two months, the FDA may have questions for the company. If these are answered in good time, the initial review may be completed within the allotted time, in which case the NDA is "filed" and given an application number. The detailed review commences when the application is filed and takes approximately 10 months. If the information is incomplete, or if questions were not satisfactorily answered by the company within the allotted time, the FDA can make a "refusal to file" action and the application will not be reviewed.

The electronic submission makes reviewing much easier since the submission will be reviewed by many people at the FDA. Each person will review only the section of the application relevant to the reviewer's area of specialization. The reviewing section of the FDA may use an internal advisory committee to review specific aspects of the application. In addition, the FDA may use an outside advisory committee, constituted of professionals in the field of use of the proposed product, to provide input into any specific aspect of the application, for example, potential for drug abuse. The FDA could also make use of a citizen's petition, whereby citizens who do not have experience in drug product development or regulation can make comments on the application. For example, teachers may present their views on a drug that is to be utilized by children or nursing home staff may comment on a geriatric drug.

If the FDA is satisfied with the application documents provided to it, it will undertake a preapproval inspection of the manufacturing facility where the product is to be produced. The FDA inspectors arrive at the company without prior notice, and many companies have, in the past, been surprised by their visit. However, the approximate timing of the visit may be easily estimated. The FDA must make a decision, in terms of PDUFA, within a period of approximately 12 months from receipt of the NDA. If no negative communications were received from the FDA, company officials should expect, and be prepared for, a preapproval inspection from about 10 months after the submission of the NDA. In terms of PDUFA V (enacted under FDASIA), there is a greater transparency regarding the FDA review process. The FDA is required to communicate with the company mid-cycle and late cycle and, therefore, the company ought to have an even better indication of when to expect the inspection and surprises regarding preapproval inspections should be a thing of the past.

The purpose of the preapproval inspection is to evaluate the facility to determine whether the product can be made appropriately and as described in the NDA. The FDA determines if the equipment that was stated in the NDA for the manufacture of the batch, are indeed available and appear to be in good working order. The FDA will also review whether cGMP conditions are being met, including a review of relevant standard operating procedures.

During the preapproval inspection, the FDA will review many records of the company. For example, documents pertaining to the manufacture and testing of clinical supplies may be requested to enable the FDA inspectors to answer the following question: do the batch manufacturing records and analytical results agree with the summaries presented in the NDA? Copies of documents that are likely to be requested by the FDA inspectors should be maintained in an easily accessible filing system and stored separately, possibly in the meeting room. A very large number of documents will be generated in the course of the development of the product, and the FDA may request any of these documents for review during the inspection. The company should make prior arrangements for rapid retrieval of documents that have not been copied and stored separately for the meeting. Such arrangements may include the nomination of one person from each of several departments, including manufacturing, analytical, and clinical, who will be available to quickly retrieve requested documents.

After the inspection, the inspectors will report their findings to the FDA. Finally, the FDA will either issue an approval notice to the company or provide a "Complete Response Letter" (CRL). The latter is provided when the marketing application is not approvable in its current form. As the name implies, all FDA comments pertaining to the NDA are included in the latter document. When the FDA grants a marketing license, the approval will include the label language and the specific claims that the company is allowed to make. These claims would have been discussed and negotiated between the company and the FDA in the course of the NDA review. The company must confine its claims to the language approved by the FDA. This language is to be used in the labeling (this includes the package insert) and in any advertisements to the public, as well as statements that representatives of the company make to physicians and other prescribers. For example, if the approved claim language was, "… for the relief of mild to moderate pain," the company would not be entitled to advertise that the product "cures all pain," nor is a representative allowed to make such a statement when talking to prescribers.

POST-APPROVAL

The company may continue to conduct clinical studies postapproval, sometimes in terms of a commitment to FDA to undertake such a study, for example, a study in a special patient population. Since the drug may not have been assessed in all patient populations as part of the NDA, it may be in the company's interests to continue testing in other population groups. This would give the company more information and data about their product, whether or not this was part of a commitment to the FDA. These studies, both those that are a part of a commitment and those undertaken by choice, are referred to as phase 4 studies. The company would, usually, also have made a commitment to continue stability testing of the so-called "commitment batches" as described in Chapter 15, Dosage Form Stability.

Often, interactions with other drugs that the patient takes, or new adverse reactions are observed after approval. The question is sometimes asked: why were these issues not observed during the testing of the product and such information incorporated into the submitted data? The answer frequently lies in the number of subjects used for clinical testing. Typically, the product is tested in a few thousand patients in phase 3. Some adverse reactions occur in a very small percentage of the population and a serious adverse reaction may be rare, for example, it is seen in 1 in 100,000 patients. With a few thousand, or even tens of thousands, of patients exposed to the drug, such an adverse reaction may not be observed during clinical studies.

On the other hand, when the drug is sold to the general population, it may be used by millions of patients and it is, therefore, possible to observe rare adverse reactions. It is in the company's interest to continue to study the drug product and to be aware of the potential for adverse reactions, the mechanisms that cause these adverse reactions, and the patient populations that are at risk for their occurrence. Armed with such information, the company may be better able to advise how to avoid such adverse reactions, or to inform clinicians not to administer the product to specific patient populations. Information about adverse events observed with the use of drugs may be obtained from the FDA adverse event reporting system (FAERS) which is a part of the FDA's post marketing safety surveillance program. Reports on individual drugs may be obtained from http://www.fdable.com/

Companies are obliged to report safety formation that is reported to them by healthcare providers. This information is submitted via a safety reporting portal. Individual health providers as well as patients, each using a different form, may report adverse events at https://www.accessdata.fda.gov/scripts/medwatch/index.cfm?action=reporting.home.

Companies are also required to provide an annual report on each product that they manufacture. This document reports such information as the number of batches manufactured throughout the year, and any problems associated with the manufacturing, including minor deviations from the method of manufacture. In this report, adverse events that were reported to the company by practitioners or the public are also summarized. Death and life-threatening adverse events must be reported to the FDA immediately after the company learns of these events, apart from inclusion in the annual report.

The batch size of a product that is the subject of an NDA has to be stipulated in the application documents. Since the company cannot accurately predict how much product they will sell (and therefore the appropriate batch size), they frequently stipulate two batch sizes. Suppose the sizes were 500,000 tablets and 1 million tablets. For each of these batch sizes they would describe the manufacturing process and name the equipment to be used. If alternate equipment is used for any step because of the batch size difference, this has also to be stipulated. Data will have to be provided to demonstrate the equivalence of the batches, despite the different equipment used for one particular step of the manufacturing process, as dictated by batch size. An example of such a situation is the blending of the powders prior to tableting. A different blender may be used for the large batch, compared to the smaller batch. Apart from this type of difference, which is mentioned upfront in the application, from time-to-time changes may be necessary for various reasons, some of them unforeseen. The regulatory environment for handling such changes is complex. Some very minor changes, as alluded to above, can be undertaken by the company and simply reported in the annual report. In respect of other changes, the FDA has to be notified before the change is made. The rules governing changes are contained in a voluminous document, the Scale Up and Post-Approval Changes (SUPAC) guidelines. This document also covers changes that may be needed due to a change in the batch size ("scale up"), for example, if a batch size of 2 million tablets was needed, due to increased sales, in the example given above in which a maximum batch size of 1 million tablets was mentioned in the NDA.

OTHER ACTIONS THAT FDA MAY TAKE

Apart from their role in pre-approval inspections, FDA inspectors also conduct regularly scheduled inspections at pharmaceutical manufacturing companies. After any inspection, the FDA can issue Form 483 (observations) to the company. This is the mildest form of response from the FDA. For more serious GMP, or other violations, the FDA can also issue warning letters, seize products, seek a civil injunction on sales of a particular product, block imports of drugs, or pursue criminal liability against the company or individual employees.

Suppose that serious GMP or other violations have occurred at a company and were documented in Form 483s and warning letters, etc. Suppose, also, that the company has not responded satisfactorily to the FDA and these violations are ongoing. Under these circumstances, the company may be placed under a consent decree which is a formal arrangement, agreed to in a court of law, in terms of which the company undertakes to remedy the systemic problems resulting in continued GMP, or other, violations. The company may be required to undertake to stop research on new products, to appoint a third party to perform its QA functions, or to have a third-party monitor certain functions undertaken at the company.

A consent decree is a very serious step and may be applied in addition to having the company pay a fine. However, it allows the company to remain in business, as long as the company complies with the consent decree. While these measures appear drastic, they are better than the FDA shutting the company down. Some large companies, including multinationals, have been in consent decree. The FDA also has a bioresearch monitoring program which conducts on-site inspections of clinical studies performed in support of marketing applications. Their function is to check for adherence to good clinical practice (GCP) guidelines.

Recap Questions

1. How long does the FDA take to review an NDA?
2. What is the next step in the approval process after the review of an NDA?
3. What action does the FDA take if an NDA is not approvable?

4. Does a company stop all clinical research on the drug product upon the approval of its NDA? Explain.

5. If a pharmacist notes adverse reactions of a drug that are not mentioned in the literature, how could this pharmacist make the information known to other medical personnel?

6. What is the mildest action the FDA inspectors can take after visiting a company and finding items that needed improvement?

7. What is the strongest action that the FDA can take against a company?

8. As a clinical pharmacist, you have seen Mr. Smith for several years. He feels that the potency of the medication he receives varies each time he collects his medication for a chronic ailment. He appears to know that the FDA must approve all drugs before they can be sold but wonders how much control the FDA has on production thereafter. He thinks companies are left to do as they please after product approval, resulting in the variable doses he believes he is receiving. What would you tell Mr. Smith? Ensure that your explanation is in layman's terminology.

ABBREVIATED NEW DRUG APPLICATION

An abbreviated new drug application (ANDA) is submitted to request approval to market a generic product. Since the drug is well known and has been used extensively, knowledge of its toxicity and adverse effects are expected to also be well known. Therefore, the company wishing to file this application does not need to conduct toxicity and other preclinical studies that the innovator was required to complete. Hence, the 505(j) application, named for the section of the FDCA under which it falls, is shorter, or abbreviated. The application must, however, contain sufficient information to demonstrate that the proposed product is identical in active ingredient, dosage form, strength, route of administration, labeling, quality, performance characteristics, and intended use, to a previously approved product, the RLD. If this equivalence holds, the generic is expected to be similar with respect to therapeutic responses and adverse reactions. For this reason, if the generic product is demonstrated to be equivalent with respect to the above factors *and* achieves a blood level profile similar to that of the innovator product, the two products are said to be equivalent. Hence, a human bioequivalence study is the major feature of the human testing of a generic product; efficacy studies are not required.

The guidelines provide direction on how the study should be conducted, the number of subjects to be used, etc. In consideration of the fact that there is an acceptable level of variability in a manufactured product between batches and even between units (such as tablets or capsules) of the same batch, as well as variability in tests involving human subjects, an allowance for this variability must be built in to the test methods. Therefore,

for equivalence to the RLD, the guidelines allow the generic to be within 80% to 125% of the values of certain key pharmacokinetic parameters. This allowance has implications for the equivalence between two generics. Each of two generic products (A and B) may be declared equivalent to the innovator's product because they are in the desired 80% to 125% range. However, these generics may not be equivalent to each other. This can occur if generic A is on the lower end of the allowed equivalence range, while generic B is closer to the upper end of the range. This effect could be of major importance when switching between generics, each of which is equivalent to the branded product but may not be equivalent to each other.

An innovator company is required to specify the patents upon which the company depends for patent protection. The patent numbers and other details will be published by the FDA in the "Orange Book," upon approval of the drug. This name is a holdover from the time when this information was published in a physical book and distributed to interested parties. The cover of the book was orange and, although paper publication has been replaced with Internet information, the name has endured. The company may have several patents relating to a product, covering different attributes of the product. The company must choose those patents that are essential, for listing in the Orange Book. Therefore, a company wishing to manufacture a generic formulation has to look up the Orange Book to know which patents protect the product. Development of the generic, prior to the expiration of the Orange Book patents for the RLD, is allowed in terms of the Hatch-Waxman Amendment, as previously mentioned. It is important to realize that the research may be conducted but the product may not be offered for sale until after the expiration of the patents (and the approval of the product by the FDA). The generic manufacturer has to provide "certification" for these products, as explained below.

At the time of the ANDA, the manufacturer of a proposed generic must provide to the FDA a patent certification document which informs the FDA how the generic company claims to overcome the patent protection of the innovator company. One of the following four reasons is offered, with supporting evidence:

1. The innovator company has not submitted patent information to the FDA and therefore it is not published in the Orange Book.

2. The innovator's patent has expired.

3. The company states the date on which the innovator's patent(s) will expire, with an assurance that the marketing of the generic product will only commence after this date.

4. The patent is invalid, unenforceable, or will not be infringed by the proposed generic.

Each of these reasons is outlined in a separate paragraph of the code of federal regulations governing content and format of an ANDA (21 CFR 314.94). If the generic company, for example, references the fourth reason listed above, it is said to have provided "paragraph 4 certification." If the Orange Book patent covers the method of manufacture of the drug product and a generic manufacturer has found a way to produce a similar product in a different manner, then they may claim not to infringe the patent. If the generic company claims that the patent is invalid or unenforceable, they must offer an explanation for their contention.

When providing the FDA with patent certification, the generic company must simultaneously inform the innovator company (patent holder) of their intention to market a generic product, providing the same information regarding patents that they provided to the FDA. In their letter, they invite the innovator company to take legal action, if the company disagrees with the generic company's contention regarding the innovator's patents. Paragraph 4 certification is the most common type of certification.

505(B)2 APPLICATION

Since much of the rationale for the development of a drug product by the 505(b)2 process hinges on what constitutes a new drug, it is appropriate to consider the definition of a new drug at the outset of this description.

Definition of a New Drug

In terms of the FDA regulations, any of the following are considered a new drug:

- A new active pharmaceutical ingredient (API) or a *new excipient*
- A new condition of use: a new dose, a new method of administration (a new dosage form), a new route of administration or a new duration of administration, *as stated in the labeling*
- A new indication, *as stated in the labeling*
- A new combination of known drugs
- A new proportion of a previously used combination

Bullets 2 and 3 mention "as stated in the labeling." This statement differentiates a prescriber (usually a physician) ordering a new use of an existing drug *for a specific patient*, and a pharmaceutical manufacturer providing dosing instructions *for all users*. The pharmaceutical manufacturing company conducts studies to show the benefits (and lack of unacceptable adverse reactions) of the prescribed method of administration (dose, frequency, etc.,) and the FDA grants approval for such use after considering the evidence. This data-driven method of use is then applicable to all users of the drug. Many physicians are likely to prescribe, and potentially millions of patients eventually will use, the drug product in this manner. Nevertheless, a physician may instruct individual patients to take the medication in a manner that is different from the label directions (different dose, frequency, etc.) or even for a different indication relative to that stated in the prescribing information. In this case, the physician prescribes the medication for a specific patient's condition and circumstances.

The NDA and the ANDA may be considered extremes, with respect to marketing applications, since the former relates to a new API that has not previously been used as a drug product, and the latter refers to a generic of an existing drug product. The 505(b)2 application, on the other hand, may be considered in between these two extremes. It is so named because of the section of the FDCA which provides the legal authority for its development. It describes a new drug product that contains a known drug or API, which has previously been marketed for human consumption. In spite of the latter, it is considered a new drug product. This apparent contradiction can be explained by examples, making reference to the appropriate section of the definition of a new drug.

Suppose that drug X, in the form of a 20-mg oral (swallowed) tablet, has previously been available for the relief of pain. The following hypothetical examples would constitute new drug products and be eligible for registration under the 505(b)2 mechanism (the reasons, in each case, for considering the formulation a new drug are given in parentheses):

a. 20 mg of drug X in an orally disintegrating tablet (a new method of administration or new dosage form)
b. 10 mg of drug X taken as a new sublingual tablet formulation (a new dosage form, a new route of drug administration, and a new dose)
c. 20 mg of drug X taken as a conventional tablet for mild sedation prior to dental treatment (a new therapeutic indication)
d. 20 mg of drug X combined with 200 mg of ibuprofen (a new combination of known drugs)

The major differences between an ANDA product and a 505(b)2 product are the following:

a. The 505(b)2 product is a new drug product and may be subject to three years exclusivity. In fact, the application is an NDA, simply falling under a different subsection of the NDA requirements. For this reason, these products are sometimes referred to as 505(b)2 NDA products.
b. Safety and effectiveness data for the application may be obtained in part from published literature. The extent to which the applicant may do this depends on the product in question and, also, the route of administration since a different route of administration may display different adverse events and efficacy.

To illustrate the proviso made under point b above, the following hypothetical examples are given. Suppose that a new suppository formulation is being developed for use as a treatment for nausea at the same dose as a previously marketed nausea treatment presented as a swallowed tablet. This is a new route of administration for the same indication as the innovator product. Equivalent pharmacokinetic data would indicate that the new product and the innovator's product have equivalent efficacy and safety. Published literature may be provided by the 505(b)2 applicant in support of efficacy and safety. It is important to understand, in this case, that the FDA is not approving a product without efficacy and safety data. This data is *provided* in terms of the published literature since the new product is connected to this data via the equivalent pharmacokinetic data.

Legislation expressly permits the FDA, for the purpose of approval under 505(b)2, to rely on data not obtained by the applicant, or on behalf of the applicant. An example of the latter is a contract research organization or university conducting research for the applicant. This provision in the law promotes innovation since there is no repetition of studies for which data is already available. In this case, any adverse events at the site of administration, and in the tissues through which the drug is absorbed (rectal tissues), may still be required by the FDA and would have to be experimentally determined by the company.

On the other hand, if the drug is being used for a new indication, phase 3 clinical studies must be performed to determine efficacy. This was the case with the first fentanyl oral transmucosal dosage form that was developed for breakthrough cancer pain (at this time, there were fentanyl products for anesthesia and long-acting transdermal pain medication). The company had to demonstrate that the product provided relief of breakthrough pain in cancer patients. For those 505(b)2 applications that require clinical studies, three years exclusivity is usually granted by the FDA upon product approval.

Since the 505(b)2 product involves a new drug application, similar meetings as described for NDAs may be requested. This includes the pre-IND meeting which is an extremely useful meeting to have in order to reach consensus with the FDA regarding which literature data the company may rely upon, and which data the company must obtain by laboratory or clinical studies. Since the contemplated product would bear some similarity to an existing, marketed product, patent certification is also required, that is, the sponsor must certify that the product does not infringe the patents of an existing product that utilizes the same drug substance, or they may provide one of the other certifications mentioned under ANDA above.

FEES

Historically, the FDA has been understaffed and the review of applications has, consequently, been slow. In 1992, PDUFA was signed into law. It provided for NDAs to be reviewed in a defined, short period in exchange for a fee. The PDUFA fees allow the FDA to employ additional staff and to complete reviews in a shorter time. In terms of PDUFA, the FDA commits to providing a response to NDAs within the time frames previously mentioned, that is, two months for the preliminary review to decide whether the application will be registered, and then 10 months for the actual review (90% of reviews completed in 10 months). Therefore, applicants can expect to receive a final action from the FDA within approximately 12 to 14 months from the date of submission.

Sometimes a provision is made in law for a certain period after which the provision must be renewed to prevent it "sun setting," and this was the case with the PDUFA provisions which have been renewed every five years. Renewal occurred with the signing of the Food and Drug Administration Reauthorization Act (FDARA) on August 18, 2017, which included a reauthorization of PDUFA until September 2022 and a further renewal, for fiscal years 2023 to 2027, was signed into law by President Biden on 30 September 2022. The NDA fee for an application with clinical studies is approximately $3.2 million, whereas an application without clinical studies is approximately $1.6 million. In this context, "clinical studies" does not include human bioavailability or bioequivalence studies. Applications for orphan drugs, that is, drugs for rare diseases that have been granted orphan drug status in terms of legislation, are exempt from the application fee. Also exempt from the application fee are 505(b)2 applications for certain positron emission tomography (PET)

drugs, in which case the applicant must waive its rights to market exclusivity to which it may be entitled under the act.

The establishment fee is paid by each pharmaceutical company that either has a human drug application pending at the FDA, or that manufactures one or more pharmaceutical products for human use. Each company pays one establishment fee of approximately $500,000 annually. In addition, companies pay a product fee of approximately $100,000 annually for each drug listed in the Orange Book (with some exceptions).

It is possible to qualify for a reduced fee or a complete waiver in terms of FDARA. These provisions are in place to promote innovation and may occur under the following circumstances:

- The product is important for public health, for example, a vaccine that is developed to curb the spread of a serious infectious disease.
- An innovative product or technology is contemplated for which the fee would be a barrier to a company with limited resources.
- The fee exceeds the total costs that the FDA would incur in reviewing the application.

If the company is a small business (less than 500 employees), the application fee for the first marketing application submitted is waived in full. This is for the first application only and the full fees, as noted above, will have to be paid for all subsequent applications. This waiver applies to the application fee only. There are no waivers for small businesses in respect of the establishment fee and the product fee.

Analogous to PDAFU is GADUFA which deals with generic drugs. President Biden also signed GADUFA III[1] into law on September 30, 2022.

Recap Questions

1. What does the acronym, ANDA stand for?
2. What is the major difference between an ANDA and an NDA?
3. What is the "Orange Book"?
4. In which way is a 505(b)2 application different from other NDAs?
5. How do application fees for a product that does not need clinical studies differ from the fee for one that requires these studies?
6. In which way is a new, small pharmaceutical company given some financial relief and the opportunity to develop its first product?

SUMMARY POINTS

- The history of the regulation of drug marketing is outlined from a state of practically zero control, to control of labeling, then safety, to the later requirement for evidence of efficacy.

- Presently there are more than 200 laws covering all aspects of the development and marketing of drug products.
- The steps toward developing a new drug application are described including:
  - The IND and IRB applications (and the documentary and other requirements for each)
  - Phases 1, 2, and 3 study outlines; their purpose and information to be derived from the results
  - The most significant meetings between the applicant and the FDA
  - The preparation and submission of the NDA
- The FDA conducts a detailed review before approval and may conduct a pre-approval inspection to verify information provided, inspect equipment, and SOPs and other documents.
- Post-approval requirements include phase 4 studies and ongoing stability studies; there are post-approval reporting requirements, including those related to SUPAC.
- The FDA may take actions ranging from the issuing of Form 483s to facilitating court-ordered consent decrees and recommending criminal action.
- The ANDA is an abbreviated and simplified application pertaining to generic drugs.
- The 505(b)2 application is for new drugs, as defined in the legislation, but the application process is less onerous than the NDA and more complex than the ANDA; an exclusivity period may be applicable.
- Fees that the FDA may charge are mentioned as are reductions and exemptions to promote innovation.

What do you think?

1. The number of new excipients coming to market is very few. Why do you think that is the case?
2. If the Shirley Amendment of 1912 prohibited the labeling of medicines with false claims, why was it eliminated in 1938?
3. What provisions are there in the law to ensure that participants in a clinical study are treated fairly?

4. Dr. Smith has 20-years experience as a physician and his colleagues consider him to be one of the best in his field. Explain why an investigators' brochure needs to be provided to Dr. Smith to read before he participates in a clinical study.
5. If plans for phase 3 testing of the drug are discussed with the FDA during the EOP2 meeting, why is there a special protocol assessment to discuss phase 3 studies?
6. Why is it necessary for the FDA to do a pre-approval inspection?
7. Propofol is an anesthetic. If a low dose of this drug was suggested for use as a sleep aid, and *it was properly researched*, what type of application, containing appropriate supporting data, would be made to the FDA to market this product?
8. Two manufacturers wish to market products containing bupropion. In each of the cases below, state what type of marketing application would be made to the FDA:
   a. Company A wants to market 100-mg-immediate-release tablets of this drug for depression.
   b. Company B wants to market this drug for weight loss.

REFERENCE

1. https://www.fda.gov/industry/generic-drug-user-fee-amendments/gdufa-iii-reauthorization. Accessed October 8, 2022.

BIBLIOGRAPHY

https://www.fda.gov/drugs/developmentapprovalprocess/howdrugsaredeveloped andapproved/ucm209647.htm. Accessed September 3, 2017.

https://www.fda.gov/AboutFDA/WhatWeDo/History/Milestones/ucm128305.htm. Accessed September 4, 2017.

https://www.fda.gov/forindustry/userfees/prescriptiondruguserfee/default.htm. Accessed September 6, 2017.

https://www.fda.gov/downloads/Drugs/Guidances/ucm079345.pdf. Accessed September 7, 2017.

https://www.fda.gov/downloads/drugs/guidancecomplianceregulatoryinformation/guidances/ucm498793.pdf. Accessed September 9, 2017.

https://www.fda.gov/industry/prescription-drug-user-fee-amendments/pdufa-vii-fiscal-years-2023-2027. Accessed October 8, 2022.

Pulmonary Drug Delivery

19

PREVIEW

- Two common conditions that can be treated by pulmonary delivery are asthma and chronic obstructive pulmonary disease
- The pressurized metered-dose inhaler has been the mainstay of treatment since the 1950s
- The lung has a large surface area and a very good blood supply, making efficient absorption possible
- Dry powder inhalers produced in the 1990s—required the development of advanced particle technology
- Particle size is important for the delivery of the drug to the correct part of the lung
- A research trends to deliver systemic drugs by inhalation

INTRODUCTION

Inhaled therapies have existed for at least 5000 years, although it is probable that there was no mechanism to deliver accurate doses of the drug. Modern drug therapy via the lungs started with nebulizers which dispersed fine droplets of drug solution for inhalation. This was followed by the development of pressurized metered-dose inhalers (pMDIs), driven by propellants, in the 1950s and by propellant-free dry powder inhalers (DPIs) in the 1990s. The pMDI and the DPI attempted to provide an accurate dose to the patient. However, the accuracy of the device only ensures the accuracy of the dose delivered out of the device. The amount of drug reaching the desired sites of absorption is an entirely different matter, influenced by many factors. These include the patient's ability to correctly use the mechanical device which requires manual dexterity. In addition, the coordination of manual action with breathing is required in the case of pMDIs. Some young children and geriatrics may lack the coordination required. A frequently encountered problem that is beyond the patient's conscious control is the inability to forcefully breathe in. Forceful inhalation is required to draw the medication deep into the lungs but many patients are unable to exert sufficient inspiratory force. The problem is especially relevant to DPI which requires more forceful inhalation than pMDI. The forceful inhalation is needed to liberate the drug particles. Most patients using pulmonary drug delivery, do so as a treatment, or prophylaxis, of asthma and chronic obstructive pulmonary disease (COPD) and the most common drug categories are bronchodilators and corticosteroids. The bronchodilators help to relieve wheezing or bronchoconstriction whereas the corticosteroids reduce inflammation in the bronchi and bronchioles.

In some of these patients, the lung function may be severely compromised, resulting in the low force of inspiration mentioned.

Many active older children and adults, who take inhaled medication prophylactically, may not invest the time and attention to taking their medication correctly. Such medication is usually taken once or twice a day, every day, and attention to detail may fall off over time. Considering these factors, an accurate dose may be delivered to the site of action less frequently than desired. Many newer devices have been developed, in recent years, in an attempt to minimize this problem. Such devices have become more user-friendly by reducing the extent of coordination required between inspiration and a manual action by the patient, and by requiring less forceful inspiration to correctly administer a dose. During the discussion of the mechanisms by which inhalers work, it will become clear why more forceful inspiration is required for DPIs.

LUNG DEPOSITION

As alluded to in the introduction, the correct deposition of an inhaled drug in the lungs is vitally important for appropriate pharmacological action. The factors affecting lung deposition are:

1. The physicochemical properties of the aerosolized droplets or particles containing the drug.
2. The mechanical aspects of the delivery device.
3. Physiological and anatomical considerations associated with the lungs.

Physicochemical Factors

The size of inhaled particles is very important for delivery of the drug to the correct part of the lungs. Particles having a diameter approximately in the 1- to 5-μm range will reach the correct parts of the lung where they are needed for bronchodilation or an anti-inflammatory effect on the lung mucosa. As mentioned in Chapter 5, Pharmaceutical Powders, the solid particles encountered in pharmaceutical processing have an irregular shape. For this reason, their size may not be accurately described by one unique measurement, such as the diameter or radius, as is the case for spherical particles. The concept of equivalent diameters was introduced in Chapter 5. For example, the Coulter counter method of particle size analysis gives the diameter of a sphere that is equivalent in volume to the irregular particle being measured. If an irregular particle, in a specific case, is said to have a diameter of 5 μm when measured by this method, it means that the irregular particle displaced the same amount of liquid that a spherical particle with a diameter of 5 μm displaces, when both particles are submerged in a liquid. On the other hand, when a particle measured by the HIAC light obscuration method is said to have a diameter of 5 μm, it means that the irregular particle has the same cross-sectional area as a spherical particle with a diameter of 5 μm. HIAC Products is the company name intended to convey the image of "hi(gh) accuracy". For lung delivery, another equivalent size is important, as explained below.

Since inhaled particles must settle on lung tissues, the terminal settling velocity is important and particles are described by their aerodynamic properties as an indication of the settling velocity. The aerodynamic diameter is the diameter of a spherical particle of unit density (density = 1 g/cm³) which settles at the same settling velocity as the irregular particle under consideration. If an irregular particle (such as one intended for pulmonary delivery) has an aerodynamic diameter of 5 μm, it means that its terminal settling velocity is equivalent to that of a 5-μm spherical particle with a density of 1 g/cm³. In this case, the settling behavior is used to find an equivalent, although the irregular particle may have a different size when measured directly, by a microscopic technique, for example.

An adaptation of Stokes' equation is used to determine settling velocity. To accommodate deviations from the spherical shape, shape factors are included in the equation. The equation also contains slip correction factors. These factors make the equation complex. However, when the shape is very similar to a spherical shape, the particle may be approximated with a sphere and the shape factors may be eliminated from the equation. The slip factors are relevant to particles less than 1 μm in diameter. For larger particles, for example, 2 to 5 μm, the slip factors may also be eliminated. When this is done, the resulting equation is very simple [Eq. 19-1].

$$D_{ae} = D_v \times \rho_P^{0.5} \qquad (19\text{-}1)$$

Where D_{ae} = aerodynamic diameter

D_v = volume equivalent diameter

ρ_P = density of particle

This equation states that the aerodynamic diameter is equal to the diameter of the particle determined by a method that gives an equivalent volume, such as the Coulter counter method, multiplied by the square root of the density of the powder. The Coulter counter can be used to easily determine the volume-equivalent diameter and using Eq. (19-1), this diameter can be converted to the aerodynamic diameter. However, lung deposition can be more complex. The size factor is complicated by the fact that solid particles may expand in high-humidity environments. In addition, very small particles are characterized by having a significant fraction in the submicron size range. Particles in the size range of 0.5 to 1 μm are subject to Brownian motion. If such particles land on the mucosa, Brownian motion may, eventually, cause them to diffuse into the mucosa and be absorbed. However, if they do not land on the mucosa, the alternate disposition of these very small particles is to stay afloat in the air and to be simply exhaled.[1] Therefore, aerosols with a large proportion of very small particles will not give good lung deposition since some of the sub-micron particles will be exhaled and be of no pharmacological value.

On the other hand, inhalation aerosol therapies are administered as liquid droplets, with the drug dissolved or dispersed in an organic liquid. In the dispersed phase, the individual droplets constituting the fine mist lose some of the solvent by evaporation. Therefore, the droplet size becomes progressively smaller with time and this also affects the area of deposition within the lungs.

Mechanical Aspects of the Delivery Device

The mechanical device provides fine particles or droplets for pulmonary absorption upon activation by the patient. The device controls the dose and, to some extent, the particle or droplet size of the released medication. In the case of inhaled solid particles, they are provided in a device or inhaler as small drug particles adsorbed onto larger carrier particles, frequently lactose. Upon forceful inspiration, the drug and the lactose are separated. The larger lactose particles are largely left within the device whereas the finer drug particles can be inhaled. The device, by design, creates turbulence on inspiration which helps with the separation of the carrier and the drug. A higher force of inspiration positively affects the ease of separation, while a larger adhesive force between the drug and the carrier negatively impacts separation. The efficiency with which the device helps to separate the drug from the carrier may also affect deposition efficiency. On the other hand, liquid droplets released from a device have a range of droplet sizes, the largest of which are typically too large for correct deposition. During transit from the device to the patient's lungs, the droplet size gradually decreases, due to evaporation of some of the propellant. As a result, some droplets become sufficiently small for transfer to the bronchioles. If the fraction of such droplets is very small, an insufficient proportion of the dose reaches this part of the lungs and the dose may be less effective than desired. The fraction of very fine droplets is determined by the functionality of the mechanical device.

Physiological and Anatomical Considerations

The lung may be considered a series of dividing tubes, with the alveolar sacs attached to the smallest tubules (Figure 19-1). The trachea divides into the main bronchi (the left main bronchus and the right main bronchus) and smaller bronchi, and then progressively into smaller bronchioles before reaching the alveolar tissue. This structure may be compared to a tree with a trunk and dividing branches that become progressively smaller. The trachea and bronchi have cartilage rings that provide support; the rings becoming more widely spaced in the smaller bronchi. The bronchioles do not have cartilage rings, but are supported by elastin and muscles. The bronchi secrete mucus whereas the bronchioles do not possess the glands that secrete mucus. The trachea has a diameter of 2 to 2.5 cm, whereas the bronchioles have a diameter of approximately 0.2 to 0.5 mm. There are approximately 23 branches from the trachea until the alveoli are

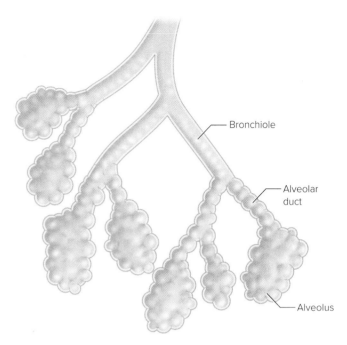

FIGURE 19-2 **Branches of the bronchial tree.**

reached (Figure 19-2). The last few subdivisions of the bronchioles are as follows: terminal bronchioles, respiratory bronchioles, and alveolar ducts. All parts of the tubular system up to the terminal bronchioles are described as being "conducting," that is, their main purpose is to conduct air through the system. Distal to the terminal bronchiole, all tubules show the presence of alveoli, that is, they are involved in gaseous exchange. There are a few alveoli in the respiratory bronchiole and more in the alveolar duct. At the end of the latter, is an alveolar sac containing the alveoli. The velocity of air varies in each of these parts of the lung, being fastest in the trachea and main bronchi, and becoming progressively slower further down the bronchial tree.

Breathing parameters, such as the rate of breathing and the tidal volume, play a key role in the deposition of drugs in the lung. The tidal volume is the amount of air inhaled, in one breath, during normal breathing. These parameters vary with the individual, and also within the individual depending on lung function at a particular point in time. Lung deposition also varies with the level of effort that the patient makes when taking the medication. This effort can be diminished by the disease condition being treated. These factors play a role in the extent to which aerosolized particles (or droplets for the remainder of this section, unless "solid" particles are specifically mentioned) are deposited into the lungs of a particular patient and the part of the lungs that these particles reach.

In practice, the particles do not have a single size but there may be a range of sizes. Some particles will be deposited in the trachea and bronchi but it is desirable that particles also reach the bronchioles. For this pattern of pulmonary deposition, a significant portion of the particles should be in the 1- to 5-μm size range. Very large particles will be deposited in the mouth and throat; large particles will reach the trachea and not go beyond. Somewhat smaller particles will reach the bronchi, and still smaller particles, the bronchioles. Hence, anatomy dictates the region of the lungs in which particles of different sizes will

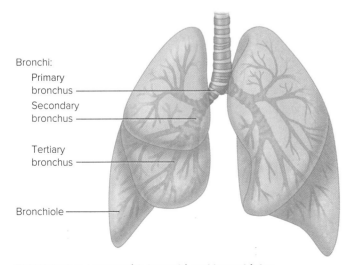

Bronchi:
  Primary bronchus
  Secondary bronchus
  Tertiary bronchus
Bronchiole

FIGURE 19-1 **Lungs with bronchi and bronchioles.**

be deposited. It also assumes that inspiration will be sufficiently deep to get the small particles to the bronchioles. The particles should be small but not too small. Particles smaller than the minimum of the size range may be deposited in the alveoli which is not desired for asthma and COPD drugs. These sub-micron particles may not be deposited at all, in any part of the lung. They may remain in air suspension for the full length of the inspiration and expiration time and, hence, will be exhaled.

In the airways, the relative humidity is approximately 99.5% at 37°C. This very high humidity causes the dispersed solid particles to expand, after administration, and deposition characteristics are altered because of the larger particle size. If in vitro testing, in a typical laboratory environment, demonstrated that a pulmonary delivery system contained particles in the ideal size range, the particles may not have this size in vivo. Therefore, the manufacturer must consider the size to which the particles are likely to expand, within the lung, when setting particle size specifications for in vitro testing of the product.

Recap Questions

1. Name the two types of inhalers that are currently used in medical practice. Provide the full names as well as acronyms.
2. Name one patient factor, one device factor, and one physicochemical factor that affect lung deposition.
3. Why is the particle size, measured in the lab, not the same as the particle size within the lung?

NEBULIZERS

A nebulizer is a device that turns a liquid into fine droplets (a mist) for inhalation (Figure 19-3). Nebulizers have different mechanisms to produce the fine mist. The mist is not steam

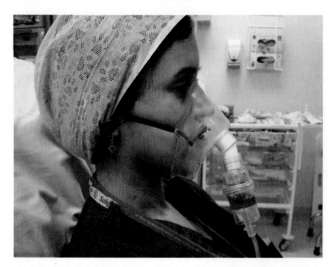

FIGURE 19-3 Nebulizer. (Reproduced, with permission, from Hadzic A. *Hadzic's Textbook of Regional Anesthesia and Acute Pain Management.* 2nd ed. New York, NY McGraw Hill; 2017.)

and, therefore, does not carry the risk of burning the patient. A mask is worn to direct the mist to the patient's mouth, or mouth and nose. The older nebulizers were large and noisy. The latter proved to be a distraction to children using the equipment. Newer equipment is smaller and far less noisy, and there are also small, battery-operated devices that are easily portable. The major advantage of the nebulizer is the fact that nebulized droplets are inspired during normal breathing (while the mask is in place). For patients who, for any reason, have difficulty taking deep inhalations, the nebulizer is a good option. There are different types of nebulizers, depending on the mechanism by which the mist is created. The jet nebulizer uses a jet of air to disrupt the liquid into fine droplets. The air is provided by a compressor. The ultrasonic nebulizer has a piezoelectric crystal that vibrates at high frequency to create fine droplets in the lower part of the apparatus. A small fan then blows the mist into the patient's mouth and nose. Alternatively, the patient's inspiration can be used to draw the droplets to the patient. In the vibrating mesh nebulizer, high-frequency vibrations of the mesh, while the liquid is flowing through it, create the fine droplets. The mesh has a large number of holes that are tapering, in profile, to assist in the formation of the mist.

The medication, diluted with water (if necessary), is added to the liquid container in the nebulizer. The mask is fitted to the tube that carries the mist from the nebulizer, and the nebulizer is turned on. Once the mist can be seen to be coming through the mask, the patient can be fitted with the mask. Typically, there is a strap to attach the mask to the patient's head. The nebulizer is a convenient way to administer medication, especially to children, for the prophylaxis and treatment of asthma and other conditions, such as cystic fibrosis, which have lung involvement. Children may have difficulty coordinating the use of a pMDI and the nebulizer is a very convenient alternative in such cases. The major disadvantage of the nebulizer is the fact that there is little control over droplet size. Hence, the percentage of very fine droplets that are capable of reaching the deep lungs is limited. Where deposition in the deep lungs is required, and the patient is capable of using an inhaler, the latter should be used.

Since surface tension is the force holding the liquid together and resisting the formation of droplets, a surfactant may be included in the liquid formulation. The surfactant lowers the surface tension and makes it easier to form fine droplets. The medication is often provided as a ready-to-use solution in single-dose containers. These solutions are usually sterile and do not contain preservatives. Multidose containers of nebulizer solution usually contain sufficient preservatives for the volume of solution in the bottle. When the medication has to be diluted, the pharmacist should provide clear instructions to the caregiver on the method of dilution, but solutions should not be pre-diluted at the pharmacy. This is because the diluted solution would not contain adequate preservatives to keep the solution free from microorganisms until used.

AEROSOLS

An aerosol is a dispersed system consisting, essentially, of an active, a liquid dispersion medium in which the active is dispersed, and a propellant. In some systems, the medium to disperse the active is the liquid propellant. The term *active*, used in the context of aerosols, means the ingredient that is to be emitted from the aerosol in dispersed form and which is the reason for the formulation of the aerosol. For inhalation aerosols, the active is a drug or active pharmaceutical ingredient (API) but, in the general context of aerosols, the active could be a perfume, an insect repellent, or a sunscreen ingredient. Several different types of aerosols are available commercially and they are differentiated in terms of their components and manufacturing procedures. Some of these are described below to provide a brief introduction to the general subject of pharmaceutical aerosols, and for comparison to the pMDI, used for pulmonary delivery.

The active, dispersion medium, and propellant are contained in an aerosol canister to which a dip tube, a valve, and an actuator are attached (Figure 19-4). The dip tube serves as the means of transporting the liquid from the canister to the valve. It extends from the liquid component containing the active to the valve. In the three-phase system shown in the figure, the dip tube extends to the concentrate, which is the active dissolved or dispersed in a liquid (frequently water). This is shown as the upper liquid layer in the figure, as most liquefied propellants have a high density and would be at the bottom of the canister. If a hydrocarbon is used as the propellant, it would be the top layer of liquid in such a system, because hydrocarbon propellants are less dense than water. When an aerosol is intended to be used in the inverted position, there is no need for a dip tube, and it is omitted. The valve stem then serves as the entry point for the liquid. The actuator depresses and opens the valve, allowing the pressurized contents to leave the canister. The top part of the actuator is the "button" that the user depresses to produce a spray, or other output, of the canister.

In some instances, the active is contained in a second liquid (as described above) whereas, in other cases, it is contained in the liquid phase of the propellant (Figure 19-4). The aerosol always contains a gaseous component (the propellant in the vapor state) which provides the pressure to expel the contents of the aerosol canister. If some of the propellant vapor is lost, an equivalent amount of the liquid propellant is converted to the vapor phase to maintain the vapor pressure. There is an equilibrium between the propellant in the liquid state and that in the vapor state. This equilibrium is maintained until most of the liquid propellant is exhausted, at which time there may be

insufficient propellant, in the liquid state, to replenish the gaseous propellant to maintain the initial vapor pressure.

An aerosol may be a two-phase or a three-phase system. In a two-phase system, the phases are the active dissolved or dispersed in liquid propellant, and the gaseous propellant. In a three-phase system, the phases are the liquid propellant, the gaseous propellant, and a second liquid containing the dissolved or dispersed active. This liquid is immiscible with the first liquid and together with the drug and other additives is known as "the concentrate." The concentrate may be water-based and contain co-solvents and surfactants to assist in solubilizing the active. The concentrate may also be an emulsion. When the active is in suspension, either in the liquid propellant or in the liquid concentrate, the output of the canister consists of droplets with active particles suspended in the droplets. When the drug is dissolved in the propellant, surfactants and co-solvents are usually added to this liquid phase. The surfactant may also lubricate the shaft of the valve to enable it to move up and down freely. Frequently, the co-solvent is ethanol which, apart from improving solubility, also contributes to the vapor pressure of the gaseous phase.

The output or product of the aerosol canister is dispersed in the gaseous propellant. The product is frequently fine liquid droplets but, by the use of special valve and actuator designs, the output could appear as a continuous stream of liquid (eg, the aerosol used to destroy a wasp's nest), a foam (shaving cream), fine droplets (hairspray), or a mist (deodorant). The concentrate used for shaving foam is an emulsion with the propellant in the internal phase. Upon depression of the actuator, the concentrate rises up the dip tube into an expansion chamber, present within the special valve developed for this purpose. The small volume of concentrate within the large chamber allows the liquefied propellant to expand and begin to form a foam. As it leaves the canister, the foam can be observed. It then expands further when exposed to the atmosphere which has a lower pressure than the expansion chamber. The same concentrate when used in a conventional valve-actuator system (with no allowance for expansion) produces a thin stream of emulsion which subsequently expands to a foam. Any non-emulsion liquid concentrate can be emitted as a stream of liquid, coarse droplets, a fine spray, or a mist, depending on the configuration of the valve. This includes the presence or absence of an expansion chamber and its size, and the size and configuration of the nozzle aperture (eg, round or semi-circular) in the actuator.

Pharmaceutical Aerosols Not for Pulmonary Delivery

Some examples of pharmaceutical aerosols that are not used for pulmonary delivery include nasal aerosols. These deliver corticosteroids, for example, to the nasal cavity for the control of allergic rhinitis. Beconase is a pMDI that delivers beclomethasone to the nasal mucosa. Other examples are rectal and vaginal foams, medicated topical aerosols, and cosmetic aerosols. Vaginal foams include contraceptive foams such as vaginal contraceptive foam (VCF) and Delfen foam, both of which contain the spermicide, nonoxynol-9. Vaginal cleansers in the form of

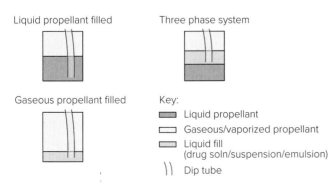

FIGURE 19-4 Aerosol Fill Types. A valve and an actuator are attached to the dip tube at the top, as a pre-assembly with the mounting cup, but are not shown in the figure for simplicity.

an aerosol foam may be considered cosmetic products. Uceris rectal foam contains 2 mg budesonide per dose. The foam is delivered using a fairly long applicator. The foam expands significantly after delivery and moves up the rectum, filling it and the sigmoidal colon, up to 40 cm from the anus. This aerosol is a convenient way to provide the medication needed for ulcerative colitis, especially in areas that are not close to the anus.

Olux topical foam contains clobetasol for the short-term treatment of dermatological conditions of the scalp and for non-scalp psoriasis. Eramaxin topical foam contains 20% urea and ammonium lactate and is used for removing hyperkeratotic skin in conditions such as psoriasis and calluses. Fabior foam (0.1% tazarotene, a retinoid) and Benzepro foam (9.8% benzoyl peroxide) are used as keratolytics in the treatment of acne. Evoclin foam is also used for acne but it contains an antibiotic, clindamycin 1%. Rogaine foam contains 5% minoxidil and is used for hair regrowth.

One of the first cosmetic aerosols to be developed was shaving foam, which was first produced in the 1950s; then followed hairspray, and then deodorants and antiperspirants in the 1960s. Later, pump sprays were used for hairspray and the aerosol canister, for this purpose, was used to a lesser extent. Perfumes were also popular in aerosol form, using glass containers instead of the aluminum aerosol canister. A plastic exterior coating was used to reduce the explosion risk (the plastic prevents the glass bottle from shattering). At present, pump sprays are more commonly used for perfumes than aerosols. Sunscreens are also provided in aerosol form but the FDA does not recommend this format. This is presumably because there is less control over the amount applied (some aerosol is lost to the atmosphere), and also the fact that there may be droplets of spray on the skin and not a continuous coating of sunscreen, which is needed for adequate sun protection. The extent to which a continuous coating is applied depends on the application procedure. In addition, there is atmospheric contamination.

Propellants

Propellants that may be used consist of chlorofluorocarbons (CFCs), hydrofluoroalkanes (HFAs), and alkanes such as butane, isobutane, and propane. Because the chlorine component of CFCs damages the ozone layer, these propellants should not be used except where there is no alternative for a medically necessary aerosol. In the place of CFCs, HFAs are used in modern aerosols. The alkanes are used in pharmaceutical aerosols for external use, such as in cosmetic applications. Since the output from an aerosol canister is intimately dependent on the propellant and the amount of pressure that it develops, the switch from CFCs was not a simple matter of replacing one propellant with another. Companies had to engage in reformulating their aerosol products to find a balance between ingredients, components such as valves, and the propellant to produce a desirable end product. Inert gases such as CO_2 and N_2 may also be used to fill aerosols.

To attain the required pressure for an aerosol, the formulator may have to combine two propellants, one with a low vapor pressure and another with a high vapor pressure. The vapor pressure of the resultant mixture is given by Raoult's law. This law states that the vapor pressure of a mixture of two ideal liquids that are totally miscible with each other is the sum of the individual values of a particular factor for each component of the mixture. This factor is the mole fraction times the vapor pressure of the pure liquid. This is represented in Eq. (19-2) below.

$$P = (X_A \times P_A^o) + (X_B \times P_B^o) \qquad (19\text{-}2)$$

Where P = total vapor pressure,

X = mole fraction,

P^o = vapor pressure of the pure liquid, and

A and B refer to the constituents of a two-component mixture.

Aerosol Filling Operations

Aerosol canisters may be filled by two basic types of fill processes which are dependent on the physical state of the propellant being filled: gas fill or liquefied gas fill. The filling process is dictated by the nature of the fill material and each process is described below.

Gas Fill

The simplest type of aerosol is one in which the active ingredient is dissolved or dispersed in a solvent and the resulting drug concentrate is filled into the canister; next, compressed gas is filled into the canister to serve as the propellant. The gas is filled into the aerosol canister from a separate container, where it is under pressure, but still in the gaseous state. This is different from the situation where so much pressure is applied to the gas that it liquefies.

The steps required to carry out this filling procedure are as follows. The product concentrate is placed into the container and the valve assembly is crimped into place. Crimping is performed as follows: the actuator, valve, housing, and dip tube are received at the assembly point as a unit (Figure 19-5). This is placed over the canister and a machine is used to squeeze the flange over the edge of the canister. The air is evacuated from the container, through the valve, by a vacuum pump so that a larger amount of propellant can be filled into the canister. The compressed gas is then transferred from a large steel cylinder into the aerosol canisters. This is done through a pressure-reducing valve attached to the gas cylinder because the pressure in the gas tank is very high. The pressure of the gas coming from the gas tank is higher than the pressure in the aerosol canister (in spite of the pressure reduction). Therefore, it pushes the valve of the aerosol canister open. The gas, then flows from the steel cylinder, into the canister. When the pressure within the aerosol canister is equal to the delivery pressure (set on the pressure-reducing valve), the aerosol valve is restored to the closed position, and the gas flow stops.

Gases like carbon dioxide (CO_2) and nitrous oxide (N_2O) are slightly soluble in the product concentrate, which is usually water. Therefore, the container is manually, or mechanically, shaken toward the end of the filling operation. This distributes the gas with the concentrate, allowing more of the gas to dissolve in the liquid. Dissolution of gas into the liquid reduces some of the gas in the headspace and, consequently, the pressure is reduced. This allows more of the propellant to be filled into the canister to achieve the desired pressure in the headspace. If these steps were not taken, the CO_2 and N_2O would dissolve in

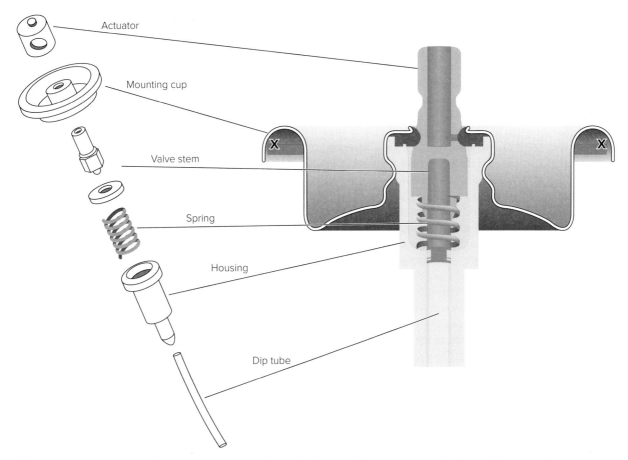

FIGURE 19-5 Actuator, valve, and dip tube pre-assembly and crimping. The areas marked with an X (around circumference) are crimped into place over the lip of the aerosol can, using a crimping device that applies pressure.

the concentrate slowly over a period of time, and the pressure in the canister would be reduced, giving the user a lower-pressured aerosol.

Liquefied Gas Fill

It is possible to fill a liquefied propellant into the canister instead of a gas. The liquid is formed by converting the propellant gas into a liquid referred to as a "liquefied gas." Fluorinated hydrocarbon gases may be liquefied by cooling below their boiling point or by compressing the gas at room temperature, that is, without cooling. Obviously, a much higher pressure is needed to convert the gas to a liquid, than the pressure used to prepare pressurized gas to fill into a canister. There are two methods of liquefied gas filling which are described below. The features of each filling process are controlled by the way in which the gas was converted into a liquid.

Cold Filling. In the cold filling method, the propellant is cooled to −34.5°C to −40°C (−30°F to −40°F) in order to liquefy the propellant gas. The cooling system may be a mixture of dry ice and acetone or a more elaborate refrigeration system. When this filling method is used, the product concentrate and the aerosol canister must also be chilled to about the same temperature as the liquefied gas. If this step is not undertaken, the liquefied gas would vaporize rapidly after it is added to the canister. The actual filling procedure begins with the addition of a measured amount

of the chilled product concentrate to the cold aerosol container. Next, the liquefied gas is added by gravitational flow to the open container, that is, the valve is not crimped into place before this step. When sufficient propellant has been added, the valve assembly is inserted and crimped into place, as described before.

During the process of cold filling, the heavy vapors of the cold liquid propellant, arising from the liquid propellant in the partially filled canister, will normally displace the air in the container. In the process, some of the propellant vapors will also be lost. Only drug concentrates in organic solvents may be filled by this mechanism. Aqueous systems cannot be filled by this process because the water will turn to ice. However, even for nonaqueous systems, some moisture usually appears in the final product due to the condensation of atmospheric moisture within the cold containers while they are open.

Pressure Filling of Liquefied Gas. The liquefied gas is obtained by applying high pressure to the propellant gas. In this filling method, the product concentrate is quantitatively transferred to the aerosol container. The valve/actuator assembly is then crimped into place onto the canister, as previously described. The canister is then moved under a pressure burette. The point of attachment to the bottom of the pressure burette has a mechanism to depress and hold open the valve of the aerosol canister. When the valve is opened, the liquefied gas, under pressure, is metered through the valve stem. The propellant is allowed to enter the closed container under its own vapor pressure (through the valve). When the pressure in the container equals that in the burette, the propellant stops flowing. The development of a vapor pressure in the burette is explained below.

The burette, also known as a pressure burette, contains liquefied propellant in a tall cylinder. Some of the liquefied propellant in the burette is converted to gas as the filling room is at a significantly higher temperature. The gas rises to the top of the burette and, due to it being in a closed system, the gas is trapped at the top and exerts a pressure on the liquid beneath it.

If a higher pressure is required in the canister, in general, then additional propellant needs to be added to it. However, the point at which filling stops, as mentioned above, is when the pressure in the canister and the burette are equal. Therefore, to increase the pressure in the canister, the pressure in the burette must be increased. This can be done by adding compressed air or nitrogen to the burette. The added compressed gas rises to the top of the burette and increases the pressure on the liquefied propellant below it. The addition of a compressed gas achieves a higher pressure than is possible from the vapor pressure of the propellant alone. While this results in the original propellant being filled at a higher pressure, there may also be some trapped air, or nitrogen, in the aerosol package. Usually this can be ignored since it does not interfere with the quality or stability of the product. If it does, the air or nitrogen may be evacuated from the canister using a special apparatus.

After the container is filled with sufficient propellant, the valve actuator is tested for proper function. This spray testing also removes pure propellant from the dip tube prior to consumer use. Tests are also subsequently conducted to check for leaks. Pressure filling of liquefied gas is used for most pharmaceutical aerosols. It has two advantages over cold filling: there is less danger of moisture contamination of the product, and less propellant is lost in the process.

Recap Questions

1. What is the difference between a two-phase and a three-phase aerosol system?

2. How does the valve change the nature of the product from an aerosol?

3. What is the advantage of a rectal foam produced by an aerosol in the treatment of ulcerative colitis?

4. Name the propellant type that has, currently, largely been phased out, as well as the recommended replacement. In both cases provide the full name as well as the acronym.

5. In the gas filling process, what determines the endpoint of filling?

6. When CO_2 and NO_2 are used as propellants, why is the filling process interrupted to shake the canister?

7. During the cold filling process, why must the aerosol canister as well as the concentrate be cooled to the same temperature as the liquefied propellant?

PRESSURIZED METERED-DOSE INHALERS

The metered dose inhaler, a small handheld aerosol, contains the drug in suspension in a liquefied propellant, or a mixture of propellants. In a few instances, the drug is in solution in the liquefied propellant. Since the dosage form is pressurized, the descriptive term used for this device is a pMDI. It has been in use since the mid-1950s and was the first inhalation dosage form that was both convenient to use and provided a reasonably accurate dose. The first product was developed by Riker Laboratories and appeared to have been an epinephrine dosage form. It followed closely after the commercial production of cosmetic aerosols. The invention of a metering valve that could provide precise, and reproducible, doses was an essential prior development.

The propellant generates a high pressure within the canister and the material of which it is made must be able to withstand this pressure. Generally, aluminum is used and has the added advantages of being inert and light proof. The pMDI is used in the inverted position and, as such, a dip tube is not required. The system has two chambers, a main chamber and an auxiliary chamber. The latter has a volume of 25 μL to 100 μL (Figure 19-6). It has a special valve that operates as follows: when the chamber is open to the atmosphere (patient's mouth), the opening into the main chamber is closed, and vice versa.

When the inhaler is not in use, the outlet to the atmosphere is closed by the valve, and the valve between the main chamber and the auxiliary chamber is open. This allows the liquefied propellant containing the drug to enter the auxiliary chamber. The correct orientation for use of the pMDI is the inverted position relative to most other aerosols that have the canister at the bottom and the nozzle at the top. In the inverted position, it is the canister that is depressed to activate the inhaler. When the pMDI is held in this position, the pressure of the vapor is the force that drives the liquid into the auxiliary chamber, and gravity also assists with the filling. When the patient opens the valve to dispense a dose, by pressing on the canister, the auxiliary chamber is opened and the liquid propellant moves to the expansion chamber in the actuator, where expansion begins. The expanded vapor then leaves via a nozzle to the atmosphere/the patient's mouth. Due to the pressure difference, 3 to 5 atm within the canister, and 1 atm outside of the nozzle, the expansion of the gas is rapid. The gas carries the droplets (of liquified propellant, containing the drug) forward into the mouth, the oropharynx (back of the throat), and into the airways of the patient. The droplets become progressively smaller due to vaporization of some of their propellant content and, therefore, they are capable of reaching further into the bronchial tree.

The arrangement described above provides for the auxiliary chamber to be filled while the inhaler is not in use, and to be ready to deliver a dose when the patient depresses the canister. However, this assumes that the pMDI is stored in the correct orientation, as described above. In any other alignment, the liquid propellant will slowly drip out from the auxiliary chamber into the main chamber. For this reason, the first dose, after a

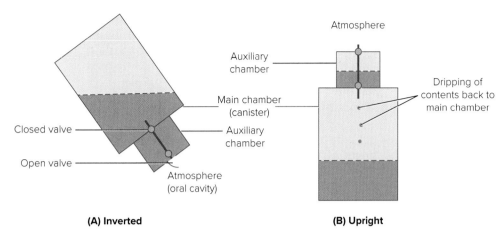

FIGURE 19-6 Metered dose inhaler. (A) Inverted position for administration and **(B)** upright position. Figure 19-6A shows that when one valve is open to the atmosphere (for administration) the second valve is closed to prevent continued filling of the auxiliary chamber. Figure 19-6B shows that there is a slow leak of contents from the auxiliary chamber to the main chamber even though both valves are closed. Hence, the need to prime if the inhaler has not been used for long.

long period of the inhaler not being used, is likely to be less than a full dose.

A surfactant is typically included in the formulation to prevent agglomeration of the drug particles. In consideration of the latter, the concentration of the drug in the propellant must also be kept low. The surfactant also lubricates the shaft of the valve. Evaporation of the propellant from residual droplets of suspension remaining on the nozzle results in precipitation of particles. The buildup of particles on the nozzle can block the aperture and reduce its effectiveness in delivering a dose.

CFC Versus HFA

In the past, all propellant-driven metered dose inhalers (pMDIs) contained CFCs. These compounds disturb the ozone layer, due to the release of chlorine, and are partly responsible for the increase in UV-related medical issues, such as skin cancer. Hence, there was a push to eliminate CFCs in medical devices. This has largely been successful in that many inhalers have been converted to HFA propellants. This was not simply a replacement of one propellant for another, since each exerts its own pressure and develops a unique spray pattern. Therefore, a great deal of research went into developing HFA aerosols that gave appropriate lung deposition. Where it is not possible to eliminate the CFC (eg, if adequate lung deposition could not be achieved) and the medication is vitally important for therapy, the FDA will waive the requirement. This is done on a case-by-case basis.

Upon the change over from CFC to HFA propellants, there were complaints from patients along the lines that the product "does not work." There were many factors that contributed to this incorrect perception. These included the fact that the taste and mouth feel of the new propellant was different from that of the old propellant. Over time, the acceptance of the new formulations by patients became widespread. In many instances, HFA is actually a better propellant than CFC. For example, upon vaporization, CFC becomes quite cold and the sensation of cold in the oropharynx had the effect of momentarily

stopping inspiration in some patients. This was known as the "Freon effect," which is not encountered with the use of HFA propellants. HFA also achieves droplets in the correct size range more easily. For this reason, the dose may be more effective than the equivalent CFC product. Some companies actually lowered the dose of their HFA product to make it equivalent to the old CFC product.

CFC damaged the ozone layer and was discontinued for this reason; but HFA is not without issues since it is a greenhouse gas. While HFA from inhalers probably has a small impact on global warming (relative to other sources of greenhouse gases), this source of contamination will probably also come under scrutiny at some time in the future.

Use of a Spacer

A major problem of all pMDIs is the fact that a significant proportion of droplets are large. When this fact is coupled with the speed at which the droplets travel, the result is a great deal of drug deposition in the mouth and oropharynx. The greater the droplet's speed, the higher the rate of impaction with these tissues. In addition, the spray may initially be very turbulent which causes deposition in the front part of the mouth. The use of a spacer between the aerosol and the patient's mouth (Figure 19-7) improves deposition to the lungs. The mouthpiece of the inhaler device fits into one end of the spacer, while the other end has a mouthpiece for the patient to use. Within the spacer the speed of the droplets is reduced, decreasing the tendency for deposition in the oropharynx. Size reduction of the droplets also occurs, by evaporation of the propellant. Reduced droplet size improves lung deposition. A further benefit of the spacer is the fact that coordination between depressing the canister and inhaling is far less critical than it is when no spacer is used.

A downside of the spacer is the fact that adsorption of drug particles on the wall of the spacer, due to static charge buildup, decreases the amount of drug available for inhalation. During continued use, the patient may see a buildup of particulate material on the wall of the spacer. Appropriate washing of the

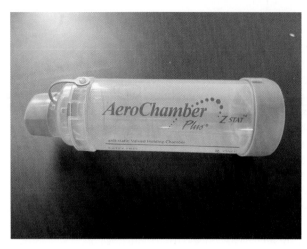 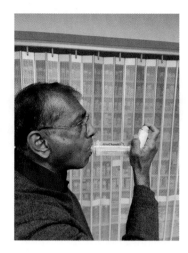

FIGURE 19-7 **Spacer for use with aerosol.**

spacer can reduce static and, consequently, the buildup of particles on the walls of the spacer. Reduced static and particle buildup is also observed in a metal spacer, available in Europe (Nebuchamber).[2] The first inhalers that were developed in the 1950s had significantly longer mouthpieces indicating, perhaps, that the issue was understood at that stage. Later, inhalers with shorter mouthpieces were developed, probably, for the convenience of being easily carried in the patient's pocket or purse.

If a patient has not obtained relief of bronchoconstriction, for whatever reason including poor administration technique, a second dose of a short-acting bronchodilator, such as albuterol, may be taken. An immediate response is not expected with corticosteroid therapy and with long-acting bronchodilators, as it is with short-acting bronchodilators. Because of the potential for overdosing, in the case of corticosteroids, long-acting bronchodilators, or combinations of these drugs, a second inhalation should not be taken when the adequacy of the first is in question. The fact that an inhalation dose may be inadequately administered due to poor technique or low inspiratory force, and that a second, compensatory dose is not advised, is a limitation of inhalation therapy. This is especially important as it applies to long-acting medication. A poorly administered dose of a long-acting medication represents sub-optimal therapy for 12 h, or more, under these circumstances.

Recap Questions

1. Name one major difference, apart from drug content, between a pMDI and other aerosols, such as a deodorant.
2. "CFC had problems and was withdrawn but HFA is the perfect propellant." Comment on this statement.
3. Why is a spacer used with a pMDI?
4. Why does poor inspiratory force lead to poor drug delivery with pMDI, and why is poor inspiration a likely factor with patients using pMDI?

DRY POWDER INHALERS

Devices that allow patients to inhale dry, micronized, solid particles distributed in air, for delivery of therapeutic substances to the lungs, are known as DPI. The DPI delivers dry particles, not a suspension of the drug particles in liquefied propellant droplets, as is the case with pMDI. To enhance the distinction from the latter, the devices for inhalation of powders are referred to as DPI since the powder does not become wet at any point. Fine particles (1-5 μm) are needed for deposition in the bronchioles. If smaller particles were provided, some could reach the alveoli and this is not desired for the treatment of asthma and COPD, the main uses of inhalation therapy at present.

In the development of the DPI device, consideration had to be given to the fact that particles in the required size range would clump due to the presence of high electrostatic forces. On the other hand, it would be difficult to package and handle individual low drug doses, such as 200 μg. Both of these issues are resolved by using special powder technology referred to as "ordered mixing." In this process, fine drug particles are mixed with the carrier, for example, lactose. The lactose particles are much larger than the drug particles and they contain active adsorption sites to which the fine drug particles adhere. There are a finite number of active sites per carrier particle of a specific size, and drug particles are mixed in a fixed proportion with the carrier particles, such as 6:1, so that the drug particles do not exceed the number of active sites (Figure 19-8). In this

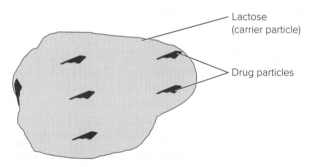

FIGURE 19-8 **Ordered mixture.** Drug particles adhere to a carrier particle in an approximately fixed ratio.

hypothetical example, six fine particles of the drug are mixed with one much larger lactose particle. As the powders are mixed, the fine drug particles adhere to the lactose particles entirely by physical forces; no chemical bond is involved. The physical forces involved are mainly those due to static and van der Waals forces. Since the particles are not held together by chemical bonds, their association can be disrupted using physical forces, such as rapid, turbulent agitation. The ordered mixture may also be referred to as an adhesive mixture, or an interactive mixture.

In ordered mixtures for pulmonary delivery, the adhesive forces should be strong enough to maintain the association between carrier and drug during storage and handling. When the drug is administered, the force of the inspired air should be strong enough to separate the drug particles from the carrier, taking into account, also, the turbulence created in the device. The inhalers are specially engineered to create turbulence for this purpose. The surface texture and other properties of the carrier affect the strength of the adhesive forces. Research is ongoing to develop carriers in which low adhesive forces develop when they interact with drug particles, so that the drug is easily released upon inspiration. The shape of the drug particle (apart from its physical size) affects its aerodynamic diameter. For example, elongated particles generally have a smaller aerodynamic diameter and are therefore more desirable for pulmonary delivery. The modifications to the carrier particle, as well as those to the drug particle properties, are referred to as particle engineering and this science plays a large role in the development of pulmonary drug delivery.

Keeping the above mechanisms in mind, patients are required to inhale forcefully from the beginning of inspiration, to inhale as deeply as possible, and for as long as possible. The forceful inspiration and high airflow rate within the inhaler create the turbulence to separate the fine drug particles from the carrier.

This is an essential step to create fine particles that are respirable. A negative effect of high airflow rates is to cause the rapidly moving powder particles to impact the mucosa of the mouth and that of the oropharynx. Therefore, such particles do not reach the deep lungs. In spite of this loss, it is still required that inspiration be forceful to separate carrier particles from drug particles in order to make the latter available for lung deposition. The device geometry helps to create turbulence within the device and it is this turbulence that is the prime factor in disassociating drug particles.

In some types of DPI, the drug is presented in capsules for insertion into the inhaler. Subsequent piercing of the capsules by pins makes the drug available. The turbulence in the device causes the capsule to spin which creates centrifugal force, causing the powder to be thrown outward and to exit the capsule through the pinholes. This action may further assist with the dissociation of drug and carrier particles. There are two types of powder inhalers, single dose inhalers and multidose inhalers and, in this description, the latter group is subdivided further into reservoir inhalers and non-reservoir inhalers (Mind Map 19-1).

Single-Dose DPI

In this type of device, individual doses are provided in capsules, in a separate container, usually packaged within a foil blister. The patient removes a capsule to insert into the device each time a dose is to be taken. At any one time, the device can only hold a single capsule or one dose. The device has a mechanism to make the powdered contents of the capsule available for inhalation. Upon forceful inspiration, the finer particles, referred to as the respirable fraction, are separated from the carrier particles and are ultimately transferred into the lungs. Just as for MDIs, the part of the lung that the particles reach depends on the particle size, with smaller particles reaching deeper into the lungs. The

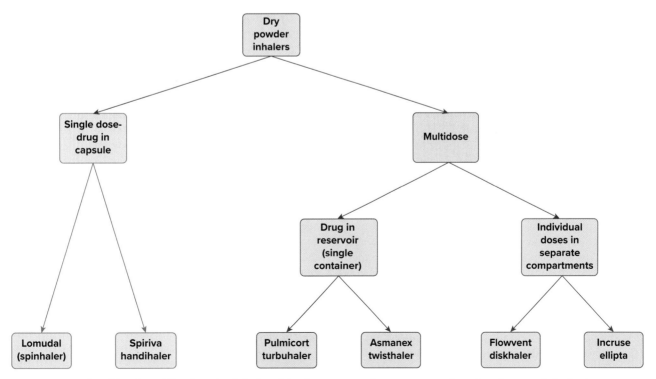

MIND MAP 19-1 Classification of Dry Powder Inhalers (The lowest row gives two examples of each type of device.)

majority of the respirable fraction should be deposited on the bronchi and bronchioles. Extremely small particles may remain suspended in the air and be exhaled, resulting in ineffective drug delivery.

The first inhalation product containing powder in a capsule was Lomudal, manufactured by Fisons plc, a British pharmaceutical company which is no longer in business. The capsules were inserted into a handheld device, the Spinhaler. Next, the patient or caregiver (many patients were children) exerted pressure on the buttons on the device. The mechanical pressure was transferred to pins to pierce the capsule. The next step was inhalation through the device which caused the capsule to spin. This allowed the drug, sodium cromoglycate, to leave the capsule through the pinholes, be separated from its carrier, and be inhaled by the patient. This product was used for the prophylaxis of asthma.

The Spiriva Handihaler device opens more-or-less in half for the patient to insert a capsule. The device functions in a similar manner to the Spinhaler. The capsule is also pierced in two places by pressure exerted by the patient on two buttons on the sides of the device. The capsule also spins upon inspiration, releasing tiotropium bromide for the control of COPD. The Spiriva patient instructions include a statement that a second inhalation through the device should be used if the powder has not been completely emptied from the capsule.

The Foradil aerolizer, made by Merck but now discontinued, had a device that operated on a similar principle. It contained formoterol fumarate for long-acting control of asthma. In announcing the discontinuation of the product at the end of 2015, the FDA stated that this step was being taken for reasons that were "business-related." The product was not widely accepted by consumers, probably because the capsules had to be stored in the refrigerator. The Onbrez Breezhaler (Novartis) also uses a device and a capsule containing the drug. Similar to the foregoing examples, the capsule is also punctured upon the application of pressure onto two buttons on the device.

All of the above devices work on the principle of puncturing the capsule with pins, followed by the inhalation of the powder by the patient. It is, therefore, important that the capsule is able to be punctured easily and cleanly, to allow the powder to leave the capsule shell. Under high humidity conditions, the capsule shell may absorb moisture and soften and swell, making it more difficult to puncture. Conversely, the capsule shell should not be very brittle in order to prevent it from fracturing into pieces when pierced. Brittleness is also a function of moisture content and capsules that are stored in an environment of low relative humidity (RH) are more brittle. Capsule properties as well as the type of capsule material for inhalation capsules are more fully described in Chapter 10, Capsules. If the capsule is shattered, most capsule shell particles will be trapped by a wire mesh in the device but there is a small potential for particles to be entrained in the inhaled air. In addition, if the patient attempts to puncture the capsule multiple times, by repeatedly pressing the buttons, the tendency for the capsule to shatter becomes greater. The patient may repeatedly press the buttons out of a mistaken concern that the capsule may not have been punctured fully the first time and, therefore, may not release the drug adequately. Inhaled capsule particles will impact the mouth or oropharynx where they will dissolve and be swallowed. If any particles reach the trachea, they will be removed by mucociliary clearance, as described later in this chapter.

Forceful inhalation withdraws the powder from the capsule, by some mechanism. First, the structure of the device creates turbulence in the airstream through the device upon inhalation. The turbulence causes the capsule to spin about its long axis. In the spinning capsule, the contents are forcefully thrown outward. In a capsule that has already been punctured by pins, the contents leave through the holes in the capsule. Since the drug and carrier are attracted to each other by physical forces, and not covalent chemical bonds, the turbulence causes the drug particles to separate from the carrier. The fine drug particles are mostly carried, with the air, out of the device, whereas the large-sized carrier particles are mostly left behind in the device. Due to the speed at which the drug particles leave the device, some may impact the mouth and others may impact the oropharynx, with higher speed resulting in greater impaction. The remaining particles enter the lungs and a fraction of these reach the deep lungs, where they are most needed. Most of the drug particles and a small amount of the carrier are transferred out of the device.

A mesh is in place within the device and, due to the size of the mesh, the finer drug particles are allowed to pass through. The mesh is intended to hold back the carrier particles. It does this effectively, with most particles remaining within the device. However, a small amount of the carrier particles may escape into the mouth, resulting in the patient experiencing a slightly sweet taste. It is also possible that a few particles go beyond the mouth and will be trapped in the oropharynx. The distance that a particle is carried is related to its particle size, such that large particles are carried a shorter distance. In evaluating "size," it is the aerodynamic diameter that is important, as previously mentioned.

The administration of a dose from a DPI is a very different experience from taking many other dosage forms: there is little sensory perception of the medication being taken. In this sense, it is very different from swallowing a capsule, or even from using a pMDI, where the propellant produces a tactile sensation. The Onbreze and Spiriva capsules (and possibly others) make a whirring sound as they spin. The patient may also experience the slightly sweet taste of a small amount of lactose. The sound and taste may provide affirmation of the administration of the dose. A legitimate concern may still be whether all of the powder has left the capsule, and whether inspiration was sufficiently forceful. In fact, many patients require two inspirations to remove all the powder from the capsule. Onbreze has clear capsules and, upon opening the device, the patient can see whether the capsule has been emptied. This, however, does require the additional steps of opening the device to check, closing, and repeating the inhalation, which some patients find bothersome.

The Rotahaler was a device manufactured by Allen and Hanbury and was marketed for many years from the 1960s onward. It was used in connection with Ventolin rotacaps which were inserted into the device. Interestingly, the device opened the capsule (rather than piercing it) and the body fell into a chamber from which the drug was inhaled. The device was large and did not achieve significant patient acceptance, and is now discontinued. More recently, the Cipla pharmaceutical company, based in India, produced an inhalation device, the Revolizer, which appears to be based on the Rotahaler design but is smaller and has some other patient-friendly attributes. To use the device, the patient inserts a capsule which has a clear body and a colored cap. The color-coding serves as an aid to correct insertion of the capsule into the device. After closing the device, the patient rotates its bottom half to remove the body of the capsule from the cap. The drug is available from the opened capsule body which falls into a lower, clear plastic compartment. Upon inspiration, the drug is inhaled. This system avoids any potential issues with the piercing of the capsule. All that is required, to make the drug available, is that the capsule open correctly. Since a clear plastic portion of the device holds the open capsule body, the patient can observe that the capsule has been opened. The clear plastic also allows the patient to see if there is any remaining powder in the capsule body, in which case a second deep inhalation is recommended. Since both the correct opening of the capsule and the complete administration of the dose can easily and clearly be affirmed by observation, this device has an advantage over other devices. The Revolizer is claimed to be "generic," meaning that capsules containing various drugs may be used in the same device. Since there is an interplay between device characteristics, such as airflow rate and turbulence, and the properties of the powder within the capsule, this is not an easy claim to fulfill and evaluation of the delivery of multiple drugs is needed to support this claim.

All capsule-containing devices suffer from a problem: it requires several steps to open the device, remove a capsule from the blister or other container, insert it into the device, puncture or open the capsule, and then inhale deeply. While this does not appear to be complicated, or to consist of too many steps, it must be borne in mind that the patient who is not well may find the steps overwhelming. This indicates one of the difficulties in bringing an inhalation product to market: after overcoming many scientific hurdles in carrier powder technology, drug particle aerodynamics, packaging, stability, and others, the resulting product must still be user-friendly for commercial acceptance.

Multidose DPI

This type of device has multiple doses contained within the device, as supplied by the manufacturer, and it is not necessary for the patient or caregiver to insert a capsule each time a dose is needed. Given the concern of some patients regarding the multiple steps required to use a single-dose DPI, the multidose inhaler is certainly easier to use and probably more patient-acceptable. Multidose DPIs are of two types: those having a reservoir of drug (in a single container) within the device, from which individual doses are metered out, as needed; and those with individual doses in separate compartments within the device.

Reservoir Devices

The first marketed reservoir device was probably the Turbuhaler, commercialized by AstraZeneca. The drug formulation is contained within a storage container and individual doses are dispensed from this container into a dosing chamber immediately before inhalation by the patient. This is done by a back-and-forth twisting action of the base of the device. In the United

States, the only product available is budesonide, marketed as Pulmicort Turbuhaler. There are other formulations supplied in this device in Europe. The Asmanex Twisthaler (Schering-Plough) is another reservoir device available in the United States. It contains mometasone furoate and removal of the cap brings the next dose into the air path for inhalation by the patient. While this arrangement may be considered convenient to the patient, any inadvertent removal of the cap wastes a dose since it cannot be returned to the reservoir.

Devices with Individual Doses in Compartments

Diskhaler. This device was introduced by Glaxo in the late 1980s and contains a disc with either four or eight drug-containing chambers along its periphery. Indexing rotates the disc, bringing a new dose in line with the mouthpiece. The aluminum blister is then pierced and its contents drop into a dosing chamber. When the drug contents of all the blisters have been used, the disc is removed and a new one is inserted. In the United States, this device was used for the delivery of fluticasone propionate to pediatric patients. Each disc held only 1 or 2 days' drug supply and the discs were perceived to be not very easy to load. Probably for these reasons, Diskhalers were not very successful in the United States and, consequently, were taken off the market. Advair Diskhalers (salmeterol and fluticasone propionate), Flovent Diskhalers (fluticasone propionate), and Serevent Diskhalers (salmeterol xinafoate) are still available in other countries, such as Canada.

Diskus. The external view of the Diskus device is that of a thick disc (Figure 19-9). Within the device, there is a foil strip with the individual doses. These are contained in compartments in a single row along the length of the strip. Lidding material seals the compartments, and the strip is rolled up around a spool for placement into the device (Figure 19-9C). In use, an indexing lever is pressed to unwind the roll of foil in order to bring a fresh drug-containing compartment in line with the mouthpiece. The indexing step also causes the lidding material to be removed from the compartment, making the dose accessible. The foil with spent compartments is taken up by another spool. A well-known formulation of this type is the Advair Diskus (GSK). It contains salmeterol xinafoate (a long-acting bronchodilator) and fluticasone propionate (a corticosteroid), making it a multidose, as well as a combination, inhalation product. Flovent Diskus contains only fluticasone propionate while the Serevent Diskus contains only salmeterol xinafoate. The Ventolin Diskus (albuterol) is available in Canada. The Diskus device has found wide acceptance amongst patients, contributing in large measure to its commercial success. When all doses have been used, the device is trashed unlike the Diskhaler which has replaceable drug-containing discs.

Ellipta. This is the next generation of devices produced by GSK, with the stated aim of making the device easier to use. The device is smaller than the Diskus. Within the device there is space for two reels of strips with drug-containing compartments that are lidded (Figure 19-10). Each reel contains a different drug so that various combinations of two drugs may be supplied in the same device. If only one drug is used, one reel within the device would be empty. Upon opening the device, the

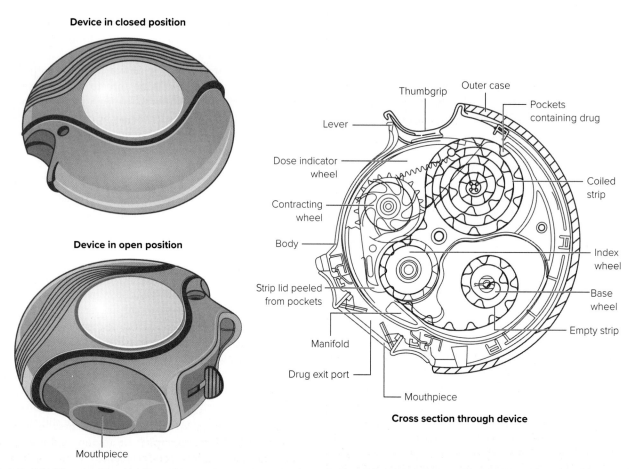

FIGURE 19-9 Diskus. (A) In closed position. **(B)** Open position. **(C)** Cross section. (Reproduced, with permission, from Atkins PJ. Dry powder inhalers: an overview. *Respir. Care.* 2005;50(10); Crompton GK. Delivery systems. In: Kay AB, ed. *Allergy and Allergic Diseases*. London: Blackwell Science; 1997:1440-1450.)

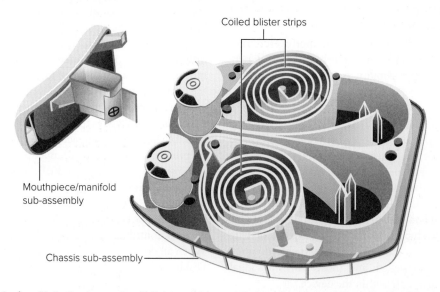

FIGURE 19-10 Ellipta device. Note the two coils of blisters which contain two drug formulations for dual therapy. For monotherapy, one coil is omitted.

reels are advanced to bring one drug-containing compartment from each reel in line with the mouthpiece and airflow path. At the same time the lids are removed from the compartments. Upon inhalation by the patient, the powder from each compartment is inhaled simultaneously, providing one dose of the combination product. The one step of opening the mouthpiece brings about all the functions mentioned above in addition to rolling up the strips containing spent compartments from the previous inhalation. The different pulmonary drugs delivered via the Ellipta inhaler are shown in Table 19-1.

TABLE 19-1	Drugs Delivered Using Ellipta Inhaler		
TRADE NAME	DRUG 1	DRUG 2	INDICATION
Incruse	Umeclidinium	–	COPD
Anoro	Umeclidinium	Vilanterol	COPD
Arnuity	Fluticasone furoate	–	Asthma
Breo	Fluticasone furoate	Vilanterol	Asthma and COPD

COPD, chronic obstructive pulmonary disease

All DPIs require that the patient inhale forcefully to remove the powdered dose. The issue with this requirement is the fact that a patient whose lung function is compromised may not have sufficient inspiratory force to withdraw the dose adequately. In this regard it should be mentioned that the inhaler itself offers some resistance to the flow of air. The extent of resistance and the ease with which a dose may be adequately inhaled differs with each DPI. Adequate inhalation refers to the inhalation of a significant percentage of the respirable dose. Those inhalers that require less inspiratory force to inhale an adequate dose are preferable. A measure of a patient's inspiratory force may be obtained by testing the patient's inspiratory flow rate, a test which is routinely conducted to help assess the patient's condition. This involves breathing through a device which measures flow rate. The flow rate is variable during the course of one deep inspiration, and the peak inspiratory flow is the highest rate measured (L/min). The reservoir inhalers require the most inspiratory force whereas the Diskus appears to require forces within the ability of patients with compromised lung function.

All DPIs may be perceived by patients as complicated to use. Each device has its own instructions for use which may be different from the next device. Therefore, when patients are switched from one device to another, it may be viewed as confusing. It is essential that the pharmacist instruct the patient thoroughly on the method of use of each device.

Recap Questions

1. Of the types of DPI discussed above, which one most closely resembles a pMDI? Why?
2. Besides the drug, what other ingredient is incorporated into the DPI?
3. Why is turbulent airflow through the device important?
4. What is the problem with the patient attempting to puncture the capsule multiple times in a DPI in which the drug is supplied in a capsule?
5. What is the function of the mesh within a DPI device?
6. In which way is the Revolizer different from other single-dose DPIs?
7. What is the difference between a reservoir-type multidose DPI and the Diskus?
8. What is the major difference between the Diskus and Diskhaler?

INHALATION THERAPY BEYOND ASTHMA AND COPD

There are many successful inhaler products on the market for treating asthma and COPD that work by means of a local effect on the lungs. Subsequent interest was, first, in the development of inhaled drug products for other lung diseases; and, second, in using the pulmonary route to obtain systemic drug delivery. The lung is ideally suited for this purpose considering that it has a large surface area for absorption of drugs (100 m²), is very well supplied with blood vessels, and the fact that the absorption barrier is very thin. In addition, the lung has low enzymatic activity and it is not a harsh environment for drugs (compare to the stomach). There are also fewer patient variables, for example, the amount and type of food consumed has no effect. The development of antibiotics as DPI for the treatment of lung infections was an obvious choice. The impetus for the development of systemic drugs by pulmonary delivery is the advent of several biotechnology-based treatments. These products, in general, are poorly absorbed orally and the injection route is the major route available for administration. The injection route is not ideal for several reasons including the fact that it causes pain, there may be a fear of the needle and injections are difficult to self-administer. These problems lead to poor compliance with regard to injectable drugs that have to be used chronically, especially when self-administered.

To reduce dependence on injections, alternate routes of drug delivery are under consideration and the pulmonary route is a leading contender for the reasons previously mentioned: the lungs have a large surface area, are well supplied with blood vessels and there is a very thin absorption barrier. The pulmonary route avoids the gastrointestinal-hepatic first-pass effect and is being considered for the delivery of the protein and peptide products of biotechnology. Vaccination is another area of interest. Inhalation of macromolecular antigens for mucosal immunization has the potential to eliminate many of the difficulties associated with parental vaccinations.

In spite of showing much promise, the first attempt at delivering a biotechnology product via the pulmonary route was unsuccessful. Exubera (Pfizer), formulated as an insulin inhaler, was marketed but later withdrawn. The device was large and said to be cumbersome to adjust doses. Diabetics frequently have to adjust doses in relation to their measured blood glucose levels and at mealtimes. The product withdrawal appears to be due to poor sales and the fact that some patients experienced pulmonary edema. Eli Lilly stopped an advanced inhaled insulin project after Pfizer withdrew its product from the market. In 2014, Afrezza (Mannkind Corporation) was approved as inhaled insulin therapy. The device is much smaller than the Exubera device and considered to be far more user-friendly. The product was licensed to Sanofi Aventis who, within a short time, withdrew from the license arrangement due to poor sales. Mannkind Corporation is presently marketing the product itself and it is yet to be determined if this product will be successful.

CLEARANCE FROM THE LUNGS

Many drugs are provided adsorbed onto lactose or other carrier particles (DPI). When substances are delivered to the lungs, the clearance of both drugs and excipients must be considered. While it is anticipated that most carrier particles, due to their large size, will be trapped within the inhalation device, some will reach the mouth, or the oropharynx, by high-speed impaction against the mucosa. Here, they will dissolve and be swallowed. After inhalation using a DPI, therefore, there will be drug particles in the lungs. Due to their large particle size, lactose particles are not expected to be in the bronchi or bronchioles. A pMDI delivers drug particles and propellant but the latter will be exhaled. Consequently, the focus must be on the elimination of drug particles whichever type of inhaler was used.

While there are several mechanisms by which the drug particle may be removed from the point at which it contacts pulmonary tissue, three main mechanisms of clearance are: absorption, cell-mediated translocation, and mucociliary transport. The composition of the particle will influence its mechanism of clearance. When we breathe, foreign substances in the inhaled air get trapped in the mucus continually secreted by the bronchi. A wave-like action of the cilia (hairs) on the mucous membrane pushes the particles, with the mucus, up toward the pharynx where they are either swallowed, and go into the stomach, or coughed up. Cilia are found on the mucosa of the trachea, bronchi, and bronchioles. The respiratory bronchioles have fewer cilia. The mucociliary action is said to "sweep" the material outward. Undissolved drug particles may experience a similar fate. It takes approximately 24 h to move particles from the edge of the lung up to the epiglottis, in the throat. This is a natural, protective mechanism to rid the body of foreign particles.

The terminal bronchioles are the last section of the bronchial tree where *active* mucociliary clearance takes place. The respiratory bronchioles have a few cilia and may participate in mucociliary clearance to a lesser extent. Particles that are deep in the lung, beyond the terminal bronchioles (ie, in the respiratory bronchioles, alveolar ducts and alveoli) will be cleared by macrophages. These cells are phagocytic and are responsible for clearing debris from the alveolar region of the lungs. Cellular clearance may take weeks to months depending upon the nature of the particles. These cells are also the primary immunological defense, presenting the initial response to microorganisms.

For drugs that have a local action, such as bronchodilators and corticosteroid drugs, it is desirable that clearance is not rapid so that the patient obtains the maximum benefit from the local effect. Drugs can be easily absorbed through the epithelial cells of the bronchioles and the drug must be predominantly delivered to this part of the lung. The rate and extent of absorption depend on the chemical properties of the drug, such as its solubility, molecular size, hydrophobicity, or hydrophilicity. These factors determine the extent of absorption and whether the transcellular or paracellular routes are utilized, as described in Chapter 3, Oral Route of Drug Delivery.

The situation is different for drugs that are administered for their systemic effect. In this case, rapid absorption into the blood stream is the desired form of clearance from the lungs and rapid absorption can be achieved through the thin walled alveoli. To achieve alveolar absorption, the drug must be delivered to a significant extent to the alveoli. The actual rate of absorption will depend on the physicochemical properties of the drug. The absorbed drug will be distributed by the blood, bringing about systemic effects.

ADVANTAGES AND LIMITATIONS OF INHALERS

Inhalers are a convenient way to deliver drugs to the lungs, in the cases of asthma and COPD. The pMDI devices are easy to carry and may be used at any time or place. Some DPI (eg, the Diskus) are somewhat larger, whereas the smaller DPI devices that are used in conjunction with capsules require that a supply of capsules be carried in a separate container. Nevertheless, all inhalers are portable and a dose is immediately available when needed, compared to a nebulizer, which has to be set up and may take a few minutes before drug delivery to the lungs is actually achieved. The pMDI canister is excellent at protecting the drug from light, moisture, oxygen, and pathogens. DPIs typically have the drug either in lidded blisters within the device or in capsules within foil blisters which also provide good protection to the drug. The reservoir type of DPI has the drug in the reservoir within the depths of the device. This arrangement also offers protection for the drug.

For all inhalers, deposition of the drug and carrier in the oropharynx may be irritant, and deposition of corticosteroids can cause candidiasis in the mouth and oropharynx. Additionally, when the drug is deposited in these areas, there may be some systemic absorption which could cause undesirable effects. When using pMDI, the coordination required between breathing and depressing the canister may prove to be difficult for children, geriatrics and even for younger adults who are experiencing bronchoconstriction. The lack of coordination can result in sub-optimal therapy for seriously ill patients. Poor therapy can also occur with any inhaler, if shallow inspiration and insufficient duration of breath-holding occur.

Recap Questions

1. Which scientific developments led to the consideration of pulmonary delivery for systemic drug effects?
2. Which product was the first insulin-inhaled product?
3. Where do most carrier particles, used in DPI, end up after a dose is administered?
4. How are foreign particles removed after deposition on the bronchi and bronchioles?
5. How are foreign particles removed from the alveolar regions of the lungs?

SUMMARY POINTS

- Nebulizers, pMDI, and DPI are currently used for administration of drugs to the lungs.
- Droplet or solid particle size is important for good lung distribution: 1 to 5 μm is ideal.
- Trachea, bronchi, and bronchioles—get progressively narrower—some drug delivery to the bronchioles is needed for effective treatment of asthma and COPD.
- pMDIs are used in an inverted position: each dose is measured into an auxiliary chamber and is ready for the next administration.
- DPI—powder is dry; there is no propellant; requires forceful inspiration to separate drug particles from carrier.
- There are single-dose DPI (capsule contains drug) and multidose DPI (drug may be in a reservoir, or individual doses may be premeasured into cavities/compartments).

What do you think?

1. Mr. Hernandez, a 45-year-old asthmatic, tells you he gets a sweet taste in his mouth after using his powder inhaler. He thinks he may have received a placebo inhaler from your pharmacy. Which of the following is most appropriate to tell him?
   a. You will check with the pharmaceutical manufacturer and get back to him. He should give you the batch no. of his inhaler.
   b. Tell him that everything is ok, providing a brief explanation in layman's terms.
   c. Tell him he is imagining the sweet taste.
2. Mr. Hernandez, from the previous question, suggests he would rather use a nebulizer. He used one as a child and he thinks it worked better. What would you say to him? Provide reasons for your response.
3. What is the optimum droplet size for the product from a pMDI?
4. Explain the effect of a spacer used with pMDIs.
5. Why does a DPI require more inspiratory force than a pMDI?
6. What are the differences between a reservoir DPI and a multidose DPI which does not contain a reservoir?
7. What are some of the problems encountered with the use of DPIs that contain powder within a capsule?

REFERENCES

1. Fröhlich E, Salar-Behzadi S. Toxicological assessment of inhaled nanoparticles: role of in vivo, ex vivo, in vitro, and in Svilico vtudies. *Int J Mol Sci.* 2014;15:4795-4822. doi:10.3390/ijms15034795.
2. Kenyon CJ, Thorsson L, Borgström L, Newman SP. The effects of static charge in spacer devices on glucocorticosteroid aerosol deposition in asthmatic patients. *Eur Respir J.* 1998; 11:606-610.

BIBLIOGRAPHY

Atkins PJ. Dry powder inhalers: an overview. *Respir Care.* 2005;50:1304-1312.

Chrystyn H. The DiskusTM: a review of its position among dry powder inhaler devices. *Int J Clin Pract.* 2007;61:1022-1036. https://doi.org/10.1111/j.1742-1241.2007.01382.x.

Grant AC, Walker R, Hamilton M, Garrill K. The ELLIPTA dry powder inhaler: design, functionality, in vitro dosing performance and critical task compliance by patients and caregivers. *J Aerosol Med Pulm Drug Deliv.* 2015; 28:474-485. https://doi.org/10.1089/jamp.2015.1223.

Kenyon CJ, Thorsson L, Borgström L, Newman SP. The effects of static charge in spacer devices on glucocorticosteroid aerosol deposition in asthmatic patients. *Eur Respir J.* 1998; 11:606-610.

Lavorini F, Pistolesi M, Usmani OS. Recent advances in capsule-based dry powder inhaler technology. *Multidiscip Respir Med.* 2017;12:11. doi:10.1186/s40248-017-0092-5.

Mehta P. Dry powder inhalers: a focus on advancements in novel drug delivery systems. *J Drug Deliv.* 2016:Article ID 8290963,17. http://dx.doi.org/10.1155/2016/8290963.

Newman SP. Principles of metered-dose inhaler design. *Respir Care.* 2005;9:1177-1190.

Buccal and Sublingual Drug Delivery

20

PREVIEW

- Advantages and disadvantages of the buccal and sublingual routes of drug delivery
- Brief historical perspective
- Ways to promote absorption through the buccal mucosa
- Some currently marketed products
- Future potential

INTRODUCTION

As mentioned in the introductory chapter, many drugs are not well absorbed in the gastrointestinal tract (GIT). This may be due to the drug's chemical structure which permits only slow diffusion from the gastrointestinal (GI) lumen into the GI tissues. In addition, the degradation of certain drugs in the GIT results in a smaller amount of the drug being available for absorption and, hence, less drug will be absorbed. Degradation of acid-labile drugs may be caused by the strong acidic conditions prevalent in the stomach. Enzymes, present in various portions of the GIT, could also inactivate sensitive drugs. Alternatively, the drug may be well absorbed from the lumen but may be metabolized during passage through the gastrointestinal membrane, or during its first pass through the liver. The latter may be responsible for extensive metabolism. This results in a very small amount of the drug being transferred into the general circulation and, consequently, a lower therapeutic response.

The delivery of drugs through the oral mucosa (the lining of the mouth), especially the buccal and sublingual mucosa, has received a great deal of attention over several years recently. This interest has stimulated many academics to perform basic research dealing with drug permeation through the oral mucosa, and to develop novel dosage forms. The mechanistic approach of these researchers led to the study of permeation enhancers and mucoadhesion, two techniques that could increase the permeability of poorly permeable drugs. In addition, several pharmaceutical companies are actively involved in the development of oral transmucosal drug products. Due to the properties of the drug, or the nature of the disease condition that it is desired to treat, the oral transmucosal formulation may be the sole delivery route under investigation. It is also possible that, due to the properties of the drug, it cannot be delivered via the GIT and the company wishes to explore several alternative routes. Once the data regarding absorption via the different routes become available, the company will choose one route for further development. Ultimately, a product may be developed and a new drug application (NDA) will be submitted to the FDA for approval to market the product. This chapter focuses on oral mucosal delivery and mentions the reasons for developing dosage forms that are suitable for this route, and the advantages and disadvantages of this form of drug delivery. It also mentions some products that have recently been introduced to the market.

ADVANTAGES AND DISADVANTAGES

The oral mucosa may be viewed as an attractive site for drug delivery for several reasons. The oral cavity is the most accessible cavity of the body. This makes the administration of drugs very easy. Since it is akin to eating, it is also very acceptable to the patient. A dosage form can easily be placed under the tongue or into the buccal cavity. Some dosage forms are mucoadhesive, that is, when correctly applied, they will adhere to the mucosal membrane. A dosage form can be attached to the oral mucosa without any pain or discomfort. This type of dosage form, used mainly for long-acting medications, may also be easily removed if necessary. When symptoms, such as pain, subside or if adverse reactions are experienced, it may be desirable to discontinue drug administration. Such discontinuation of treatment is not easy to achieve with most other routes of administration.

The buccal mucosa is well vascularized and blood vessels drain from the mucosa directly into the jugular vein. Therefore, drugs penetrating the epithelium are delivered directly into the systemic circulation, avoiding drug loss due to acid degradation or enzymatic hydrolysis in the GIT. The hepatic first-pass effect is also avoided. The buccal mucosa provides an environment free from strong acidity and with limited protease activity, unlike the conditions encountered elsewhere in the GIT.

New cells are estimated to be produced in the buccal region of the oral cavity every 4 to 14 days. This rate is intermediate between the slow turnover rate of the skin and the fast GI turnover rate. Very rapid cell division would disturb a mucoadhesive device. Since cell division is not rapid, a mucoadhesive device may be worn for many hours, or even days, without disturbing its adhesion. On the other hand, if slight tissue damage occurs due to the wearing of a dosage form, fairly rapid recovery is possible.

For drug delivery purposes, it is often advantageous to alter the microenvironment around a dosage form that is within the body. For example, if the pH in the immediate vicinity of a tablet can be altered, it is possible that the drug may dissolve faster. The microenvironment of a dosage form placed into the oral cavity can be directly and easily modified. This is an often-overlooked advantage of oral mucosal delivery. Furthermore, this can usually be done with little to no damage to the mucosal tissues.

There are also disadvantages associated with this route of drug delivery, mainly the low permeability and the smaller absorptive surface area in comparison to that of the small intestine. Additionally, the continuous secretion of saliva (0.5-2 L/day) leads to dilution of the drug resulting in a slower rate of permeation. In addition, salivation, and resulting swallowing, effectively removes the drug from the preferred absorptive region. Conversely, for patients secreting too little saliva ("dry mouth syndrome"), there may be insufficient saliva for dissolution to occur at the desired rate. The taste of the drug may also present difficulties to patients and decrease compliance with the dosing regimen. This problem may be greater with certain patient populations such as the young, the elderly, and patients experiencing nausea. The latter may be due to their illness or to concomitant medications. If the buccal delivery system is mucoadhesive, movements of the mouth or tongue may displace the dosage form, or otherwise affect it in an adverse manner. It is also an inconvenience when the patient is eating or drinking. Moreover, the hazard of choking by involuntarily swallowing the delivery system is a concern.

Where a dosage form is to be held for any length of time in the oral cavity, with specific instructions, it becomes increasingly difficult to adhere to the instructions over time. For example, an instruction may be to avoid detaching the dosage form with movements of the tongue. Additionally, the instruction to avoid swallowing of saliva may be difficult to follow by some patient populations, for example, the young, the elderly, and some physically or mentally impaired patients. If food or liquid consumption occurs post-application of mucoadhesive dosage forms, the temperature and pH of the consumed material may affect drug release. The patient may be instructed to eat or drink using only one side of the mouth, the one opposite to the attached drug. For some drugs, mucositis may be a contraindication to the use of oral transmucosal dosage forms due to potentially faster absorption. An additional reason for the contraindication is the pain that may be experienced by these patients at the site of application.

MUCOADHESIVES AND PENETRATION ENHANCERS

In certain instances, it may be useful to hold a delivery system in a specific position, against the oral mucosa, for an extended period. One example is when there is a local adverse condition, such as a mouth ulcer. In this instance, it would be beneficial to maintain the drug-containing dosage form close to the problem area. A second example is the situation where the drug is only slowly absorbed, due to the drug's properties, but a higher permeation of the drug is desired. It would be possible to attain such higher total permeation by maintaining the dosage form in close proximity to the mucosa for an extended time. This affords more opportunity for absorption, with the rate of absorption remaining the same. Another approach to improve absorption, in order to achieve the desired therapeutic levels of a drug, is to incorporate a penetration enhancer into the formulation. In this case, the rate of absorption increases.

Sometimes, the drug may be relatively rapidly absorbed and also quickly eliminated. If a longer duration of drug action is desired for such a drug, the drug may be placed within a matrix which slowly releases the drug for correspondingly slow absorption. The slowly-releasing matrix is used in conjunction with a mucoadhesive dosage form. In such a case, the delivery system is held in place while it slowly releases the drug in order to facilitate slow absorption over a long period. From the foregoing, it can be seen that mucoadhesive dosage forms may be used for local treatment as well as for systemic drug delivery. Mucosal adhesion is obtained by the use of mucoadhesive polymers. These are essential to maintain an intimate, and prolonged, contact of the formulation with the oral mucosa.

When a drug is placed in a sustained-release (SR) matrix, in the situation described above, the ideal release rate from the matrix should be less than, or equal to, the absorption rate of the drug through the mucosa. If the release rate is faster than the absorption rate, the excess drug will be lost to swallowing.

The "excess drug" refers to the difference between the amount of drug released in a unit of time and the amount that can be absorbed through the oral mucosa in the same unit of time.

Mucoadhesives

As mentioned, the SR matrix is usually used in conjunction with a mucoadhesive excipient which holds the dosage form in a fixed location while it slowly releases its drug content. Examples of mucoadhesives are carbomer (Carbopol®), chitosan and derivatives, cellulose derivatives, and polycarbophil. These mucoadhesives offer a reasonable mucoadhesive strength and duration of effect. The first step of the mucoadhesive reaction is the spreading of the applied polymer over the mucous membrane. The mucous found on the mucous membrane also contains a polymer, called mucin. The subsequent step of the mucoadhesive reaction is the penetration of the mucoadhesive polymer strands into the mucous. Next, the polymer strands and the mucin strands may intertwine to form a stronger interaction. After this stage, the two polymers may interact to form a covalent bond, if such a covalent interaction is possible. This depends on the types of functional groups present in each of the two polymers.

Thiolated polymers are polymers containing SH groups. These groups are the sulfur equivalents of hydroxyl functions. The thiol-group is capable of reacting with other S-containing compounds to form disulfide bonds. Mucin contains cysteine groups (S-containing). When thiolated polymers intertwine with mucin polymers, a disulfide bond can form between the two polymers. This is a relatively strong bond which results in a stronger mucoadhesive reaction than is the case with non-thiolated polymers. The strength of the interaction could be 2 to 3 times as strong as that with conventional polymers.

The SR matrix material may, itself, provide mucoadhesion and, therefore, only one additive is necessary for the SR effect and mucoadhesion. An example of such a material is the gum from the plant, Hakea gibbosa. Some drug delivery systems, with an adhesive, deliver the drug unidirectionally, that is, toward the mucosal side of the dosage form only. In the case of a tabletted-delivery system, only one surface of a flat-faced tablet releases the drug: the face that is exposed to the mucosa. The surfaces of the tablet not exposed to the mucosa (those facing the lumen of the mouth) are coated with a wax, or other impermeable substance in research studies (Figure 20-1). This eliminates drug diffusion through the other surfaces of the tablet. In this way, significantly less drug is swallowed with the saliva.

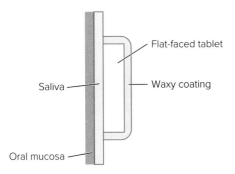

FIGURE 20-1 Diagram of tablet coated on all-but-one surface.

Permeation Enhancement

If a drug is inadequately absorbed for it to be useful in drug therapy, its permeation through the biological barrier (oral mucosa, in this instance) can be enhanced by the incorporation of certain chemicals into the formulation. Alternately, physical methods that utilize energy to drive molecules across the biological barrier can be used. Even in cases where the drug is absorbed reasonably well, permeation enhancers could be used to bring on a faster onset of action (decrease the lag phase) or to increase the degree of the pharmacological effect. Physical methods of enhancement for oral mucosal use are still in the research stage and will be mentioned briefly (products for transdermal delivery using such enhancement have already been commercialized). On the other hand, chemical enhancers for oral mucosal delivery have been researched for long and are present in commercial products. Hence, the latter will be discussed in a little more detail.

Physical methods to promote permeation involve the use of a device as the energy source. The types of physical enhancement include sonophoresis (ultrasound energy), electrophoresis (electrical energy to move charged molecules or ions), and electroporation. The latter involves the use of high-voltage energy for a very short duration (microseconds to milliseconds) to induce transitory nanosized pores in the tissue for improved permeation. The short-lived nature of the pores means that toxins do not have much opportunity to permeate the membrane whereas the relatively large quantity of the drug placed adjacent to the pores will have adequate opportunity to permeate.

The ideal chemical enhancer should provide sufficient enhancement using relatively small amounts so that a reasonably-sized dosage form may be developed. Tissue damage from the enhancer should be minimal and recovery should be quick, especially for drugs that require repeated administration. Ideally, there should be no side effects from the enhancer which should also not be absorbed systemically. The enhancer should have no taste and should not upset the taste sensitivity of the patient, or in any other way interfere with the patient's lifestyle.

Bile salts have been used traditionally to enhance the absorption of drugs administered to the GIT. Subsequently, they were used in attempts to enhance oral mucosal delivery in research studies. The bile salts were found to damage mucosal tissues in in-vitro experiments. They are also very irritating to mucosal tissues which preclude their use in products for human use. A number of studies have shown the permeation-enhancing effect of fatty acids. The exact mechanisms have not been clearly elucidated but they are thought to interact with the phospholipids of cell membranes. By insertion of a monomer of the fatty acid between alkyl chains of the cell membrane phospholipids, the fluidity of the membrane increases. This allows greater drug permeation via the transcellular route.

Chitosan has been used as a mucoadhesive and permeation enhancer. It is a chemical obtained from crustacean shells by treating them with sodium hydroxide. This polysaccharide is thought to enhance absorption by several mechanisms, and in some instances, multiple mechanisms may be at play. The exudate from the Hakea gibbosa plant has also been shown to enhance permeation by more than one mechanism. One of the ways by which surfactants enhance drug absorption is by interacting with cell membrane lipids. This disrupts the regular packing of the lipids and, therefore, compromises their integrity. Thus, drugs included in the same dosage form as the surfactant may permeate the cell membrane more easily. Surfactants may also extract proteins from cell membranes which compromises the integrity of the membrane. Sodium lauryl sulfate is probably the surfactant that has been tested the most. Its permeation-enhancing effect occurs at very low use levels. In its experimental application, often low enhancement was accompanied by toxicity.

Inclusion complexes, dendrimers, and micelles hold drug molecules within the interior of a chemical structure. They may carry a drug molecule across a biological membrane where it may be released. Hydroxypropyl-β-cyclodextrin is probably the most studied inclusion complex. The pH control and effervescence have been found to be very effective in enhancing the permeation of fentanyl through oral mucosal tissues.

Some drugs, such as peptides, are metabolized by enzymes present in the mucosal membrane. By including an enzyme inhibitor, the permeation of the peptide across the oral mucosal membrane can be enhanced. It should be noted that the level of peptidases in the oral mucosa is far lower than in other routes of drug administration. Nevertheless, the presence of an enzyme inhibitor can improve the inherently poor permeation of a peptide through this membrane.

STRUCTURE OF THE ORAL MUCOSA AND ROUTES OF ABSORPTION

When a pharmaceutical dosage form is placed into the oral cavity, for oral mucosal delivery, the drug is released and crosses the mucosa, to then penetrate blood capillaries. To understand this process, one must be familiar with the structure of the oral mucosa.

The lining of the mouth, or mucosa, is not the same throughout the oral cavity: it is differentiated according to function. In some regions of the mouth, the mucosa is subject to the mechanical forces associated with mastication. In these areas, the mucosa is covered by a keratinizing epithelium resembling that of the epidermis of the skin. This mucosa is known as masticatory mucosa and is found on the gingiva (gums) and hard palate. The mucosal lining of the floor of the mouth and the buccal regions must be flexible to accommodate chewing and speech. This mucosa is termed a lining mucosa and is covered with a nonkeratinizing epithelium closely resembling that of the esophagus and uterine cervix.

The epithelium arises from a basal layer of cuboidal cells (Figure 20-2). From this actively dividing layer, cells are pushed to the surface. They become more flattened toward the uppermost layers and these cells are described as squamous, stratified cells. The epithelium consists of 40 to 50 layers. For simplicity, only a few of these layers are shown in Figure 20-2. The function of the epithelium is to protect the underlying tissue from mechanical and chemical injury. While all areas of the epithelium provide a mechanical barrier, some areas are particularly well adapted to this function, as mentioned above. Connective tissue supports the epithelium and consists

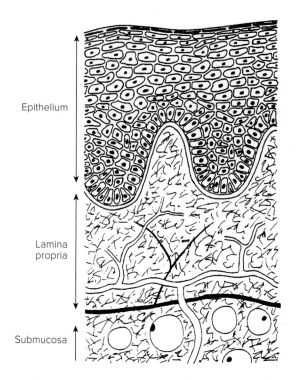

FIGURE 20-2 Structure of the buccal mucosa. (Reproduced, with permission, from Harris D, Robinson JR. Drug delivery via the mucous membranes of the oral cavity. *J Pharm Sci.* 1992;81(1):1-10.)

of a lamina propria and submucosa (Figure 20-2). The lamina propria contains a network of capillaries.

The barrier functions of the epithelium are highly effective. The mechanical barrier enables one to chew on rough food without significant damage to the mucosa, while the chemical barrier prevents noxious chemicals from entering the systemic circulation. The latter is important since blood flowing from the oral cavity bypasses the liver and flows directly into the systemic system. Since the barrier also limits the permeation of drugs, its efficiency is one of the major obstacles to the oral transmucosal delivery of drugs. The development of oral transmucosal delivery systems must take this barrier function into account.

It is difficult for drugs to permeate the tightly-bound cell layers of the epithelium, especially the outermost layers. However, once a drug has permeated the epithelium and the basement membrane, it can easily penetrate the capillaries and enter the general blood circulation. Hence, the epithelium is the barrier to drug permeation and, since it is an effective barrier, only certain drugs are able to permeate the mucosa. Such drugs have the correct physicochemical properties, as described later in this chapter. In order to deliver a wider range of drugs across the mucosa, reversible methods of reducing the barrier potential must be employed. This would permit the permeation of more drugs, including those with a less-than-ideal chemical structure. This requirement has fostered the study of permeation enhancers. A permeation enhancer should safely increase the permeability of the buccal mucosa for a sufficient length of time to allow selected permeants to pass through the barrier. Thereafter, the permeability of the barrier should revert to its original level. If the latter did not occur quickly, unwanted chemicals (including noxious substances) would penetrate the barrier and the use of the penetration enhancer would be considered undesirable. In addition, it is important to examine the irritation potential and the compatibility of the enhancer with the mucosa.

Saliva continually bathes the surface of the oral mucosa to maintain a moist environment and a stable, slightly acidic pH. This environment is maintained constant, to a large extent, by the continual secretion of saliva into the oral cavity from the salivary glands. There are three major salivary glands and numerous minor salivary glands located in, or beneath, the mucosa. Compared to the secretions of the GIT, saliva has less mucin which makes it relatively less viscous. It also has limited enzymatic (protease) activity.

The basic drug transport mechanism for the oral epithelium is the same as for other epithelia in the body. There are two major routes involved: the transcellular route (directly through the cells or intracellularly) and the paracellular route (through the spaces between the cells or intercellularly). These routes are illustrated in Figure 20-3. For some drugs, permeation across the buccal epithelium is thought to occur via the paracellular route by passive diffusion. This pathway is favored especially by small hydrophilic drugs. They dissolve more readily in the aqueous fluids filling the intercellular spaces. Figure 20-3 also illustrates the transcellular pathway. While it looks simpler than the paracellular pathway, closer examination reveals that it involves a drug permeating the cell membrane and then going through the cell's cytoplasm, each of which represents a very different environment. It then encounters the opposite cell membrane, which it penetrates, and then permeates the intercellular fluid before it enters the next cell. This continues until the drug has passed through the epithelium. An example of a drug known to penetrate via the transcellular pathway is fentanyl. Some drugs probably penetrate via both pathways. This may occur with drugs that have approximately balanced hydrophobic and hydrophilic properties, with a slight predominance of hydrophobicity. Such drugs will usually penetrate the fastest. Most often, however, one pathway predominates. In addition to these major pathways, other transport mechanisms (eg, carrier-mediated transport) play a role in the transport of some drugs across the oral mucosa.

The transcellular pathway is direct, with drugs tending to move in a straight line across the cell layers. There is little lateral diffusion. Drugs using the paracellular pathway move in a tortuous fashion around the cells. For this reason, this is a longer pathway. In addition, there is also a greater tendency for the drug to diffuse laterally during paracellular diffusion. This results in the drug passing over a wider area of the mucosa. This may help to explain the longer lead time to a steady-state with paracellularly absorbed drugs. Drug absorption, in general, is initially slow and then gradually increases until a steady-state, when the rate of absorption remains approximately constant. Caffeine is an example of a drug absorbed via the paracellular route and it is used as a marker of paracellular absorption in experimental studies.

While the transcellular route is more direct, the drug has to traverse the lipophilic cell membrane, the hydrophilic interior of the cell, and then pass through two cell membranes to reach the cytoplasm of the next cell (Figure 20-4). Between cells there is also the hydrophilic interstitial fluid. Therefore, a predominantly hydrophobic drug should have some hydrophilicity, if permeation through multiple cell layers and, finally, absorption into the systemic circulation is required. If the drug is extremely hydrophobic, there would be a tendency for it to be retained in the more hydrophobic components of the mucosal tissue, such as the cell membranes of the superficial epithelial layers. In this case, the drug would not reach the blood circulation in significant amounts. Retaining a large amount in the mucosal tissue is not desirable if a systemic effect is sought. Of course, such retention would be desirable for a topical effect, for example, anti-inflammatory action.

Recap Questions

1. Why do we use oral mucosal delivery?
2. If oral mucosal permeation is low, how can permeation be improved?
3. What is the biological reason for a chemical barrier in the mucosa?
4. Why are some parts of the oral mucosa keratinized?

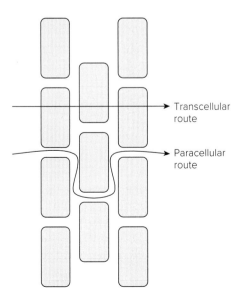

FIGURE 20-3 Drug delivery pathways schematic.

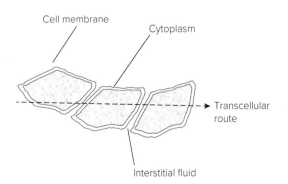

FIGURE 20-4 Detailed pathway followed by a drug permeating via the transcellular route. (From Pather SI, Rathbone MJ, Senel S. Current status and the future of buccal drug delivery systems. *Expert Opin Drug Deliv.* 2008;5(5):531-542.)

PROGRESS IN BUCCAL DELIVERY SYSTEMS

The first recorded use of oral transmucosal delivery appears to be an 1879 paper describing the use of glyceryl trinitrate for the sublingual treatment of angina. This drug penetrates the mucosa easily and does not require any enhancement. In spite of this early success, not much further development of this route occurred during the next 70 to 80 years. Then there were a series of papers from Beckett and coworkers in London in the 1960s and 1970s that demonstrated the ability of the oral mucosa to absorb the drug contained in a solution held in the mouth. This work is described in somewhat more detail in the section on Permeation Studies, later in this chapter. While it would not work for any drug, drug permeation of the mucosa was demonstrated for certain carefully selected drugs. This appeared to have spurred the development of oral mucosal formulations and, thereafter, a few easy-to-develop products were marketed. An example of such a product is nicotine used as an aid to smoking cessation. Nicotine also permeates the mucosal tissues well and several products containing this drug were developed, each in multiple strengths. The historical development of oral mucosal dosage forms is illustrated in Mind Map 20-1.

The fentanyl Oralet™ was the first FDA-approved opioid children's formulation, developed in 1996, for painless administration via the oral transmucosal route. One opinion holds that opioids for children should have an unpleasant taste as a disincentive to unauthorized self-administration. Adherence to this view would disallow the use of fentanyl Oralet which has a pleasant taste. On the other hand, taste remains one of the major determinants of mucosal contact time for the reasons mentioned below. In general, poor taste may cause the patient to either spit out the dosage form or swallow quickly in an effort to reduce the taste sensation. This is an automatic response to the unpleasant stimulus. On the other hand, good taste also has a major disadvantage: it promotes salivation and swallowing of saliva. The drug that is dissolved in the saliva will, therefore, be removed from the preferred absorption site. The swallowed drug may not be well absorbed in the GIT, or it may be destroyed in the environment encountered. Since swallowing the drug is disadvantageous, a bland taste is preferred.

In general, taste is very important for children's oral mucosal products. In addition, these products often have more complicated administration procedures. If the child does not cooperate fully during the drug administration process with a caregiver or has difficulties in coordination during drug self-administration, the administration becomes difficult. The utility of these pediatric dosage forms generally depends on the age of the child with older children coping better with administration procedures. There is also the risk of choking and aspiration. In addition, the accuracy of dosing is suspect if the oral mucosal dosage form is swallowed or spat out.

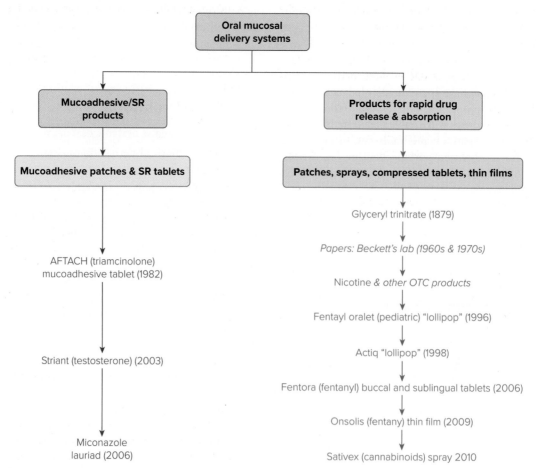

MIND MAP 20-1 **Historical Development of Oral Mucosal Dosage Forms.** (Only selected products which, in the author's view are milestones, have been mentioned.)

In 1998, the fentanyl transmucosal lozenge, Actiq was introduced to the market. The concept originated from the Department of Anesthesiology at the University of Utah and the product was developed by Anesta Corporation, later bought out by Cephalon and now part of Teva, Inc. This was the first product labeled for breakthrough cancer pain although other products, such as oral morphine, had previously been used off-label for this purpose. It was also the first oral transmucosal product of this type for adults. In September 2006, the fentanyl effervescent buccal tablet, Fentora, was introduced by CIMA LABS (later bought out by Cephalon and now also part of TEVA). It was the second fentanyl oral transmucosal dosage form with an indication for breakthrough cancer pain. The product is suitable for this purpose since significant blood levels may be attained within 15 minutes. This was a large improvement over Actiq and a significant development for oral mucosal delivery, keeping in mind that fentanyl is not well absorbed through the GIT. Actiq and Fentora were scientific and commercial successes and spurred the development of other mucosal dosage forms.

Fentora contains effervescent agents which promote oral transmucosal absorption by eliciting a series of reactions (Figure 20-5). The effervescent couple reacts in the presence of an aqueous medium, releasing CO_2 which dissolves in the saliva present in the oral cavity. This makes the medium more acidic and promotes the formation of the ionic (salt) form of the drug. Since this form is more soluble than the non-ionic form of the drug, dissolution is enhanced. The dissolved CO_2 is released from the saliva, after some time, making the solution more basic. This causes the formation of the non-ionic form of the drug. The latter is more permeable and, hence, permeation into buccal tissues is rapid. The system is thus ideal for drug delivery since it presents an acidic aqueous medium initially to favor drug dissolution and later promotes the formation of a basic aqueous medium in conjunction with an additional pH adjusting substance. The latter facilitates rapid permeation of the lipid cell membrane, leading to rapid drug absorption. For this reason, the effervescent dosage form has a much higher bioavailability than the same dose of Actiq. Fentora should be used at half the dose of Actiq for a similar effect. Prescribers and pharmacists

should be aware of this fact in view of the serious side effects of fentanyl. Dosing is further complicated by the fact that different doses may be required by different patients, and even the same patient as the pain gets worse. In general, treatment starts with the lowest dose and is titrated upwards until the patient is comfortable and has minimal side effects. The most noteworthy side-effect is respiratory depression which, if uncontrolled, leads to death.

Subsequent to the US approval of Fentora, Cephalon, Inc., obtained marketing approval from the European authorities and the product is now available in 29 European countries as "Effentora." The tablet is placed in the buccal cavity (above the upper molar tooth, between the gum and the cheek) or under the tongue. It disintegrates over approximately 10 minutes, releasing the drug. More recently, the product was approved for breakthrough neuropathic pain. The product can only be administered to patients who have previously had opioids and are tolerant to it. In opioid nontolerant patients, life-threatening respiratory depression could occur. This may happen at any dose, including low doses. For this reason, this product is contraindicated in the management of acute or postoperative pain, where the patient might not have had an opioid before. Since the amount of fentanyl contained in these preparations can be fatal to children, great care should be taken to restrict the access of these medications to children. Since the development of Actiq and Fentora, other fentanyl products with similar indications have been developed.

Oral mucosal delivery is now an area of active research with many companies involved in developing new products. In addition, many university researchers are studying mechanisms of drug transport, developing novel ideas for drug delivery, and conducting other aspects of basic research. This provides the scientific basis for new formulation developments, using this route of drug delivery. The combination of academic and industrial research represents a significant investment of time and resources.

Dosage forms for oral mucosal delivery may be of two types: those for rapid oral transmucosal permeation; and those intended for slow release of the drug, and correspondingly slow permeation, providing a prolonged action. When rapid absorption is required, the drug may be presented as lozenges, patches, sprays, or compressed tablets. The latter must have a fairly rapid in-mouth disintegration time (15 minutes or less). Where prolonged action is required, the dosage form is usually mucoadhesive, that is, it contains a chemical substance which causes the dosage form to adhere to the mucosa for a significant, predetermined time. A patch, or a mucoadhesive tablet with a very long disintegration time, may be used. The drug is released slowly from such dosage forms for slow absorption through the oral mucosa. The mucoadhesive nature of the dosage form ensures that it will stay in place, on the absorbing membrane, for a prolonged time. Professor Nagai, working in Japan, was among the first to pioneer the bioadhesive drug delivery system in the early 1980s. The first product developed by him contains a steroidal anti-inflammatory, triamcinolone acetonide, and is still on the market for the treatment of aphthous stomatitis (AFTACII by Teijin Pharma Ltd, Japan).

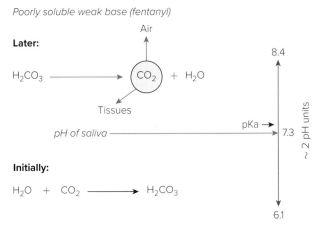

FIGURE 20-5 Fentora chemical reactions.

Thin films were initially developed for local effects in the mouth. An example of such a product is the Listerine strip, used to freshen the breath. It may also be used for dosage forms where the release of the drug occurs in the mouth. The drug-containing saliva is then swallowed, for subsequent absorption in the GIT. Utilizing this type of formulation, many over-the-counter (OTC) products were marketed for the treatment of colds and influenza. As mentioned, the drug is swallowed and absorbed by conventional mechanisms in the small intestine. The Triaminic and Theraflu range of products were claimed by the manufacturer to be the first therapeutic products of this type. Subsequently, there has been much interest in developing thin film formulations that release the drug in the oral cavity for absorption through the oral mucosa. One of the best known of these was the fentanyl thin film, Onsolis®. This product is now discontinued, possibly due to widespread abuse.

In contrast to what is commonly believed by the lay population, releasing a drug in the oral cavity does not necessarily mean that it will be absorbed through the lining of the oral cavity. Much research is usually done to enhance the penetration of the drug through the oral mucosa. There is also no evidence that homeopathic products, placed in the oral cavity, can deliver the active ingredient through the oral mucosa.

In 2002, the FDA approved Subutex (buprenorphine) and Suboxone (buprenorphine and naloxone), both tablet formulations. The former product is used for initiating treatment of opioid dependence, and the latter for continuing treatment of addicts. Opioid dependence involves addiction to opioid drugs, including heroin (a street drug) and opioid analgesics which are often obtained legally. In 2016, opioid overuse or misuse was responsible for most drug-related deaths in the US. Subutex is used under very controlled conditions in the doctor's office until such time as the patient has become accustomed to its effects. Suboxone is a take-home product. The naloxone it contains is intended to be a deterrent against the intravenous injection, by drug abusers, of the active ingredient, buprenorphine, in this transmucosal dosage form. Suboxone is the only centrally acting product approved for the treatment of opioid dependence in the European Union (EU). These drugs were introduced by Reckitt and Colman in an attempt to address the wave of opioid abuse sweeping Europe and America. Suboxone films have replaced Suboxone tablets in order to better control misuse and accidental pediatric exposure. The individually-packaged films are more difficult for children to open.

Oral mucosal testosterone has been shown to be useful to elevate male hormone levels. In comparison to oral medication, it avoids the drug degradation that occurs due to the acidic contents of the stomach and the metabolism that occurs mainly due to the hepatic first-pass effect. Columbia Pharmaceuticals' Striant buccal delivery system was approved by the FDA in 2003. It offered a novel treatment option for men who required testosterone replacement therapy. The need may have arisen due to an age-related deficiency, or to the absence of endogenous testosterone associated with hypogonadism. The tablet was placed against the gum above an incisor and the drug is claimed to be absorbed through both the gum and closely located buccal mucosa. The tablet was worn for 12 hours before being replaced by another tablet on the other side of the mouth,

which was worn for a further 12 hours. The product has been discontinued and it is unclear to what extent the lack of comfort in keeping a tablet in place for 24 hours a day contributed to its decline.

In 2005, Health Canada conditionally approved Sativex (GW Pharmaceuticals, PLC, and marketed by Bayer, Inc., a subsidiary of Bayer AG), a cannabis-derived pharmaceutical buccal spray for the adjunctive treatment of neuropathic pain in adults with multiple sclerosis (MS). The pain arises from the muscle spasticity experienced by these patients. The formulation, which is said to provide symptomatic relief, is a yellow-brown solution made from two extracts of Cannabis sativa L., folium cum flore (leaf and flower). The extracts contain, respectively, 27-mg delta-9-tetrahydrocannabinol and 25-mg cannabidiol. It is recommended that the spray be directed at different sites on the oromucosal surface each time the product is used.

In 2007, Health Canada conditionally approved Sativex for a new indication, the adjunctive analgesic treatment of moderate to severe pain in adult advanced cancer patients already being treated for persistent background pain with the highest tolerated dose of a potent opioid. In 2010, Sativex was fully approved in Canada to treat spasticity associated with MS, a third indication. Sativex is also approved in Europe for spasticity. At the time of writing, it was undergoing phase 3 clinical trials in the US. The US application is for the cancer pain indication; relief of spasticity in MS is not an indication that is presently being sought. The FDA has noted that the application has been granted "Fast Track" status, which basically means faster review. This designation indicates that the FDA believes that this medication, if approved, would fulfill an important unmet medical need. However, it will still have to undergo a rigorous review process.

Middle-of-the-night (MOTN) insomnia is characterized by difficulty returning to sleep after awakening either in the middle of the night or too early in the morning. This type of insomnia is different from initial, or sleep-onset, insomnia which refers to difficulty falling asleep at the beginning of the sleep period. Due to the disrupted sleep patterns caused by MOTN insomnia, the symptoms of the condition are fatigue and an inability to concentrate. In the case of some tasks, such as driving, this may prove to be dangerous. Intermezzo® was a sublingual tablet containing zolpidem tartrate, sold in two strengths (3.5 mg and 1.75 mg) for the indication of MOTN insomnia. Zolpidem is a well-known drug that has, traditionally, been used for insomnia at a dose of 10 mg (Ambien®). An extended-release tablet formulation (Ambien CR®) containing 6.25 mg or 12.5 mg of the drug is also available. Until the advent of Intermezzo, Ambien or its generic forms, taken at bedtime, appear to have been commonly used to treat MOTN insomnia. Intermezzo was specifically labeled for MOTN insomnia. This means that the FDA had approved its use for this condition. It dissolved fairly rapidly and a large portion of the dose was absorbed sublingually for a rapid effect.

MOTN affects a large percentage of the population but was undertreated prior to the development of this product by Transcept Pharmaceuticals. Most sleep aids, such as Ambien, are designed to put the patient to sleep at bedtime and to maintain sleep until the next morning, a period of approximately

8 hours. Since there were no products (prior to Intermezzo) specifically for this indication, a patient with MOTN had to take a full dose at the beginning of the sleep period. A further problem is the fact that patients generally do not experience MOTN every night. Hence, the patient had to guess whether they would experience MOTN on a particular night. If they thought this was likely, they would take a full dose. It is probable that they took medication on nights on which it was not needed. A greater problem occurred if they did not take medication at bedtime and awoke in the middle of the night. The dilemma, then, was whether to take a full dose with the probability that they would have difficulty awakening at their regular time in the morning. An even greater issue was whether they would be drowsy while performing tasks such as driving or operating machinery the next morning.

The sublingual Intermezzo tablet contains zolpidem tartrate and other ingredients to promote absorption through the oral mucosa. It may be taken when a MOTN awakening results in difficulty falling off to sleep again. Due to the formulation which enhances sublingual permeation, the drug is rapidly absorbed through the sublingual mucosa, thus allowing the patient to fall asleep rapidly. Due to the low dose, the patient awakens after approximately 4 hours, without undue daytime drowsiness. In a study comparing the 3.5-mg sublingual formulation with the 10-mg immediate-release (IR) swallowed tablet, it was demonstrated that the mean plasma concentration at 15 minutes and the AUC from 0 to 15 minutes was higher for the sublingual formulation despite the much lower dose (3.5 mg compared to 10 mg). This illustrates the higher absorption rate for the sublingual formulation which translates to more rapid sleep onset. A lower dose is recommended for women.

The requirement of the FDA, at the time of approval, was that the packaging be designed to emphasize:

1. that the drug should not be taken when there is less than 4 hours bedtime remaining; and

2. that the package help guard against the patient inadvertently taking a second dose on the same night.

This is a good example of what is referred to as compliance packaging and is discussed further in Chapter 14, Packaging. While it was innovative, the product has been discontinued due to poor sales, probably a result of poor marketing.

Miconazole Lauriad 50-mg bioadhesive buccal tablets (Loramyc, BioAlliance Pharma SA) was approved in October 2006 by France's regulatory body, AFSSAPS. It is indicated for the local treatment of oropharyngeal candidiasis in immunodepressed patients, particularly those with head and neck cancers who have undergone radiotherapy. It is also indicated for patients infected with HIV. Loramyc (miconazole) is formulated using the company's patented Lauriad drug delivery technology which permits the tablet to adhere to the mucosal membrane. This allows the delivery of the therapeutic agent onto the site of the disease. In the US, the product is known as Oravig.

The tablet is applied between the inner cheek and upper gum, that is, a buccal application. Alternate sides of the mouth should be used for each successive application. The tablet is held in place by slight pressure on the upper lip for about 30 seconds. During this time, the polymers hydrate, and this provides adhesion to the proteins of the mucous surface. Early drug release is followed by a period of slower, extended release of the therapeutic agent onto the site of the disease. The same technology is being used to develop a second product, Acyclovir Lauriad, for the treatment of oral herpes (herpes labialis) which affects many people and for which there is no vaccine.

Buccal–midazolam (Epistatus) is becoming an accepted option for the treatment of status epilepticus and serious tonic-clonic seizures in community settings in the United Kingdom (UK). Although currently unlicensed, this treatment option is advocated by certain official organizations in the UK. It is more convenient to use, and less embarrassing for the child, than rectal diazepam, the previous treatment of choice. However, the introduction of this liquid buccal formulation a few years ago raised the possibility of dose confusion as it is twice the strength of the injection that was initially used for this purpose. A licensed midazolam oromucosal product, Buccolam, has become available in the UK in pre-filled syringes. Each syringe contains 2.5 mg, 5 mg, 7.5 mg, or 10 mg of midazolam. The product was developed by Viropharma, now part of Shire.

Since orally disintegrating tablets (ODT) have become popular, it is important to distinguish them from oral transmucosal dosage forms. In the case of the latter, the drug is released in an absorbable form within the oral cavity. An absorption enhancer may be incorporated to facilitate drug absorption within the oral cavity. Conversely, the drug released from an ODT is not intended to be absorbed by the oral mucosa. Instead, it will be absorbed in the GIT mostly. In ODT, the drug may be contained within coated microcapsules (or other small units). These are released from the dosage form into the oral cavity after rapid disintegration of the tablet. The microcapsules are then swallowed and, when the coating dissolves, the major portion of the drug is released. This occurs distal to the oral cavity. The purpose of the coating is to prevent the patient from experiencing the bad taste of the drug which may only be perceived once the coating dissolves. Since coating dissolution generally occurs after the microcapsules have left the mouth, taste perception is minimal. For these reasons, ODT should not be considered as buccal, or sublingual, delivery systems. Some recently approved products are listed in Table 20-1.

Recap Questions

1. What do Actiq and Fentora have in common?

2. How are Actiq and Fentora different?

3. What is the purpose of naloxone in an oral mucosal product?

PERMEATION STUDIES

Having considered some recently marketed products for oral mucosal drug delivery, attention is now focused on the rates at which drugs cross the mucosa for penetration into blood

TABLE 20-1	Some Recently Approved Oral Mucosal Drug Delivery Systems		
Drug	**Trade Name**	**Dosage Form & Route**	**Manufacturer / Marketer***
Fentanyl citrate	Subsys	Sublingual Spray	INSYS Therapeutics
Fentanyl citrate	Fentora	Tablet – sublingual & buccal	Cephalon
Fentanyl citrate	Effentora	Tablet – sublingual & buccal	Cephalon
Fentanyl citrate	Onsolis	Buccal film	Meda
Fentanyl citrate	Breakyl	Buccal film	
Zolpidem tartrate	Edluar	Sublingual tablet	Orexo AB
Zolpidem tartrate	Intermezzo	Sublingual tablet	Transcept
Zolpidem tartrate	Zolpimist	Oral spray	ECR
Buprenorphine	Subutex	Sublingual tablet	Reckitt Benkiser
Buprenorphine and Naloxone	Suboxone	Sublingual film	Reckitt Benkiser
Ondansetron	Zuplenz	Oral film	Strativa
Asenapine	Saphris	Sublingual tablet	Schering Plough
	Sycrest	Sublingual tablet	Lundbeck A/S
Miconazole nitrate	Oravig	Buccal mucoadhesive tablet	BioAlliance Pharma
Miconazole nitrate	Loramyc	Buccal mucoadhesive tablet	BioAlliance Pharma
Midazolam	Buccolam	Oromucosal solution	Shire
Tetrahydrocannabinol & Cannabidiol	Sativex	Buccal and sublingual solution	GW Pharmaceuticals

*The company name may be abbreviated by the exclusion of terms such as pharmaceutical, company, Inc., etc.

capillaries, after being released from pharmaceutical products placed into the oral cavity. The permeability of the oral epithelium and the efficacy of selected penetration enhancers have been investigated in numerous in vivo and in vitro models. Since such studies may be a key component of the overall development of buccal and sublingual products, an overview of this methodology is presented here as background information to help understand how products are developed.

A drug solution that is held in the mouth will lose some of its drug content over time. Some drug is also lost from the retained solution through swallowing. The solution is also diluted due to salivation and a portion of this drug loss can be attributed to oral mucosal absorption, the magnitude of which can be determined by calculation. Absorption of drug in this manner was first demonstrated by Beckett and coworkers using human subjects. In their earlier experiments and publications, they did not account for swallowing and dilution by salivation and were criticized for this. In their later experiments, they were able to account for these factors in their calculations. A series of papers from Beckett's laboratory in the 1960s and 1970s demonstrated the buccal absorption of different drugs. They also demonstrated the fact that the pH of the solution influences the absorption of many drugs. In later research, they used specially designed cells to hold the drug solutions. These were fixed to the oral mucosae of various test animals. In some instances, perfusion cells were used in human volunteers.

This work was basic research to illustrate a scientific principle. A drug manufacturer's approach would probably be more practical. Prior to developing a commercial formulation, a drug company may wish to know if a specific drug permeates the buccal mucosa so that it could subsequently enter into the general circulation. To test the drug on human subjects is costly and difficult. Approval would have to be obtained from the Institutional Review Board (IRB) as well as the FDA or other regulatory body, as explained in detail in Chapter 18, Introduction to the Drug Regulatory Process. The FDA will not give permission for the testing in humans of a new chemical entity that has not been previously tested in animals and demonstrated to be safe. Testing on whole animals is also expensive. While permissions have also to be sought, these are generally less onerous than when performing human studies. Nevertheless, the process is not without its difficulties, and in vitro methods will likely be sought initially.

Using in vitro experiments, it is relatively easy to obtain an early indication of whether a specific drug will permeate the buccal mucosa. Likewise, such experiments can be used to readily determine the extent of permeation. If permeation is low, the degree to which permeation enhancers will need to be used can also be determined. The in vitro model has largely supplanted human or whole animal studies when a researcher needs to obtain initial information of this nature. In later experiments, whole animals may be used. Before a drug application can be submitted to the FDA for marketing approval, data from human studies are needed. The purpose of such studies is to demonstrate efficacy and a lack of serious side effects and, as mentioned, such studies are expensive to conduct. Hence, the initial in vitro work, which is relatively inexpensive, is done to give an indication of the probability that the drug will permeate the mucosa.

The setup of the in vitro experiment is as follows: a carefully prepared piece of mucosal tissue is placed between two glass cells of the diffusion apparatus. While there are different designs to this apparatus, each having somewhat different properties and advantages in specific situations, the Frantz diffusion cell and the Ussing chamber are two types that are commonly used. A Frantz diffusion cell is illustrated in Figure 20-6. A known volume of a drug solution, of known concentration, is placed in the donor chamber or cell of the apparatus. The drug is allowed to diffuse from the donor cell through the mucosa to the receiver cell. An aliquot of the solution in the receiver chamber is removed, at a specific time, and replaced with the aqueous medium. The concentration of the drug in the small, removed sample is measured, and from this, the amount of drug that is within the receiver compartment can be calculated. This is the amount that has diffused from the time of starting the experiment to the time at which the sample is withdrawn. This is repeated at fixed time intervals.

The cumulative amount diffused at each time point is plotted against time to obtain the time course of permeation. Permeation is slow initially, gradually increases, and then the rate of permeation is relatively constant. When the rate is constant, the curve is approximately linear. The apparent permeability coefficient is determined from the slope of the linear portion, using a mathematical equation. The permeability coefficient may be obtained in this way for several drugs that are being studied. This factor may then be used to compare the permeability of different drugs. The potency of several permeation enhancers may also be compared. In a series of experiments, the permeability of the selected drug is measured upon the addition of each permeability enhancer being tested. The permeation coefficients, thus obtained, are used to compare the effectiveness of the different enhancers. However, the results of such experiments do not always lend themselves to unambiguous interpretation as mentioned below.

Variations in the tissue preparation method can lead to differences in the observed permeation rate. Each laboratory should, therefore, standardize its method of tissue excision and preparation. Differences in preparative methods should also be taken into account when comparing results from different laboratories. It is best to use fresh membranes whenever possible, as the method of storage of the membrane can also lead to observed differences in the permeation rates. Variability in permeation rates obtained from experiments, as described above, is high even in well-controlled experiments. There are many reasons for this, some of which have been mentioned above. Therefore, this type of experiment can only be used to get an initial idea about permeation, or about the rank order of permeability of a series of drugs that are being compared, or the rank order of permeability enhancers.

It is usual to use a surrogate for human oral mucosal tissue, such as porcine buccal tissue, in such experiments. In countries where the use of pigs is not culturally acceptable, bovine buccal tissue with a non-keratinized epithelium has been used. The tissue may be excised from sacrificed animals or the local abattoir may provide a ready supply. Such experiments are commonly performed in the course of developing oral transmucosal dosage forms. Recently, cultured epithelial cell lines have been developed as an in vitro model for studying drug transport. They may also be used to study drug metabolism and to elucidate the possible mechanisms of action of penetration enhancers. Non-keratinized buccal cells (EpiOral™) available in six-well plates may be obtained from MatTek Corporation, and other brands are available from other companies as well. The use of these tissue plates involves a cost greater than that associated with obtaining excised buccal tissue from the local abattoir. However, the tissue is less variable and a more controlled experiment may result.

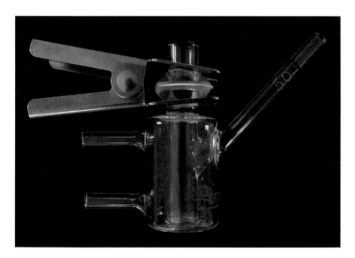

FIGURE 20-6 Frantz diffusion cell. (Used with permission from Permegear.)

Recap Questions

1. When using excised mucosal tissues, how can a lab reduce variability in in-vitro testing?
2. In vitro testing, using excised tissues may produce variable results. Should a scientist, therefore, go directly to human testing? Give reasons for your answer.
3. If porcine buccal mucosa is culturally unacceptable in a specific country, name two other methods that could be used for permeation testing.
4. What is a Frantz diffusion cell?
5. What does the acronym IRB refer to?

RESEARCH

Apart from the types of dosage forms mentioned above, several new approaches to the utilization of the oral mucosa for beneficial effects are currently being researched. These will be briefly discussed in order to give the student an idea of research directions, and the types of products that will likely be available in coming years when the student is a practitioner.

Oral Mucosal Vaccines

Vaccination has been one of the most important discoveries promoting the health of mankind. Most vaccines have been administered parenterally. In the past two decades, however, a growing body of research has shown that the administration of vaccines through the mucosal routes is viable in several instances. Transmucosal vaccination is different from parental vaccination for a number of reasons. The skin is a mechanical barrier that protects the body in different ways including the fact that it keeps out noxious chemicals and pathogens. To obtain an immune response via the skin, the skin has to be pierced and antigenic material introduced. Mucosal tissues, on the other hand, form part of the usual port of entry of pathogens which enter the body under normal circumstances encountered every day. The exposure to microorganisms does not require the presence of a disease condition, or of tissue damage. One example of such a situation is the act of swallowing food which may contain microorganisms. Therefore, these tissues have an arsenal of immunological mechanisms to deal with the normal load of microorganisms. The antigenic substance is engulfed by M cells on the surface of the mucosa and, thereafter, underlying specialized cells bring about the immunologic response. Since the mucosa is well-equipped to deal with antigens, it is logical that scientists make attempts to use the mucosal routes, including the oral mucosa, to develop mucosal vaccines.

One of the basic problems to be faced, in an attempt to develop an oral mucosal vaccine, is the fact that the mucosa comes into contact with a large number of epitopes every day. An epitope is the part of the antigen that the immune system recognizes. The immune system has created a mechanism to ignore the majority of them since they are not harmful. The immune response occurs only when an antigen is recognized as a threat. The problem in vaccine development, therefore, is to ensure that the antigen of interest is duly recognized by the immune cells and elicits an immunological response. It would, indeed, be a pity if, after much scientific development, the cells of the immune system chose to ignore the antigen that was presented in a vaccine as part of an elegant delivery system!

Generally, much larger doses of mucosal vaccines are required to elicit an immune response as compared to injectable vaccines. Since live, attenuated, and inactivated vaccines may present toxicity issues, the administration of a portion of the antigen (subunit vaccines) has been investigated. Since this type of vaccine has reduced immunogenicity, it became necessary to potentiate subunit vaccines for mucosal administration. This allows the administration of a low dose. One way to do this is through the use of adjuvants. The antigen is adsorbed onto the adjuvant and this potentiated combination is then incorporated into a vaccine delivery system. Unfortunately, an adjuvant that is useful for parenteral vaccines may not be efficient for mucosal vaccines. The adjuvant may help to modify the nature of the human response so that cell-mediated (TH1) and antibody-mediated (TH2) responses are produced. There are regulatory hurdles to bringing new adjuvants to market, just as there are with the use of new excipients for pharmaceuticals. The adjuvant-antigen combination is the subject of the regulatory application. Often companies would elect to use an approved adjuvant in their new antigen formulation instead of risking regulatory failure of the product due to FDA concerns about a new adjuvant. This approach has held back the availability of new adjuvants as well as the development of new vaccines.

Photodynamic Therapy

Two relatively new techniques which may be used for treating the oral mucosa are photodynamic therapy (PDT) and photodynamic antimicrobial chemotherapy (PACT). Both these techniques use a photoactive dye, or photosensitizer, which is activated by exposure to light of a specific wavelength. Once activated, the dye kills cancer cells or the microorganisms responsible for an infection, respectively. The dye itself is nontoxic, or has minimal toxicity, before activation by light energy. In addition, the photosensitizer is selectively attracted to the cancerous cells or microbial cells. Therefore, these unwanted cells are preferentially killed, whereas normal body cells are largely unaffected.

A wide range of medical conditions, including neoplastic conditions, may be treated. PACT has been shown to eradicate a wide range of pathogens in the oral cavity and is useful for those infections that respond poorly to conventional antibiotics and antifungal treatments. As may be expected, special formulations of the photosensitizer are required to deliver it accurately to the desired cells. A simple formulation, such as a mouthwash, may result in the photosensitizer staining the teeth and gums. This therapy is in the research stage at the time of writing, and no formulations have reached the market.

Physical Methods to Enhance Drug Delivery

The oral cavity is a convenient route for the administration of drugs. However, it offers resistance to the passage of many drugs. Various chemicals have been used to promote the absorption of drugs that are inherently poorly permeable, and research to study such enhancers, or to find additional enhancing compounds, has occurred over many decades. More recently, physical methods to promote transdermal permeation of drugs have been tried with some success. Considering these successes, it was natural for scientists to begin thinking of using physical methods to aid the delivery of drugs through the oral mucosa. For several reasons, including the fact that the oral mucosa is much thinner than the skin, these techniques have greater potential for success on the oral mucosa, than on skin. However, the skin is exposed, whereas the oral mucosa is within a cavity and more complex devices are needed to apply this technique to the mucosa than to skin. The patient acceptability of such delivery systems has yet to be established.

Iontophoresis is the physical technique that has been most studied with respect to the skin as well as the oral mucosal. It involves the creation of charged drug molecules due to the presence of an electric field created by the device used with this technique. The drug is applied to the permeating tissue (skin or mucosa) as a constituent of an electrolyte solution. Next, the device creates transient electric fields on the tissue in the area of the applied drug. The electric field causes the charged drug molecules to repel each other and pass through the tissue. The devices used to achieve these effects have become increasingly smaller as electronics and microchip fabrication have evolved. For this technique to work, the drug must be ionized or ionizable. While there are marketed transdermal products utilizing iontophoresis, this technique is in the research stage with respect to oral transmucosal drug delivery.

Sonophoresis is a physical method of enhancing drug delivery using sound waves. This technique has not been developed as much as iontophoresis. Research, however, is further advanced for transdermal delivery than for oral mucosal delivery. Physical methods of enhancing drug delivery have greater applicability to the transdermal route of drug administration and, for this reason, are discussed in greater detail in Chapter 22, Dermal and Transdermal Drug Delivery.

Recap Questions

1. Why do oral mucosal vaccines have to be potentiated?
2. What is the difference between PDT and PACT?
3. Why do you think physical methods of enhancing drug delivery have been tried on the skin before they were tried on the oral mucosa?

SUMMARY POINTS

- The need for oral mucosal drug delivery is mainly due to the fact that some drugs are destroyed in the GIT, or have poor bioavailability, yet may be sufficiently absorbed by the oral mucosa.
- Issues and problems:
  - Drug permeation is often inherently poor.
  - Mucoadhesive products have to be developed for prolonged action or for improved absorption.
  - The swallowing of the drug in the saliva is equivalent to a drug loss.
  - Complex patient instructions may be difficult to follow.
- Due to these issues, development includes permeation enhancement, dosage form development (taste may be an issue), and animal and human testing.
- Therapeutic advantages:
  - Non-invasive delivery
  - Reduced first-pass effect

- Fast attainment of clinically relevant blood levels may be possible
- Useful for drugs not well absorbed, or destroyed, in GIT
- The fentanyl products, Actiq and Fentora, by their scientific and commercial successes appear to have stimulated interest in basic research and in product development.
- Potential future new areas of research and development: oral transmucosal vaccines, photodynamic therapy and photodynamic antimicrobial chemotherapy, iontophoresis, and other physical methods of enhancing drug delivery

What do you think?

1. Why would one perform permeation studies using porcine buccal tissue (or other animal tissue) when the product is intended to be administered to humans?
2. Which characteristics of the oral mucosa impede the delivery of drugs via this route?
3. Which characteristics of the oral mucosa facilitate the delivery of drugs via this route?
4. A physician asks you to recommend either the oral route (swallowed drug) or the oral mucosal route, for a specific drug. What are the drug characteristics that you would need to know about in order to provide a reasoned answer?
5. Compare drug delivery through the skin and through the oral mucosa.
6. What is breakthrough pain as related to cancer?
7. Why is the oral mucosa suitable for the treatment of breakthrough pain?
8. Why should two doses be given: one for background treatment and one for breakthrough pain? Could the patient be given a higher dose of drug to cover both needs for pain medication?
9. What is MOTN insomnia? What is the rationale for using a special dosage form for treating this condition? Why not simply use a regular hypnotic?

BIBLIOGRAPHY

The author has abstracted and simplified, in part, several publications of which he is a coauthor.

Senel S, Rathbone MJ, Cansiz M, Pather I. Recent developments in buccal and sublingual delivery systems. *Expert Opin Drug Deliv.* 2012;9(6):615-628.

Rathbone MJ, Pather I, Senel S. Overview of oral mucosal delivery. In: Rathbone M, Senel S, Pather I, eds. *Oral Mucosal Drug Delivery and Therapy* (Book Series: *Advances in Delivery Science and Technology*). Springer (for Controlled Release Society); 2015.

Rathbone MJ, Senel S, Pather I. Design and development of systemic oral mucosal drug delivery systems. In: Rathbone MJ, Senel S, Pather I, eds. *Oral*

Mucosal Drug Delivery and Therapy (Book Series: *Advances in Delivery Science and Technology*). Springer (for Controlled Release Society); 2015.

Pather SI, Rathbone MJ, Senel S. Current status and the future of buccal drug delivery systems. *Expert Opin Drug Deliv*. 2008;5(5):531-542.

Pather SI, Rathbone MJ, Senel S. Introduction to oral mucosal drug delivery. In: Rathbone MJ, Hadgraft J, Roberts M, eds. *Modified-Release Drug Delivery Technology*. 2nd ed. New York, NY, and Basel: Marcel Dekker; 2008:53-73.

Pather SI, Hontz J, Khankari RK, Siebert J. OraVescent™: a novel technology for the transmucosal delivery of drugs. In: Rathbone MJ, Hadgraft J, Roberts M, eds. *Modified Release Drug Delivery Systems*. New York, NY, and Basel: Marcel Dekker; 2003:463-469.

Alur HH, Pather SI, Mitra AK, Johnston TP. Transbuccal sustained-delivery of chlorpheniramine maleate in rabbits using a novel, natural mucoadhesive gum as an excipient in buccal tablets. *Int J Pharm*. 1999;188:1-10.

Nasal Drug Delivery

PREVIEW

- Why nasal delivery is not only for conditions in the nose?
- Major anatomical and physiological features of the nose
- The physiological role of the nasal valve and how it impacts drug delivery
- Biopharmaceutical factors impacting drug delivery
- How are drugs absorbed through the nasal mucosa?
- What are the advantages and limitations of nasal drug delivery?
- A review of the major nasal drug delivery systems

INTRODUCTION

The nasal delivery of drugs has long been utilized for the alleviation of local conditions in the nose. Such conditions include allergic rhinitis, colds, and the nasal manifestations of influenza. The latter includes either a stuffy nose or a runny nose. Nasal delivery is a logical choice for the treatment of such conditions and largely prevents exposure of the entire body to the pharmacological agent. Most topical nasal treatments from the 1950s and earlier were vasoconstrictor formulations used to treat a stuffy nose, resulting from one of the above conditions. A number of these products contained ephedrine. The variety of topical treatments for these conditions has increased tremendously since their initial development. Starting initially with analogs of ephedrine as vasoconstrictors, additional treatments for these conditions now include a range of antihistamines, corticosteroids, and vasoconstrictors. In addition to the administration of locally acting drugs, it is now recognized that the nose may be utilized for the delivery of systemically acting drugs. This recognition arose from the observation that the nasal passages are lined with mucosal surfaces that have a good potential for drug absorption. This route is useful as an alternative to the oral route, for example, when a drug formulation cannot be easily swallowed. This could occur in very young children or in geriatrics, several of whom have difficulty swallowing.

Nasal delivery is important for the treatment of nausea which may arise as a side effect of certain treatments, such as chemotherapy. Oral anti-nausea medication is frequently administered prior to chemotherapy, as a preventative, and may be effective delivered in this manner. When a patient is already experiencing nausea (after chemotherapy, for example), it is frequently futile to offer the patient oral medication. This is because the patient is either unable to swallow the medication or unable to hold down the medication after consumption, without vomiting. In such a case, nasal drug administration is very useful. The nasal route is also useful in those disease states in which nausea is a complicating factor. Migraine is a significant condition displaying this characteristic. For this condition, the nasal route of

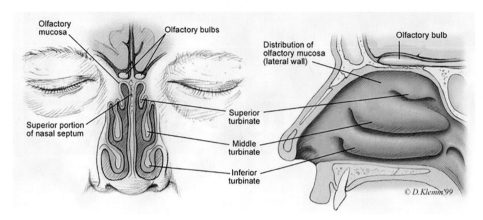

FIGURE 21-1 **Structure of the nose showing the olfactory bulb and olfactory mucosa.** (Reproduced, with permission, from Loscalzo J, Fauci AS, Kasper DL, et al. *Harrison's Principles of Internal Medicine.* 21st ed. New York, NY: McGraw Hill; 2022.)

drug administration is very useful. Because of the large nasal surface area, and its good absorptive properties, nasal delivery may also be used for other drugs, which are intended to exert their effect systemically. There is, presently, an intense research effort to formulate nasally delivered drugs for the systemic treatment of disease conditions (in contrast to local conditions within the nose). Some products in this category have already reached the marketplace.

A more recent discovery is the fact that certain drugs may be delivered directly to the brain via the nasal cavity. The olfactory neurons extend into the middle meatus of the nasal cavity and drug molecules that are brought to this region, deep within the nasal cavity, may be absorbed directly into the brain (Figure 21-1). Nasal drug delivery, therefore, serves three important functions: first, the delivery of drugs to treat local conditions within the nose; second, an alternate route for the systemic delivery of drugs; third, a mechanism to deliver drugs directly to the brain. The latter is very much in the research stage at present but provides an extremely useful potential for future drug delivery and has attracted a great deal of interest from researchers.

ANATOMY AND PHYSIOLOGY

The nose is the primary entrance to the respiratory tract in that air enters through the nose and passes into the lungs. The nasal cavity continues from the openings of the nostrils, or nares, at the front of the face to the nasopharynx, deep within the head. It is divided into a left and a right, half by the septum which is made of cartilage. The nose has a total surface area of around 160 cm² and a total volume of 16 to 19 mL in the average person. Since cold, dry air is not ideal for the lungs, the nose serves a useful function to warm as well as to humidify the air we breathe. Since particulate entry into the sensitive structures of the lungs, especially the alveoli, would be harmful, the nose serves the important function of filtering out particles in the inspired air. This is achieved by means of the cilia which trap such particles. In these ways, the nose serves to protect the delicate structures of the lungs by filtering and conditioning the air that reaches it. Considering the fact that thousands of liters of air are inhaled

daily, even in the resting state, the nose serves an important protective function. In addition, the nose helps with moisture retention during exhalation, thus preserving valuable body fluid.

The nose can be divided into three main regions: the vestibule, the turbinates, and the olfactory region (Figure 21-1). The vestibular region is the first (anterior) part of the nose and it is also the narrowest of the three major regions. Most of this area is covered by hairs (or vibrissae) which are responsible for the filtering function. Inhaled particles with an aerodynamic diameter of more than 10 μm will be trapped by these hairs, thus reducing the number of particles that reach deeper airways. (See Chapter 19, "Pulmonary Drug Delivery," for a description of aerodynamic diameter.) The surface lining of the vestibular region changes from one that is similar to the epidermis of the skin (in the proximal region close to the nares) to stratified squamous epithelium more distally. The turbinates are large bony structures, shaped like cones stretching backward into the deeper part of the nose. It is divided into the superior, the middle, and the inferior turbinates. Each turbinate encloses a space or cavity referred to as a meatus, that is, the three turbinates are associated with three meatuses. This region is covered by a highly vascular mucosa, the upper layer of which is a pseudostratified columnar epithelium composed of the following cell types: mucus secreting, ciliated, non-ciliated, and basal cells (Figure 21-2).

Each ciliated cell is covered with approximately 100 motile cilia. Their wave-like action transports mucus toward the pharynx. Inhaled particles are trapped in the mucus and are, therefore, removed from the nose by ciliary action. Since the cilia treat all particles alike, both pollutant particles as well as drug particles, from nasally administered medication, are transported to the posterior part of the nasal cavity. Since a drug solution, administered as either drops or a spray, will become mixed with mucus, such solutions will also be transported by mucociliary action. This limits the interaction of the drug with the mucous membrane and, hence, reduces the potential for drug absorption. Both the ciliated and the non-ciliated cells are covered with microvilli. These extensions of the cell membrane are not motile, and they are not responsible for clearing matter out of the nasal passage. These microvilli are responsible for vastly increasing the surface area available for drug absorption.

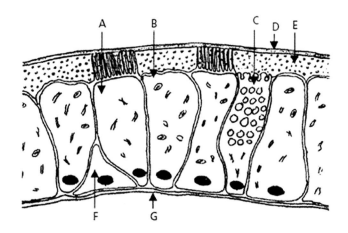

FIGURE 21-2 Cell types of the nasal mucosa showing:
A. ciliated cell; **B.** non-ciliated cell; **C.** Goblet cells; **D.** mucous gel-layer; **E.** sol layer; **F.** basal cells; and **G.** basement membrane. (Reproduced, with permission, from Ghori MU, Mahdi MH, Smith AM, Conway BR. Nasal drug delivery systems: an overview. *Am J Pharmacol Sci.* 2015;3(5):110-119; Ugwoke MI, Verbeke N, Kinget R. The biopharmaceutical aspects of nasal mucoadhesive drug delivery. *J Pharm Pharmacol.* 2001;53(1):3-22.)

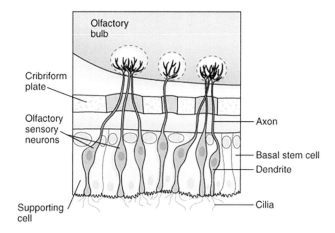

FIGURE 21-3 Olfactory sensory neurons. (Reproduced, with permission, from Kandel ER, Schwartz JH, Jessell TM, eds. *Principles of Neural Science.* 4th ed. New York, NY: McGraw Hill; 2000.)

Close to the end of the vestibular region, at the boundary with the inferior turbinate, is the internal nasal valve. The external nasal valve originates close to the internal nasal valve and extends toward the nares. These valves, especially the internal nasal valve, limit airflow into the nose. The two nasal valves are in close proximity to each other, and their function is also coordinated. When the general term, "the nasal valve" is used, it refers to both valves. The limitation of airflow is also a protective mechanism as large volumes of cold or toxic air, which would be harmful, cannot be inhaled rapidly into the lungs. The nasal valve is dynamic and its dimensions can increase by the action of dilator muscles to allow more rapid airflow. During rapid inhalation, the openings narrow progressively, again to control inspiratory airflow rate. In addition, the rate at which air is exhaled is also controlled by the nasal valve, so that warm, moist air is not rapidly lost. Retention of fluid and heat, as well as an extended time for gaseous exchange in the lungs, are the results of this limiting effect on the expiration rate.

The olfactory region consists of a neuroepithelium and olfactory sensory neurons located in the neuroepithelium[1] (Figure 21-3). The neuroepithelium covers the cribriform plate and other closely related regions at the back of the nose. Each neuron has a dendrite, the end of which projects into the nasal cavity. The end of each dendrite has 6 to 12 cilia that protrude into the mucus which covers the neuroepithelium. The mucus layer is approximately 5 μm thick and can trap drug particles. The mucus contains mucin, salts, proteins, and water, as well as some lipid material and has a pH that ranges from 5 to 6.5. Each sensory neuron expresses only one of approximately 450 receptor proteins.[2] Each protein reacts with more than one chemical. Odorous chemicals dissolve in the mucus and diffuse to the receptors located on the cilia. The mucus provides a good environment, in terms of molecular and ionic content, for odor detection. These chemicals may also be actively transported to the receptors by specialized proteins as an alternate mechanism

to diffusion. The axons of the sensory neurons pass through the Cribriform plate to the olfactory bulb which contains a few cell types. Certain cells of the olfactory bulb are directly connected to the brain.

From the above description, it can be seen that there is a direct connection from the nose to the brain. It is possible for drugs administered to the nose to reach the olfactory neurons and to be transported, by these neurons, into the brain. One possible mechanism is for the drug to dissolve in the myelin sheath of the axons of the olfactory neurons. The drug molecules may then be rapidly transported, along the axons, to the brain. However, the olfactory region represents only about 8% of the total surface area of the nose, and it is situated deep in the nasal cavity. Therefore, it is difficult to reach the entry point for drug administration to the brain. For this reason, this form of drug delivery may not be easy to achieve, although it may appear to be a tantalizingly good way to administer drugs directly to the brain.

Since the mucosal tissues, in general, are the major portals of entry for pathogens, mucosa-associated lymphoid tissues (MALT) are scattered along mucosal linings. It is the most extensive component of human lymphoid tissue and serves the purpose of protecting the body from an enormous quantity, and a very wide variety, of antigens. The mucosa which lines most of the nose, specifically, has immunologically active tissue referred to as nasal-associated lymphoid tissue (NALT). This tissue provides the opportunity for an early immunologic response to allergens contained in the air.

A component of NALT, the M cells, are scattered throughout the mucosa and are located at the epithelial surface. Under the M cells, are a variety of subepithelial lymphoid cells. All of these cell types function in a coordinated fashion to produce the immune response. The role of the M cells is absorption of antigen-containing material via the process of endocytosis. Next, the M cells process the material and transport specific fractions in order to present antigens to the subepithelial lymphoid cells. A cascade of events involving these subepithelial mucosal cells occurs which finally results in cell-mediated (Th1) and humoral (Th2) responses. Nasal mucosal tissues form a part of the nasal port of entry of pathogens, under normal circumstances, and these tissues have immunological mechanisms in place to confront and disarm entering pathogens. Immunological memory is also created.

Nasal vaccines may be produced, after appropriate scientific research and development, to protect against specific pathogens and allergens. While influenza nasal vaccine is already marketed, this is an area of intensive research to produce additional vaccines. Such vaccines are intended to induce both mucosal and systemic immunity. Nasal vaccines are potentially cheaper to produce and distribute than injectable vaccines. Injectable vaccines must consistently be maintained under refrigerated conditions, even when transferring from an aircraft to a truck, for example. Since there is no need to maintain such a "cold chain" during transport of nasal vaccines, costs are reduced. Nasal vaccines are also needle-free and eliminate the risk of needle reuse.

Recap Questions

1. Name three local conditions for which nasal delivery is useful.
2. Name the three major areas of the nasal cavity.
3. What is the major physiological function of the nasal valve?
4. Considering that the nostrils are not very large, how is it possible that nasal drug delivery can be effective?

BIOPHARMACEUTICAL CONSIDERATIONS

The high surface area of the nose makes it an attractive organ for drug delivery, and the easy accessibility to this absorptive surface is an added advantage. Drug absorption is affected by adequate deposition on the nasal mucosa, and by retention on the mucosa for a sufficient time. The latter is required for the drug to diffuse through the mucus layer to reach the mucosal cells. Therefore, several formulation factors must be taken into account to promote these desirable attributes. With regard to deposition, consideration should be given to the fact that the medication must be introduced into a tubular structure which has bends. For creams, gels, and other semisolids, this may be achieved by using a tube with a long, thin nozzle for deeper administration. In the case of a liquid, small drops (or a fine mist) should be administered into the nasal cavities so that the drug is dispersed over a large surface area to enhance absorption. Such administration must occur some way up the nostrils and not at their openings, or nares. The medication is administered in this way to prevent the liquid from simply leaking out of the nostrils and over the upper lip of the patient. Incorrect administration reduces the amount of drug available and is also inconvenient and cosmetically unacceptable to the patient. For improved delivery, special delivery devices may be needed to ensure that at least a portion of the medication reaches the absorptive mucosa. Such a device must be able to consistently deliver the liquid in the chosen format (ie, fine droplets of a specific size range), the nozzle should not clog easily, and residual liquid that has not left the delivery tube, should be able to flow back into the container.

The container must be of a suitable size to hold a sufficient number of doses, but it should not be bulky since the device may have to be carried in the patient's pocket or purse. The container must also help to keep the product stable over the shelf life of the product. For example, it should reduce light penetration if the drug is light sensitive. The fine mist may be achieved by applying pressure on a squeeze bottle, or by using a pump spray which has a mechanical device (such as a piston) to deliver the spray. In other instances, a fine mist may be achieved by using a pressurized aerosol device.

The greatest factor affecting the delivery of drugs to the absorptive surfaces of the nose is the presence of the nasal valves. As mentioned, they serve the physiological function of limiting rapid air entry into the lungs, and rapid exit of air and moisture from the lungs. Since the valves are narrow apertures, they also limit the volume of aerosolized droplets that may enter the deeper nasal passages. The openings of the sinus cavities (or ostia) are also located in the region of the superior and middle turbinates, and limited amounts of drug reach this area of the nasal cavity due to the presence of the nasal valves. In connection with this, consideration must also be given to the shape of the spray emitted by spray bottles or pressurized metered-dose inhalers (pMDI). This 3-dimensional shape, also known as the plume geometry (Figure 21-4B), is radically different from the narrow, slit-like aperture through which the medication must pass to reach the deeper parts of the nose. In in vitro testing, the plume has been shown to be a few centimeters wide. In contrast, the aperture allowing passage into the deeper structures of the nose, the nasal valve, is only a few millimeters wide. Furthermore, there is a tendency for droplets or particles to be, predominantly, at the periphery of the plume. Therefore, there is

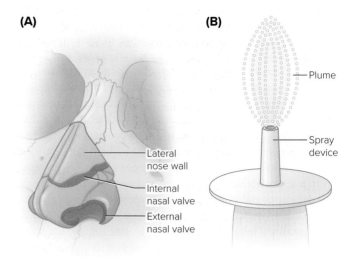

FIGURE 21-4 **A.** The nasal valves. **B.** The spray pattern or plume shape from a pump spray. Due to the width of the plume, much of the dose may reach the walls of the nostril and not pass the internal nasal valve. (**A:** springer.com.)

no alignment between the physical attributes of the spray plume and the aperture through which it must pass.

The selection of excipients frequently influences both the stability of a liquid product and its delivery characteristics. The latter includes the production of either droplets, or a mist, and the droplet size range. The solubility of the drug determines the concentration of the solution that can be produced. If the solubility is poor, a solution of sufficient concentration, to promote good absorption, cannot be formed. In such a situation, a solubility enhancer may be required. In other instances, a permeation enhancer is required because the drug is not very permeable through the nasal tissues. The latter two characteristics of the drug, namely, solubility and permeability, are dependent on many attributes of the drug such as its pKa, partition coefficient, and molecular weight.

Polar drugs and some macromolecules are not absorbed in therapeutic amounts due to poor membrane permeability and the presence of drug-degrading enzymes in the nose. The nasal cavity differs from the oral cavity in this respect: the nasal cavity displays much greater enzymatic degradation than is the case for the oral cavity. Since enzyme degradation in the nose is very significant, a (nasal) first-pass effect during absorption through the nasal mucosa has been described in the literature. This is similar to the first pass effect in the GIT. The "first pass" refers to the initial passage of the drug through the absorptive membrane when its high drug concentration can be greatly reduced by the action of metabolizing enzymes present in the membrane. This is in contrast to the lower level of metabolism that occurs in the oral cavity. The nasal blood flow rate and the mucociliary clearance rate affect absorption: an increase in the former improves absorption, whereas an increase in the latter reduces absorption since the drug is removed from the absorption site.

The physical condition of the nose is a person-to-person variable and, within the same individual, there may be changes in the physical condition from day to day. Some conditions, such as severe vasomotor rhinitis (chronic sneezing, congestion, or runny nose without the involvement of allergens; also known as non-allergic rhinitis) and atrophic rhinitis (a form of rhinitis involving atrophy of the nasal mucosa) can reduce nasal drug absorption. Allergic rhinitis or the common cold can cause a dripping of nasal secretions out of the nostrils, or down the back of the throat (post-nasal drip). When drugs are administered via the nose, under such circumstances, a loss of instilled drug may result in reduced bioavailability. Drugs that reach the back of the throat will eventually be transported to the stomach where the drug will experience the rigors of the GIT, as described in Chapter 3, Oral Route of Drug Delivery. Consequently, only a fraction of the swallowed drug may be absorbed in some instances. Knowledge of such degradation may have dictated the utilization of nasal administration, in the first place, for the drug in question.

Due to its viscosity, the mucus layer may limit diffusion and, thereby, act as a barrier to drug absorption. Mucus contains elongated strands of mucins to which drugs may bind, thus also limiting absorption. Colds and influenza may increase the viscosity of mucus, which further decreases absorption due to either mechanism: reduction of drug diffusion or enhanced binding to mucin. In either case, the effect is to decrease the bioavailability of administered drugs. On the other hand, the increased viscosity of the mucus, due to colds and influenza, can decrease mucociliary clearance, so allowing a longer time for absorption. These disease conditions can also affect the permeability of the membrane itself (apart from the effects mediated via the mucus) and such membrane alteration can influence the efficacy of the medication. Notwithstanding such limitations, the rate and extent of drug absorption, for several drugs, is rapid. In some instances, the plasma concentration versus time curve is comparable to IV drug administration curves.

Delivery of drugs from the nose directly to the brain, overcoming the blood-brain barrier (BBB), may be achieved by transport of certain drugs via the olfactory neuroepithelium. Considering that the brain is a very sensitive organ, nature has provided it with a barrier to drug penetration. This is largely made up of a membrane, surrounding the brain, which has tight junctions that seriously limit permeation of drugs. This barrier prevents substances circulating in the blood from entering the brain (apart from nutrients). In this way, the permeation of toxic substances into the brain, is limited. For example, if environmental pollutants were able to get into the blood stream, the BBB prevents them from entering the brain. This means that drugs, intended to treat brain conditions, are also prevented from penetrating the brain tissue since the BBB regards them as foreign, potentially toxic substances. Considering these limitations to drug delivery, the olfactory bulb presents an important route for drug administration to the brain. Drugs may be transmitted very rapidly along the neuronal axons directly to the brain. See Mind Map 21-1 for a summary of the functions and utility of the nose in drug delivery.

MECHANISMS OF DRUG ABSORPTION

After a drug is delivered to the nasal cavity, it must reach the mucous membrane before absorption can occur. To reach this membrane, the drug must diffuse through the mucus layer. Small molecules pass easily but large molecules may experience difficulty in diffusing through this barrier. As mentioned in Chapter 4, "Pharmaceutical Solutions, Diffusion, and Dissolution," a larger molecular size decreases the diffusivity of the molecule. In addition, mucus may also retard the diffusion process, as previously explained. Subsequent to diffusion through the mucus layer, absorption occurs by a few mechanisms, including:

1. Transcellular diffusion: diffusion across the cellular membrane and through the cytoplasm of the cell before passing through the opposite cell membrane and into the next cell, and so on.

2. Paracellular transport: diffusion of molecules between and around cells (through the interstitial fluid).

3. Transcytosis: the formation of vesicle carriers to transport drug molecules across the cell, involving the expenditure of energy (active transport).

In addition, tight junctions may be opened to allow enhanced diffusion. Transcellular and paracellular transport are the main mechanisms by which drugs move across the nasal membranes. These mechanisms are described in more detail in Chapter 20, Buccal and Sublingual Drug Delivery.

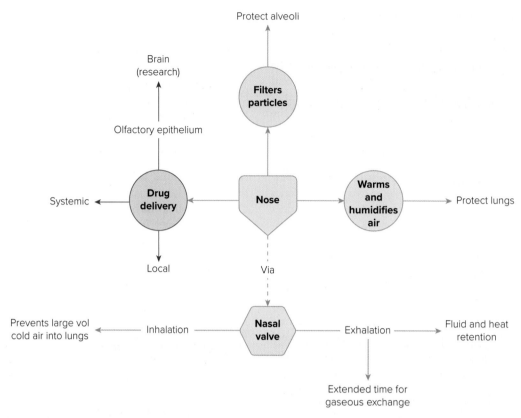

MIND MAP 21-1 Functions and Utility of the Nose

Lipophilic molecules are transported via the transcellular route. Generally, the greater the lipophilicity, the faster the transport. However, very highly lipophilic drugs may penetrate the upper layers of the squamous epithelium rapidly but may not permeate into deeper tissues which are more hydrophilic, that is, they display a tendency to remain in the hydrophobic regions. Paracellular transport is the mechanism of choice for highly water-soluble compounds. Such compounds do not penetrate the lipophilic cell membrane easily. The higher the molecular weight, the slower the diffusion of these compounds via the paracellular route. Lower bioavailability values have been reported for drugs with molecular weights higher than 1000 Daltons.

Many drugs, especially water-soluble drugs, display poor permeability across the nasal mucosa. To achieve reasonable absorption and bioavailability of such drugs, permeation enhancers must be used. These, generally, work by changing the structure of the mucosa temporarily. The rationale is to disrupt the permeation barrier for long enough that the drug may pass through and, thereafter, to reverse the changes fairly quickly. In this way, the barrier is interrupted for a short time only, limiting the opportunity for the permeation of noxious substances. While the exact mechanism of permeation enhancement, for a specific enhancer, is frequently not known, it is postulated that changes to the phospholipid bilayer of the cell membrane are often responsible for improved permeability. The subject of mucosal permeation enhancement is an area of intensive ongoing research with the aim of finding the ideal absorption enhancer. Some good enhancers were found to have unacceptable side effects. These include a reduction in the motility of the cilia and a temporary loss in the ability to smell, both

undesirable characteristics. The ideal permeation enhancer should not influence the nasal mucosa adversely in any way.

ADVANTAGES AND LIMITATIONS OF NASAL DRUG DELIVERY

With regard to the delivery of drugs to the systemic circulation, the nasal route has several advantages and some limitations.

Advantages

1. With certain drugs, very rapid absorption via the nasal route is possible. In such cases, the plasma concentration versus time profile may resemble that of an IV injection. Thus, the nasal route offers a rapid response without resorting to the invasiveness of an IV injection, in selected cases.

2. Nasal drug administration may be used to achieve therapeutic goals, in some instances where oral administration provides only sub-therapeutic blood concentrations. This includes drugs that are not well absorbed in the GIT, are degraded, or undergo extensive gut-wall, or hepatic first pass, metabolism.

3. The nasal route may also be utilized in cases where the GIT is not the preferred route, but also not a contraindicated route. Such situations include:

   a. Patients with nausea and vomiting, including those who have undergone chemotherapy, in whom the administration of an oral medication is likely to worsen the nausea; or migraineurs for many of whom the placement of a dosage form in the mouth, or even the thought of doing so, may induce nausea. Salivation from the placement of a dosage form in the mouth, in these patients, may act as the physical trigger for vomiting.

    b. Patients with swallowing difficulties including children and geriatrics

4. A major advantage of nasal delivery is the fact that the olfactory route may be utilized to deliver drugs directly to the brain. While this aspect of nasal delivery is very much in the research phase at present, it holds great potential. The magnitude of the olfactory advantage cannot be overstated because it is very difficult to deliver many drugs to the brain. Even IV injections are not very successful due to the BBB.

Limitations

1. The major limitation is the fact that the nasal route is not applicable to all drugs.

2. For several drugs, appreciable absorption is only possible with the use of permeation enhancers which have side effects, sometimes serious enough to preclude their use.

3. Many drugs administered for their local effects are also partially absorbed and may display unwanted systemic effects. Vasoconstrictors which are administered to relieve nasal congestion, elevate blood pressure in this manner (eg, pseudoephedrine).

4. While attempts have been made to make nasal drug delivery devices portable, they are not very small, and their size may be a limitation to some patients. This observation excludes nebulizers which, by their nature, are large.

5. For chronically administered drugs, the application procedures may not be as discreet as some patients prefer.

6. Nasal delivery was initially promoted as totally avoiding first-pass metabolism (through the gut wall and liver). It is now recognized that drug molecules passing through the nasal membrane also experience enzymatic degradation in the nose. While nasal "first pass" metabolism is less in extent than GI first pass metabolism, this effect is significant in many cases.

7. The nose is a sensitive organ and the drug as well as excipients can cause irritation. Irritation may also be due to the pH of the medium, its ionic strength, or the fact that a relatively large volume of medication is delivered.

8. Absorptive conditions within the nose are not static but may change with various common conditions such as allergic rhinitis, colds, and influenza.

Recap Questions

  1. What is the "plume" of a pump spray?

  2. What is the blood-brain barrier?

  3. Is the first pass effect limited to the GIT?

  4. What limits the utility of corticosteroid pump sprays used for relief of conditions in the nasal sinuses?

NASAL DRUG DELIVERY SYSTEMS

While it is theoretically possible to use a wide variety of delivery systems in the nose, only a few are commonly marketed dosage forms. Several others, such as nanotechnology delivery systems, are in the research phase at the present time. This section will emphasize delivery systems in common usage and very briefly mention a few that are in the research phase. Mind Map 21-2 presents a summary of nasal dosage forms.

Aqueous Drops

Aqueous nasal drops are probably the simplest dosage form for drug delivery to the nose. The fact that many drugs are not soluble in water is a limitation. However, this may be partially overcome by the addition of cosolvents and solubilization enhancers, as long as such additives are not irritating to the sensitive nasal mucosa. Two commonly used cosolvents are glycerin and propylene glycol. Nasal drops are delivered by means of a pipette or by the use of a squeeze bottle which is inverted and gently squeezed to deliver individual drops. Neither of these presentations delivers very accurate volumes.

The lack of precision of the dose is one of the major disadvantages of nasal drops. Delivery of the drops to the nasal passages is also largely dependent on gravity, which may be insufficient for the drops to reach deep into the nasal cavity, beyond the nasal valve. The risk of contamination of the pipette tip, or the nozzle of a squeeze bottle, by nasal secretions is an additional disadvantage. This could result in contamination of the contents of the bottle and consequent microbial growth. These are inherent risks associated with the use of drops.

Nasal drops are usually used for the symptomatic relief of local conditions but the leakage of the liquid from the front of the nose (onto the upper lip), or down the back of the throat, removes the drug from the required therapeutic area. Multiuse drops have, to a large extent, been replaced by metered-dose pump sprays. However, medications filled into inexpensive single-dose disposable pipettes are still offered for OTC products, such as decongestants and saline drops. In such products, there is no need for a preservative. Some common nasal drops are listed in Table 21-1.

Sprays from a Squeeze Bottle

Squeeze bottle sprays are largely confined to OTC products such as topical decongestants. The squeeze bottle is only partly filled with the product. As a result, a mixture of air and the drug solution is emitted when the bottle, held in the upright position, is squeezed. The formulation of nasal sprays is similar to that of nasal drops, with the additional requirement that the viscosity of the solution must be controlled at a low value. This is to ensure efficient passage through the nozzle of the device. In addition, the surface tension should be such that droplets of the optimal size are delivered. Droplet size is affected primarily by the orifice diameter of the nozzle of the bottle, and the surface tension of the liquid. The surface tension of a liquid pulls surface molecules inward and may be considered to be acting like a "skin," holding the liquid molecules together. A high surface tension in the formulation resists breakup of the

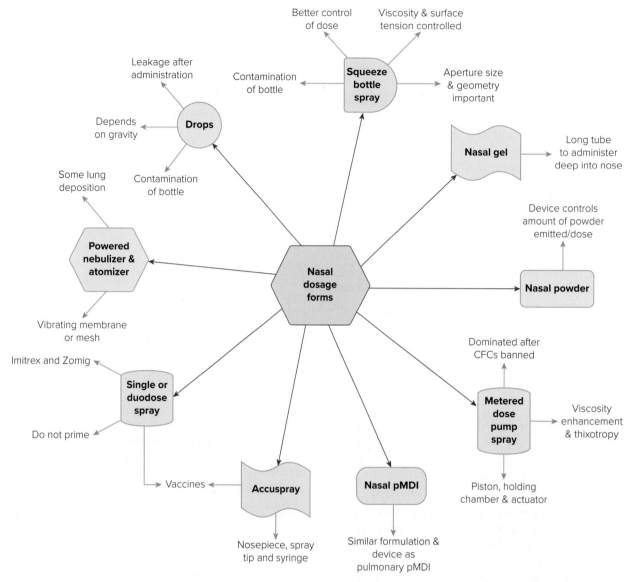

MIND MAP 21-2 Nasal Dosage Forms

liquid, resulting in large drops. Of the solvents used for nasal formulations, water has a high surface tension and forcing it through small apertures helps to overcome the surface tension to form fine droplets. Surface tension may be reduced by the use of surfactants. However, they must be used judiciously because the surfactant is likely to be irritant to the sensitive nasal mucosa.

Nasal sprays may be delivered by means of a squeeze bottle or a spray system. Squeeze bottles for sprays differ from those for drops in terms of the orifice size and geometry. Spray bottles have finer apertures and more complex geometry is required to create a fine-droplet spray. Spray bottles deliver more accurate volumes than can be achieved with drops. However, the volume delivered, as well as the droplet size, may vary with the

TABLE 21-1	Some Common Nasal Drops and Squeeze-Bottle Nasal Sprays		
TRADE NAME	**ACTIVE INGREDIENT**	**INDICATION**	**MANUFACTURER**
Little Remedies Saline Drops/Spray	NaCl	Nasal allergy	Novartis
Afrin Nasal Spray	Oxymetazoline HCl	Nasal decongestant	Bayer
Neo-Synephrine Spray	Phenylephrine HCl	Nasal decongestant	Walgreens
Otrivin Spray	Xylometazoline HCl	Nasal decongestant	GSK (Canada)
Flixonase Nasal Spray	Fluticasone	Nasal polyps	Allen and Hanbury's (UK)

force applied to create the spray. Furthermore, when the pressure on the squeeze bottle is released, air is sucked back into the bottle to make up the total volume of the (undepressed) bottle. If the pressure on the bottle is released while the tip of the squeeze bottle is still within the nasal cavity, nasal secretions (in addition to air) will be sucked into the bottle, leading to contamination. Some squeeze bottle nasal delivery products are listed in Table 21-1.

Metered-Dose Pump Sprays

Metered-dose pump sprays achieved prominence in the nasal market after their introduction in the early 1970s. With the elimination of chlorofluorocarbons (CFCs) for aerosol use, the domination of metered-dose pump sprays has been even more extensive. When CFCs were banned, aerosols for pulmonary delivery were largely changed from CFC to hydrofluoroalkane (HFA) propellants. On the other hand, nasal pMDIs were largely converted to propellant-free, metered-dose pump sprays. The aqueous drug solution is delivered by means of a device consisting of a chamber, a piston and an actuator. In the typical pump spray, the emitted dose is replaced with air that goes into the main chamber of the device.

Factors such as surface tension and viscosity can influence droplet size which has an impact on the dose delivered. In this context, thixotropy may also have an impact on the delivered dose since any changes in viscosity may influence the droplet size. Thixotropy is the ability of a solution, of a certain viscosity, to reversibly change viscosity as a consequence of being subjected to a shearing stress. A common example of a shearing stress is observed when a liquid is stirred. In general, it is possible for rapid stirring to decrease the viscosity of some solutions (containing plastic or pseudoplastic polymers), and to increase the viscosity of others. The solution slowly reverts to its original viscosity when stirring is stopped. This behavior, of undergoing a reversible viscosity change under shearing stress, is referred to as thixotropy. While stirring has been given as an example of a shearing stress, other examples can be observed in pharmaceutical technology. The force required to push a liquid through a narrow aperture is a shearing stress, analogous to stirring and is of relevance to the present discussion.

Formulators may consider adding small amounts of polymers to solutions for nasal delivery in order to enhance the viscosity of the solution. This is done to reduce drip from the nose after the dose is delivered. Upon administration, the polymer-containing solution is subjected to a shearing stress and the viscosity of the solution is reduced. After delivery of the droplets, there is no further shearing stress, and the viscosity gradually increases to its original level which is effective in reducing drip. Such viscosity changes must be taken into account when estimating droplet size, since viscosity influences the droplet size produced after forcing a liquid through a small aperture. The delivered droplet size impacts the magnitude of the delivered dose.

The design of the pump, the applied force and the orifice size can also affect the droplet size. A typical metered-dose pump spray is depicted in Figure 21-5. To operate the pump spray, the index and middle fingers are placed on the shoulders of the device, with the thumb placed onto the base of the liquid

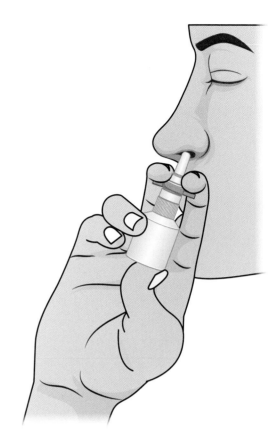

FIGURE 21-5 A typical metered-dose pump spray.

container. The pump spray is activated by pressure between the thumb and the two fingers. This forces liquid through a narrow aperture in the nozzle and the liquid is emitted as a fine spray. The shape of the emitted spray, referred to as the plume geometry, can also affect the deposition of droplets within the nasal cavity. For example, whether the plume is broad or narrow can affect how efficiently the spray droplets are deposited within the nasal cavity. A narrow plume is better for penetration beyond the nasal valve.

The manufacturer decides the volume to be delivered based on the formulation. Typically, the delivered volume is in the 25 to 200 μL range to match commercially available pump spray components. Each volume requires a different holding chamber and valve assembly. The latter has two valves: when one opens, the other is closed, and vice-versa. The holding chamber is designed to hold the specified volume of liquid needed for dosing. The first time the actuator is depressed by the patient, no spray is emitted because the holding chamber is empty. However, when the pressure is released, the piston rises and the predetermined volume is filled into the holding chamber from the bulk liquid container. At this time, the lower of the two valves is open, allowing the liquid to flow from the bulk container into the holding chamber. The next time the spray is activated, the volume of liquid in the holding chamber is forced out through the fine aperture of the nozzle. During actuation, the upper valve opens to allow the liquid to be forced out of the holding chamber under pressure, while the lower valve remains closed. When the pressure on the bottle is released, the lower valve opens and the holding chamber is filled once more. During this time, the upper valve is closed and no spray is emitted. If the spray is not used for an extended time, the liquid in the holding chamber gradually leaks out into the main chamber. However, the loss is negligible if the pump spray is used within a short time, that is, the volume of liquid in the holding chamber will be intact for practical purposes.

Priming refers to the actuation of the pump without inserting the nozzle into a nostril, with the emission of some spray into the air. This first spray, executed in this manner, may not be the equivalent of a full dose. However, it allows for the transfer of the correct volume of liquid, from the bottle, into the pumping system when the pressure between the thumb and fingers is released. This ensures that a more accurate dose is delivered when the spray is applied to the nostrils, immediately after priming. It is for this reason that the pump spray must be primed again, if it has not been used for some time. If the pump spray is used again within a short time (for example, the next day), there is no need for re-priming because the dose is maintained in the pump system. It is only when the pump spray has not been used for long that there may be significant loss of liquid from the metered (measured) dose.

Within the volume range of commercial pump spray components (25-200 mL), the selected volume is fairly accurately delivered. In addition, plume geometry is also reproduced quite well. The plume geometry affects the deposition of the spray in the nostrils and the fact that it is reproducible positively influences consistent deposition from day to day, or from one spray bottle to the next. It does not necessarily mean that deposition is efficient. The plume is much broader than the slit representing the nasal valve and, in addition, the periphery of the plume is richer in droplets. For these reasons, the plume is not ideal for drug delivery into the deeper parts of the nose, as previously mentioned under "Biopharmaceutical Considerations." Some commonly used commercial pump sprays are listed in Table 21-2. The typical pump sprays contain many doses, enabling continued use over an extended time. For conditions such as allergic rhinitis, for example, the pump spray may be used twice daily for 2 weeks and then not used again until the next allergy season. With such intermittent use, the pump will require priming when first used, and then re-priming at the next allergy season.

Because of the need for priming, as well as to ensure delivery of the labeled number of doses, some degree of overfill is utilized in these systems. This was acceptable for the drugs used in these older pump sprays, for example, antihistamines or corticosteroids. However, nasal delivery is also suitable for the treatment of systemic diseases, often using high-potency, narrow therapeutic index drugs. Both the overfilling and the priming may not be acceptable for such drugs, especially since some are expensive. It is also not acceptable to spray potent drugs into the air. In addition, the traditional pump spray delivered a reasonably accurate, but not a highly accurate, dose. For expensive drugs, those requiring tight control of dosage, and for drugs that are administered once, or sporadically, single-dose or duo-dose spray devices are preferable (Figure 21-6). These devices control the dose very accurately and, due to their construction, do not need priming.

A potential problem with pump sprays containing one dose is the fact that the dose will be lost if the patient primes the pump. This may occur, due to force of habit, if the patient is accustomed to using multi-dose pumps. An important instruction for the pharmacist to give the patient is the direction not to prime the pump, mentioning that the single dose (or one of two

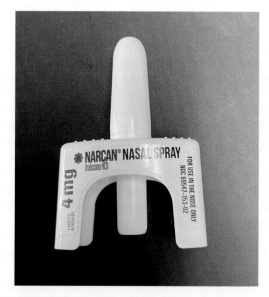

FIGURE 21-6 A single-dose, disposable pump spray.

TABLE 21-2	Some Common Nasal Mechanical Pump Sprays		
TRADE NAME	**ACTIVE INGREDIENT**	**INDICATION**	**MANUFACTURER**
Fluticare	Fluticasone proprionate	Nasal allergy	Novartis
Afrin Pump Mist	Oxymetazoline HCl	Nasal decongestant	Bayer
Rhinocort	Budesonide	Nasal allergy	AstraZeneca AB
Miacalcin	Calcitonin	Osteoporosis	Novartis
Narcan Nasal Spray (duo dose)	Naloxone	Opioid overdose	Adapt Pharma
Zomig Nasal Spray (syringe-type single dose units)	Zolmitriptan	Migraine	AstraZeneca

doses) would be lost if this instruction is not followed. Similar information needs to be provided to nursing, or other clinical staff when mass vaccinations are given using single- or duo-dose nasal vaccines.

Becton Dickinson Technologies developed a relatively simple device consisting of a nose piece with a spray tip attached to a prefilled syringe to accurately administer one or two doses (Accuspray*). It is used to deliver the influenza vaccine, FluMist* which is approved for both adults and children in the United States. The barrel of the syringe is placed between the index and middle fingers, and the actuator is depressed with the thumb (much like an injection would be administered). Pressure on the actuator depresses a piston which causes the liquid contents of the device to be emitted into a swirl chamber. Continued pressure causes the liquid to swirl within the chamber, forming the spray which is forced out through the nose piece. Nasally administered migraine drugs such as Imitrex (sumatriptan) marketed by GSK, and Zomig (Zolmitriptan) marketed by AstraZeneca (in addition to FluMist) are supplied with this type of device. With sterile filling, and the limited number of doses, the need for a preservative is obviated. However, there is still the requirement for a small overfill in order to deliver an accurate dose.

Nasal Pressurized Metered-Dose Inhalers

The construction of nasal pMDIs is similar to that of aerosols for pulmonary delivery, as described in Chapter 19, "Pulmonary Drug Delivery." Such devices were popular when the use of CFCs, to obtain the required pressure, was considered acceptable, and were also legally permissible. Such inhalers had the disadvantage of causing nasal irritation and some dryness, and some patients complained about a sensation of cold upon discharge of the inhaler. In addition, the very high velocity at which the droplets were emitted from the pMDI caused a stinging sensation. Since the velocity of emission from a pump spray is lower, this effect is not experienced. The velocity of emission from an HFA product is in between that of a CFC pMDI and a pump spray.

For these reasons, an HFA product could, theoretically, have been predicted to have been more patient acceptable than the equivalent CFC product. Nevertheless, HFA nasal products were slow to reach the marketplace. As mentioned, when CFCs were banned, many manufacturers did not convert their nasal CFC products to nasal HFA products. Instead, many products were converted to pump sprays. The first nasal HFA product to be marketed in the United States contained the steroid, beclomethasone dipropionate, with an indication for allergic rhinitis.

The pMDI has the same disadvantage as the pump spray: deposition of the drug is mostly in the vestibule, with a small amount reaching beyond the nasal valve (Figure 21-4). This is due to a similar plume shape, and the distribution of droplets within the plume, for the pMDI and the pump spray (ie, the droplets are found to a greater extent toward the periphery of the plume). However, liquid dripping out of the nostrils is less of a problem with the pMDI than it is with the pump spray, since the liquid droplets evaporate rapidly in the former because the droplets consist of liquefied propellant and not water.

Powered Nebulizers and Atomizers

Several powered nebulizers are available and they use either compressed gases or power (ultrasonic or mechanical) to distribute a solution as small aerosol droplets. The VibrENT nebulizer uses a pulsating perforated membrane to deliver the droplets while the Aironeb Solo has a vibrating mesh for the same purpose. These mechanisms result in small droplets which move at a low speed. This promotes, in theory at least, improved delivery to the middle and superior meatuses and paranasal sinuses. For this reason, these devices are attractive, and they have been demonstrated to show better deposition to the upper part of the nose compared to a metered dose pump spray. The problem of lung deposition is, however, inherent with nebulizers. Lung deposition may be significant while nasal delivery may be relatively low. A large proportion of the dose reaches the vestibule only and it is also delivered close to the floor of the vestibule. If the droplets were delivered higher up (ie, away from the floor), it would increase the probability of the droplets penetrating the nasal valve.

Several efforts have been made, in experimental studies, to decrease pulmonary delivery. These include aspiration of the contralateral nostril. This involves nebulization into one nostril and removal of the nebulized droplets from the other, while breathing through the mouth. In another study, subjects were asked to consciously push the soft palate upwards, to close off entry to the lungs. Both techniques reduced pulmonary delivery but are not practical since they involve special breathing techniques, not easily achievable for many patients.

The ViaNase atomizer is a handheld, battery-driven device intended for nasal delivery (Kurve Technology, Inc.). A vortex of flowing liquid is produced at the exit of the device and both the circular velocity as well as the direction of flow of the liquid can be adjusted. The aim is to target the sinuses and some gamma scintigraphy images suggest that there is a degree of deposition in this region, but the extent of deposition has not been quantified. This device has been used to deliver nasal insulin in patients with early Alzheimer's disease and some clinical benefits have been claimed although deposition of insulin in the lungs is likely. The consequences of pulmonary insulin deposition were highlighted with the advent of Exubera, intended for pulmonary delivery of insulin for diabetes treatment. The product had to be withdrawn due to the unacceptable side effects of insulin on pulmonary tissue.

Nasal Gels

A gel is a soft semisolid material consisting of two or more components, one of which is a liquid present in a large proportion. The other is a solid, often a polymer, although gels may also be formed from certain solid, inorganic particles. The latter become solvated and swell in the liquid, forming a network of linked particles, thus creating the gel structure. Gels are discussed in more detail in Chapter 22, Dermal and Transdermal Drug Delivery. The rheological properties of the gel depend on the type of polymer, or inorganic particulate material, and its concentration. With respect to polymers, the average molecular weight is critical. For a fixed concentration of polymer (eg, 3%), the viscosity may vary widely depending on the molecular weight of the polymeric substance, for example, 3% methylcellulose 1000 will produce a much lower viscosity than 3% methylcellulose 3000.

The primary reason for using gels in the past was the fact that they have a higher viscosity and will not easily leak out of the nose or be cleared by mucociliary action. In recent years, mucoadhesive gels have been developed with improved characteristics. In addition to the higher viscosity, there is the additional effect of mucoadhesion. The latter retains the dosage form in the nasal cavity for significantly longer than can be achieved with enhanced viscosity alone. The mucoadhesive action is a specific interaction of the polymer with the mucus. Since the mucoadhesive effect is not instantaneous, the gel may spread initially over the mucous membrane. This is referred to as the contact stage. The next stage is the consolidation stage which involves the penetration of polymer chains into the mucus. The initial intermingling of mucin strands with polymer strands progresses to entanglement of the strands with each other. Subsequently, chemical bonding between the strands further consolidates the interaction in the case of polymers which have a chemical structure that enables chemical interaction.

While mucoadhesion retains the gel at the site of application, the viscous nature of the gel controls the rate and extent of drug permeation into the mucosa. The higher the gel viscosity, the slower the permeation of drug molecules through it. Consequently, drug molecules reach the absorptive membrane slowly and continuously over an extended period, and this results in prolonged action of the medication. Since the frequency of administration is reduced, mucoadhesion has the potential to improve patient compliance. The fact that the gel is retained for a longer period means that absorption can continue for longer, resulting in improved bioavailability in many instances.

In selecting polymers to formulate mucoadhesive systems, it is essential that the polymer be biocompatible. It is also desirable that the polymer be biodegradable. Some of the polymers that have been used in nasal delivery systems are polyvinyl alcohol, Carbopol, alginate, starch, gellan gum and various cellulose derivatives (eg, hydroxypropyl methylcellulose and hydroxypropyl cellulose). The gel may be dispensed from a tube with an elongated nasal applicator, for insertion deep into the nose. Many gels are pseudo-plastic, exhibiting shear-thinning behavior. This means that they become thinner when they are subjected to shearing stress, such as when they are rapidly stirred. In light of this behavior, it was expected that they could be delivered from a spray squeeze bottle. The rationale for this is that pressure applied to the gel, as it is squeezed through a narrow aperture, represents an application of shearing stress (analogous to rapid stirring). This would result in sufficiently reduced viscosity to enable the material to flow from the squeeze bottle. In practice, however, it was found that it is not easy to deliver gels from squeeze bottles.

A solution to this problem, apart from dispensing gels in tubes with a long nozzle, is to make use of *in situ* gel-forming polymers. An *in situ* gel former is one that does not have the form of a gel in the bottle in which it is supplied but, instead, is a liquid (or sol). When administered, some condition prevailing at the administration site changes the sol formulation into a gel, that is, a sol-gel transformation occurs. Factors that may induce this transformation include temperature, the ionic strength, and the pH of the medium into which the gel is placed.

Nasal Powders

A multidose budesonide powder inhaler is marketed by AstraZeneca utilizing a Turbuhaler device modified for nasal inhalation. See Chapter 19, Pulmonary Drug Delivery for a description of the pulmonary Turbuhaler device which is mechanistically similar to the nasal device. The nasal product is marketed under the trade name, Rhinocort Turbuhaler, for allergic rhinitis and nasal polyps. It is an alternative to the liquid spray. In a study comparing aqueous budenoside spray and the Rhinocort Turbuhaler, both treatments significantly reduced polyp size, with no difference between these treatments. However, in terms of nasal symptoms experienced by the patient, the liquid spray was significantly better. In deposition studies, it was shown that the Turbuhaler displays predominantly anterior deposition in the nose, that is, deposition in the vestibule. In addition, there was some deposition in the lungs.

Several other powder devices are currently under development, including novel systems that require the patient to blow through the device, via the mouth, to release the powder that enters the nostril. The advantage of so doing is that the act of blowing through the mouth causes the soft palate to be pushed upward, closing it off from the pharynx, thus limiting pulmonary delivery of the active. Another interesting concept is the bidirectional technology which involves inhalation through one nostril, passage of the powder, or liquid, around the back of the septum and into the other nostril. Since it is generally difficult to deliver medication beyond the nasal valve, this mechanism of entering a nostril through the "back door" may have possibilities. Interestingly, such a technique for the administration of irrigation liquids to the nose has been described well over 1000 years ago. In Ayurveda, an ancient system of medicine, breath control is used for inhalation of a liquid through one nostril and expulsion of the liquid through the other nostril, without reliance upon a device.

Recap Questions

1. A squeeze bottle may be used to deliver a spray, or drops, to the nose. What is the difference in the method of administration to achieve each of these presentations from the same bottle?

2. What is the disadvantage of a squeeze bottle, the nozzle of which is inserted into a nostril before the dose is administered?

3. What is the major disadvantage with nasal drops?

4. What is the advantage of using drops from a single-use pipette compared to using them from a dropper bottle?

5. What led to the increased popularity of metered-dose pump sprays?

6. What is meant by "plume geometry"?

7. When is it necessary to prime a metered-dose pump spray?

8. Under what circumstances does a nose spray not require a preservative?

9. Why is there a reduced tendency for liquid to leak out of the nose after using a nasal pMDI compared to a metered-dose pump spray?

10. Powered nebulizers create smaller droplets that travel at a slower speed. Why is this advantageous for nasal delivery?

11. What is the major disadvantage of powered nebulizers?

12. The ViaNase atomizer is used to target the sinuses. How did the company illustrate that some of the liquid droplets reached their target?

13. What is the advantage of using a gel for nasal delivery?

14. How does the Rhinocort Turbuhaler differ from a metered-dose pump spray?

What do you think?

1. Explain the major disadvantage of nasal drops in terms of physical forces involved and anatomical considerations.

2. What is the "ideal" spray pattern from a pump spray?

3. What is the difference between "viscosity" and "muco-adhesion"? Explain the effect of each on the efficacy of drug delivery to the nose.

4. "Aerosols for nasal delivery were largely supplanted by metered-dose pump sprays for reasons that do not relate to the efficacy of the aerosol." Do you agree or disagree with this statement? Give reasons for your answer.

5. An athlete wishes to widen his normal nasal valves to improve his athletic performance. How would you advise him? Assume the surgical procedure can be relatively easily performed.

SUMMARY POINTS

- Nasal delivery was traditionally used to treat local conditions in the nose but is also used today for systemic drug delivery, while delivery via the olfactory route shows promise.
- The structure of the nose is complex revealing a large surface area for drug absorption.
- Delivery beyond the nasal valve is difficult and the subject of several research studies.
- HFA nasal inhalers did not replace CFC inhalers to the same extent as occurred for pulmonary inhalers.
- Nasal pump sprays have become popular, but they require priming and re-priming if not used for long.
- Single-dose and duo-dose disposable inhalers, which do not need priming, are coming into the market for vaccines and sporadic treatment of systemic conditions.
- Nebulizers are able to deliver a portion of the dose beyond the nasal valve but suffer from the disadvantage of some pulmonary delivery.
- The ideal nebulizer would be patient-friendly, would not require difficult breath control, and would deliver a significant proportion of the drug beyond the nasal valve with negligible pulmonary delivery.

REFERENCES

1. Smell & taste. In: Barrett KE, Barman SM, Boitano S, Reckelhoff JF. eds. *Ganong's Medical Physiology Examination & Board Review*. New York, NY: McGraw-Hill; http://accessmedicine.mhmedical.com/Content.Aspx?Bookid=2139&Sectionid=160312294. Accessed January 06, 2018.

2. Doty RL, Bromley SM. Disorders of Smell and Taste. In: Loscalzo J, Fauci A, Kasper D, Hauser S, Longo D, Jameson J. eds. *Harrison's Principles of Internal Medicine, 21e*. McGraw Hill; 2022. https://accessmedicine.mhmedical.com/content.aspx?bookid=3095&sectionid=263546447. Accessed January 08, 2024.

BIBLIOGRAPHY

Djupesland PG. Nasal drug delivery devices: characteristics and performance in a clinical perspective: a review. *Drug Deliv and Transl Res*. 2013;3:42-62. https://doi.org/10.1007/s13346-012-0108-9. Accessed 22 September 2017.

Ghori MU, Mahdi MH, Smith AM, Conway BR. Nasal drug delivery systems: an overview. *Am J Pharmacol Sci*. 2015;3(5):110-119. Accessed 29 September 2017.

https://www.medicines.org.uk/emc/files/pil.5503.pdf. Accessed December 15, 2017.

https://www.narcan.com/. Accessed December 17, 2017.

Dermal and Transdermal Drug Delivery

22

PREVIEW

- The difference between dermal and transdermal delivery systems
- A brief outline of the more important types of dermal dosage forms
- Why transdermal drug delivery is important
- A brief history of the transdermal route of drug delivery
- The different types of transdermal drug delivery
    - Passive diffusion
    - Chemically enhanced
    - Energy enhanced
    - Poration methods
- Future developments in transdermal drug delivery

INTRODUCTION

Substances purported to provide beneficial results to human health have been applied to the skin for thousands of years. Among the earliest records of dermal treatments are those of traditional Chinese medicine, and those of Ayurveda, the

317

traditional Indian system of medicine. The latter provides many examples of massaging the body with unmedicated oils, or oils infused with herbal medications. Interestingly, massage with oils is prescribed for the penetration of medicinal agents into, and for the removal of toxins from, the body. In modern Western medicine, ointments, creams, gels, etc., have been used for topical effects. These include the relief of muscular pain by the counter-irritant principle, the local treatment of infections, soothing burns and minor injuries, and other skin conditions such as eczema.

Following anecdotal reporting that several drugs crossed the skin to exert desirable systemic effects, a systematic approach to the study of transdermal drug delivery was adopted in recent decades. The delivery of drugs through the skin into deeper tissues continues to be an area of great interest. When a permeated drug is further absorbed into the blood circulation, it will be delivered throughout the body. Such a drug has an even greater interest because it can enable systemic effects. This research interest has spawned the development of several products for human use. Intensive research into this subject continues today, both in academia and in the pharmaceutical industry. Mind Map 22-1 illustrates dermal products as well as the development of transdermal products.

DERMAL DRUG DELIVERY

Local actions of drugs on the skin include effects on the surface, that is, effects exerted on the stratum corneum, as well as those on the epidermis, or the dermis. Product types used for local action are numerous, with a nomenclature that is frequently poorly defined. These include powders, creams, ointments, gels, pastes, lotions, foams, and sprays. They are typically referred to as topical products to distinguish them from transdermal products. The latter deliver drugs to the circulation for systemic pharmacological effects.

Ointments

Ointments contain ingredients with an oily or waxy feel as a large percentage of the formulation (usually over 50%). Such components usually consist of hydrocarbons, waxes, or polyols (or mixtures thereof). While the polyols are not hydrophobic, they usually have a waxy feel and are, hence, included in this group. An ointment consists of the active ingredient(s) and an ointment base. Since the base is the major component, ointments may be categorized by reference to the type of base that it contains. The following classes of bases are recognized:

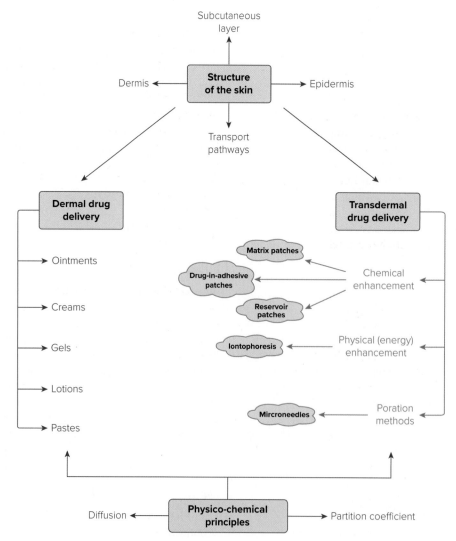

MIND MAP 22-1 **Dermal and Transdermal Drug Delivery**

hydrocarbon bases (also known as oleaginous bases), absorption bases, water-removable bases, and water-soluble bases.

Hydrocarbon Bases

Two well-known examples of hydrocarbon bases are White Petrolatum, USP and White Ointment, USP. Because of their oleaginous (oily) nature, only a small amount of aqueous components can be incorporated into these bases. Since they are difficult to wash off, they keep the medicament in close contact with the skin for a prolonged time. Perspiration, for example, will not easily remove the base. They also act as occlusive dressings, because of their oily nature. Substances cannot pass out of occluded skin easily, nor can external substances penetrate the occlusive barrier. In addition, water vapor cannot leave the skin easily and therefore such ointments have an emollient function, that is, they increase the hydration of the skin. A piece of cellophane stuck onto the skin is an example of an everyday material that is occlusive.

The resistance to washing off keeps the drug in close contact with the skin. These preparations do not dry out or change noticeably during storage because of their low water content. Generally, they age well and their stability will usually be determined by the stability of the drug and not by changes in the ointment base. This is different from creams, for example, where the stability of the formulation may be dependent, significantly, on the stability of the cream base. The latter is subject to physical changes such as creaming and breaking (see Chapter 15, Dosage Form Stability).

Absorption Bases

As the name implies, these hydrophobic bases absorb water. One subcategory is ointments that can absorb water to form a cream of the water-in-oil (W/O) type, examples of which are hydrophilic petrolatum, USP and lanolin, USP. The other subcategory consists of bases that have already absorbed water and, therefore, exist in the form of W/O emulsions where such emulsions have the ability to absorb more water or aqueous solutions. An example of this type is hydrous lanolin, USP. Both classes of absorption bases are good emollients since they contain water, in a finely distributed state, which they can release to penetrate into the skin.

Water-Removable Bases

Water-removable bases are oil-in-water (O/W) emulsions and, for this reason, ought to be called "creams." The latter terminology is only mentioned here for completeness, since these bases are referred to as ointments due to their waxy or oily feel. Emulsions are miscible with their external phase, that is, an O/W emulsion is miscible with water, explaining why this base is water removable and the reason for the name of this class of base. See Chapter 7, Emulsions, for an explanation of the different types of emulsions. These bases are more consumer acceptable because they can be easily washed off the skin or clothing with water.

Some medications may be more effective in these bases, as compared to hydrocarbon bases. This is due to the fact that a hydrophobic drug will more readily leave such a base, compared to a more hydrophobic base, to enter the skin. The latter type of base has a greater affinity for the hydrophobic drug which it retains to a greater extent. These bases will absorb aqueous

discharges, for example, from wounds. Hydrophilic ointment, USP is an example.

Water Soluble Bases

Water-soluble bases have a greasy or waxy feel though they are actually hydrophilic. They are also called "greaseless" ointment bases. They can also be removed by water and, in addition, are soluble in water. They contain no water-insoluble substances, such as lanolin, which distinguishes them from the water-removable bases. Polyethylene glycol ointment is the only preparation of this type mentioned in the USP. (They may be more correctly referred to as gels.)

Choice of Base

After the nature of the different bases has been briefly described, the parameters pertaining to the choice of base may now be considered. These parameters include the stability of the medication in the base, the need for occlusion versus water washability, and the influence of the base on drug absorption. The latter is extremely important and may have been underestimated in earlier formulation work. Consider a minute portion of the base, with its dissolved drug. The dissolved drug has a certain affinity for the base. When an aliquot is placed onto the skin, the drug molecules may now remain with the base, but they also have the opportunity to diffuse into the skin. The extent to which the drug molecules diffuse into the skin depends, to a large extent, on the strength of its association with the base versus its potential to associate with the chemical components of the skin. If the drug is dispersed in the base as particles, the solubility of the drug in the base is an added factor to consider, when determining the drug's potential for skin permeation.

If the drug degrades in the presence of water, then any base that contains water (or that has the ability to absorb water) may be unsuitable. The rate of drug degradation is an important factor in such cases. If the rate of degradation is so slow that a reasonable shelf life can be assured, it may be possible to develop the drug in such a base. If water washability is the prime concern (and drug stability is not), then a water-washable base should be chosen.

Creams

Since creams are a subset of emulsions, it is appropriate to mention emulsions first. An emulsion is a two-phase liquid system consisting of oil and water. One of the phases (the internal phase) is distributed as fine droplets within the other phase (the external phase). Two basic types of emulsion are possible: the W/O type where the water is the internal phase; or the O/W type where oil is the internal phase. Creams are semisolid emulsions and may be of the W/O or the O/W type. Emulsions are discussed in detail in Chapter 7, Emulsions, and will not be further described here. The tendency to describe W/O creams as ointments, due to their oily feel, has been mentioned in the section on ointments.

Gels

Gels are semisolid systems and may be of two types. One type of gel, the more common type, consists of fine inorganic particles dispersed as a network throughout an external liquid.

The vast majority of particles are not agglomerated, that is, they are present in the gel as individual particles. However, they are not randomly distributed in the gel, but they form strands of particles. The dispersion medium is distributed between the strands and this structured network confers some rigidity to the mass of material consisting of liquid and particles (Figure 22-1).

Lotions

The term "lotion" is used in a generic sense to describe liquid formulations for application to the skin over large areas of the body. This term includes cosmetic lotions (such as "body lotion" used as a moisturizer) and medicated lotions. While solutions for external use have been described as lotions, this is not correct. Lotions are distinguished by their higher viscosity which prevents them from dripping off the skin. Most often, a lotion is an emulsion that is more fluid than a cream. In addition, a lotion may be a suspension, an example of which is Calamine Lotion, USP. This lotion contains calamine, zinc oxide, and bentonite as fine particles. Hence, this formulation is more correctly called a suspension but it has become accepted to call it a lotion. In addition, it contains calcium hydroxide (a solution) and a small quantity of glycerin. Of the suspended particles, bentonite is in the largest concentration. The suspended particles confer increased viscosity to the lotion.

Pastes

Pastes are suspensions which contain a very high concentration of finely dispersed powders, often greater than 50% of the entire formulation. The high solids content gives pastes their stiffness. Pastes serve as protective coatings on the areas of the skin to which they are applied. They remain on that area and do not spread easily to adjacent areas, because of the very high viscosity of the product. Fatty pastes have a high concentration of fine powder dispersed in a viscous, fatty ointment. The ointment, itself, is sufficiently viscous that it would not flow at body temperature. The incorporation of the solids increases the viscosity further, forming a stiff paste. An example of this type of preparation is zinc oxide paste, USP which is a mixture of zinc oxide and starch (25% of each) in white petrolatum. Another type of paste consists of a single powder component in water, an example of which is carboxymethylcellulose sodium paste, USP which contains 16% of this powdered ingredient.

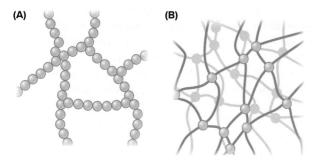

FIGURE 22-1 Gel structure. A. Spherical particles aggregated into strands, which cross each other to form a network. The individual particles may also be slightly elongated, or rod shaped. **B**. Intersecting fibrous particles may form a gel network.

Powders

Powders consist of finely divided solids, frequently a combination of more than one type, for application to the skin. Often, a major constituent of a powder for external use is talc which is free-flowing and has a pleasant, slippery feel when applied to the skin. This feel may be augmented by the addition of a small amount of magnesium stearate. Non-medicated powders are used for their pleasant feel which is enhanced by the fact that they absorb moisture. The use of this type of powder has received a great deal of adverse press recently since talc may contain a trace of asbestos. This, it is claimed, led to ovarian cancer in women who had used the powder in the vaginal area over many years. It was further claimed that manufacturers were aware of the asbestos content, of some batches of talc, but did not disclose this fact.

Medicated powders are a second class of powder for external use. In addition to the ingredients mentioned above, they may contain a medicinal agent. For example, foot powders may contain an anti-fungal agent to control the growth of fungi. They are usually not effective, on their own, for treatment of fungal infections. They may exert a complementary effect to other antifungal treatments. They also serve a cosmetic purpose since they keep the feet drier and feeling "fresh."

Topical Aerosols

Topical aerosols deliver fine liquid droplets, or fine powder particles, upon the depression of the actuator. The latter opens a valve to release the contained material which is under pressure from a propellant. The formulation of aerosols is dealt with in Chapter 19, Pulmonary Drug Delivery, and will not be discussed in this chapter. The major advantage of an aerosol delivery system, for topical or dermal use, is the fact that there is no actual contact with the affected area, except for the medication itself. This means that the hand (or the glove) of the person applying the medication will not be contaminated. Nor is the remainder of the medication contaminated, as might be the case with a liquid formulation dabbed on repeatedly with the same piece of cotton wool. Likewise, the application causes the least amount of pain to an injured area.

A disadvantage of this delivery mechanism is the fact that some of the emission invariably misses its target with resultant wastage. There is also some level of air pollution, from the propellant and the drug, both of which could be concerning depending on the nature of the latter. A major disadvantage of aerosols has been stated to be the cost. However, with bulk production, the cost has decreased greatly as evidenced by low-cost aerosols, such as shaving foams. By appropriate choice of the valve mechanism, the aerosol may be made to deliver a fine spray that dries rapidly on the skin. This leaves the active ingredient as a fine coating on the sprayed area. Spray-on bandages are of this type. The valve can also be replaced by one that creates foam. When the foam subsequently breaks, it leaves the area moist.

Sprays

Topical sprays also deliver fine droplets, or a mist, on the target area according to the choice of valve design. The drug may be dissolved or dispersed in the liquid. As distinct from an aerosol, the pressure to deliver the liquid does not come from a propellant gas but from mechanical pressure. The user squeezes a bottle or presses a device that applies pressure on the liquid to force it through a fine aperture in the nozzle. While the device (sometimes also referred to as an "atomizer") subdivides the liquid into fine droplets, the maintenance of the droplets, in this state, depends on the surface tension of the liquid. Some sunscreen formulations are available as sprays. While the spray presentation offers ease of application and is less irritating to sun-burned skin, there is also the loss due to overspray that must be considered in terms of waste and contamination of the atmosphere.

Recap Questions

1. Name the two major types of drug delivery to the skin and explain the difference between them.
2. What is the difference between a spray and an aerosol; and an emulsion and a cream?
3. What is the difference between an O/W cream and a W/O cream?
4. How does an absorption base differ from a washable base?
5. How does a gel differ from a paste?

TRANSDERMAL DRUG DELIVERY

Historical Development

The history of drug application to the skin has been briefly described in the introductory section of this chapter. Over and above topical actions, a need was recognized for using the skin to absorb drugs for systemic effects. This would require the drug to penetrate the skin, be taken up by blood vessels, and be distributed by the blood circulation. Transdermal drug delivery is desirable for many reasons. Some reasons pertain to problems related to absorption from the gastrointestinal tract (GIT), while others are related to the convenience of having prolonged drug delivery from one dosage form. As mentioned in greater detail in Chapter 3, Oral Route of Drug Delivery, some drugs irritate the sensitive lining of the GIT (especially the lining of the stomach). Other drugs are poorly absorbed or, after good absorption, are passed directly to the liver, via the portal vein, where they are metabolized to various degrees. This results in a smaller fraction of the absorbed drug reaching the systemic circulation. By contrast, one modern patch applied to the skin can, in some instances, provide several days of therapy.

Drugs that undergo extensive hepatic metabolism are preferably administered by a parenteral route, that is, a route of administration other than oral. Prior to the advent of transdermal patches, several of these drugs were administered by injection. This route of administration has many disadvantages including the pain of administration, the difficulty experienced with self-administration, the requirement for sterility of the injection formulation, and the maintenance of sterility throughout the shelf life of the product. For such drugs, a transdermal patch is a good alternative.

While the development of transdermal patches is relatively new, beginning in the 1970s, the concept, and the ability, to deliver drugs via the skin for systemic effects is not new. There were a few drugs, prior to 1970, which were delivered via the skin utilizing simple, well-known dosage forms such as ointments and gels. While adequate delivery could be obtained in some instances, these dosage forms were considered inelegant. It was generally difficult for the patient to control the quantity of medication applied, and the area of skin exposed to the medication. Since these are two primary parameters that control, respectively, the amount of drug administered and the rate of drug absorption, drug delivery by these mechanisms showed variability. The variation in the extent of drug effect, and in its duration, were frequently well beyond acceptable limits. For these reasons, such dosage forms were generally considered inefficient for systemic drug delivery.

The development of transdermal patches was initiated, in large part, by the Alza Corporation headed by Dr. Alejandro Zaffaroni. Such a patch, or transdermal drug delivery system (TDDS), contains the required amount of drug and delivers it at a reliable rate for an extended therapeutic effect. The fixed dimensions of the patch eliminate the variability in the drug-absorbing surface area of the skin. In addition, problems with the application of a cream or gel are eliminated. Furthermore, elements can be incorporated within the patch to effectively control the rate of drug delivery for a far more prolonged period than is feasible with a cream or gel.

The first TDDS, Transderm-Scop, was developed by Alza Pharmaceuticals. The scopolamine patch (as it is commonly called) is used for motion sickness. This small patch is applied to the thinner skin found behind the ear. This is typically done the night before travel to account for the lag time before pharmacological effects are observed. Consequently, the applied patch affords protection against nausea and vomiting beginning the morning after application. The three-day duration of action of the patch is sufficient for a short cruise, for example. This patch was approved in 1979. Nicotine patches were the next advancement in this type of therapy and are used for assistance with smoking cessation. Starting from approximately 1989, nicotine patch formulations became extremely popular and, subsequently, generic patches became commercially available. The fact that it is an over-the-counter product, contributed to the nicotine patch's widespread use. The success of this formulation demonstrated that transdermal patches could be a commercial success.

The fentanyl patch gave three-day relief from pain, such as cancer pain, and also became a bestseller, and several generics followed. The combination patches for either hormone replacement therapy or for contraception also became popular with a great deal of effort expended to make the patches smaller and, therefore, more cosmetically acceptable. Not all drugs will permeate the skin of their own accord, or naturally. Therefore, scientific endeavors to improve permeability proceeded down several avenues. Before discussing the different approaches, it may be instructive to review the advantages and disadvantages of transdermal drug delivery.

Advantages

The advantages of transdermal drug delivery are the following:

1. The drug is delivered at a controlled rate into the systemic circulation.

2. Effective plasma levels are maintained from 1 to 7 days.

3. Due to the ease of use, patient compliance is improved.

4. Hepatic first-pass metabolism is avoided.

5. More reliable, consistent blood levels are obtained due to advantages 3 and 4.

6. Increased efficacy is obtained and the potential for toxicity is decreased, in comparison to oral drug delivery.

7. Therapy can be terminated by the removal of the patch, for example, in the event of untoward reactions; effects will not terminate abruptly due to unabsorbed drug present in the skin.

Disadvantages

This drug delivery mechanism in its simplest, diffusion-dependent form (not enhanced) has certain limitations:

1. Only relatively potent drugs may be used; typically, the dose is less than 20 mg, and for an ideal formulation less than 10 mg, per day.

2. The molecular size of the drug should, ideally, be small (<500 Da).

3. With large molecules and hydrophilic drugs, poor diffusion is observed; this delivery system is not useful for peptides and other products of biotechnology.

4. Skin irritation and contact dermatitis have been observed and are often related to the adhesive in the formulation.

5. Poor adhesive properties, with resultant poor absorption, have been observed with certain TDDS; conversely, the application of occlusive dressings to counteract poor adhesion has, in some instances, resulted in undesirably rapid drug absorption due to increased local temperature at the site of application.

6. These formulations are more expensive than typical oral drugs.

Recap Questions

1. What is the name of the first transdermal patch developed? What drug did it contain?

2. Mention two reasons why transdermal drug delivery is important.

3. Give two disadvantages of transdermal delivery related to the dose and the type of drug.

4. Compare a self-administered injection to the application of a transdermal patch, from the patient's perspective.

STRUCTURE OF THE SKIN

Before studying the construction of TDDS and the formulation of the drug-containing component, it is important to understand the structure of the skin. Any released drug intended for systemic effect must permeate the skin and reach its deeper layers in order to penetrate blood vessels. In the blood circulation, the drug is carried to the different parts of the body to elicit a systemic effect at the sites of action.

The skin is approximately 1.5 to 4 mm thick, depending on its location, and it performs a containment and protective function. Body fluids, for example, do not simply diffuse out of the body in an uncontrolled fashion. With respect to the protective function, the skin provides several barrier types: microbial, chemical, mechanical, and heat. Distinct from the heat barrier function is the temperature regulation function. The former is a passive heat-insulating barrier preventing excessive transmission of heat into the body on a hot day, or loss of heat from the body on a cold day. By contrast, thermal regulation is an active mechanism with feedback loops that maintain the body at, or close to, 37°C. It is brought about, for example, by increasing the blood flow to the skin for convective heat loss when the body is hot and, conversely, reducing blood flow to the skin on a cold day; or by carrying water to the external surface of the skin (perspiration) for the evaporation of this water. The latter process causes heat loss since the conversion of water to vapor requires the provision, by the body, of the latent heat of vaporization. Perspiration also serves an excretion function in that certain compounds are eliminated through this mechanism. The microbial, chemical, and mechanical barrier functions are largely afforded by the tough outer layer of the skin, referred to as the stratum corneum. Figure 22-2 shows the different layers of the skin.

An important function of the skin is the biosynthesis of vitamin D_3 in the presence of ultraviolet (UV) light, most commonly provided by sunlight. This fact has important implications for the use of sunscreen formulations, especially those with a very high sun protection factor, that block the penetration of UV light to the skin. The epidermis of the skin also contains a small population of immune cells (epidermal dendritic cells or Langerhans cells) that play an important role in initiating the immune response. These cells are targeted in dermal vaccinations. The skin also performs an important sensory function, with the sense of touch being particularly acute in important locations, such as the fingertips. The sensory nerve endings are located close to, but not at, the surface of the skin. The different layers of the skin are briefly described below.

Epidermis

The epidermis is made up of stratified squamous epithelial cells that are keratinized, that is, they contain the protein, keratin, that gives strength and structure to the epidermis. The epidermis does not contain blood vessels and obtains its nutrition from the dermis by virtue of diffusion. A basement membrane separates the epidermis from the dermis. The epidermis consists of several layers. From the deepest to the most superficial layer, these are basal layer (consisting of cells that actively divide and are pushed upwards), the stratum spinosum, the stratum

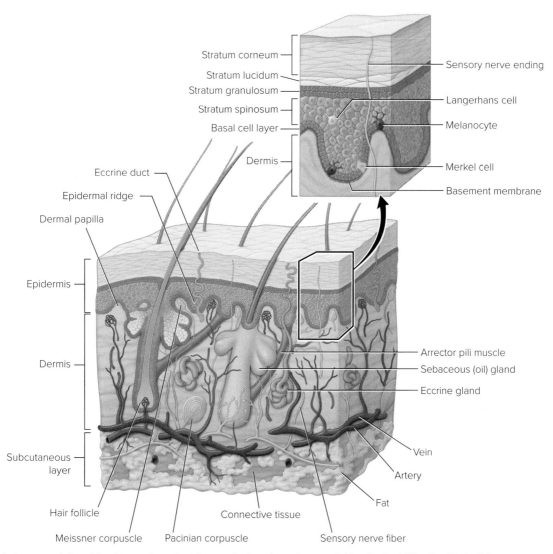

FIGURE 22-2 Layers of the skin. (Reproduced, with permission, from Soutor C, Hordinsky MK, eds. *Clinical Dermatology: Diagnosis and Management of Common Disorders*. 2nd ed. New York, NY: McGraw Hill; 2022, Fig. 1-1.)

granulosum, the stratum lucidum (only present in thick skin), and the stratum corneum. The basal layer is tightly attached to the basement membrane. The basal layer also contains cells, referred to as melanocytes, which produce the pigment melanin. Granules of pigment, called malanosomes, are transferred to the keratinocytes in which they locate around the nucleus to protect the DNA from the effects of UV light. A few tactile cells are also found within the basal layer. These are sensitive to touch.

Only the first three (deepest) layers listed above are composed of living cells (keratinocytes) which are capable of forming keratin. The last two layers (stratum lucidum and stratum corneum) contain dead cells. The stratum lucidum, which is thin and contains translucent cells, is only present in thick skin, which is the type of skin on the soles of the feet and the palms of the hands. Thick skin lacks hair follicles and sebaceous glands but contains sweat glands. The epidermis of thick skin can be from 400 to 600 μm thick. Thin skin is structurally different and is found on the rest of the body and its epidermis is only 75 to 150 μm thick. The descriptive term "thin skin" comprises a twofold difference from the lower to the higher thickness value.

Thus, it is possible that certain parts of the body may have "thin" skin which is thicker than the thin skin in other regions. The area behind the ears, for example, contains especially thin skin and this location is recommended for the application of the scopolamine patch, the first patch to be marketed.

Dermis

The dermis lies below the epidermis and its thickness is between 0.5 mm and 3 mm. There are two major regions of the dermis, namely, a superficial papillary layer and a deeper reticular layer. The papillary layer (adjacent to the epidermis) is composed of loose (areolar) connective tissue. This layer has prominent projections called dermal papillae which project outwards toward the epidermis. These projections interlock with deep projections of the epidermis called epidermal ridges. These two sets of ridges increase the area of contact between the epidermis and the dermis and, in combination with the interlocking effect, result in a stronger connection between these layers. Within each dermal papilla are capillaries which, by diffusion, supply nutrients to the cells of the epidermis. The dermis also houses sensory receptors. For example, nociceptors or pain receptors are found in the dermis. This location has important implications for the development of several types of drug delivery systems which utilize controlled damage to minute areas of the uppermost layer of the skin, the stratum corneum. Had the sensory nerve endings and associated receptors been more superficially located, such delivery systems could not have been contemplated.

The deeper second layer of the dermis is the reticular layer which forms the major portion of the dermis, that is, it is much thicker compared to the papillary layer. The reticular layer consists mainly of dense irregular connective tissue: large bundles of collagen fibers project in all directions. The bundles of fibers surround, and physically support, the structures found in the dermis. These are hair follicles, sebaceous glands, sweat glands, nerves, and blood vessels. Some collagen bundles are continuous with the subcutaneous layer of collagen.

Subcutaneous Layer

The subcutaneous layer is also referred to as the hypodermis. It is not actually a part of the skin. It is considered in conjunction with descriptions of the skin due to its proximity and functional relationship to the skin. This relationship is also relevant with respect to drug absorption. The subcutaneous layer is composed of areolar connective tissue as well as adipose connective tissue. The latter predominates in some areas of the body in which case the tissue is referred to as subcutaneous fat. Some fibers of connective tissue of the reticular layer of the dermis are interwoven with the fibers of the subcutaneous layer. This serves to bind the skin to the underlying tissues, making it more difficult to separate. The subcutaneous layer acts as a pad which protects the underlying tissues and organs, insulates the body, and also serves as an energy reservoir.

With particular reference to drug delivery, it is important to note that the subcutaneous tissues are well supplied with blood vessels. A drug that is able to permeate the various layers of the skin will reach the subcutaneous tissues. If it is, additionally, able to permeate blood vessels, it will be distributed throughout the body by the general circulation. Highly lipophilic drugs may remain in the fat stores for an extended time and will only slowly perfuse the blood vessels. It is also true that hydrophobic drugs (however administered) can reach the circulatory system and diffuse from the capillaries into the subcutaneous fat layer and be retained there for a period. They are then slowly absorbed back into the circulation. This effect may be responsible for the longer duration of action of some drugs (such as anesthetics) and, correspondingly, for a longer duration of side effects. Since women, in general, have more subcutaneous fat, such drug effects may be felt for a longer time in women.

Considering the structure of the skin, as briefly described above, it has been stated (and is currently accepted) that the stratum corneum is the major barrier to permeation. Once a drug molecule moves past the stratum corneum, according to the current thinking, the remaining layers present little resistance to the passage of the drug to the subcutaneous layer and, finally, to the blood vessels. This has been shown to be largely true for small molecules. However, consideration should be given to the tight basal layer as well as its binding to the basement membrane. This structure may provide some resistance to permeation, especially in the case of larger molecules. Proteins and peptides, which are very large, show strong resistance to permeation through the skin.

Transport Pathways

The transport pathways through the stratum corneum are illustrated in Figure 22-3. The stratum corneum is the major barrier to permeation through the skin. The transcellular pathway is the more direct pathway whereby drug molecules traverse the keratinized cells in a more-or-less straight line. The paracellular pathway, as the term indicates, is the pathway around the cells of the stratum corneum. The area around the cells is filled with an aqueous medium which contains packed lipid bundles. For paracellular transport, molecules must diffuse through this aqueous/lipid matrix.

The overall structure of the stratum corneum may be compared to bricks and mortar, where the cells are the bricks and the intercellular spaces, filled with tissue fluid, can be compared to the mortar around the bricks. The transcellular pathway is directly through the bricks, whereas the paracellular route is via the mortar. When the latter mechanism is utilized, the drug spreads out over a wider area of the skin. For this reason, a lag time may be observed before drug effects are noticed. The transappendageal pathway refers to transport via hair follicles and sweat ducts. As shown in Figure 22-3, this mechanism takes a

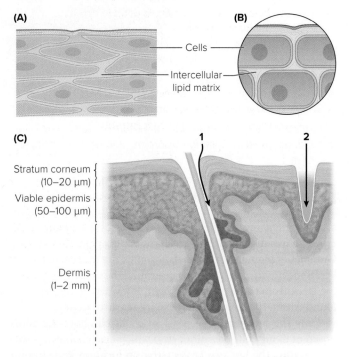

FIGURE 22-3 Transport pathways through the stratum corneum. Part **A** shows the cells and intercellular lipid matrix of the stratum corneum. Part **B** is an idealized diagram showing the brick and mortar model. (in the paracellular pathway, drug permeates the intracellular lipid and passes around the cells as it permeates through the skin; in the more direct transcellular pathway, the drug moves through the cells to the deeper layers of the skin.) Part **C** illustrates (1) the transappendageal pathway; and (2) the microneedle pathway. Note that the microneedle does not penetrate the dermis where nerve endings are located.

drug in solution on the surface of the skin directly to the subcutaneous tissue where the blood vessels are located. Systemic effects may begin shortly after uptake of the drug molecules into these vessels.

SYNOPSIS OF SOME RELEVANT PHYSICO-CHEMICAL PRINCIPLES

As mentioned in the introductory chapter, this book is not intended to describe physico-chemical principles of relevance to pharmacy. However, an understanding of how to enhance drug absorption from transdermal products is so intimately connected to certain physico-chemical principles that an explanation of absorption enhancement would be difficult if the reader did not grasp these principles. Therefore, a few salient principles that are particularly relevant to transdermal drug delivery will be mentioned here.

Diffusion

Diffusion is the passage of the substance from a region of high concentration to a region of low concentration. Typically, in biological systems, diffusion through a membrane is of importance. Usually, there is a lag time before diffusion begins. Then, the rate of diffusion increases to a steady state and then the rate falls off. The rate at which a molecule diffuses during the steady state, referred to as the flux, is defined by Fick's first law. According to this law, the flux (J) is proportional to the concentration gradient across the membrane. It is equal to the diffusivity of the molecule (D) multiplied by the concentration gradient, where the latter is the change in concentration with distance. This relationship is reflected in Eq. (22-1); the negative sign simply indicates that diffusion occurs from a region of high concentration to a region of low concentration.

$$J = -D\frac{dC}{dx} \qquad (22\text{-}1)$$

The diffusivity is a function of the molecular structure of the diffusant (or drug, in this case), the properties of the barrier material (skin) and the temperature. It is considered a "constant" but it is a constant only for a narrow set of conditions. Thus, the size, and the shape, of the drug molecule in question has an influence on its diffusivity. In general, small molecules diffuse faster than large molecules of a similar type. For molecules of equal weight, the shape of the molecule can have an influence and a highly branched structure may have a lower diffusivity than a compound with less branching. Furthermore, temperature affects the rate of diffusion (by increasing the diffusivity).

It is clear that a higher concentration of drug will give a faster diffusion rate. This can be achieved by incorporating more drug, than is needed, into a transdermal patch (and removing the patch before the drug load is depleted). It may be less obvious that removal of the drug from the side of the membrane to which the drug is diffusing (in a lab experiment or under physiological conditions) also increases the concentration gradient. This is because the concentration gradient is the difference between the concentrations on either side of the membrane. Therefore, if a portion of the drug that has diffused through the skin is

removed, it allows more drug to diffuse through the skin. As drug molecules pass into the circulatory system and flow away with the blood, the drug concentration on the "receiving" side of the skin is reduced greatly. This factor increases the diffusion rate because the drug concentration on the "receiver" side is lowered to essentially zero. It can be said that sink conditions prevail. While this effect facilitates diffusion of the drug from the region within the skin to the bloodstream, the subsequently lowered skin concentrations, in turn, enhance drug diffusion from the dosage form into the skin.

Partition Coefficient

Consider two immiscible liquid phases, such as oil and water, at equilibrium. When these two phases are placed in to a container, such as a beaker, they form two separate layers since they are immiscible. Usually, the oily layer is less dense and would be the top layer. Now, if a solute was mixed with these two immiscible liquids for a time and then the liquids were allowed to separate, a portion of the solute will be dissolved in each phase. (This model system will be referenced again later in this section.) The ratio of the molar concentrations of the solute in the oil, and in the water, is referred to as K, the partition coefficient (Eq. [22-2]).

$$K = \frac{C_o}{C_w} \qquad (22\text{-}2)$$

where C_o is the concentration in the oil phase, and
C_w is the concentration in the water phase

Partition coefficients can have a very wide range: values of 0.01 to 100,000 are not uncommon. To cater to this large range of values, a log scale (log P) is commonly used. The above values, on the log scale, would be log P = −2; and log P = 5. For oral drug delivery log P values in the range 2 to 3 are ideal. However, for transdermal drug delivery somewhat higher values are desirable because of the lipophilic nature of the stratum corneum. Obviously, other factors play a role in absorption and having the ideal log P does not guarantee optimal absorption of a drug.

Whereas the above example of partitioning used two liquid layers, oil and water, a partition coefficient can be determined for any two immiscible phases. For example, the partition coefficient between the drug-containing layer of a transdermal dosage form and the skin could be determined. Changes in either of the two immiscible layers, in the model system, could change the partition coefficient, K, of the system. For example, if a hydrophobic drug is considered, making the oil phase more hydrophobic will change the distribution of the drug in favor of the oil phase. Similarly, making the skin more hydrophobic changes the distribution of the hydrophobic drug in favor of the skin. The ratio of the concentrations, or the K value, will be a larger number. On the other hand, changes in the water phase of the model system (or in the drug-containing layer of the transdermal dosage form) will also influence the partition coefficient. For example, making the dosage form more hydrophilic will also change the partition coefficient in favor of the skin (again considering a hydrophobic drug).

Consider a hydrophobic drug that is administered by means of a TDDS. If other non-drug compounds, that are more hydrophobic than the drug, were included within the dosage form in a way that allowed them to *diffuse easily*, these compounds would migrate rapidly into the skin. As a consequence, the skin will be made more hydrophobic than in its natural state. This mechanism increases the partition coefficient of the hydrophobic drug. Therefore, by the inclusion of such non-drug hydrophobic compounds, drug diffusion from the dosage form will be made more rapid. Conversely, if the dosage form, after application to the skin, were to become more hydrophilic (than its initial state), then the partition coefficient of a hydrophobic drug would also be altered in favor of more drug penetrating into the skin. In both cases mentioned above, there is a change in either the skin or the dosage form after the application of the dosage form to the skin. For these techniques to work, the substance that brings about the change must diffuse easily and quickly. Both of these techniques have been utilized in transdermal drug delivery and are discussed in the examples given in the section below.

Recap Questions

1. Which layer of the skin is largely responsible for providing its barrier function?

2. Which layer of the epidermis is responsible for its growth?

3. What makes the connection between the epidermis and dermis strong?

4. What does Ficks' law describe?

5. Why does removal of the drug, via the circulation, result in faster diffusion from the dosage form into the skin?

CHEMICAL ENHANCEMENT OF TRANSDERMAL DRUG DELIVERY

Before describing chemically enhanced systems for drug delivery through the skin, it is important to understand delivery systems in which the drug leaves the device to pass into the skin by passive diffusion. This provides a background to understanding chemically enhanced drug delivery.

Dosage Forms for Passive Diffusion

Some drugs, by their nature, are able to permeate the skin by passive diffusion. These drugs are generally lipophilic and of small molecular size and may be effectively utilized in TDDS without the incorporation of a substance to enhance permeation. Fentanyl (for relief of pain) and nicotine (an aid to smoking cessation) are examples of drugs that behave in this manner.

The most common specialized dosage form for transdermal drug delivery has the superficial appearance of a small, square, or rectangular adhesive bandage, or "band-aid" and such dosages forms have, therefore, been called "patches." However, they are more correctly referred to as TDDS. The latter terminology implies complexity in the dosage form. In this chapter, patch and TDDS will be used interchangeably. The patch contains a drug within a complex system consisting of multiple layers of material, one of which contains an adhesive substance. The adhesive

allows adherence to the skin upon application, requiring some pressure to facilitate adhesion.

Most patches have an area of 45 cm² or less, and some are considerably less than this size. The size of the patch must take into account the intended site of placement. Tokuhon-A Plaster® (which contains camphor, menthol, and methylsalicylate) and Salonpas Plaster (which contains menthol and methylsalicylate) are notable exceptions. They have a much larger surface area and are applied to the back, or to joints, for the relief of pain. Interestingly, these products were available long before the recent intense development of patch formulations and they may be considered as topical, rather than transdermal, formulations even though they are in patch presentations. The recent wave of "heat" patches that provide soothing warmth to the area of application are also larger than the size mentioned for a typical patch and these may, similarly, be considered to be "topical" patches.

Skin tolerability is a concern that must be kept in the mind when formulating patches: all currently marketed formulations list skin irritation as a possible side effect. The irritation is often from the adhesive that is used in the formulation but other aspects of the formulation may also be responsible. In fact, merely applying a patch to an area of skin will cause, in sensitive individuals, reddening of the area and an uncomfortable sensation of heat. Excipients in the formulation may also cause sensitivity, if not outright irritation. In addition, several drugs may show sufficient irritation that they cannot be administered topically. These include some drugs that are not irritant when taken orally. In vivo testing for irritancy potential, starting with animal studies first is usually required for all transdermal products.

Two major types of transdermal dosage forms utilize the principle of passive diffusion: matrix TDDS and reservoir TDDS. The former contains the drug within a matrix which may be a gel. Diffusion through the matrix controls the rate of drug release from the dosage form. On the other hand, a reservoir TDDS has a rate-controlling membrane to control the release of the medication. Without this membrane, the drug would diffuse out of the reservoir too rapidly for effective transdermal delivery. Each of these dosage forms consists of several layers as shown in Figure 22-4. Starting from the layer furthest from the skin, these are a backing layer (which prevents drug loss to the external surroundings); a drug matrix (in matrix TDDS) or a drug reservoir

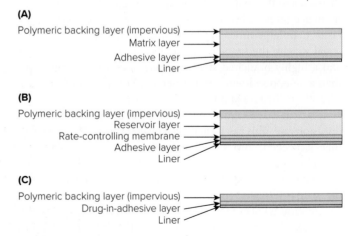

FIGURE 22-4 Block diagrams showing structure of (A) matrix TDDS, (B) reservoir TDDS, and (C) drug-in-adhesive TDDS.

(in reservoir TDDS); a porous rate-controlling membrane (in reservoir TDDS); an adhesive layer which helps the patch adhere to the skin; and a protective film over the adhesive layer to prevent the patch sticking to anything before application to the skin.

A relatively new development is the combination of the drug matrix layer and the adhesive layer, thus achieving a reduction of one layer in the formulation. The formulation still has a matrix, but the adhesive is now part of the matrix. This type of formulation is also shown in Figure 22-4. In a conventional matrix system (individual matrix and adhesive layers), a period of time may elapse before the drug effect is felt. This lag time occurs because the drug must diffuse from the matrix layer through the adhesive layer, and then through the skin, prior to permeation into blood vessels. For this reason, some instances of this type of formulation have incorporated a novel mechanism to reduce the lag time: a small portion of the dose is incorporated into the adhesive. This portion of the dose is absorbed more quickly and allows for a faster onset of action. Beyond the initial period, the matrix is the source of the drug that permeates the skin in such formulations. The drug-in-adhesive type of formulation may be considered an extension of this idea. Examples of commercial products of the three types are listed in Table 22-1.

Chemical Enhancers

In many instances, the drug being formulated does not diffuse through the skin, on its own or in an unenhanced formulation. In some cases, the drug does permeate the skin but it does so at a rate that is too slow for effective treatment. One approach to enhance drug delivery, in such cases, is to incorporate a chemical permeation enhancer. Chemical enhancement of drug delivery has been the subject of intense research for several decades. This area of research includes the development of suitable non-toxic enhancers, their testing in vitro and in animal models, and the elucidation of their mechanisms of action. A large number of compounds have been tested in laboratories, both in academia and in industry. In spite of such intense activity, few enhancers have been found to be effective, yet safe. As a consequence, very few have passed FDA scrutiny and reached the marketplace as enhancers included in approved TDDS. It is important to understand that the utilization of an enhancer is an attempt to overcome the substantial barrier function of the skin. What follows is a short description of a model of drug permeation followed by a brief synopsis of some enhancers, with an emphasis on those used in approved products.

Drug permeation from a TDDS into the deeper layers of the skin, from which they can be absorbed into blood vessels, may be considered a two-step process. This division also helps to understand the mechanism of action of enhancers. These steps are permeation of the stratum corneum which is a more hydrophobic layer than the deeper layers of the skin, and diffusion from the stratum corneum to the deeper layers of the skin. In many instances, permeation of the stratum corneum occurs relatively readily and a depot of drug forms in this skin layer. From this depot, diffusion into deeper skin layers may, thereafter, occur at a slower rate. Keeping this two-step model of drug permeation in mind, and for convenience of description, enhancers may be divided into two major categories:

1. Those that alter the barrier nature of the skin, usually by perturbation of stratum corneum lipid structures, that is, by upsetting the orderly arrangement of lipid molecules to permit drug penetration into the skin, beyond the stratum corneum; and

2. Those that, by some mechanism apart from perturbation of stratum corneum lipids, increase the drug content of the

TABLE 22-1	Examples of Transdermal Drug Delivery Systems Available on the US Market			
ACTIVE	**TRADENAME**	**PATCH TYPE**	**INDICATION**	**MANUFACTURER**
Clonidine	Catapres-TTS	Reservoir	Elevated Blood pressure	Boehringer Ingelheim
Estradiol	Vivelle-DOT	Matrix	Hormone replacement Therapy	Novartis
Nicotine	Nicoderm CQ	Reservoir	Smoking cessation	Sanofi Aventis US LLC
Fentanyl	Duragesic	Reservoir	Moderate to severe pain	Janssen
Rivastigmine	Exelon	Matrix	Dementia associated with Parkinson's and Alzheimer's	LTS Lohmann Therapie-Systeme AG for Novartis Pharmaceuticals Corp.
Rotigotine	Neupro	Drug in adhesive	Parkinson's & restless leg syndrome	UCB, Inc.
Nitroglycerin	Nitro-Dur	Drug in adhesive	Angina	Merck Sharp and Dohme Corp.
Oxybutynin	Oxytrol	Drug in adhesive	Overactive bladder	Watson Pharma.
Asenapine	Secuado	Reservoir	Schizophrenia	Hisamitsu Pharmaceutical Co., Inc.
Scopolamine	Transderm-Scop	Reservoir	Motion sickness	Alza Corp for Novartis Consumer Health

stratum corneum, thereby leading to a higher concentration gradient between this layer of the skin and the deeper layers. Consequently, faster diffusion occurs into the deeper skin layers and the blood vessels.

Examples of enhancers in category 1 include glyceryl monolaurate, methyl laurate, and ethanol, which are used in combination to enhance the permeation of glyceryl trinitrate (Minitran S). Andropatch (testosterone) contains glyceryl monolaurate, methyl laurate, and ethanol. In addition to reduced irritation, the skin changes brought about by these commercially used enhancers are reversible. This is important and ensures that toxins in the environment do not permeate the skin after the use of a TDDS. These enhancers are very different from those initially tested ex vivo and in animal studies, as described below.

Compounds such as bile salts, individually and in various combinations, were initially employed in research studies to enhance transdermal permeation. While they were often more successful at increasing the extent of drug absorption than the above commercial examples, the changes made to the skin were not quickly reversible. There were also instances of skin damage, in the experimental studies, which could be demonstrated microscopically in stained skin samples. Some enhancers, that were relatively milder than the bile salts, did make it to early clinical trials. However, these compounds caused non-trivial skin irritation and it was unlikely that the products would have been approved for marketing. As a result, the research studies were terminated. These test enhancers are very different from the mild hydrophobic enhancers, mentioned above, that are used in commercial products.

Turning to enhancer category 2, it is emphasized that higher drug concentrations in the stratum corneum lead to faster diffusion through the other skin layers and, eventually, to faster diffusion into blood vessels. Fick's first law of diffusion is relevant: the higher the concentration gradient, the faster the diffusion. Two subclasses of enhancers promoting high drug concentration in the stratum corneum have been identified: (a) those that effectively change the partition coefficient of the skin relative to the drug compartment of the dosage form; and (b) those that use supersaturation in the dosage form to create analogous supersaturation in the stratum corneum.

Examples of category 2a enhancers are povidone and polyvinylpyrrolidone (PVP). These compounds are hydrophilic and their incorporation into the patch causes the absorption of water from the skin, into the delivery system, after patch application. The reduction of the water content of the skin (mostly in the area under the patch) causes this area of the skin to be more hydrophobic. On the other hand, the increased water content of the patch causes it to be more hydrophilic and, therefore, a less favorable environment for the hydrophobic drug. Consequently, the partition coefficient changes to one that is more favorable to the partitioning of the drug into the skin, that is, there is a greater tendency for the drug to leave the patch to diffuse into the skin. This technology is used in the rotigotine patch, Neupro®, for Parkinson's disease and restless leg syndrome.

Butrans® (buprenorphine) is a drug-in-adhesive patch which contains (among other ingredients) oleyl oleate which increases skin hydrophobicity, and povidone which enhances water uptake by the patch. Hence, this patch appears to incorporate both mechanisms. For the oleyl oleate to work, it should leave the patch rapidly to enter the stratum corneum. If it stays in the patch for an extended time, the patch would have increased hydrophobicity and this would decrease skin permeation. Oleyl oleate does, in fact, permeate the skin rapidly. The Combipatch® contains estradiol and norethisterone acetate as a drug-in-adhesive patch and has oleic acid and povidone as inactive ingredients. It, thus, appears to have a similar dual enhancement mechanism to Butrans®.

In 2b enhancers, a high drug content, or even supersaturation, in the patch may be used to create a similar effect, in place of alteration of the partition coefficient. This is achieved by modifying the manufacturing process as follows. A drug and a polymeric adhesive are dissolved in an organic solvent. This solution is deposited as a layer onto the patch and a controlled drying process is used to evaporate a portion of the solvent, resulting in supersaturation of the drug in the remaining adhesive/solvent. When applied to the skin, the supersaturated solution causes a rapid diffusion of the drug into the skin since the driving force for diffusion is the concentration gradient. Since the stratum corneum is hydrophobic, it will have an affinity for the hydrophobic drug which will pass into the stratum corneum. Usually, the supersaturation in the patch results in supersaturation of the drug in the stratum corneum. The underlying tissues are more hydrophilic, and they do not rapidly equilibrate with the stratum corneum. The stratum corneum, as a consequence, provides a source of drug for diffusion at a steady rate, over an extended period, into the deeper layers of the skin, and then into the blood circulation, that is, the stratum corneum acts as a drug reservoir.

This technique may appear simple at first glance, but it should be remembered that it is critical to maintain the metastable, supersaturated state until the patch is applied to the skin. Therein, lies the difficulty which is overcome by drying at a highly controlled rate. Additionally, substances that stabilize the supersaturated drug solution may be incorporated into the patch. If the drug crystallizes out of solution (as is its natural tendency), then the supersaturated state is lost and, with it, the high concentration in solution. The latter provides the large gradient necessary for this enhancement mechanism to work. As a consequence, the rapid diffusion advantage is lost.

The maintenance of high drug levels in the patch has also been assisted by developments in adhesive technology. An example is the development of the DOT-matrix technology for TDDS. The acronym, DOT, represents "delivery optimized thermodynamics." In this technology, an acrylic adhesive is loaded with the drug and the mixture is then dispersed into a second adhesive consisting of silicone. The drug is very soluble in the acrylic polymer (or other selected compound) and is less soluble in the silicone adhesive. This creates areas of high acrylic intensity (or spots) in which the drug concentration is high, whereas drug concentration is lower in the largest area of the patch, the silicone-containing area. Because of its large surface area, the latter area is the prime source of drug for diffusion into the skin. As it gets depleted, the high-drug-content acrylic spots serve as reservoirs to maintain the drug content of the silicone-containing area. This formulation approach results in good drug absorption and this technology is used in hormone-containing patches for the control of hot flashes in postmenopausal women (eg, Vivelle DOT). It is also used in Daytrana (methylphenidate) for attention deficit hyperactivity disorder (ADHD) control in children.

Recap Questions

1. What are the two basic types of patch formulations currently on the US market?

2. How has patch design been simplified in recent years, eliminating one layer of the patch?

3. Distinguish between passive diffusion and chemically enhanced diffusion.

4. What is the chemical principle involved with the improvement of drug permeation through the skin when supersaturated patches are used?

5. How does a highly hydrophilic substance like povidone contribute to the enhancement of hydrophobic drug permeation by transdermal drug delivery?

6. Your client at a community pharmacy is very concerned about the cost of the patch that has been prescribed for him. He asks if you could make an ointment containing the drug for him to apply to his skin. It would "still go into the skin" and be a lot cheaper. How would you respond to this client?

PHYSICAL (ENERGETIC) ENHANCEMENT OF DRUG DELIVERY

Many of the physical methods of enhancing drug delivery through the skin are in the research stage at present. The notable exception is iontophoresis, examples of which have been commercialized. The non-commercialized examples are briefly mentioned for completeness and because products, using these technologies, may appear on the market in the near future. Unless a marketed product is specifically mentioned in connection with a technology in this section, it may be assumed that no product was commercially available in the United States at the time of writing.

Iontophoresis

Iontophoresis is the use of low-voltage electricity to drive charged molecules across the skin. The principle of iontophoresis has been known for long but not much progress was made toward the development of a drug delivery system based on this technology. In the 1970s and 1980s, there was a resurgence of interest in using this technique for transdermal drug delivery.

The iontophoretic device consists of a source of electricity, two electrodes and two chambers for the drug and salt, respectively (Figure 22-5). The latter is needed to complete the electrical circuit. The iontophoretic mechanism involves the application of a small electric current through the skin. The cationic drug is placed in contact with the anode (positively charged) and a salt solution is placed in contact with the cathode. The drug molecules are repelled by the positive electrode and are propelled toward the skin which they penetrate under this electrical driving force.

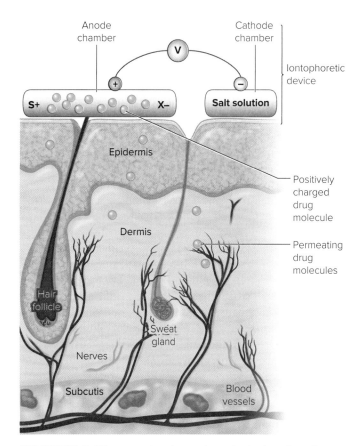

FIGURE 22-5 Diagram of an iontophoretic device placed on skin. Note that the positively charged drug molecules are repelled at the positively charged electrode and permeate the skin to be absorbed into the blood vessels.

Analogously, a negatively charged drug is placed in contact with the cathode (negatively charged) and a salt solution is placed in contact with the anode. The repulsion between the negatively charged drug and the cathode propels the drug toward the skin. While the above implies that the drug should be in a charged state, that is, ionized, or becomes charged in the presence of the electric current, uncharged drugs in solution may also be transported across the skin by the following mechanism. The electrical charge, in addition to moving ions through the skin, also causes water to penetrate the skin due to a phenomenon referred to as electro-osmosis. If the uncharged drugs are in solution, they will be carried with the flowing water, a process referred to as solvent drag. At the present time, no more than 0.5 mA/cm^2 is permitted by the FDA in iontophoretic devices. Iontophoresis is the only physical method that has been commercialized, at the time of writing.

The Vyteris and E-TRANS iontophoresis systems are probably the market leaders. The Vyteris lidocaine delivery system is used for local dermal anesthesia. It eliminates pain and has a much more rapid onset of action than conventional (non-iontophoretic) transdermal systems. The Vyteris system contains two reservoirs in a flexible adhesive pad. The main reservoir is filled with lidocaine and epinephrine, the latter being used to cause vasoconstriction which limits the spread of the administered lidocaine within the tissues. The second reservoir contains saline. The Alza Corporation developed the E-TRANS system. The transdermal patch is applied, by means of the self-adhesive backing, to the patient's upper chest or outer arm. The mechanism of operation is similar to the Vyteris system. Fentanyl is effectively delivered by this system which incorporates patient-controlled delivery, that is, the patient controls the pulse of electric current. In this way, a dose can be administered only as needed. This is in sharp contrast to other long-acting pain medication administration methods which utilize a slow, constant delivery of drug irrespective of the pain status of the patient.

Lidocaine, fentanyl, and sumatriptan have been approved as iontophoretic products. However, due to technical problems and/or lack of commercial success, several products were withdrawn from the US market, leading to skepticism about this delivery mechanism. While it has been attempted, in research studies, to deliver larger molecules such as peptides by this mechanism, such attempts have not been sufficiently successful to prompt commercialization. Iontophoresis has been used in glucose monitoring since the level of glucose in interstitial fluids parallels that in blood and can be used to adjust the insulin dose of diabetics. This allows for fine control of their blood glucose levels. Any system of monitoring that does not require frequent finger pricks saves patients a repeated painful experience. The FreeStyle Libre is an example of a device of this type that is very popular, eliminates painful finger pricks, and also provides continuous monitoring (as opposed to monitoring at a few discrete times a day). The expanded use of iontophoresis for the monitoring of other physiological compounds indicative of disease states, and for drug monitoring, is a reason for cautious optimism.

Temperature

The surface temperature of skin is 32°C and any elevation in temperature, at the site of drug application, will enhance drug delivery. There is an approximately two- to threefold increase in flux for every 7°C to 8°C rise in temperature. This increase in flux is attributed to increased drug diffusivity in the dosage form and in the skin. The skin diffusivity increase is due to increased lipid fluidity. The higher temperature also causes an increase in blood supply to the surface of the skin with a consequent rapid removal of the drug from the absorption site. This creates sink conditions and plays a role in increasing transdermal permeation.

The temperature effect on drug release rate may be concerning if a patient, wearing a patch, spends an extended time in a sauna or hot tub. On the other hand, this effect could be exploited to improve the transdermal delivery of slowly-permeating drugs. Zars, Inc., developed the CHADD delivery system. The acronym refers to controlled heat-aided drug delivery. The heat source is a chemical reaction which is initiated at the time of application of the patch. A developmental deal was entered into between Zars and Johnson & Johnson Company for a system which, essentially, consists of a CHADD disk placed over a Duragesic (fentanyl) patch, to form the so-called Titragesia patch. This commercialized patch provides improved fentanyl delivery compared to the Duragesic patch.

Non-cavitional Ultrasound

Ultrasound occurs at a frequency too high for humans to hear. Nevertheless, it is an oscillating pressure wave which is similar to sound waves that humans are capable of hearing. The pressure increases, and then decreases or ablates. Ultrasound may be divided into high-frequency, or low-frequency, ultrasound. For medical purposes, 20 to 60 kHz is considered low frequency but high power, whereas frequencies above 60 kHz are considered high frequency. Low-frequency ultrasound causes cavitation. Cavitation involves the formation of bubbles, their oscillation, and, eventually, their collapse due to the ultrasonic pressure field.

High-frequency (low-power) ultrasound does not cause the formation of bubbles in media containing a liquid and, for this reason, it is referred to as non-cavitational ultrasound. The unintentional enhancement of drug permeation by non-cavitational ultrasound was noticed as follows. High-frequency ultrasound is used for relief of pain in specific areas of the body, such as the back or knees. It causes a pleasant, warming effect on tissues, while increasing blood flow to the area of application. Physical therapists applying ultrasound generally use a gel to reduce friction between the handheld ultrasound device and the skin. When an anti-inflammatory gel (instead of the usual unmedicated gel) was used for this purpose, it was noticed that the beneficial effect was far greater than that from the ultrasound, or the anti-inflammatory (and pain-relieving) gel, alone. The dominant effect of this irradiation is to disrupt the stratum corneum lipid structure, thereby increasing the permeability of small, lipophilic compounds. More intense use of non-cavitational ultrasound causes heating of underlying tissues, resulting in their damage, and is contraindicated.

Cavitational Ultrasound

At low frequency, ultrasound does not generate significant heat, as is the case for high-frequency ultrasound, but it is capable of generating cavitation (the formation, oscillation, and collapse of bubbles). The cavitation bubbles concentrate energy which can be used to bring about certain effects at the site of bubble activity. Bubbles form, swirl, and oscillate more easily in less dense media. Hence, they will form preferentially in the gel between the ultrasound transducer and the skin, rather than in the skin itself. When bubbles oscillate and then collapse at the skin surface, localized shock waves are created and liquid micro jets are directed at the stratum corneum. These micro jets disturb the stratum corneum lipid structure and increase skin permeability for several hours. Low-frequency ultrasound does not penetrate deeply into tissues. Therefore, the energy effects are not felt in the subcutaneous region.

The SonoPrep is an example of a handheld device that is used to generate cavitational ultrasound. The device creates an electrical signal at the ultrasonic frequency of 53 to 56 kHz. This signal is transmitted to an ultrasound transducer which converts it into mechanical vibration. This device has been used as the source of cavitational ultrasound in research studies. One such study involved rapid delivery of lidocaine through the skin so that venous cannulation, after 5 minutes of pretreatment, was virtually pain-free.[1] Lidocaine applied to the skin, without any energy input, takes much longer to permeate the skin and is less effective at reducing pain during cannulation.

PORATION METHODS OF DRUG DELIVERY ENHANCEMENT

When it became clear that an extremely small number of drugs, having a narrow range of properties, could permeate the skin by passive diffusion, attention was turned to chemical enhancers. However, these had limitations and only increased the spectrum of permeable drugs in a limited way. Attention was then focused on the application of external energy to the skin to serve as the driving force for drug permeation. These, too, had limitations: the only product type to reach the market is iontophoresis and, even with this technique, there have been significant developmental challenges. In addition, some drug products were withdrawn from the market after commercialization. While iontophoretic research and product development is ongoing, the next wave of effort is currently directed to creating minute pores in the stratum corneum (only), so that drugs can be delivered across this barrier. Since the major barrier to drug permeation is removed by such treatment, the remaining journey of the molecule into the depths of the skin and into the blood vessels is easier. Other mechanisms, largely diffusion, come into effect to transport the molecule over this, easier, part of its journey.

Numerous small pores create the means for the passage of a reasonable amount of drug across the skin. The drug is incorporated into a patch. Since the area of the patch is small, the dose cannot be large. The pores created in the skin are closely spaced in a small area and heal rapidly after application of the proration method. Little pain is experienced since the poration takes place through the stratum corneum only. The next dose is applied to a different location on the body, allowing the first area of application to completely heal before it is used again, if necessary.

Chemical enhancers and physical methods utilize mechanisms aimed at achieving the permeation of drugs through the skin, in spite of the barrier function of the stratum corneum. Poration methods, on the other hand, cause skin damage, albeit to minute areas, in order to create drug transport passages. While every effort is made to reduce irritation and skin damage when using chemical enhancers or when applying physical methods to enhance permeation, poration methods actively seek to damage minute areas of the skin.

Since the drug will flow in through a "pore," the need for the drug to be lipophilic is removed. In fact, water-soluble drugs are preferred since they can dissolve in the tissue fluid of the deeper layers of the skin. For this reason, the soluble salt form of the drug is typically used, in contrast to passive diffusion methods of transdermal drug delivery where the hydrophobic form of the drug is preferred. The molecular weight of the drug is no longer a problem since each pore is much larger than molecular dimensions. However, there are still dose limitations, as mentioned above, due to the small patch size. Several proration methods have been used experimentally and are briefly described below. Microneedles, at the present time, appear to be at the forefront of these poration methods.

Electroporation

Electroporation, unlike iontophoresis, uses high-voltage electricity in very short pulses to produce transient pores. The voltages, typical of this technique, exceed 100V but they are applied for milliseconds only. The pores created allowed the permeation of drugs that are resistant to diffusion through untreated skin.

Thermal Ablation

In this technique, heat is applied, with little or no discomfort, to create pores in the epidermis. A very high temperature (130°C) is used over a short duration (eg, 30 ms). Numerous, minute heat sources are combined into a device covering a small area of skin, comparable to the size of a patch. After the short burst of energy, numerous micrometer-sized areas of the stratum corneum evaporate. The arrangement of the multiple heat sources and the level of energy imparted cause damage to a small area of the stratum corneum only, and little to no pain is experienced.

Laser-Assisted Ablation

Laser treatment is frequently used in modern dermatology practice. The laser radiation can be targeted accurately to certain cells to kill them with very short exposure of the order of 300 ns. This technique can be used to improve acne, for example. Laser treatment has been used for this purpose for decades and its effects on the skin are, therefore, well understood. When used correctly, ablation of the stratum corneum can occur without significantly damaging deeper tissues. This process has been used to enhance the delivery of lipophilic as well as hydrophilic drugs in research studies.

Radiofrequency Ablation

The effect of radiofrequency electrical current is to increase temperature and this effect has been used in thermal ablation as a part of electro-surgery. It is used, for example, to remove malignant tumors. Radiofrequency currents have also been used to ablate nerve endings, so that pain signals cannot be transmitted. This technique has been used as a treatment for chronic pain, such as back ache. Similarly, the skin can be exposed to high-frequency alternating current (approximately 100 kHz) to create heat-induced micro-channels that are similar to those created by laser radiation. Transpharma Medical has developed the ViaDerm device, which contains an array of micro electrodes, for this purpose. It is a handheld electronic device used in conjunction with a drug. The device has a feedback mechanism to inform the operator when the micro-channels have been created. After treatment for less than one second, a drug-containing patch is placed onto the treated area of the skin. Work with this device is still in the experimental stage.

Microdermabrasion

Microdermabrasion is a cosmetic technique used to remove some layers of stratum corneum in order to give a "rejuvenated" appearance to the skin. The technique has been used for long in spas and beauty salons. Removal of any portion of the thickness of the stratum corneum should enable easier permeation of drugs through the skin and this has been the focus of experimental studies. A small template with fine, evenly-spaced holes is placed over the area of skin to be treated. Once in place, microdermabrasion is applied over the template so that small spots of skin (of micrometer dimensions) are abraded. When a drug formulation is placed over the treated area, the abraded spots serve as the drug delivery channels. By the use of dyes as the permeating agents, it can be demonstrated that penetration occurs preferentially through the abraded areas.

Microneedles

Microneedles technology consists of the application to the skin of a small patch containing an array of very small needles (Figure 22-6). The height of the needles used in experimental studies ranges from 25 μm to approximately 1500 μm. Most microneedles are much shorter than the maximum in this range and they do not reach the dermis where the pain receptors (nociceptors) and nerve endings are located. Thus, pain experienced with the application of microneedles is of low intensity, increasing with both the microneedle length and their density on the patch. Some erythema (redness) is observed in the local area but disappears quickly. This is probably due to the rapid closing, usually within hours, of the created pores. Repeated dosing uses different areas of the skin. Therefore, repeated insults to the skin do not occur and no increased risk of infection, at the application site, has been noted. For these reasons, microneedles are attractive to patients and healthcare workers: it is far easier to administer than an injection.

The needles themselves may consist of silicon, metals, polymers, or ceramics. Insoluble needles release their drug load after piercing the skin. After a predetermined length of time, the patch with the attached microneedles is removed from the skin. The drug load in such cases may be in the coating applied onto the needles. The coating solution consists of the drug and a second material to help adherence to the needles. The drug may also be present as a solution in hollow-core needles. After puncturing the skin, the solution flows into the skin. The pathway for absorption of the drug after microneedle administration is shown in Figure 22-3. An interesting innovation is the construction of microneedles from a soluble material, such as maltose. These needles break off after application. When the patch is removed, the broken needles remain within the skin where they dissolve and release their drug load. Polymers loaded with drug may be used to form solid breakable microneedles. Again, the drug is released into the interstitial fluid as the polymer dissolves.

Microneedles may be made by a printing process (lithography), etching, laser cutting, and by use of molding methods. Microneedles may be used to deliver small-molecular-weight drugs. Since drug molecule size is not an impediment, they may also be used for high-molecular-weight biopharmaceuticals, including peptide and protein drugs. In addition, they may be used for vaccine delivery which, currently, appears to be the foremost application of microneedles in human trials. However, none has reached the market at the time of writing.

Vaccination is an attractive application since the dose required is very low, it is usually a "once-off" application and, typically, the therapeutic window is large. The skin has been used for vaccination, by conventional methods, for a very long time. Apart from the easy access, the skin provides excellent amplification of the immune response due to the presence of epidermal dendritic cells, or Langerhans cells, situated close to the skin surface. Vaccine delivery by microneedles, therefore, appears to be relatively easy and is likely to be successful. The fact that a large portion of the interest in microneedles is directed to vaccines, at the current time, may also be a question of picking the "low-hanging fruit." With future product approvals and marketed vaccines, manufacturers may be more confident and inclined to invest money and time in the delivery of other substances by this technology.

FUTURE DEVELOPMENTS

The initial successes with TDDS, which were remarkable, led to over-exuberance and exaggerated claims of the potential of this route of drug delivery. However, it soon became clear that systemic delivery of drugs by this mechanism has some severe limitations. In particular, delivery was limited to low-dose, potent drugs of relatively low-molecular weight. Most frequently such molecules have balanced hydrophilic and lipophilic properties, with a slight tendency to be more hydrophobic. When a drug does not comply what the requirements for transdermal drug delivery, it is extremely difficult, if not impossible, to utilize formulation approaches to enhance drug absorption. There has to be some tendency for a drug to be absorbed, in the first place, for the utilization of formulation approaches to improve the extent of absorption. If the drug has none of the required properties, only a harsh enhancer, or mixture of such enhancers, may be able to achieve the required permeation. Such a formulation would be unacceptable from regulatory, and from patient acceptability, perspectives.

It should be remembered that the perfusion barrier is a protective mechanism and perturbation of this barrier can be dangerous, if such modification is not reversed fairly quickly, that is, if the enhanced permeability is not reversed, many toxins could permeate the skin. This could lead to undesirable effects even if a relatively small area of the skin is modified. Given these limitations, there have been some failures. For example, the particular properties of testosterone, and the dose required for amelioration of low hormonal levels in older males, have led to several failed attempts to produce an effective transdermal patch containing this hormone. This has led to the idea that a patch dosage form of this drug, given the dose requirements, cannot be successfully formulated.

The delivery of larger molecules and those that are hydrophilic have been a major difficulty for long. Much research has produced only limited success and no commercialized products at the time of writing. However, poration methods offer some hope, as mentioned in the section on this topic. Since minute sections of the stratum corneum are removed, molecular size and drug hydrophilicity are no longer issues. Nevertheless, delivery of such drugs is still in the research phase.

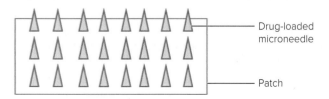

FIGURE 22-6 Diagram of a microneedles-containing patch.

In spite of such limitations, transdermal drug delivery is presently a multibillion-dollar market. In fact, sales of the fentanyl patch alone have consistently exceeded $1 billion annually for several years. Therefore, despite the limitations and failures of the early years, patches as a delivery system are a success. Consumer familiarity with, and acceptance of, patches have probably been aided by the widespread availability of over-the-counter (OTC) nicotine patches. This author suggests that a delivery system may be considered to have "come of age" when a new drug is offered, for the first time, as this delivery system. (The typical commercial route for a new drug is to be first offered as an oral, or an injectable, dosage form with subsequent development of novel dosage forms utilizing alternate routes of drug administration.) Neupro® (rotigotine) is the first product to go directly to a TDDS and this event may be an indication of the significance of this form of drug delivery. Several generic patches, of other drugs, have also been available for a few years. Some came to market only after legal battles over the right to produce a generic. This was the case with the fentanyl patch. The availability of OTC and generic patches are further indications of the developmental progress of this route of drug administration.

Recap Questions

1. Name two methods of enhancing drug delivery through the skin that use electricity.
2. How does cavitional ultrasound differ from non-cavitional ultrasound?
3. Which is the most advanced physical method of enhancing drug delivery, as assessed by the earliest achievement of marketing approval?
4. How do poration methods enhance drug permeation?

- Microneedles for vaccine delivery appear to be close to commercialization and this may be the forerunner of drug administration by this technique.
- While initial successes with TDDS led to euphoria, it is clear that any one mechanism of drug delivery will not be universally applicable and will probably only work with a narrow range of drugs.

What do you think?

1. "A person who is nervous may sweat profusely. While their hands may be wet, they will not be oily from the perspiration." Do you agree, or disagree, with this statement? Explain your view.
2. Scientists have expressed the idea that chemical enhancers should do no harm. However, poration methods intentionally damage the skin. When the first poration technology is commercialized, would transdermal drug delivery be viewed as having achieved great success, or be viewed negatively for having to cause damage in order to deliver a drug? Explain your answer fully.
3. Is there potential for microneedles to be misused for drugs of abuse and, if so, should further development be halted?
4. Mr. Lee, a patient that you see at the hospital where you work as a pharmacist has been prescribed the Duragesic patch. He is very concerned about getting adequate medication for his pain. He thinks the patch is just a gimmick. How could a small patch be equivalent to 3 days' pain medication and how will it go through his skin? What will you say to Mr. Lee to re-assure him?

SUMMARY POINTS

- Transdermal drug delivery is important because some drugs cannot be effectively delivered orally, and injections are uncomfortable and are not convenient for self-administration in contrast to transdermal delivery which can provide extended therapy from one dosage form.
- The structure of the skin is designed to keep out noxious substances (including drugs) and special measures must be used, in most cases, to promote drug delivery through the skin.
- While chemical enhancers can damage the skin, or at least cause unacceptable irritation, some formulation techniques, including supersaturation of the drug in the delivery system and altering the partition coefficient between the delivery system and the skin, have improved transdermal drug delivery significantly.
- While many physical methods have been explored, only iontophoresis, that is, the use of a low-voltage electrical current, has been successful thus far and several systems have been commercialized.

REFERENCE

1. Becker BM, Helfrich S, Baker E, Lovgren K, Minugh PA, Machan JT. Ultrasound with topical anesthetic rapidly decreases pain of intravenous cannulation. *Acad Emerg Med.* 2005;12:289-295.

BIBLIOGRAPHY

Brown MB, Martin GP, Jones SA, Akomeah SK. Dermal and transdermal drug delivery systems: current and future prospects. *Drug Deliv.* 2006;13:175-187.

Prausnitz MR, Langer R. Transdermal drug delivery. *Nat Biotechnol.* 2008;26(11):1261-1268.

Walter JR, Shuai X. Therapeutic transdermal drug innovation from 2000 to 2014: current status and outlook. *Drug Discov Today.* 2015;11:1293-1299.

Wiedersberg S, Guy RH. Transdermal drug delivery: 30+ years of war and still fighting! *J Control Release.* 2014;190:150-156.

https://www.fda.gov/drugs/drug-approvals-and-databases/orange-book-data-files. Accessed July 18, 2023.

Ophthalmic Drug Delivery | 23

PREVIEW

- The eye is an extremely sensitive organ which is protected from noxious substances in the air and those that are blood-borne—this makes drug delivery to the interior of the eye difficult.

- Historically, medications were applied topically to the eye; a few medications penetrated to some extent.

- The structure of the eye reveals an anterior segment and a posterior segment: drug delivery to the posterior segment is difficult.

- To overcome poor permeation, topical devices were developed for slow release of a drug to the eye for a prolonged time—successful for anterior segment.

- Several serious diseases affect the posterior segment and may cause loss of sight.

- To target this region, invasive, radical therapies were developed; these have side effects, but may save the patient's sight.

- New nanotechnology therapies being developed offer the potential for good permeation from "conventional" dosage forms and may, in the future, provide drug delivery to the posterior segment without resorting to invasive techniques.

INTRODUCTION

Drug delivery to the eye may be divided into topical administration (drugs administered onto the surface of the eye) and internal administration, that is, the placement of the drug into the interior of the eye by means of injections or surgically inserted drug delivery systems. It is obvious, from even a superficial reflection, that internal administration is inherently risky, carrying with it the danger of damage to the eye during repeat injections or surgical procedures. Such damage may be serious and include injury resulting in blindness. Topical administration to the eye has a long history, whereas drug administration into the interior of the eye is relatively recent. In terms of the complexity of *pharmaceutical technological* development, some topical drug delivery devices parallel those for insertion into the eye.

Drugs delivered topically to the eye may be required, in some instances, for the treatment of superficial conditions on, or close to, the surface of the eye. In other cases, the drug from a topical delivery system may be required to penetrate the eye, to some extent, in order to bring about its pharmacological effect on an eye structure that is not superficial. For this reason, a basic understanding of the structure of the eye is required for both internal and topical drug administration. While drug penetration into the eye is generally poor, some drugs administered topically may permeate the tissues of the eye, to some extent, to be effective in the area of penetration. This classification emphasizes the placement or administration of the drug rather than its location of effectiveness.

STRUCTURE OF THE EYE

The structure of the eye (Figure 23-1) can be approximated to a gel-filled sphere where the wall of the sphere consists of three layers. These are, from the outside to the interior, the sclera, the choroid, and the retinal layer. These layers go all around the surface of the sphere (except for the front), and not simply around the periphery of a circle, as depicted in the two-dimensional drawing. The front of the eye has specialized structures instead of the continuation of the three layers. Within the eye, toward the front, the ciliary body is formed as a thickened outgrowth of the choroid layer. The iris (the colored part of the eye) can be viewed as an extension of the ciliary body. The lens, which is located behind the iris, is attached to the ciliary body by the ciliary muscles. The iris and ciliary muscles are not two structures (upper and lower) as the two-dimensional drawing implies, but they go all the way around the circular lens. The interior of the eye is divided into the anterior segment (in front of the lens) and the posterior segment (behind the lens).

The inner surface of both the upper and lower eyelids is lined with conjunctival epithelium which extends onto the eyeball itself, adjacent to the sclera. The portion of the conjunctival epithelium that is on the eyeball is continuous with the corneal epithelium, which covers the area in front of the iris and the lens. Therefore, there is a continuous epithelial layer covering the entire region from the lower eyelid, over the eyeball, and over the upper eyelid (interior surface of eyelids). This conjunctival epithelium is a mucous membrane, that secretes mucus, keeps the eye moist in conjunction with the tears, and protects the internal structures. The lower eyelid may be pulled down by placing a finger slightly below the eyeball, and applying gentle downward pressure. This creates a conjunctival pocket which may, conveniently, be used for the administration of ophthalmic medications. This space has been described by various terms including the conjunctival cul-de-sac, the conjunctival pocket, or simply the pocket. The term "conjunctival pocket" will be used in this chapter.

At the juncture of the membrane covering the inner eyelid and the membrane covering the eyeball, there are several folds of the conjunctival epithelium. The anatomical advantage of having these folds is to allow movements of the eyeball since the epithelial connections are not rigid. These folds are referred to as the "fornix." In anatomy, a fornix is a vault or arched structure. In drug delivery, advantage may be taken of this location to place a small drug-containing device between the folds for extended periods. This may be visualized as placing a small coin between multiple folds of a towel. The drug is slowly released from the device and this form of drug administration provides a long duration of action.

The space between the cornea and the lens is filled with aqueous humor, whereas that behind the lens is filled with vitreous humor, which is more viscous than aqueous humor. Drug delivery into the eye may be divided into two major areas: regions in front of the lens (anterior segment), and regions behind the lens (posterior segment). The latter is also known as "the back of the eye" or the vitreous. While each of these areas has barriers which impede the permeation of drugs, drug delivery to the vitreous is much more difficult.

SOME OPHTHALMIC CONDITIONS REQUIRING DRUG TREATMENT

Some ophthalmic conditions that require drug treatment are briefly described to provide a perspective on why drug absorption into the eye is needed, and the regions of the eye to which the drugs should permeate to treat the respective condition. The seriousness of the condition is mentioned, in some instances,

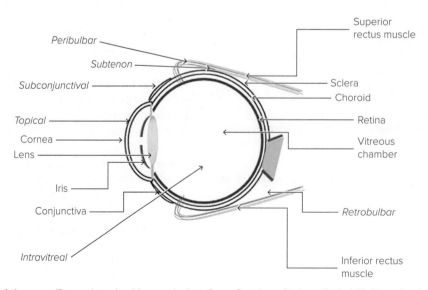

FIGURE 23-1 **Structure of the eye.** (Reproduced, with permission, from Gaudana R, Ananthula HK, Parenky A, Mitra AK. Ocular drug delivery. *AAPS J.* Springer Nature, 2010;12(3):348–360.).

to illustrate the urgency with which enhanced drug delivery to these regions is necessary. Only as much detail, as required for the above purposes, is provided and this is done only for those diseases that are referenced later in this chapter. Mind Map 23-1 summarizes the diseases of the eye that are amenable to drug treatment at present.

Conjunctivitis

Conjunctivitis is an inflammation of the conjunctiva. The symptoms of conjunctivitis are usually mild and, with proper treatment, the condition will usually be of short duration. It may be caused by an allergy in which case it is called allergic conjunctivitis and treated with antihistamine or vasoconstrictor eye drops or combination products. The vasoconstrictor reduces symptoms, such as redness. Conjunctivitis may also be caused by an infection, in which case, it is treated with antibiotics.

Dry Eye

Dry eye is caused by reduced tear production. This condition becomes more common as patients get older. One of the problems with a dry eye is the fact that it could lead to corneal abrasion due to rubbing of the dry, itchy eyes. In addition, they may be a tendency for the lids to stick to the mucosa of the eye, including the corneal mucosa. When the eyelids are opened, some abrasion to the corneal mucosa may occur. A clinical test used to assess dry eye is the tear film breakup time. For this test, a drop of fluorescein dye is inserted into the eye which is then observed by means of a cobalt blue light. The patient is asked not to blink, and the length of time is noted from the last blink until signs appear of tear film breakup. Breakup appears as dark patches in areas where the previously uniform film is disturbed. Tear film breakup times less than 10 seconds are indicative of

dry eye. If, during the patient's normal activities, the tear film breaks up before the patient's next blink, the eye would feel dry and uncomfortable. Each blink distributes the tears and forms the film once more.

Dry eye is treated by the administration of aqueous drops to replenish the liquids lost and to provide a soothing feeling to the eyes. Drops in which the viscosity is enhanced have a longer duration of effect because they are not drained from the eye rapidly. In some cases, gels may be prescribed for nighttime use since they keep the eyes moist for a prolonged period. Eye drops which are in the physical form of an emulsion are desirable for reasons described under "Topical Drug Administration."

Corneal Abrasion

Corneal abrasion refers to damage to the cells of the cornea, typically the mucosal layer of the cornea. This is commonly known as "scratching" of the cornea. This can occur in various ways such as injury due to walking into a branch (or similar accident), abrasion due to a contact lens that is not perfectly smooth, or which has been worn too long. Abrasion resulting from dry eye has been mentioned above. Minor abrasions cause discomfort with eyesight remaining intact. More severe manifestations of corneal abrasion, involving deeper layers, can affect the patient's eyesight as the cornea is responsible for the refraction of light (together with the lens).

Corneal abrasions are treated by the application of tear replacement drops which are soothing to the damaged tissues and allow natural healing to occur. Antibiotic preparations may be applied if the corneal abrasions become infected. They may also be applied, as a preventative measure, in the absence of any infection. If left untreated, more severe corneal abrasions can turn into corneal ulcers, a much more serious condition. When corneal ulceration is severe, blindness results.

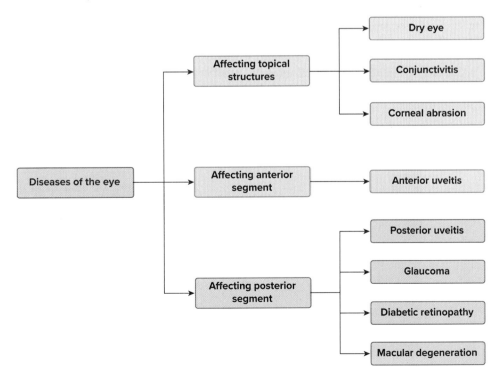

MIND MAP 23-1 Some Diseases of the Eye Amenable to Drug Treatment

Glaucoma

Glaucoma is a condition in which there is increased ocular pressure. The increased ocular pressure may result in damage to the optic nerve, a condition which affects eyesight. Progressively worsening glaucoma results in increased damage to the optic nerve, which results, eventually, in blindness. Glaucoma may be caused by diabetes.

Diabetic Retinopathy

Diabetic retinopathy is a disease of the micro-vasculature of the retina. The disease is characterized by leakage of fluid (edema) and the growth of new blood vessels, both of which may cause visual disturbances. New blood vessels may form at the optic disc which is located at the back of the eye, on the nasal side (the macula, which is described later, is closer to the temple). The optic disc is the point on the retina at which various nerve fibers collect to become the optic nerve which leaves the eye at this point (Figure 23-2). The optic disc is also the point at which the central retinal artery enters the retina and where the central retinal vein exits the retina. The abnormal growth of blood vessels may cause retinal and vitreal hemorrhage and detachment of the retina. Progression of the disease causes loss of visual acuity and, if untreated, leads to blindness. Since the growth of new blood vessels is promoted by vascular endothelial growth factor (VEGF), anti-VEGF factors are hypothesized to reduce proliferation and to improve the condition. Certain anti-VEGF factors are approved for use in treating ocular disorders, while others have been approved for treating certain neoplasms (new and abnormal growth of tissue). Some of the latter drugs have been used, off-label, by intravitreal injection, and appear to improve diabetic retinopathy.

Macular Degeneration

The macula is a circular area of the retina at the back of the eye, a little toward the temple. It is an area rich in cones (rather than rods), responsible for focusing vision and for distinguishing fine detail and color. By contrast, the rods which are found in other areas of the retina distinguish basic shapes and movements, and are responsible for lowlight vision, which is devoid of color. When the cells of the macula are not functioning correctly, the image becomes distorted. Deterioration of the state of the macula is referred to as macular degeneration. In the initial stages of macular degeneration, the patient may not experience much disturbance in vision. As deterioration continues, images in the center of the field of vision become blurry and, ultimately, sight in this area is lost and is replaced by a black disc. Although peripheral vision may be intact, people with severe macular degeneration are considered legally blind.

Macular degeneration may be wet or dry. The dry form of macular degeneration is far more prevalent than the wet form and is characterized by atrophy and the presence of yellow pigment deposits, called Drusen. Minimal-to-moderate visual loss is associated with this form of the disease. In the wet form, there is an overgrowth of blood vessels in response to VEGF, a secreted protein. The latter binds to receptors on vascular endothelial cells (the cells of the internal lining of blood vessels). The receptors are activated to form new blood vessels, a process referred to as angiogenesis. The rapidly growing blood vessels are imperfectly formed and leaky, hence this condition is described as being "wet." Since new blood vessels are formed, the descriptive term, "neovascular" is also used. Macular degeneration may be age related in which case it is referred to as age-related macular degeneration (AMD).

When leakage of blood or serum into the space below the retina occurs, it may result in retinal detachment. The neovascular form of AMD has been treated with laser phototherapy (to reduce blood vessel growth) or with antibodies against VEGF. Lucentis (ranibizumab) and oligopeptide pegaptanib (Macugen) are approved for this indication whereas Avastin (bevacizumab) has been used off-label.

Anterior Uveitis

Anterior uveitis is an inflammation of the anterior structures of the eye, including the uveal body. It may be recognized by the presence of inflammatory cells floating in the aqueous humor. Treatment consists of medications to reduce inflammation and scarring, most commonly the application of topical glucocorticoids.

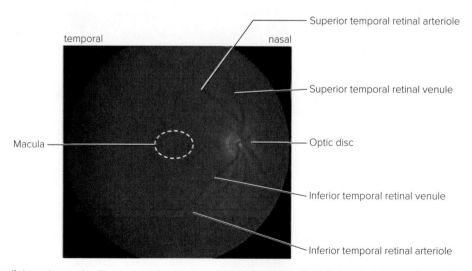

FIGURE 23-2 **Optic disk and macula.** (Reproduced, with permission, from Putz R, Pabst R. *Sobotta: Atlas of Human Anatomy: Head, Neck, Upper Limb, Thorax, Abdomen, Pelvis, Lower Limb.* 14th ed. Munich: Urban & Fischer; 2008.)

Posterior Uveitis

The characteristics of posterior uveitis are inflammation of the vitreous, retina, or choroid. It is more likely to be associated with a systemic disease, than is the case for anterior uveitis. Some patients have panuveitis which is an inflammation of both the anterior and posterior segments of the eye. The presence of this condition may be evidence of an autoimmune disease.

DRUG PERMEATION INTO THE EYE

Drug permeation into the eye may be divided into three types: drug permeation to the superficial structures of the eye, into the anterior segment, and into the posterior segment. The superficial structures of the eye include the conjunctiva and the cornea. Drug permeation to the conjunctiva, as a superficial mucous membrane, is relatively straightforward in contrast to permeation through the cornea, which is described next. Allergic conjunctivitis is treated with antihistamine and vasoconstrictor eye drops which are readily absorbed by the conjunctival membrane. Infective conjunctivitis is treated with antibiotics such as sulfacetamide eye drops and eye ointment, from which sulfacetamide also permeates relatively easily into the conjunctival membranes.

The cornea has alternating layers of hydrophobic and hydrophilic membranes which are described in the next section, Drug Permeation into the Anterior Segment. Considering these alternating barriers, permeation into the cornea is extremely difficult. In addition, the pool of available drugs, for example, antibiotics to treat infected abrasions, will rapidly be eliminated by drainage through the nasolacrimal ducts. For these reasons, infections of the cornea may require treatment with repeat administration of antibiotics at very short intervals, for example, every 2 hours.

Drug Permeation into the Anterior Segment

Even a cursory observation of Figure 23-1 will indicate that permeation into the anterior segment must involve passage through the cornea. The first barrier to drug permeation is, however, not the cornea, but the tears. It may be surprising to learn that the passage of a drug through the tears may not be as fast as presumed. The reason for this is related to the specific constituents of tears and the structure of the tear film. Blinking spreads the tears and forms a liquid film over the eye. This liquid film is not simple or uniform: it has different layers, each containing different components. As shown in Figure 23-3, these layers, going from the outermost inward, are the following:

1. a lipid layer: this is comprised of two sub-layers, the outermost being a layer of nonpolar lipids, whereas the next is a polar bilayer;

2. an aqueous compartment containing soluble mucin and free lipid; and

3. a coating of mucus which is attached to the corneal epithelium by means of microvilli extending from the epithelial cells.

The difficulty in penetrating this liquid layer is the fact that a molecule must first pass through a hydrophobic layer, which is easy for hydrophobic drugs but difficult for hydrophilic drugs. Next, it must pass through an aqueous layer, which is easier for

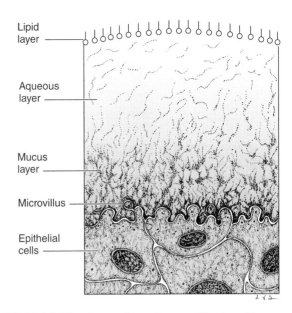

FIGURE 23-3 **The three primary layers of the tear film covering the superficial epithelial layer of the cornea.** (Reproduced, with permission, from Riordan-Eva P, Augsburger JJ, eds. *Vaughan & Asbury's General Ophthalmology*. 19th ed. New York, NY: McGraw Hill; 2018.)

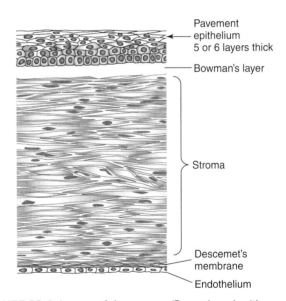

FIGURE 23-4 **Layers of the cornea.** (Reproduced, with permission, from Riordan-Eva P, Augsburger JJ, eds. *Vaughan & Asbury's General Ophthalmology*. 19th ed. New York, NY: McGraw Hill; 2018.)

a hydrophilic drug than for one that is hydrophobic. Finally, the molecule must pass through the mucus layer which has the potential for physical entrapment of the drug.

If a permeating molecule is able to penetrate the tear film, it must then cross the next barrier to permeation, the cornea. The cornea also consists of different layers which are shown in Figure 23-4. These layers are hydrophobic and hydrophilic, alternatively, which increases the barrier function:

1. The outermost layer is the epithelium which consists of five or six layers of cells, the most superficial of which is differentiated into different regions, including tight junctions.

The lipophilic nature of the epithelial cell membranes, in conjunction with the tight junctions, makes it difficult for drugs to pass through this barrier. The greatest resistance is to hydrophilic drugs.

2. Bowman's membrane is a much thinner structure without cells.

3. The stroma is the next layer. It consists mainly of water, together with collagen, mucopolysaccharides, and proteins, giving it a gel-like structure. As can be seen from the diagram, it is the thickest layer of the cornea.

4. The Descemet's membrane is a thin, tough membrane supporting the endothelium.

5. The endothelium is a single layer of cells regulating stromal hydration. For the stroma to remain clear and transparent, hydration is important.

A molecule that was not drained out of the eye via the nasolacrimal system, and has permeated the tear film, must next permeate the five layers of the cornea, described above, in order to get to the aqueous humor. For this reason, a very small proportion of the drug content of instilled drops actually reaches the aqueous humor. To increase the chances of drug permeation to therapeutic levels, solubility enhancers may be added to the formulation. Given that the volume of drops that may be instilled into the eye is limited, this technique achieves a higher concentration of drug in the instilled drops. Since the extent of diffusion is proportional to concentration, drug diffusion is improved.

Drug Permeation into the Posterior Segment

If drug delivery to the anterior segment is difficult, it is much more so to the posterior segment of the eye. There are additional structural barriers which inhibit permeation to this region of the eye. There are also clearance mechanisms that remove drugs that have permeated into the anterior segment, or which are attempting to permeate into deeper structures of the eye. For example, any drug molecules that have permeated the ciliary body may be taken up by blood vessels in that region, for transport away from the eye. Figure 23-1 shows mechanisms of clearance from the anterior and the posterior segments. This figure also shows various routes of possible drug administration into the eye. While the above are some of the problems associated with delivering drugs to the posterior segment, there is a great need for drug delivery to this region in the light of several important diseases of the posterior segment of the eye. These include AMD, diabetic retinopathy, and related ocular neovascular diseases, as previously discussed.

Orally administered drugs cannot be used for delivery to the posterior segment for several reasons, including the fact that there is a blood-retinal barrier. Due to this barrier, systemically administered medication does not reach the posterior segment in significant amounts to be therapeutically useful. This is one of the situations mentioned in Chapter 1, Introduction, with regard to the use of systemic drug administration to get medication to a specific organ. Toxic systemic blood levels would have to be attained, in order to provide reasonable drug levels within the organ, in this case, the eye. The blood-retinal barrier, which is the major reason for this situation, has a protective function, that is, it isolates the retina, a sensitive structure, from toxins that may arrive via the blood. As discussed under the anterior segment, drugs cannot easily permeate the tear film and cornea, and this, also, is a protective mechanism keeping noxious chemicals from the atmosphere away from the eye. For these reasons, drug delivery to the posterior segment, up to the present time, requires invasive delivery. This takes the form of injections or drug-releasing devices placed into the eye. The latter have mostly been achieved by special surgical techniques although some recent devices are so small that they may be injected into the eye through a needle.

Drug administration to the eye may be divided into topical administration (onto the surface of the eye) and invasive drug administration (into the eye), as previously mentioned. These administration techniques are described in more detail in the following sections. The different forms of drug administration to the eye are summarized in Mind Map 23-2.

Recap Questions

1. Name three conditions involving superficial structures of the eye, which can be treated with topical medication (eye drops, ointments, etc.)

2. The eye may be described as a sphere with three outer layers. What are these layers?

3. What is the fornix and why is it important for drug delivery to the eye?

4. Briefly describe corneal abrasion and glaucoma.

5. Name the layers of the tear film.

6. Why is permeation through the cornea so difficult?

TOPICAL (NONINVASIVE) DRUG ADMINISTRATION

Noninvasive drug administration to the eye may be divided into two groups: the conventional, "simple" formulations and drug delivery systems or devices. Conventional formulations include eye drops, gels, and ointments. Drug delivery devices are placed into the upper or lower conjunctival pocket, into the upper or lower fornix, or directly onto the cornea. Drug delivery systems act as a drug reservoir, providing a continuous, slow release of the contained drug. The pharmaceutical development of such devices is complex, involving an understanding of the anatomy and physiology of the eye, polymers and material science, novel sustained-release technology, and in vitro and in vivo testing methods. Possibly by comparison to devices, the traditional topical dosage forms have been considered "simple"; but this term is deceptive as there are many considerations to take into account in the development of conventional formulations.

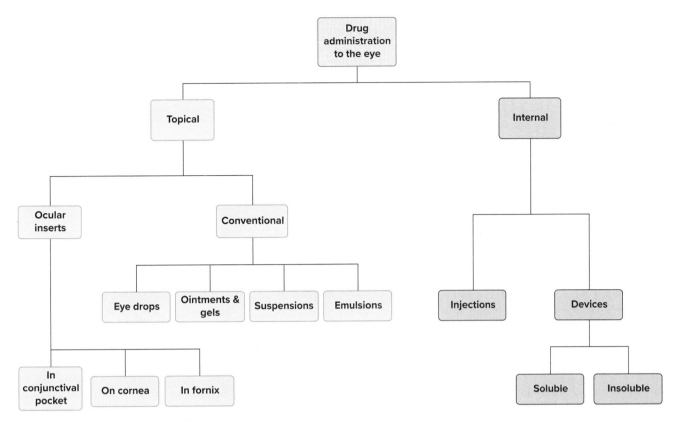

MIND MAP 23-2 Drug Administration to the Eye

Conventional Formulations

Formulations of a type that have been well established, and are commonly used, are considered conventional. Drugs for topical application to the eye are presented as ointments, gels, suspensions, and eye drops. Commonly used medications include formulations to treat conjunctival infections, vasoconstrictors to reduce redness of the eyes, and artificial tears to treat dry eye syndrome. Antibiotics are available as drops, ointments, gels, or suspensions. The eye is an extremely sensitive organ and topical drug delivery products must be formulated taking this fact into consideration. These products must be non-irritant, sterile, isotonic, and both convenient and cosmetically acceptable to use. Formulations that are developed specifically to extend contact with ophthalmic tissues are desirable since drug formulations are rapidly removed from the conjunctival pocket in the absence of such formulation strategies.

The two major sources of irritancy are the chemical nature of the medication, or additives, and particulates in the formulation. Since the eye is a highly sensitive organ, chemicals that are routinely applied topically to the skin, or even taken internally, may not be suitable for application to the eye. Any new chemical that a formulator wishes to incorporate into an ophthalmic formulation must be tested using a standard test for eye irritancy. The Draize test has been applied historically to test ingredients for ophthalmic use. It has also been used to test ingredients that are intended to be used in cosmetics. Interestingly, it was shown in the 1930s, that some types of mascara contained irritant chemicals, which served as the stimulus to include cosmetics in this test.

The Draize test, developed in 1944, involves the application of the test material to the eyes of albino rabbits, which are then observed and scored for signs of irritation. The latter can occur in different parts of the eye, and to different degrees. This is a test for acute toxicity where different ranges of score values indicate the level of hazard to humans. There have been many objections to this test methodology, stating that it is cruel to the animals and arguing that there are several differences between rabbit and human eyes. The application of the test has been modified over the years, making it less cruel to the test animals. The theme of the test modifications is to exclude those substances that will cause gross irritation and pain to the test animals. Whereas a wide range of chemicals were tested in rabbit eyes previously, the selection of chemicals for testing is now much more judicious: there is little point in testing substances that are very likely to be irritant, based on a knowledge of the nature of the substance. After proper, stepwise screening, as briefly described below, those chemicals that are not rejected may be tested in the eyes of several rabbits.

In vitro test methods have also been developed and substances that display gross irritancy *potential*, in these tests, are not tested in rabbit eyes. In addition, a chemical must first be tested on rabbit skin. Those substances that have been shown not to be irritant, in this test, may proceed to ophthalmic testing. The latter is done, initially, in the eyes of one rabbit only. A full 24-hour observation time must pass before further testing, in additional rabbits, can be considered. If there are obvious signs of irritation, the study is discontinued (with a positive outcome for irritation).

TABLE 23-1 Examples of Preservatives Used in Eye Drops

PRODUCT	PRESERVATIVE	CONCENTRATION (%)
Dexamethasone sodium phosphate ophthalmic solution, USP	Sodium bisulfite Phenylethyl alcohol Benzalkonium chloride	0.1 0.25 0.02
Cromolyn sodium ophthalmic solution, USP	Benzalkonium chloride	0.01
Cetirizine hydrochloride (Zerviate®)	Benzalkonium chloride	0.01
Ciprofloxacin hydrochloride ophthalmic solution, USP	Benzalkonium chloride	0.006

The ultimate purpose of the test is to exclude the intentional application of irritants to human eyes. It is important to realize that it is not only the drug substance that may be irritant but also any excipient that is incorporated into an ophthalmic formulation. For this reason, all ingredients have to be tested for irritancy potential before they can be used in ophthalmic preparations. Such ingredients include viscosity-enhancing agents, co-solvents, and buffers. It is a very common experience that dust particles on the surface of the eye are extremely irritant. Therefore, drops inserted into the conjunctival pocket of the eye should be free from particulate matter. The USP states that ophthalmic solutions should be "essentially free from foreign particles."

To prevent infections of the conjunctiva and other eye tissues, medications applied to the eye should be sterile. Since heat increases the instability of many drugs, sterilization by autoclaving eye drops is not the preferred method. For example, alkaloids, which are frequently used in eye drop formulations, are unstable at elevated temperatures. The instability is worse at pH values close to that of tears (pH = 7.4). Pilocarpine hydrochloride, an alkaloid, is commonly used in eye drop formulations, for the treatment of glaucoma. Pilocarpine eye drops degrade rapidly when autoclaved, especially at pH values approaching 7. For this reason, the USP states that the preferred method of sterilization of eye drops is membrane filtration under aseptic conditions. Single-use, pre-sterilized filter systems are preferred for aseptic filtration. Small units can be used in a compounding pharmacy. The outer wrapper should be opened, and the filter system is used, under a laminar flow hood. In cases, where it can be demonstrated that the stability of the eye drop formulation is not adversely affected, autoclaving may be used.

The sterilization techniques applied, in the course of manufacture, can be expected to maintain sterility until the seal on the container is broken and the medication used by the patient. With repeated opening and closing of the container, and the possible touching of the applicator tip to the eye or eyelids, the sterility may not be maintained. For this reason, a preservative is usually added to the formulation. The type of preservative(s) used and the amount(s) depend to some extent on the nature of the formulation. Some formulations, by their nature, are self-preserving and do not need an additional preservative.

Many preservatives are poorly soluble in water. Rapid dissolution of these preservatives, for non-ophthalmic use, is achieved by heating or by the addition of a small amount of a good solvent for the preservative, such as ethanol or certain surfactants. In many types of formulations, such as oral or topical formulations, the addition of a small amount of selected organic solvents is pharmaceutically and biologically acceptable. Such solvents cannot be used in ophthalmic formulations. The preservative, benzalkonium chloride, is a quaternary ammonium salt and, as such, is water-soluble (polar compound). Partly for this reason, it is a commonly used preservative in eye drops. Table 23-1 lists some ophthalmic products with the preservative that they contain. The preservative used in a formulation may be especially irritant to tissues damaged as a result of physical injury or surgical trauma. For this reason, eye drops to be used during, or after, surgery, are sterile, single-use sachets, which contain no preservatives. Similarly, preservative-free eye drops should be used on eyes that have sustained an injury.

The volume of tears in the eye at any time is approximately 7 to 8 μL (Table 23-2). This is a very small volume, considering that a microliter is one-thousandth of a milliliter. This gives an indication of the volume of medication that may be applied to each eye, without a large volume flowing over the eyelids. The liquid that cannot be retained within the conjunctival pocket will flow out in this manner.

Any medication should be convenient to use, since convenience improves patient compliance which, ultimately, leads to an improvement in the clinical condition. Generally, eye drops are convenient to use, even in a work situation. The fact that eye drops will run out over the eyelids may not be cosmetically pleasing, if the patient is using eye makeup. Ointments and gels are, typically, for nighttime use since the presence of a semisolid material on the surface of the eye will obscure vision. The semisolid products are used because they remain in contact with the eye for a longer period. The gels referred to in this context are traditional gels, administered from a tube. This distinction is important in terms of the next type of product to be described. After such use, the patient may find, in the morning, that some of the product is on the eyelashes and the outer surfaces of the eyelids. While this may be cosmetically unacceptable, the excess material can easily be cleaned off the eyelids in the morning, and this factor is not a major concern.

TABLE 23-2 Volumes Related to Eye Drops

OBJECT	VOLUME (μL)
Typical drop from conventional dropper	50
"Ideal" drop	5-10
Volume of tears	7-8

Sol-gel transformation is the process by which a nonviscous liquid is converted into a gel due to a change in the environment of the formulation. Such changes include temperature, ionic strength, and pH. The temperature difference, when a drop is instilled into the eye, is the difference between body temperature and the temperature of the bottle of liquid (room temperature). Similarly, once a drop is instilled into the eye, it will experience a difference in ionic strength and pH. In the case of products that undergo sol-gel transformation, the disadvantages of a gel during administration are eliminated. This arises from the fact that a single drop of liquid (sol state) can be easily instilled into the eye. It is converted to a gel, upon contact with the eye, due to differences in the environment. Polymers are selected for inclusion into eye drops based on their ability to undergo such phase transitions.

Since the quantity of gel is very small, having originated from a single drop in the sol state, it is less messy and also obscures vision to a lesser extent. As mentioned in the next section, even a single drop is too much to hold in the eye, but this amount is less than the smallest amount of gel that may be easily squeezed out of a tube.

Eye Drops

Eye drops are by far the most common ophthalmic dosage form: 70% of prescriptions for ophthalmic products are for eye drops. The volume dispensed by a typical dropper is about 50 µL. Therefore, a single drop of liquid instilled into the eye consists of a far larger volume than may be held in the eye at any one time. The excess liquid spills out over the eyelids and runs down the cheek.

Viscosity Enhancement. The portion of the eye drops remaining (ie, that has not spilled out) also has a short lifetime bathing the eye due to the system of lacrimal ducts (Figure 23-5) that drain liquids from the eye sockets. These originate from the inner corner of each eyelid and eventually drain into the nose. The effectiveness of instilled eye drops is reduced due to the very small volume held in the eye, as well as the rapid drainage of this small volume through the lacrimal system. Therefore, pharmaceutical interventions are necessary to prolong their effectiveness. One approach is to incorporate viscosity-enhancing agents in the drops. When the more viscous liquid is instilled, the portion that exceeds the volume that can be retained will still flow out over the eyelids. However, lacrimal drainage of the remainder will be slower due to the increased viscosity. As a separate characteristic, some viscosity-enhancing materials are also bioadhesive. This means that they are able to interact with the mucous membrane, as well as the mucus layer that is present on the membrane. The instilled liquid, consequently, is retained for a longer time. Viscosity enhancement and mucoadhesion allow a longer time for the drug to exert its pharmacological action.

Some examples of eye drops which contain viscosity-enhancing agents are the following:

1. Viscosity-enhanced tear replacement formulations, used for dry eye syndrome. Chronic dry eye is a common problem that is treated with tear replacement formulations which consist of an isotonic aqueous medium with a demulcent (ocular

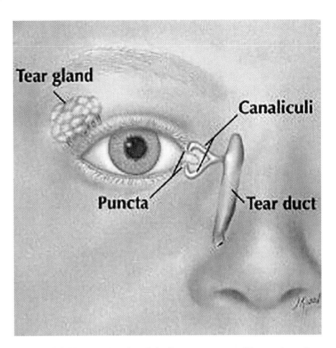

FIGURE 23-5 Nasolacrimal drainage system. (Reproduced, with permission, from Glossary: Nasolacrimal duct obstruction. American Association for Pediatric Ophthalmology and Strabismus, Roseville, MN. https://aapos.org/glossary/nasolacrimal-duct-obstruction. Accessed May 16, 2023.)

lubricant). The latter provides a soothing feeling to the eyes. Title 21 section 349.12 of the Code of Federal Regulations (CFR) lists substances that are approved by the FDA for use as ophthalmic demulcents in over-the-counter (OTC) formulations. The list includes cellulose derivatives, liquid polyols, glycerin, PEG 300 and PEG 400, polysorbate 80, propylene glycol, polyvinyl alcohol (PVA), and povidone, amongst others. The CFR also states the concentration range of each substance that may be used. If a concentration higher than stated in the regulations is used, the product will not be classified as OTC.

There are numerous "tear replacement" formulations on the market that comply with the above description. These formulations are nonviscous and leak out of the eye rapidly. Other formulations include viscosity-enhancing agents, which prolong the effect of the eye drops. An example is Systane Ultra which contains polyethylene glycol 400 (0.4%) and propylene glycol (0.3%) as lubricants (demulcents), and a hydroxypropyl derivative of guar gum as a viscosity enhancer. Some artificial tear formulations contain more than one demulcent. In terms of the regulations, up to three demulcents may be combined in one formulation (within the concentration ranges stated for each). If a formulation contains two or three demulcents, each having a concentration toward the upper end of the allowed range, these demulcents will enhance the viscosity of the formulation to some extent.

2. Timoptic XE is a solution formulation that contains timolol maleate (0.25% or 0.5%). The drug is a β-blocker and is used to reduce intraocular pressure in glaucoma patients. For this effect, it has to permeate the anterior segment. Since permeation is slow, increased contact time improves

permeation and makes the product more effective. The viscosity-enhancing agent, in this formulation, is gellan gum. This polymer, in the presence of anions (only), is not viscous. The naturally occurring gum is purified for use in eye drops by the removal of cations and the resulting material is incorporated into the eye drop formulation. When the drops are instilled into the eye, the liquid comes into contact with tears which contain cations, such as calcium, which convert the liquid into a gel. The sol-gel transformation, in this case, is brought about by the presence of ions.

3. AzaSite is an eye drop formulation that contains the antibiotic, azithromycin (1%), in a viscous medium. Unlike Timoptic, it does not undergo sol-gel transformation; the contents of the bottle are viscous at all times. As a result, the container needs to be first held inverted to allow the viscous drops to flow into the integrated dropper. Second, the container has to be squeezed to allow the drops to flow into the eye. A proprietary medium, called DuraSite®, is used for viscosity enhancement. The system contains polycarbophil as the thickening agent. Azithromycin is not stable for extended periods in an aqueous solution and the developers of this product, InSiteVision, claim that the drug is chemically stable in the DuraSite base. The product is marketed by Akorn, Inc.

The increased viscosity results in reduced drainage of the drops through the nasolacrimal system. It is also bioadhesive and the combined effect results in prolonged antibiotic action, claimed to last for 4 to 6 hours. The drops are used for specified bacterial infections of the conjunctiva with a 7-day treatment plan: one drop twice a day for the first two days and, thereafter, one drop a day for 5 days, giving a total of 7 days' treatment.

Buffered. Tears are buffered to pH 7.4 and eye drops instilled into the eyes should, ideally, be at a similar pH to reduce irritation. The buffer capacity of tears is low. Considering that only one drop is usually instilled into the eye, and the fact that tears are constantly produced, the pH of the instilled drop is fairly quickly adjusted toward pH 7.4, in spite of the low buffer capacity of tears.

An eye drop product is considered unstable if the drug precipitates out of solution, within the bottle, prior to the expiration date. The pH of the solution is important in this regard. Consider poorly soluble weak bases, such as alkaloids, which are frequently used for ophthalmic conditions. By the addition of an acid, the manufacturer converts the weak bases to acid salts, for improved solubility of the salt form. For example, pilocarpine is converted to pilocarpine hydrochloride, by the addition of HCl, and this is the form in which the drug is supplied. With regard to precipitation, the drug product is stable during its shelf life, that is, the patient will not see an insoluble precipitate at the bottom of the container. Consider the behavior of this acidic salt in different media. In an acidic medium, the ionization of the weakly acidic salt is repressed, and this form persists (pilocarpine.HCl). In basic media, the ionization of the salt is favored and, after reaction with the basic medium, the free base form of pilocarpine is formed.

The base form of the drug (differentiated from the acidic salt) may exist in the ionized and the unionized form. The unionized form is more permeable than the ionized form while the latter is more soluble. The ratio of the unionized, to the ionized, form of this base is related to pH, in terms of the Henderson-Hasselbach equation [Eq. (23-1)].

$$pH = pKa + log \frac{[Unionized]}{[Ionized]} \qquad (23\text{-}1)$$

By rearranging Eq. (23-1) and inserting the pKa value of pilocarpine:

$$log \frac{[Unionized]}{[Ionized]} = pH - pKa$$

$$log \frac{[Unionized]}{[Ionized]} = pH - 7.2 \qquad (23\text{-}2)$$

Consider, first, the situation within the bottle of eye drops during storage, and what would occur at different, hypothetical, pH values. At a pH of 7.2, the right-hand side of the equation equals zero, that is, the log of the ratio of [Unionized]:[Ionized] = 0; and the ratio of [Unionized]:[Ionized] = 1. This means that the unionized and ionized forms of this drug would be present in equal concentrations, that is, approximately 50% of the drug would be in the unionized form. Similarly, at pH values greater than 7.2, more of the drug would be in the unionized form. This form of the drug is poorly soluble and, the greater its concentration, the greater the possibility that some of the drug would precipitate within the container. This is an undesirable situation since the concentration of drug in solution would be lower than intended and, second, if the bottle were shaken before administration, particles may be dispensed, causing irritation.

If the drops were adjusted to a pH of 6.2 it could be determined, by similar calculations, that the ratio of the unionized drug to the ionized would be 1:10, that is, the ionized form of the drug would predominate in a 10:1 ratio. This pH adjustment allows stability from precipitation during storage of the eye drops. Next, consideration must be given to whether this eye drop formulation should be buffered to a low, or a high, buffer capacity.

The eye drops should, ideally, be buffered to a *low* buffer capacity for the following reason. When instilled into the eye, the buffers in the tears slowly raise the pH of the instilled solution toward the pH of tears. Since the pH of tears is 7.4, some of the ionized drug would be converted to the unionized form. The latter is more permeable and, hence, drug permeation through the tissues will occur more readily. As a result, more of the ionized drug will be converted to the unionized form (within the eye conjunctival pocket). This occurs in order to maintain the ratio of the two species at the level dictated by the prevailing pH value, in accordance with Eq. 23-2. As this process continues, it promotes the absorption of the unionized form of the drug.

It is important to note that all of the drug is not converted to the unionized species at once. If this were the case, some of the drug may precipitate. However, the conversion is progressive and the unionized form is removed from solution by the absorption process. Therefore, the probability of precipitation is low. The overall effect of supplying the drug in the manner described, is the fact that the drug is maintained in solution in the container during storage, and is converted to the more permeable form upon instillation into the eye.

Isotonic. Liquids that are intended to be instilled into the eyes should have the same osmotic pressure as tears. Osmotic pressure is a colligative property, that is, it depends on the number of particles in solution. From a knowledge of the concentration of substances in a liquid, and also their propensity to dissociate, it is possible to calculate a theoretical value for osmotic pressure. Osmotic pressure may also be measured using instruments designed for this purpose (osmometers). The term "isotonic" is analogous to iso-osmotic but refers specifically to blood in which the erythrocytes (red blood corpuscles) are permeable to certain substances, for example, urea. This is in contrast to other cells in which only water may freely diffuse through the membrane. Isotonicity takes this difference into account: a solution containing urea may be shown, by calculation or laboratory measurement, to have the same osmotic pressure as blood, that is, it is iso-osmotic. However, when erythrocytes are placed into the solution, urea will diffuse into the erythrocytes, since diffusion occurs from a high to a low concentration. Hence, the solution will be come hypotonic, and water will permeate the erythrocyte.

Tears have the same osmotic pressure as blood which is equivalent to the osmotic pressure of 0.9% sodium chloride. For this reason, the term "isotonicity" can be used with reference to tears. Liquids that are hypotonic will cause the absorption of water into tissues, in an attempt to equalize the osmotic pressures on either side of the cell membrane. Liquids that are hypertonic cause loss of water from tissues to the surrounding fluid, again in an attempt to equalize the osmotic pressure. Both hypotonic and hypertonic solutions cause irritation and the ideal is, therefore, to have an isotonic solution for drug administration to the eyes.

Aqueous solutions for eye drops that contain low concentrations of the drug are typically hypotonic and can be made isotonic by the addition of certain substances, such as sodium chloride and boric acid. Eye drops containing high concentrations of drugs may be hypertonic. Drops containing moderately high concentrations of drugs, or other substances, may also be hypertonic, especially if the solutes ionize into multiple particles. This is because the osmotic pressure depends on the number of particles in solution, as mentioned. Such solutions would have to be used in the hypertonic state. This causes some eye irritation which becomes reduced as the eye drops are diluted with tears. The irritation caused by hypertonic solutions is less than that caused by hypotonic solutions. The hypertonic solution causes cells to lose water to the instilled solution in an effort to equalize the osmotic pressures. This causes the cells to shrink which is not a major problem. On the other hand, hypotonic solutions cause the inflow of water into cells which causes swelling that can be painful. In applications other than eye drops, hypotonic solutions can even cause certain cells to burst, for example, erythrocytes.

Emulsions

The formulation of emulsions is discussed in more detail in Chapter 7, Emulsions. As described in that chapter, emulsions

may be oil in water (O/W) or water in oil (W/O). Emulsions have also been used as eye drops where O/W emulsions are preferred because of better ocular tolerance. In W/O emulsions, oil is in the external phase and may cause more irritation during use. Apart from the better tolerance of O/W emulsions, the drug, in such formulations, is contained in the internal (oily) phase and leaves this phase relatively slowly. It then permeates the ocular tissues to provide steady uptake. Compared to a solution of the drug, longer drug activity may be expected from an emulsion. However, if the emulsion rapidly drains out of the eye conjunctival pocket, through the nasolacrimal system, there will be insufficient time for the described mechanism to have an effect. On the other hand, the mere formation of an emulsion (the physical combination of two immiscible phases by the use of an emulgent) increases the viscosity of the resultant preparation to some extent. The enhanced viscosity decreases the flow of the emulsion through the nasolacrimal duct. In addition, the nature of emulsions makes them mucoadhesive to some extent.

Restasis and Refresh Endura are two commercial emulsions that are used for eye lubrication (tear replacement). Restasis contains cyclosporine (0.05%) for its anti-inflammatory effects. While no drug is included in Refresh Endura, it does contain castor oil as the oil phase of the emulsion. This oil consists mainly of a triglyceride, a major component of which is ricinoleic acid, a polar fatty acid. The emulsifying agent is polysorbate 80, and carbomer 1342 serves as the emulsion stabilizer. The demulcent, or ocular lubricant, effect is due to the polysorbate 80 as well as to the added glycerin. The triglyceride is compatible with the oily component of tears (see Figure 23-3 for the components of the tear film). Since carbomer is incompatible with ions, upon administration, the ions in tears disrupt carbomer's emulsifying ability. This results in the breaking of the emulsion. Next, the separated oil merges with the oily layer of tears. This enhances the anti-evaporative effect of the oily layer of tears. It counteracts the feeling of dryness and keeps the eyes moist and comfortable. Soothe XP, manufactured by Bausch and Lomb, contains 1% light mineral oil and 4.5% mineral oil, for a similar function.

Suspensions

The properties of suspensions and the general methods of formulating them were described in Chapter 6, Pharmaceutical Suspensions. Ophthalmic suspensions have the added requirement of a fine particle size of the suspended matter to limit irritation. The USP requires that particles for ophthalmic suspensions must be micronized. The USP further states that any ophthalmic suspension, in which a cake or aggregation is observed, must not be dispensed.

After administration of an ophthalmic suspension to the conjunctival pocket, the suspended particles will be retained in this location and contact time with the ocular tissues is improved. Within the acceptable particle size range, smaller particles dissolve more rapidly (making the medication more rapidly available for absorption) while larger particles result in slower drug release, thereby extending the duration of action of the medication to some extent.

There are several suspensions marketed to treat ocular bacterial infections. Tobradex suspension is a combination of tobramycin (0.3%) and dexamethasone (0.1%). The latter relieves inflammation, while the former drug is an antibiotic. Neomycin and polymyxin B sulfate and hydrocortisone ophthalmic suspension, USP contains, in 1 mL, neomycin sulfate equivalent to 3.5 mg neomycin base, 10,000 units polymyxin B and 10 mg of hydrocortisone. The first two ingredients are antimicrobial while the latter is anti-inflammatory. Fluorometholone ophthalmic suspension, USP contains fluorometholone 0.1%, a corticosteroid used for its anti-inflammatory effect. Polysorbate 80 and PVA serve as the viscosity-enhancing agents which assist in keeping the particles in suspension.

A suspension formulation for dry eyes is rebamipide,[1] available as a 1% or a 2% suspension. It is an amino acid derivative of a quinolinone, first developed to treat gastric ulcers. The active increases production of a mucin-like substance which helps to heal corneal and conjunctival injuries. It effectively treats tear deficiency, and gives a feeling of comfort and relief to dry eyes. It can restore the microstructure responsible for tear stability. The aqueous layer of the tear structure contains soluble mucin, as can be seen in Figure 23-3. This product is available in Japan and other Asian countries. In a four-week study to determine the effectiveness of this suspension, it was found that there was no significant difference in tear production from baseline, but the tear film breakup time showed a significant increase, relative to placebo.

Ointments

Ointments are more fully described in Chapter 22, Dermal and Transdermal Drug Delivery. Ophthalmic ointments are intended for topical drug delivery to the eye. According to the USP, the main base for ophthalmic drugs is petrolatum which is hydrophobic. When a hydrophilic base is needed, some absorption bases and water-soluble bases may be used. These hydrophilic bases allow for better dispersion of water-soluble drugs. However, they should be non-irritating to the eyes. The base should melt at ocular temperature, 34° C. The choice of base is largely guided by compatibility with ocular tissues. Several bases, including some that are used in current ocular ointments, display some degree of ocular irritation. The ointment base can improve the bioavailability, especially of hydrophobic drugs, since a larger concentration may be contained in a fixed volume of ointment base, as compared to an equal volume of aqueous drops. The ointment is also not rapidly drained from the conjunctival pocket, as happens with drops. The ointment base may, in addition, provide controlled release of the drug to the ocular tissues, thus promoting prolonged absorption. The major problem with ocular ointments, apart from irritation potential, is the fact that after application they blur the patient's vision. For this reason, they are usually used at bedtime, in which case the ointment may be more acceptable.

The ingredients must be individually sterilized, and the ointment is then manufactured under aseptic conditions. The drug is added to the ointment base either as a solution or as a micronized powder. The finished ointment must be free from large particles which would irritate the sensitive ocular tissues. Utilizing the process of levigation during small-scale compounding reduces the tendency for lumps to remain. Since a product that is sterile at manufacture may become contaminated with repeated opening and closing of the container, the

product should contain preservative(s). As mentioned under eye drops, preservatives are irritant and are unsuitable to use post-surgically. For such an application, single-use sterile ophthalmic ointments are provided in suitable dispensers. For all ophthalmic ointments, attention must be paid to packaging. In particular, the immediate container must be sealed in a tamper-evident manner (see Chapter 14, Packaging).

Vancomycin HCl is a glycopeptide antibiotic with excellent activity against aerobic and anaerobic gram-positive bacteria, especially methicillin-resistant *Staphylococcus aureus*. On a theoretical basis, good permeability of vancomycin HCl into the eye cannot be expected. However, in the diseased eye, there appears to be good absorption. This is hypothesized to be due to the fact that a compromised ocular barrier, due to the disease condition, promotes absorption.

Topical Drug Delivery Devices

Two major areas of interest for topical drug delivery devices are drugs delivered to the cornea, since corneal diseases have a major impact on visual health, and drugs delivered to the anterior segment. The latter are mainly for the treatment of glaucoma, which is characterized by high intraocular pressure. Conventional dosage forms, which may be considered for each of these conditions, are inadequate since each application has a short duration of action. Repeat administrations are inconvenient, leading to poor compliance and, as a result, poor therapeutic outcomes.

Ocular inserts are devices that are placed either in the upper or lower conjunctival pocket, in either fornix, or on the cornea itself. They contain drugs for controlled release over an extended period, obviating the need for repeated instillation of eye drops. For patient acceptance, these devices should be easy to insert, discrete, and comfortable to wear. The devices may be soluble ophthalmic drug inserts (SODIs) or insoluble inserts. The latter require removal after a certain time in use whereas the former may be allowed to dissolve or erode in place. Ocusert®, made by the Alza Corporation, was one of the first successful products of this type in the modern era. The inserts contained pilocarpine for long-term relief of glaucoma. This product has been discontinued probably because it was not patient convenient. Patients expressed difficulty with placement of the inserts, and stated that the inserts would fold before they could be placed on the eye. The fact that the inserts were thin made unintentional folding easier during handling. Some reports mentioned that the inserts would come off at night and get "lost." It should be noted that the concept of a drug-loaded "device" had been tried more than 100 years ago. One such attempt utilized paper, previously soaked in the drug, for application to the eyes. The extent of success of such devices is unknown but patient convenience was probably minimal, and possibly a reason for discontinuation of the therapy.

Ocufit SR®, made by Escalon Medical Corporation, is a silicone elastomer device that is rod shaped. It is placed in the lower conjunctival fornix. These devices are well tolerated and inadvertent removal of the device appears to be a far less frequent occurrence than is the case with oval or flat inserts. The improved tolerance may be due to the soft and pliable nature of the silicone elastomer. In research studies with timolol maleate-loaded devices, drug release was steady for more than 30 days, after an initial burst release.

The Minidisc Ocular Therapeutic System (OTS) is manufactured by Bausch & Lomb (UK) as polymer disks, smaller than contact lenses. They reside on the sclera in the upper or lower fornix where they deliver gentamicin or sulfisoxazole over 3 to 14 days depending on the system utilized. The company produces non-erodible systems that are either hydrophobic or hydrophilic. Their erodible devices are made of hydroxypropyl cellulose (HPC), a water-soluble polymer. Most patients found the inserts comfortable to use. IOLTech, in Germany, manufactures Mydriasert® which are insoluble devices for the delivery of phenylephrine (an α-1 agonist) and tropicamide (anticholinergic) for sustained mydriasis during surgery or during examinations of the interior surface of the eye. The combination of drugs, affecting two systems, is useful for those patients in whom monotherapy does not enlarge the pupil sufficiently.

The idea of using regular hydrogel contact lenses as drug-delivery devices has been suggested. However, conventional lenses are limited by the amount of drug that may be loaded, as well as by the fact that their drug release rate was shown to be unreliable. An initial burst was followed by a rapid decline in the release rate over a short period. For this reason, research is ongoing to develop special lens materials that can be adequately loaded with the drug to provide a controlled rate of drug release over an extended time. In addition, the lens is intended to function as an optical lens. Such products are likely to be marketed in the next few years. One of the concerns for such a system is that the drug should not make the lens opaque and so disturb the vision of the patient.

Recap Questions

1. Distinguish between the placement of a drug delivery device in the fornix, and the conjunctival pocket, of the eye.
2. What is the Draize test?
3. What is the preferred method of sterilization for eye drops?
4. Mention one reason why benzalkonium chloride is commonly used as a preservative for eye drops.
5. What is meant by the term "sol-gel transformation"?
6. What is the function of viscosity enhancement in eye drops?
7. Why do some tear replacement formulations contain oil?
8. Alkaloids (weak bases) are commonly formulated as .... salts in eye drop formulations. (Fill in the blank.)
9. What is the most common base for eye ointments, as recommended by the USP?
10. Why do drug delivery companies try to develop topical drug delivery devices?

INVASIVE DRUG ADMINISTRATION

Posterior segment eye diseases are serious conditions, leading to impaired vision and even blindness. Orally administered drugs do not reach the posterior segment due to the blood-retinal barrier. In addition, it is difficult, if not impossible, to administer drugs to the posterior segment via the topical route, using conventional formulations. This is due to the successive barriers to permeation, as previously described. As drug product developers considered these factors, they could not escape the reality that invasive drug administration is necessary to treat serious diseases of the posterior segment.

The earliest form of invasive drug administration was the intraocular injection, which continues to be used in certain instances. Medications may be injected into the eye, especially the posterior segment, for treatment of serious diseases. Since an injection through the sclera is inherently risky, it is limited to treatment of serious diseases only. The path of entry into the vitreous is depicted in Figure 23-1. The injection needle, obviously, must avoid the retina. Even when performed correctly, repeated injections may be harmful, though necessary. One approach to avoid repeated injections is the use of long-acting injectable materials, for example, small sustained-release spheres. An alternate approach is to surgically implant a small device into the vitreous. The latter may provide drug therapy for many months or even years.

Intravitreal Injections

The most common way to effectively administer drugs into the posterior segment is by means of an injection into the vitreous humor. This places a high drug concentration where it is needed, while avoiding the systemic circulation. However, repeated injections are needed to treat many ophthalmic conditions and this may cause undesirable effects within the eye. These effects include cataract formation, ocular hypertension, hemorrhage, and retinal detachment. Considering the seriousness of these side effects, the question arises as to whether such injections have value. Since many of the diseases treated by intravitreal injections cause blindness if untreated, the risks are considered acceptable.

Eylea (aflibercept) is a recombinant fusion protein for intravitreal injection. It acts as an anti-VEGF agent in that it serves as a soluble decoy receptor for VEGF. Instead of VEGF acting on blood vessels, to cause growth, it reacts with this drug. There is a need for repeat injections, at approximately 1-month intervals. The treatment is expensive, especially with the repeat injections, and there are also side effects. However, patients with AMD that were progressing toward blindness have been successfully treated with this drug. It is available in several countries and is used for AMD, diabetic retinopathy, and related conditions.

Lucentis (ranibizumab) is an intravitreal injection indicated for wet AMD, macular edema following retinal vein occlusion (blockage, usually due to a blood clot), diabetic macular edema, and diabetic retinopathy. It is available in two strengths, 10 mg/mL and 6 mg/mL. Injections are generally given once per month into the eye but the dosage regimen may vary somewhat with each condition and with recommended treatment options. The drug is available in a prefilled syringe and also in a single-dose vial. In the case of the latter, the dose must be drawn up into the syringe using a filter needle, which is then removed and another needle attached for injection. The needle used for drawing up the liquid cannot be used for injection, and the size of each needle is different. In the case of the prefilled syringe, the needle cover has to be simply snapped off before the syringe-needle assembly is ready for injection (after removal of the syringe from the single unit pack). All of these procedures, for both the prefilled syringe and the vial, must be performed aseptically. It appears much more convenient to simply use the prefilled syringe.

Another drug used for similar conditions is Avastin. It is not approved for intraocular injection, but is used off-label for this purpose and is found to be effective. The injection has to be compounded and the sterility of the final product cannot be overemphasized, considering the fact that it is to be injected into the vitreous. This off-label medication is considerably cheaper than Lucentis and Eylea, which are both specially formulated and manufactured for intravitreal injection.

Macugen (pegaptanib sodium) is a sterile aqueous solution for intravitreous injection that is supplied in single-dose prefilled syringes. It is a VEGF antagonist used in the treatment of wet (neovascular) AMD. For maintenance therapy, the injection should be repeated every 6 weeks.

Ocular Implants

Ocular implants deliver high doses of the drug to the interior of the eye without the need for repeated injections. While the procedure to insert implants is invasive, it is done once for several months, or even years, of therapy. Implants may be soluble and not require removal after drug depletion, or insoluble and require removal. The latter frequently provide near-zero order release which is advantageous (see Chapter 17, Introduction to Bioavailability) and have the potential for a longer duration of action than is the case with soluble polymers. An example of a soluble polymer is PVA, while polyvinyl acetate (PVAC) and ethylene vinyl acetate (EVA) are insoluble and nonbiodegradable. Vitrasert and Retisert are devices that utilize insoluble polymers.

Vitrasert provides sustained delivery of ganciclovir, a drug used to treat cytomegalovirus (CMG) infections of the eye. The virus replicates and infects new cells, thus spreading this opportunistic infection associated with AIDS. The drug prevents both the replication of the virus and the infection of new cells, but it does not eliminate the virus from infected cells. The device is composed of a small ganciclovir tablet supplied in a holder. Its appearance is very similar to the Retisert device, described below and shown in Figure 23-6. The tablet is 2.5 mm in diameter and 1 mm thick and contains 4.5 mg of the drug. The tablet is coated with PVA and EVA.

Vitrasert was discontinued in 2016 in the USA, and in 2002 in Europe. The reason provided, in the latter case, was a "lack of demand," possibly reflecting the reduction in the number of CMG infections as AIDS cases decreased. Nevertheless, this product, as the first approved intravitreal insert, provides an interesting example of what may be achieved with targeted drug delivery. One end of a suture was attached to the holder and the device was inserted into the eye surgically. The other end

of the suture was sewn onto the (exterior) sclera after closing the incision. The drug was slowly released over a period of at least three months. The maintenance dose of oral ganciclovir, to treat this condition, is 1000 mg three times a day, which is a very high dose of a drug that has serious side effects. These include birth defects in pregnant women and, in men, reduction in sperm count and eventual elimination of sperm production. Intravitreous injection reduced this high dosing but the injections had to be repeated for maintenance therapy. In contrast to this, the intravitreous insert provided therapy for 3 months (with 4.5 mg of drug). The reduced dose that was achieved using this device represents significant progress in targeted drug delivery.

Retisert is an insert that delivers fluocinolone acetonide (Figure 23-6) used for the treatment of posterior uveitis. If untreated, this condition can result in blindness. The device releases therapeutic amounts of the drug for up to 30 months. The implant controls inflammation, reduces uveitis recurrences, and improves vision acuity. The side effects are the development of cataracts, after long-term use, and elevated intraocular pressure. Vitrasert and Retisert are nondegradable and, for this reason, require surgical removal. This is done when a new device is required to be implanted. Both devices were developed by pSiveda Corporation, using their Durasert technology, and both were licensed to Bausch and Lomb.

Iluvien was also developed by pSivida and is licensed to Alimera Sciences. It is an erodible, micro-insert that is injected into the vitreous humor with a thin gauge needle. The product releases fluocinolone acetonide for up to 3 years with a single injection. It is FDA-approved and also marketed in Europe for the treatment of diabetic macular edema in patients who had

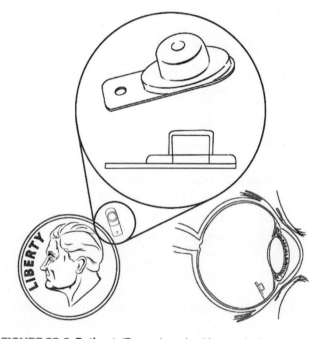

FIGURE 23-6 Retisert. (Reproduced, with permission, from García-Estrada P, García-Bon MA, López-Naranjo EJ, Basaldúa-Pérez DN, Santos A, Navarro-Partida J. Polymeric implants for the treatment of intraocular eye diseases: trends in biodegradable and non-biodegradable materials. *Pharmaceutics.* 2021;13(5):701. https://doi.org/10.3390/pharmaceutics13050701.)

previously been treated with corticosteroid therapy and who did not display an increase in intraocular pressure. Patients who did not display this side effect of the corticosteroid therapy were considered suitable candidates for this intra-ocular treatment.

Medidur, a device, developed by the same company, is also implantable and delivers fluocinolone acetonide for up to 36 months. The device consists of a narrow, hollow polyimide tube loaded with the drug. PVA-based end caps seal the tube on either end and provide rate-controlled drug delivery. It is interesting that this tiny tube (3.5 mm long × 0.37 mm in diameter) is inserted into the eye using a 25 gauge needle. The insertion is carried out under local anesthesia in the ophthalmologist's office. After removal of the needle, there is a small wound which is self-healing due to the narrow gauge of the needle. The device delivers 0.18 mg of fluocinolone acetonide over 3 years, an extremely low amount of drug compared to systemic therapy, which has also been used for the treatment of posterior segment uveitis, the indication for this device. The device, at the time of writing, was undergoing phase 3 testing in multiple centers in the USA and Europe. Iluvien and Medidur are developed by the same company, pSivida, and appear to have similar characteristics although they are intended for different applications.

Biodegradable devices have the enormous advantage that they do not have to be removed from the eye by surgical intervention and they are, therefore, of great interest. Generally, they provide a shorter duration of action which,

in some instances, is acceptable. One such example is drug therapy to counter inflammation due to surgical procedures. For this indication, there is no additional surgical procedure, as the device is inserted toward the end of the surgery. Surodex (Oculex Pharmaceuticals, acquired by Allergan) is a poly (lactic-glycolic acid) micro-device that is inserted into the anterior, or the posterior, segment at the time of cataract surgery. It delivers dexamethasone for up to 10 days and is used to treat intraocular inflammation due to the cataract surgery. It was shown that the degree of postoperative inflammation was less in patients treated with this device than in patients treated with dexamethasone eye drops. The product is marketed in China, Singapore, and other Asian countries. The Ozurdex device, marketed by Allergan Inc. in the USA, is also a biodegradable polymer device that is loaded with the drug dexamethasone (0.7 mg). It is used for the treatment of macula edema resulting from retinal vein occlusion, noninfectious posterior segment uveitis, and diabetic macular edema. Drug release is over a 4-month period.

Drug Delivery via the Suprachoroidal Space

In recent years, a few publications suggested that a potential space for small volume injections existed between the sclera and the choroid layers (Figure 23-7) and that this route could be used for delivery of drugs to the posterior eye structures. (This space is utilized physiologically for water flow to maintain intra-ocular eye pressure.) The injected solution will distribute within this suprachoroidal space (SCS) circumferentially

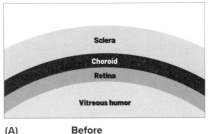 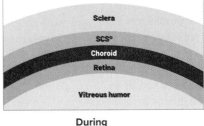 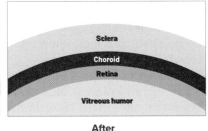

(A)   Before   During   After

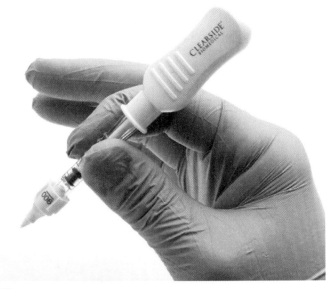

(B)

FIGURE 23-7 A. Drug delivery to the posterior structures of the eye via the suprachoroidal space **B.** Microinjector fitted with a 900 μm needle. (Part B reproduced with permission, from Kansara VS, Hancock SE, Muya LW, Ciulla TA. Suprachoroidal delivery enables targeting, localization and durability of small molecule suspensions. *J Control Release.* 2022;349:1045-1051.

and posteriorly and then diffuse into eye structures. Compared to intravitreal injections and inserts, this route provides a less invasive mechanism to supply drugs to posterior eye structures for serious eye conditions.

XIPERE, which is offered by Bausch + Lomb in the United States, contains 40 mg/mL of triamcinolone acetonide for SCS administration to treat macular edema associated with uveitis. It provides a high bioavailability to the choroid and retina with compartmentalization away from non-target tissues. The product is in the form of a suspension which is injected with a proprietary microinjector that utilizes a 30-gauge needle with a length of either 900 μm or 1100 μm, with differing lengths to accommodate for variation in patient ocular anatomy. When the needle tip is in the SCS, there is less resistance to the flow of fluid from the syringe, indicating to the clinician that they may slowly administer the injection. At the time of this writing, Xipere is the only therapy approved for suprachoroidal use although others are in development.

FUTURE DEVELOPMENTS

Conventional formulations (eye drops, gels, suspensions, and ointments) are adequate to treat topical conditions such as dry eyes, redness (vasodilation), and conjunctival allergies and infections. There are also disease conditions that affect the anterior segment of the eye for which drug penetration may not be ideal from conventional dosage forms. Either the drug penetration is too little to provide the desired drug concentrations within the anterior segment or the administration has to be repeated at very frequent intervals, leading to noncompliance. As previously mentioned, drug penetration to the posterior segment is even slower, or nonexistent. For these reasons, invasive drug delivery systems were developed.

Intravitreal injections or surgically inserted devices provided enormously improved therapy. The dosage was decreased by a large amount and the method of administration greatly helped to decrease systemic exposure. However, injections have side effects such as increased intraocular pressure, and surgical procedures are not without risk; the simple fact that they are invasive makes these treatments less desirable. For this reason, pharmaceutical scientists have re-visited the role of so-called conventional medication, in the light of recent pharmaceutical technology advancements. The aim is to improve the penetration of medications and to increase the dosing interval, while using conventional dosage forms that do not require invasive methods of administration. This may be achieved, in some instances, by using nanotechnology-based medicines in conventional dosage forms. While much of this development is in the research phase at present, and topics of research interest are generally not covered in student textbooks, it may be valuable to mention some of this research briefly, since such products may reach the marketplace in the near future.

Nanomicelles are micellar components made with amphiphilic molecules; they have diameters which allow them to be placed in the nanoparticle size range. All nanotechnology structures mentioned in this section are described in more detail in Chapter 13, Nanotechnology. A great deal of interest has been shown by pharmaceutical scientists in nano-micellar formulations which may be developed as aqueous formulations. They are relatively easy to prepare, show high drug encapsulation capability, and can penetrate ocular tissues to a much greater extent than conventional formulations. Several research studies are underway as "proof of concept" studies.

Drug-loaded nanoparticles, made from natural or synthetic polymers, have also been utilized for ocular drug delivery. The suspensions made from these particles benefited from viscosity enhancement or bioadhesion to reduce drainage from the conjunctival pocket.

Liposomes are lipid vehicles made with phospholipid bilayers and the sizes of some liposomes, especially small unilamellar vesicles (SUV), fall into nano-dimensions. They have walls consisting of one double layer of phospholipids. Hydrophilic drugs may be encapsulated in the aqueous core of the liposome, whereas polar drugs may be trapped between two polar heads of the phospholipid layers, while nonpolar drug molecules may insert themselves between the lipid tails of the phospholipid residues. Liposomes are attractive because the phospholipid layers resemble the constituents of the cell membrane and may be easily taken up by cells, while both polar and nonpolar drugs may be trapped within the liposome, as mentioned. They have been extensively researched for both anterior and posterior segment ocular delivery.

The above novel technologies are the subject of research to enable conventional dosage forms, which have simple modes of administration, to be used for drug delivery to the interior of the eye. From historical drops and suspensions (which were ineffective) to intraocular injections and implanted devices (which are effective but invasive) and back to drops and suspensions (now with novel, nanotechnology-based active ingredients), pharmaceutical development has come full circle.

Recap Questions

1. Why is it necessary to administer drugs invasively to the eye?

2. What are the major concerns with intravitreous injections?

3. What is the advantage of drug-eluting devices, inserted into the eye, over intravitreous injections?

4. What is the probable reason for the discontinuation of Vitrasert (ganciclovir)?

5. What is the advantage of dissolving or eroding devices?

6. Mrs. Drake is scheduled for a visit to her ophthalmologist to have a drug-eluting device inserted into her eye. She is concerned about the invasiveness of the procedure and wants to know if you could compound the medication into eye drops so that she can avoid the procedure. How would you respond to Mrs. Drake?

SUMMARY POINTS

- Eye drops are the most commonly used dosage form for ocular drug delivery. They surpass ointments, suspensions, and emulsions in popularity. The volume of tears in the eye at any time is very small and the volume of eye drops that may be held in the conjunctival pocket is also very small. There is a constant draining of tears and replenishing with fresh liquid. Both these factors make drug delivery difficult.

- Dry eye is a common problem that is treated with ocular lubricant(s). Viscosity-enhanced formulations remain in the eye for a longer time than non-enhanced formulations. Emulsions work effectively because the oil phase contributes to the oily layer of the tear film.

- Conventional dosage forms are effective for treating topical conditions and there may be some penetration to the anterior segment; penetration to the posterior segment is difficult.

- Many technological advancements have been made to improve drug delivery to the anterior segment so that drug delivery systems are more efficacious and more convenient to use. Devices placed onto the cornea, into one of the conjunctival pockets, or into the upper or lower fornix, provide long-term therapy.

- Many serious eye conditions affect the posterior segment and lead to seriously impaired vision and, if ineffectively treated, to blindness. These include macular degeneration and diabetic retinopathy. Hence serious efforts have been made to develop drug delivery to the posterior segment of the eye. Vitreous injections offer long-term therapy but repeated injections result in many side effects. Implants offer significantly longer-term therapy than vitreous injections.

- Nanotechnology advances may, in the future, provide topical preparations, which permeate into the posterior segment, thus providing therapy to this region in a noninvasive form having the presentation of conventional ocular dosage forms. The familiarity with the dosage forms may improve compliance.

What do you think?

1. What is meant by "structure of the tear film"?
2. Explain why drug diffusion through the tear film is different from diffusion through a film of water.
3. Ointments provide several hours of therapy. Why are all ocular medications not provided in ointment form?
4. Assume that all the ingredients of an eye drop formulation are stable for autoclaving. What are the advantages of autoclaving the final formulation in comparison to the sterilization method recommended in the USP?
5. If a weak base, such as an alkaloid, is absorbed as the free base, that is, in non-ionized form, why do manufacturers of eye drops first convert the base to an acid salt? What advantage is gained from such a conversion?
6. "The tear film and the cornea together provide a formidable barrier to the penetration of noxious chemicals into the eye." Do you agree or disagree with this statement? Give reasons for your answer.
7. Light must pass through the pupil of the eye to reach the retina for vision to occur. How is it possible to insert a device into the vitreous without it obstructing vision?
8. How is it theoretically possible to use conventional dosage forms with nanotechnology to achieve drug penetration to the posterior segment?
9. An emulsion may be used for tear replacement therapy in which the emulsion is intended to break within the eye. Why would the developer formulate an emulsion if it is going to break?
10. If nanotechnology-based eye drops have been commercialized when you are a practicing pharmacist and your patient thinks that they are conventional eye drops, would you correct their impression or not? What are the advantages and disadvantages of each position?

REFERENCE

1. Kashima T, Itakura H, Akiyama H, Kishi S. Rebamipide ophthalmic suspension for the treatment of dry eye syndrome: a critical appraisal. *Clin Ophthalmol (Auckland, NZ)*. 2014;8:1003-1010. doi:10.2147/OPTH.S40798.

BIBLIOGRAPHY

https://www.allergan.com/assets/pdf/ozurdex_pi.pdf. Accessed September 30, 2017.

https://www.gene.com/download/pdf/lucentis_prescribing.pdf. Accessed October 3, 2017.

Morrison PWJ, Khutoryanskiy VV. Advances in ophthalmic drug delivery. *Ther Deliv*. 2014;5(12):1297.

Patel A, Cholkar K, Agrahari V, Mitra AK. Ocular drug delivery systems: an overview. *World J Pharmacol*. 2013;2(2):47-64. doi:10.5497/wjp.v2.i2.47.

Rectal and Vaginal Drug Delivery

24

PREVIEW

- Why is rectal and vaginal drug delivery important?
- What are the common dosage forms used for rectal and vaginal delivery?
- The formulation of suppositories and the choice of excipients to confer specific properties are often related to the drug
- The anatomy of the rectum and the vagina; how their structures influence drug delivery
- Specialized applications of rectal and vaginal drug delivery

INTRODUCTION

The rectum and the vagina are major body cavities for which similar dosage forms may be used for the treatment of local pathological conditions. More recently, these body cavities have been used as the means to deliver drugs systemically. In several instances, similar dosage forms are used for both cavities. For this reason, drug delivery to these cavities has been grouped together and presented in this combined chapter. However, the rectum and the vagina have very different functions. The rectum stores feces and is responsible for the process of defecation, while the function of the vagina is mostly related to reproduction. Consequently, there are also distinct treatments needed for each body cavity, or to treat adjoining organs. For example, the vagina is used to deliver drugs to the uterus and the rectum for drug delivery to the colon. Orally administered, extended-release drug delivery to the colon is dealt with in Chapter 11, Modified Release Oral Dosage Forms.

The major dosage forms that are common to both cavities are ointments, creams, gels, suppositories, liquid formulations, and aerosol delivery systems. An example of the latter is the aerosol foam. The suppository is by far the most common rectal dosage form, and it is also a frequently used dosage form for vaginal administration. The USP recently stated that the term "vaginal inserts" are preferred for all solid dosage forms inserted vaginally (includes suppositories, tablets, and capsules) to reduce inappropriate rectal insertion. However, this term is not yet widely used and "suppositories" will be the term used in this chapter when intended for vaginal insertion (as well as for rectal insertion). Suppositories for vaginal use are called pessaries in the British Pharmacopoeia. Both of the above alternate terms are mentioned simply to inform the reader. Suppositories have been used for a long time, in the modern era, for the treatment of a variety of local ailments. There is some evidence that suppositories may have been used for thousands of years. In recent times, suppositories have been administered, not only for local problems in the rectum and the vagina but also for the systemic delivery of drugs. There are several reasons why these routes of administration may be more beneficial than oral administration with respect to certain clinical situations, or specific drugs.

Rectal suppositories have been used for extended-duration therapy lasting many hours. The vagina, in contrast to the rectum, has been used for ultra-long-term drug delivery. The fact that vaginal drug delivery may be used in this manner is a major distinction between the two routes. Mainly for contraception, devices such as vaginal rings can deliver drugs for 3 weeks. In addition, cervical caps have been used for the treatment, or prevention, of viral infections for extended periods.

The major dosage forms that are commonly used for drug delivery to both cavities will first be discussed before the anatomy of each cavity and its drug delivery characteristics are described.

COMMON RECTAL AND VAGINAL FORMULATIONS

Suppositories are by far the most common rectal formulation. Other formulations, including ointments, gels, creams, liquids, and foams, are also used. While it is theoretically possible for capsules and tablets to be inserted both into the vagina and the rectum, these dosage forms have only been used vaginally and these will be discussed as specialized dosage forms for vaginal use. Foams are useful for their ease of application, with an applicator tip being inserted into the respective body cavity for this purpose. The penetration power of the foam is an advantage since it spreads the contained medication into the cavity without additional effort. Foams spread upwards into the rectum and even into the sigmoid colon as the foam expands. A similar penetration occurs in the vagina. Creams, ointments, and gels have been formulated for either vaginal or rectal delivery.

Suppositories

Suppositories may take the form of elongated cylinders with rounded heads (Figure 24-1). More commonly, they are torpedo-shaped, being wider close to the pointed front end (which is inserted first) and narrower at the opposite end. The shape helps to retain the suppository after insertion. The base materials used to formulate a suppository must not irritate the sensitive rectal and vaginal tissues. The suppository must release the drug at an appropriate rate, and must not interact with a wide range of drugs, both acidic and basic, which may be incorporated into suppositories. Many of the suppository bases are fatty and melt at a low temperature, releasing the drug as they melt. Another large group of bases are the water-soluble bases. For release of the drug, they depend on the dissolution of the base in the aqueous rectal or vaginal fluids. The choice of base depends on the nature of the drug, lipophilic drugs being formulated in water-soluble bases, whereas hydrophilic drugs are formulated in fatty bases. The reason for so doing is to ensure the favorable release of the drug from the base into the body cavity fluids, as described below.

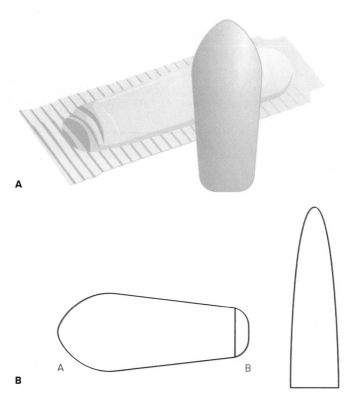

FIGURE 24-1 **Common suppository shapes: A.** torpedo and **B.** cylindrical.

Consider a lipophilic drug that is dissolved in the fatty base of a suppository. When this suppository is in contact with aqueous fluids, after administration, the dissolved drug substance experiences competing forces of attraction. There is the attraction, first, to the base in which the drug is dissolved, and also an attraction to the water molecules in the rectal or vaginal fluids. If the attraction to the suppository base is strong, drug dissolution will be slower. Even if the drug is not dissolved but suspended in the base, the lipophilic drug will still experience an attraction, albeit less, for the lipophilic base. For this reason, lipophilic drugs are formulated into hydrophilic bases, resulting in a low attraction for the base. The resulting product is likely to be a suspension since it is unlikely that a hydrophobic drug will dissolve in a hydrophilic base. As the base dissolves, it releases the drug particles into the aqueous medium where they dissolve. The rate of dissolution, after release, depends on the drug's aqueous solubility, without significant interaction with the suppository base. For hydrophilic drugs, similar reasoning can be applied to conclude that they should be formulated in a hydrophobic base (less active to base interaction). It should be noted that the fatty bases chosen for suppositories melt at body temperature to release their drug content.

Fatty Suppository Bases

Some common fatty suppository bases are listed in Table 24-1. Cocoa butter was the traditional suppository base, despite certain problems which are described below. As new bases were developed, the use of cocoa butter declined. Cocoa butter (also known as theobroma oil) is a fat extracted from the cocoa bean. It melts at approximately 35°C, that is, slightly below body

TABLE 24-1	Some Fatty Suppository Bases		
VEHICLE	**COMPOSITION**	**MELTING T°'** **RANGE (°C)**	**COMMENTS**
Cocoa butter	Theobroma oil	33–35	Changes to crystalline form when heated to a high temperature.
Witepsol E 75	Mostly triglycerides (with smaller amounts of mono-, and di-) + cera alba (E 75 only)	38	Melts at higher than body T°, Range of E-bases (E 75, E 76, E 85)—higher number, higher melting T°. These bases are used when drug lowers the melting T° of the base.
Witepsol H 5	Mostly triglycerides with about 15% di-, and <1% monoglyceride	34–36	Range of H-bases: higher number indicates higher melting T°. Low hydroxyl values.
Witepsol W 25	Higher diglyceride content and hydroxyl value	33.5–35.5	Range of W-bases.
Witepsol S 51	Triglyceride with nonionic ethoxylated emulsifier added	30–32	Range of S-bases—"special' hard fats with emulsifier
Suppocire A	Mostly triglycerides, with di- and monoglycerides	34–38	Hydroxyl value = 20–30
Suppocire AGP	As for Suppocire A but includes glyceryl monostearate and PEG-75 stearate	34.5–37.5	Hydroxyl value = 40–50
Suppocire AM	Mostly triglycerides, with very low amounts of di- and monoglycerides	34–36	Hydroxyl value <10. Recommended for acidic drugs

'T° = temperature

temperature. For this reason, there should be no issue with the suppository, melting too slowly to release its drug load at an acceptable rate. Considering this melting point, a disadvantage of cocoa butter is the fact that the suppository cannot be handled for long without it softening and, possibly, melting. Softening can occur if the insertion of the suppository is fumbled, resulting in even greater difficulty to insert the deforming mass. This problem can occur, for example, when a parent is trying to administer the suppository to a crying child, who resists insertion.

A more serious problem with cocoa butter arises if it is overheated during the preparation of the suppositories. Cocoa butter must be heated to about 40°C to melt the base. This temperature is sufficient, since the β crystals of cocoa butter melt in the temperature range of 34° to 38°C. Upon cooling, the crystals re-form in a similar temperature range. This results in the suppository solidifying very quickly, once the heat source is removed. If the cocoa butter is heated significantly higher than this temperature (eg, to 50°C), or held at an elevated temperature for a longer period, it changes polymorphic form from β crystals to β′ crystals, upon solidification. The latter do not solidify until a temperature of 28°C is reached. Therefore, a longer period is required for the suppository to cool to the solidification point.

More seriously, when handling such a suppository, it melts again at 28°C. In practice, these suppositories become soft and very easily deformed during handling. Upon prolonged standing, the crystals gradually transform back to the β crystals, which

is the stable form. If the cocoa butter is heated to an even higher temperature, γ crystals form upon solidification which occurs at 18°C, that is, the suppositories will be semisolid at room temperature. To transform γ crystals to β crystals takes several weeks. When cocoa butter is correctly heated, some β crystals remain and act as seeds for further crystallization as the material is cooled. Even heating to the correct temperature, and holding at this temperature for a longer period, will result in the melting of all β crystals, with the resulting problems as noted above.

As described above, cocoa butter is difficult to work with and it is, therefore, not the fatty base of choice at the present time. It was popular in the past because there were not many bases to choose from and cocoa butter has a melting temperature that is conveniently close to body temperature. Obviously, this only applies when it is correctly processed. Many of the newer bases do not undergo polymorphic change upon heating and cooling and, for this reason, are much easier to work with. The formulator does not have to take extreme care to prevent overheating by even a few degrees. However, compounding pharmacists are still likely to come across formulations using cocoa butter as the base in the course of their practice.

Bases such as Suppocire® may be heated several degrees beyond the melting point with no detrimental effect. There are several Suppocire® grades, with different physical properties such as melting point and hardness. The formulator may blend different grades of this material to obtain the desired melting point. If other factors (such as the drug content) are constant, the lower the melting point, the shorter the melting time for the suppository and the faster the release of the drug after administration. The latter is required for dissolution of the drug in body cavity fluids. If dissolution occurs sooner, it often results in quicker absorption, but this is not always the case.

While many of the newer bases can be heated several degrees beyond the melting point, care should be taken not to excessively overheat any base to avoid "browning" of portions of the material. The latter results in suppositories of poor appearance, with small dark areas on a light-colored background. This appearance is the result of the small amount of browned material being mixed with the remaining light-colored molten mass. Most fatty suppository bases are off-white to light tan in color.

Most of the fatty suppository bases are synthetic fats derived from glycerol using an esterification reaction. The mono-, di-, or triglyceride is formed by linking one, two, or three fatty acids, respectively, to glycerol. This is illustrated in Figure 24-2 which shows the formation of glyceryl stearates. The product is a mixture of the mono-, di-, and triglycerides, with longer reaction times favoring a larger proportion of the latter. The degree to which triglycerides are formed, relative to the di- or monoglyceride, cannot be exactly controlled. The relative proportion of each in any suppository base is approximate, as usually stated in the product literature. The reason for the lack of precise control is the fact that time is not an exact mechanism to control the reaction.

Since unreacted glycerol is washed away after the reaction, the free –OH groups present in the product arise from the di- and monoglycerides. The total number of free –OH groups in the suppository base is a measure of its chemical reactivity, if other parameters are held constant. "Free" –OH groups mean that they have not participated in the esterification reaction and are hence free, or available, to react with other molecules. In some instances, a surfactant is added to the suppository base to make it more hydrophilic or to emulsify the fatty base in the presence of water. The surfactant may contain –OH groups and such groups must also be taken into account when estimating the extent of free –OH groups. The significance of the number of free –OH groups, from a pharmaceutics perspective, is that it is an indication of the reactivity of the base. Will the base react with the drug, for example? Low reactivity is, obviously, preferred but some hydroxyl groups are needed for the reason mentioned below.

The presence of –OH groups on some glyceride molecules leads to a plasticizer effect. The base becomes more plastic with the result that the formed suppositories (after cooling) are less brittle. Generally, suppositories should not be rapidly cooled (such as, by placing the molds on ice) because rapid cooling can cause brittleness in the suppositories, resulting in the formation of cracks. Cracking occurs because of different cooling and solidification rates in different parts of the suppository after the pouring of the molten mass into the suppository molds. The presence of increased numbers of –OH groups on the glycerides lessens the tendency to crack.

On the other hand, post-hardening may increase with larger numbers of –OH groups. This phenomenon occurs when a prepared suppository, of a specific hardness, becomes increasingly harder during storage. In addition, the presence of –OH groups may lead to better wetting and dissolution of the base. Consequently, faster dissolution of a poorly soluble drug, contained in the suppository, also occurs. Probably the most

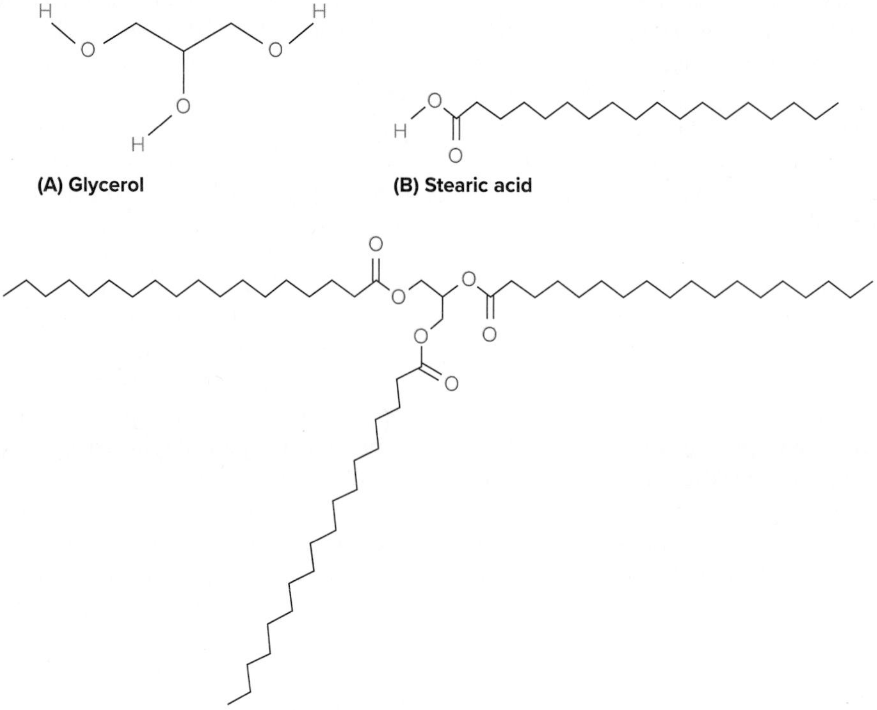

FIGURE 24-2 Chemical structures of A. Glycerol; **B**. stearic acid; and **C**. combination of the two components to form glyceryl tristearate. Note that each –OH group of glycerol has participated in an esterification reaction with one molecule of stearic acid to form the third structure; glyceryl mono stearate and glyceryl distearate are also possible.

significant effect of an increased number of –OH groups is the potential for interacting with drugs, for example, those containing carboxyl groups. The result of such an interaction is the formation of an ester linking the drug to the polymer chain of the base. This covalently bonded structure is difficult to absorb since it is large. Typically, esterases in biological media cleave the ester bond with the result that the drug is released from its binding to the polymer. The net result of ester formation is, then, the slower availability of the drug for absorption and not a lower amount absorbed. The influence of –OH groups on the properties of the base is summarized in Mind Map 24-1.

Water-Soluble Suppository Bases

In certain instances, it is preferable to use a water-soluble base. This includes the situation where the drug to be incorporated is poorly soluble. Since the base dissolves, and usually does so fairly rapidly, the drug is quickly available to the fluids for dissolution, and subsequent absorption from the drug solution. The water-soluble base that has the longest history of use is the glycero-gelatin base which, as the name implies, contains glycerin and gelatin. Glycerin is included to make the suppository more flexible and these suppositories also contain water. The concentration of gelatin may be varied to some degree: if more gelatin is included, the suppositories become firmer whereas, with less gelatin, softer suppositories result. A firmer suppository may be required in hotter climates. Interestingly, the British pharmacopeia gives a formula with 14% gelatin, whereas 20% gelatin is used in the United States pharmacopeia.

Gelatin suppositories swell in the presence of water. Packaging should reduce water ingress, for this reason, as well as the fact that the suppositories soften upon imbibing water. After the administration of a glycero-gelatin suppository, swelling will occur and the pressure that is exerted against the rectal wall gives the patient the urge to defecate. This urge may occur, to some extent, with any suppository formulation. The urge is increased with suppositories, such as glycerol-gelatin suppositories, that swell. The formula for the typical suppository of this type is given in Table 24-2 while the method of compounding the suppository is described below.

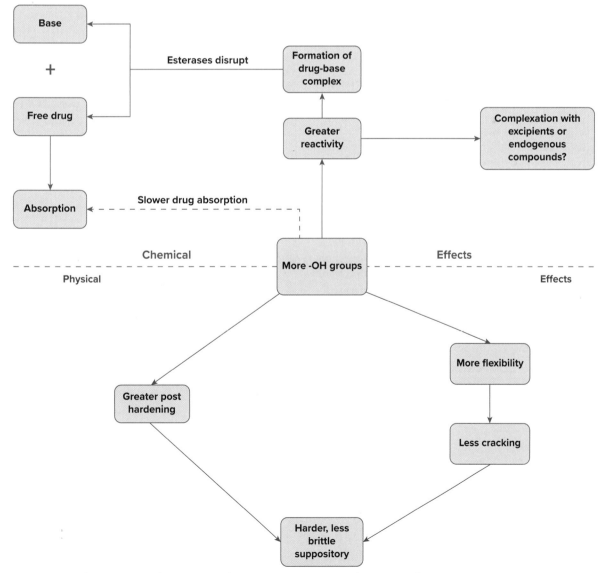

MIND MAP 24-1 Physical and Chemical Effects of Increased –OH Groups in a Suppository Base

TABLE 24-2	Glycero-Gelatin Suppositories Formula
INGREDIENT	**AMOUNT (G)**
Gelatin	70
Glycerin	20
Water	10
Total	**100**

All of the ingredients required for the formulation are first weighed. The glycerin is added to the water and stirred. The powdered gelatin is sprinkled onto the water in the container, with stirring, and the total weight of the container plus contents is obtained. The container is covered and left to stand for at least 1 h. The container is then carefully heated, with gentle stirring, to dissolve the gelatin. The water should not boil as elevated temperature discolors the gelatin. Also, stirring should not be excessive since this would cause air bubbles to be incorporated. When the gelatin is completely dissolved, the container is removed from the heat source. When partially cooled, the container is weighed again and made up to the previously recorded weight, by the addition of water, and stirred once more. The solution is allowed to cool further until it begins to thicken and is then poured into pre-lubricated molds. Light liquid petroleum, which is hydrophobic, is used as a lubricant for the hydrophilic glycerol-gelatin mixture. The method of soaking the gelatin initially brings about partial hydration. When heated subsequently, more rapid and complete dissolution results.

In recent years, other water-soluble suppository bases have been developed commercially and some common examples are listed in Table 24-3. Of these, polyethylene glycol (PEG) is probably the most commonly used water-soluble base. Macrogol® is a well-known trade name of one of the earliest commercially available brands of PEG. Numerous generic products are also available at the present time. PEG is available in different molecular weight grades. The higher the number associated with PEG, the higher is its molecular weight. Those having a very high molecular weight are hard solids, whereas those with a very low molecular weight (up to 600) are liquids, while intermediate molecular weights represent softer solids and semi-solids.

PEG 4000 and 6000 are solids that produce hard suppositories, making insertion uncomfortable. Intermediate grades produce softer suppositories that are more patient acceptable.

It is also possible to mix various grades of PEG, including liquid grades, in order to produce a suppository of the desired hardness. In addition to liquid PEGs, propylene glycol or another miscible liquid may also be added. In addition, the formula may contain water which has the effect of softening the final suppository. If water is to be included in the formulation, care must be taken to ascertain that the drug is not degraded in the presence of water. The PEGs are mixed together after melting the solid, and warming the liquid. Similarly, other liquids should be warmed before adding them to molten PEGs. Liquids are warmed to prevent localized precipitation of solid PEG. The latter could occur in the moments after the cool liquid is added to the molten solids, before the constituents are well mixed together. An example of a formula utilizing a mixture of PEGs is given in Table 24-4 and the method of compounding this formula is given below.

Suppose that 20 suppositories are required to fill a prescription. Each contains 300 mg Zinc oxide (ZnO) and a mixture of PEG 3000 (40%), PEG 2000 (40%), and PEG 400 (20%) as the base. Since the suppositories are to be used by an adult, a 2-g suppository mold should be used.

TABLE 24-4	Example of a Polyethylene Glycol Suppository Formulation	
INGREDIENT	**AMOUNT PER SUPPOSITORY (g)**	**AMOUNT FOR 22 SUPPOSITORIES (g)**
Polyethylene glycol 2000	0.770	16.940
Polyethylene glycol 3000	0.770	16.940
Polyethylene glycol 400	0.385	8.470
ZnO	0.300	6.600
Total	**2.225**	**48.950**

TABLE 24-3	Some Water-Soluble Suppository Bases		
VEHICLE	**COMPOSITION**	**MELTING TEMPERATURE RANGE (°C)**	**COMMENTS**
Macragol 400	Polyethylene glycol (PEG)	4–8	Higher the number, the higher the melting point
Macragol 1000	PEG	35–40	
Macragol 4000	PEG	53–59	
Macragol 8000	PEG	55–62	
Pluronic F68	Tri-block copolymer (hydrophobic block with a hydrophilic one on either side)	Approx. 85	"F" refers to flake (solid); other pluronics are liquid (L) or pastes (P)
Tween 61	PEG 4 sorbitan monostearate	42	
Myrj 51	PEG 40 monostearate	40	

Zinc oxide is used to soothe hemorrhoids and relieve itching. After insertion of the suppository and its melting in the rectum, the mixture of ZnO and base forms a coating over the inflamed rectal tissues. This makes defecation more comfortable. The mold size, 2 g for an adult, is a nominal size. The actual weight per suppository, obviously, depends on the ingredients to be included. Density differences between the active pharmaceutical ingredient (API) and the base can lead to difficulties in compounding suppositories with an accurate dose. This issue is particularly acute, when the density of the API is very different from that of the base. In this case, ZnO has a density of 4.4 and the density of the base, which consists of a mixture of different PEGs, can be assumed to be 1.1, for this example. To illustrate the problem at hand, suppose 300 mg of the API is added to the bottom of a mold and 1.7 g of the base is added thereafter, above the API. When this is done, it would be noticed that the mold is not filled. The reason for this is the fact that ZnO is very dense and occupies significantly less space than the same weight of suppository base. It should be noted that the nominal 2-g suppository weight associated with the mold is calculated taking into account the density of common suppository base materials.

The appropriate amount of base to use, so that the base plus 300 mg ZnO fills the mold, is calculated as follows:

$$\text{The ratio of the densities of ZnO: base} = \frac{4.4}{1.1} = 4$$

$$\text{The amount of base that ZnO displaces} = \frac{300\ mg}{4} = 75\ \text{mg}$$

Hence, the amount of base required per suppository

$$= 2000\ \text{mg} - 75\ \text{mg}$$
$$= \mathbf{1925\ mg}$$

The ratio $\frac{4.4}{1.1}$ in the above example is referred to as the displacement factor, abbreviated DF. The DF of ZnO provides the information that 300 mg of ZnO occupies the same volume as 75 mg of suppository base, that is, in connection with the extent of filling of a suppository mold, 300 mg of ZnO is considered the equivalent of 75 mg of base.

If the displacement factor had not been taken into account, the amount of suppository base that would have been added is 1700 mg (2000 mg − 300 mg). This large difference (1700 mg compared to 1925 mg) comes about because an equal weight of ZnO occupies a much smaller space than the base. If the weight of the API, in the general case, is small in comparison to the total weight of the suppository base (eg, 50 mg API in a 2000 mg suppository), the density factor is less significant, and usually need not be accounted for.

The amounts of each base ingredient can easily be determined for the formula given in Table 24-4, as follows. The total amount of base per suppository is 1925 mg (as calculated above) and the percentage of each ingredient within the base can be calculated from the table. For example, PEG 3000 constitutes 40% of the base. Therefore, 770 mg of PEG 3000 (40% of 1925 mg) is required per suppository. The final working formula is calculated for 22 capsules, that is, 10% excess. This is done to allow for wastage which arises from the overfilling of molds, as well as

from the residual material remaining in the mixing container. The container in which the ingredients were melted and mixed together cannot easily be emptied of all material due to the viscosity and stickiness of the material.

The method of manufacture is to first weigh out all ingredients. Next the solid PEG components are gently heated until melted and the pre-warmed PEG 400 is added to the PEG melt. The mixture is gently stirred and then the ZnO is incorporated with stirring. After cooling until the mixture begins to thicken, it is poured into the molds with overfilling. Compared to glycerogelatin suppositories, the overfill is greater since PEG contracts extensively on solidification. Due to the latter, some authors state that a lubricant is not necessary, contraction providing separation of the suppository from the mold. However, it is considered preferable to use a lubricant to ensure clean removal of the suppositories. Since PEG suppositories are hydrophilic, light liquid paraffin may be used as a lubricant.

Once solidified, the excess suppository material is trimmed before removal from the mold. A knife, or a spatula blade that has been warmed, is used for this purpose. The mold is then opened, the suppositories removed, and then packaged and dispensed. Vaginal suppositories are formulated in a similar manner to rectal suppositories. They mostly contain antifungal drugs or female hormones.

Aerosol Formulations

Aerosol formulations have been used for rectal and vaginal drug delivery, usually as a foam. The generation of foams by an aerosol is discussed in Chapter 19, Pulmonary Drug Delivery, while the nature of the foam product is discussed in more detail in Chapter 22, Dermal and Transdermal Drug Delivery. Briefly, an aerosol foam formulation consists of an emulsion, with the propellant (or a mixture of propellants) in the internal phase. For stability, all emulsion formulations must contain emulsifying agents which maintain the internal phase as discrete droplets dispersed within the external phase. The emulsifying agents, also known as emulgents, are a subset of a larger group of chemicals known as surfactants. The latter locate at the interface between two phases, oil and water in this case. Therefore, the emulgent must have an affinity for both phases. The concentration of emulsifying agents and the type lead to the formation, as described below, of either a quick-breaking foam or a stable foam.

When the actuator is depressed, the emulsion is forced out of the aerosol container via the dip tube. The liquefied propellant, in the internal phase, expands. It does so because its natural tendency to expand was confined by the pressure within the aerosol canister, and it now experiences the lower pressure of the atmosphere. The expansion actually begins in the expansion chamber of the actuator/valve assembly, so that the immediate output of the aerosol canister is a foam. This foam may further expand in the initial period after delivery. The expanding gas is within many bubbles. Each bubble is surrounded by the surfactants, which may be in several layers. Further expansion is limited by the strength of the surfactant layers which resist the breaking of the bubbles. In this case, the resulting foam is stable. If the individual bubbles are surrounded by a weak shell of surfactant(s), the expansion of the internal gaseous phase cannot be contained and the bubbles break. This type of foam is referred to as a quick-breaking foam. All foams eventually break, the difference between quick-breaking and stable foams is the time it takes for the foam to break.

After the application of a stable foam, the foam is retained for an extended period. On the other hand, the net result of a quick-breaking foam is a wet surface within a short time of the application. This is due to the bursting of the surfactant bubbles and the liquid external phase of the emulsion, together with surfactants and other ingredients, covering the area of application. Stable foams are more useful for rectal and vaginal delivery. The continued expansion of the foam, after emission from the aerosol canister, allows the foam to penetrate deeper into the vaginal or rectal canals. When the foam eventually breaks, a layer of the liquid components, including the medication, remains as a coating on the surfaces. From the above, it is clear that the formulation difference between a quick-breaking foam and a stable foam is the strength of the emulgent sheath. It is stronger in a stable foam and, hence, it resists the expansion of the gas for longer. A foam may be stabilized by the addition of other surfactants, known as foam stabilizers.

Cortifoam contains 10% hydrocortisone acetate in a foam formulation for rectal use. Other constituents are propylene glycol which acts as a solvent; emulsifying wax and cetyl alcohol which constitute the oil phase and also have emulsifying properties; methyl- and propyl-paraben (preservatives); the propellants, isobutane and propane; and water. The product literature lists polyoxyethylene-10-stearyl ether and trolamine as inactive ingredients. Both substances have foam-stabilizing properties, while trolamine also acts as a topical analgesic. Trolamine is more commonly known as trolamine salicylate or triethanolamine salicylate.

Spermicidal foam is an example of a foam dosage form that is used intravaginally. The foam is delivered by an aerosol device through a special applicator. The active in many spermicidal foams is nonoxynol 9. This active also has some efficacy against several sexually transmitted disease (STD) organisms and, in combination with condom use, may provide some protection in this regard. In addition, the foam (and the liquid created from the breakdown of the foam) have some lubricating properties which is advantageous in this application. An example of such a foam product is Delfen Foam.

Liquid Formulations

Liquid formulations for rectal and vaginal use frequently take the form of solutions but they may also consist of suspensions or emulsions. Liquid formulations for rectal administration are usually enemas (used for the evacuation of the rectum). This may be done for the treatment of constipation, or as a preparation for colon surgery or other medical procedures, such as colonoscopy. In the case of rectal procedures, clearing the contents from the rectum facilitates the performance of these procedures. Liquids in the rectum may also be used as so-called liquid suppositories, that is, dosage forms inserted as liquids that undergo sol-gel transformation, forming solids in the rectum. Liquid formulations may be used vaginally as a douche, that is, for cleansing purposes or for the treatment of mild infections. For the latter, mild antimicrobial solutions are administered.

Sodium phosphate solutions, which work as laxatives by an osmotic effect, have been administered both orally and rectally. The solution creates a high osmotic pressure, due to the high concentration of salts, which draws water from the surrounding tissues. When administered orally, the solution draws water from the entire gastrointestinal tract (GIT). When administered as an enema, it draws water from the rectum and distal colon. The high water content serves to soften the stool and increases the volume of the colonic contents. The expansion of the colon, due to the increased volume, stimulates contractions which expel the contents. The salts are not intended to be absorbed to a significant extent. Other soluble, non-absorbed substances will cause a similar reaction.

Such remedies have come under scrutiny by the FDA which issued a safety communication in this regard in 2014. The FDA warns, in this communication, that the use of a larger-than-recommended dose, or more than one dose in 24 h, can cause serious harm to the kidneys and heart, and even death. Both oral and rectal solutions of this type, taken in excess, can cause severe dehydration and alterations in serum electrolyte levels. The serum electrolytes that may be affected are calcium, sodium, and phosphate. The FDA warns that certain individuals may be at a higher risk for adverse events, as described above. Such individuals include young children, people older than 55 years, dehydrated patients with kidney disease or bowel obstruction, or patients with inflammation of the bowel. Caution is also needed with patients taking medications that may affect kidney function.

A range of enemas under the trade name, "Fleet," are produced by Fleet Labs, Inc. Fleet Saline Enema delivers 118 mL (adult dose) of an aqueous solution consisting of 19 g of monobasic sodium phosphate monohydrate and 7 g of dibasic sodium phosphate heptahydrate. Fleet Enema Extra is a saline enema that delivers 197 mL of a phosphate solution containing the **same** amounts of the two phosphate salts contained in Fleet Saline Enema. It is claimed, that the larger volume of this enema is effective if the stool is very hard and unusually difficult to pass. It should be noted that the dose of phosphate salts is identical whether the Fleet Saline Enema or the Fleet Enema Extra is used. Pharmacists should be alert to the possibility that patients who are switching between these two products, may use a larger volume of Fleet Saline Enema, thinking it is acceptable to do so since Fleet Enema Extra has a larger volume. This would result in the patient self-administering a significantly larger dose. Both products should be used with caution and the pharmacist should warn patients not to exceed the dose.

Fleet Bisacodyl Enema contains 10 mg of bisacodyl in 30 mL of solution. Bisacodyl is a drug that increases the motility of the rectum, thus promoting evacuation. Fleet Mineral Oil Enema delivers 118 mL of the oil from a bottle of enema. It is regarded as a stool softener and the product literature states that it reduces water loss from the stool (by reabsorption of the water into the rectal tissues). It is probable that the mineral oil also has a mild irritant or stimulant effect, thus producing the rapid evacuation noted with this product. In other enema formulations, corticosteroids and mesalamine are common ingredients. These drugs are anti-inflammatory and are used in the treatment of inflammatory conditions prevailing in the rectum and the distal colon, including ulcerative colitis, proctitis, and proctosigmoiditis.

For vaginal conditions, Betadine Feminine Wash contains 7.5% povidone-iodine. The iodine is released over an extended period from the povidone component. The latter is also known as polyvinyl pyrrolidone. This solution functions as an antiseptic, killing several species of fungi, bacteria, and protozoa. Betadine Vaginal Douche contains 10% povidone-iodine and is to be used with a special applicator as a rinse-off cleansing solution.

Gels, Creams, and Ointments

Gels, creams, and ointments are formulated in a manner similar to that for dermal preparations. The latter are described in more detail in Chapter 23, Dermal and Transdermal Drug Delivery. The one essential difference is that rectal and vaginal formulations, especially creams and gels, may contain mucoadhesive components to enable the semisolid to adhere to the mucosa. Carbopol and polycarbophil are commonly used as mucoadhesives in vaginal formulations. Replens is a mucoadhesive formulation containing no drug but the gel provides moisture to the vaginal tissue. It is indicated in conditions characterized by dryness, such as vaginal atrophy, which occurs frequently postmenopause. The ability of semisolid formulations to spread easily, after application, is more important for rectal and vaginal delivery than it is for dermal. In the latter case, the patient or caregiver can spread the semisolid dosage form during the application process. In contrast to this, spontaneous spreading is required upon rectal and vaginal administration. Semisolids for delivery to the vagina should also be pH adjusted to match the somewhat lower vaginal pH of 4.5 to 5.5.

In the case of rectal delivery, an elongated nozzle is used to deliver the medication within the rectum. The nozzle is attached to the tube containing the semisolid, and the nozzle is then inserted into the rectum. The tube is squeezed in order to administer the material. In the case of vaginal drug delivery, a special applicator (as opposed to a nozzle) is screwed onto the tube, after removal of the cap. The tube is then squeezed to fill the delivery portion of the applicator. The applicator is then disengaged from the tube and inserted into the vagina. By depressing the handle located on the opposite end of the applicator, the semisolid is expelled from the applicator into the vaginal cavity. The patient may consider these semisolid formulations messy to use, especially for vaginal delivery, in which case the patient may wish to wear a tampon to absorb any leaking material.

Vaginal creams available on the US market are mainly hormone-containing (eg, estrogen) and antifungal. Gels contain hormones or metronidazole, which is antibacterial and antiprotozoal. Most vaginal ointments contain antifungal drugs. Crinone 4% and 8% are gels that contain progesterone in the indicated concentrations. The gel is mucoadhesive and adheres to the vaginal wall for several days giving extended-release of the progesterone. Progesterone is necessary for endometrial receptivity for implantation of an embryo. After implantation, progesterone is required to maintain the pregnancy.

Crinone 8% is used in assisted reproductive technology, while Crinone 4% is used for the treatment of secondary amenorrhea.

Progesterone absorption from these formulations is prolonged with an absorption half-life of approximately 25 to 50 h. Since the elimination half-life is short (5 to 20 min), the progesterone biological levels are controlled by the absorption kinetics. Crinone 8% is administered either once or twice daily depending on the extent of progesterone supplementation required. Dosing is continued for up to 10 to 12 weeks during the pregnancy. This maintains the required levels of progesterone to sustain the pregnancy. The alternative route for administering progesterone is intramuscular injection. Therefore, this dosage form is much easier to administer.

Several creams and ointments for rectal delivery are used for the treatment of hemorrhoids. Some formulations contain a combination of phenylephrine (a sympathomimetic amine to relieve swelling) and a local anesthetic such as pramoxine (to relieve pain). Other formulations in this category also incorporate aloe extract to soothe inflamed tissues whereas some formulations contain phenylephrine alone. An anti-inflammatory steroid, such as hydrocortisone, is often combined with pramoxine. The steroid reduces inflammation and swelling effectively. The only rectal gel on the US market at the time of writing is Diastat Acudial which contains diazepam for the emergency treatment of status epilepticus. The term, Accudial, refers to the fact that an accurate dose may be administered, which is especially important when the medication is administered to young children.

Recap Questions

1. What is the most common rectal delivery system?
2. What is the difference in the duration of action of rectal, compared to vaginal, extended-release drug delivery systems?
3. Name one difference between rectal versus vaginal suppositories.
4. Why is cocoa butter no longer as popular as it used to be?
5. Mention one advantage and one disadvantage of a higher number of –OH groups in a suppository base.
6. What is the effect of increasing the gelatin content of glycero-gelatin suppositories?
7. What is the major advantage of an aerosol foam formulation designed for rectal or vaginal drug delivery?
8. Explain the difference between a quick-breaking and a stable foam.
9. What is the difference between an enema and a douche?
10. Name one similarity and one difference between Betadine feminine wash and Betadine vaginal douche.

ANATOMY OF THE RECTUM

The rectum is a continuation of the GIT and its basic structure resembles that of the colon (Figure 24-3). While there are no villi or microvilli in the rectum, there is sufficient surface area for drug absorption. Apart from motility during defecation, the rectum displays a lack of regular motility in contrast to the small intestine. The rectum usually contains 2 to 3 mL of inert mucus fluid, in the absence of any fecal matter. This small volume of fluid is usually insufficient to allow rapid dissolution of drugs contained in suppositories or other dosage forms. An exception may be observed in the case of extremely soluble drugs, especially in low doses, for which this small volume of liquid may be sufficient for dissolution. The terminal 4 cm of the rectum is referred to as the anal canal which opens via the anus to the exterior.

The rectum receives its blood supply from the superior, middle, and inferior rectal arteries. Blood is returned from the rectum through three veins (Figure 24-3). These are:

1. the superior rectal vein, which is a branch of the inferior mesenteric vein, a part of the portal system (ie, the blood entering this vein is transported to the liver);

2. the middle rectal vein which is a branch of the internal iliac vein; and

3. the inferior rectal vein which is a branch of the internal pudendal vein, which is also a branch of the internal iliac vein.

RECTAL DRUG DELIVERY

The above description of the venous drainage of the rectum provides an indication of where the drug will be transported after absorption, assuming the drug is absorbable. As can be seen from Figure 24-3, a drug that is present in the distal one-third of the rectum (closer to the anus) will be absorbed into veins that drain, eventually, into the inferior vena cava. This means that such a drug is taken up directly into the systemic circulation, bypassing the liver. On the other hand, drugs

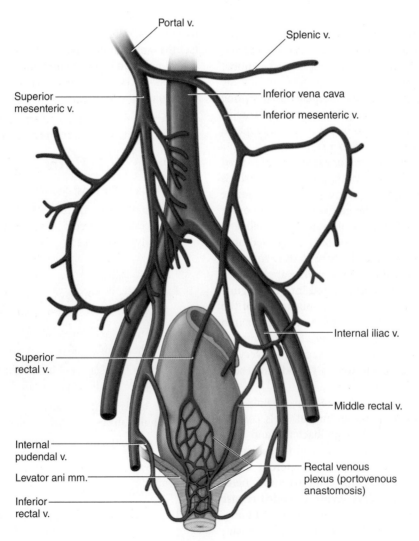

FIGURE 24-3 Structure of the rectum showing rectal veins. (Reproduced, with permission, from Morton DA, Foreman KB, Albertine KH. *The Big Picture: Gross Anatomy*. 2nd ed. New York, NY: McGraw Hill; 2019.)

placed deep into the rectum (ie, beyond the lower one-third) will be absorbed and reach the superior rectal vein. This vein leads eventually to the liver, where the drug will be subjected to first pass metabolism. The presence of the rectal venous plexus, as seen in Figure 24-3, indicates that there will be some mixing of blood flowing from different regions of the rectum. Hence, the division of venous rectal drainage into portal circulation and systemic circulation is not as clear cut as the above description implies.

Of importance to the pharmacist is the fact that the drug from suppositories placed in the external one-third of the rectum will be absorbed in a way that largely bypasses the liver, and thus the drug escapes much of the first pass effect. On the other hand, drugs placed into the upper two-thirds of the rectum will be absorbed and taken to the liver where they may be extensively metabolized. This results in a smaller amount of drug reaching the systemic circulation. Obviously, this applies equally to drugs delivered to the rectum by other drug delivery systems.

The rectum is also extensively drained by lymphatics, offering an alternate route for drug absorption, especially for large molecules such as proteins and peptides. The gaps between adjacent cells in lymphatics are larger than they are in veins. Hence, the permeability of the lymphatics to large molecules is more pronounced and these molecules are preferentially absorbed into the lymphatics. Absorption into veins may still occur but at a significantly slower rate. For this reason, there is great interest, and ongoing research, in using rectal delivery for the administration of proteins and peptides.

Suppositories that release the drug slowly have been utilized for therapy over many hours. Examples include theophylline suppositories for the treatment or prophylaxis of asthma. Such suppository formulations were popular in the past, especially for children, but are no longer in vogue. For example, aminophylline (a theophylline derivative) was popular because a high dose could be administered in suppository form. A suppository for an adult may be up to 2.5 g in total weight. This allows a large dose to be incorporated into the suppository which can be administered conveniently. In the case of aminophylline, the drug is irritating to the stomach and was preferably delivered in suppository form. Theophylline products are used much less at the present time because the drug has a narrow therapeutic index (there is a small difference between toxic drug levels and those that produce the desired result). Newer long-acting inhalation bronchodilators have replaced theophylline products (see Chapter 19, Pulmonary Drug Delivery).

Similarly, suppositories containing a barbiturate for the treatment of epilepsy over an extended period were more common previously. There are no theophylline- or barbiturate-derivative suppositories on the US market at the time of writing. However, these examples illustrate that systemic drug action could be prolonged over several hours, allowing twice-a-day administration of a suppository. Canasa 500 mg rectal suppositories contain 5-aminosalicylic acid, in a base consisting of hard fat, for the local treatment of tissues in ulcerative colitis patients. These suppositories are administered every 8 hours and each provides sufficient drug levels in the rectal tissues for treatment of the condition. While some drugs may be absorbed systemically, this suppository is not intended to deliver the drug to the systemic system. Only the local tissues need to be treated in this condition. Mind Map 24-2 summarizes the more important rectal and vaginal dosage forms.

Advantages

The advantages of the rectal delivery of drugs are summarized below:

1. Easy administration.

   a. In cases of nausea or vomiting, the patient cannot be given oral medication and a suppository is convenient to administer.

   b. For a patient who is unconscious, but in urgent need of medication, a suppository may be useful. The administration can be performed by caregivers who are not able to administer an injection. This has been used to advantage for emergency treatment of status epilepticus.

   c. It is possible to administer large doses, for example, greater than 500 mg in a convenient dosage form.

   d. A suppository avoids the objectionable taste of certain drugs and is a way to administer these drugs to children.

2. Potential for better absorption.

   a. The drug is not affected by the acid contents of the stomach and, in addition, there is less enzymatic activity in the rectum compared to the small intestine.

   b. Drugs administered rectally are not subject to the impact of delayed gastric emptying, as described in Chapter 3, Oral Route of Drug Delivery.

   c. While orally administered drugs are subject to the effects of food (increasing or decreasing the rate and extent of drug absorption), rectally administered drugs are not.

   d. The first pass effect which is prominent in orally administered drugs is significantly less when the drug is administered rectally.

   e. Diseases of the upper GIT may affect absorption, for example, hyperacidity can cause a delay in stomach emptying, which leads to delayed, and potentially decreased, absorption. Drugs administered rectally are not subject to this type of effect.

3. Rapid systemic effect.

   This is possible with rectal administration, especially if a fluid is administered. Epistaxis®, a rectally administered liquid, has been used in Europe for a long time for the emergency treatment of epilepsy.

4. Overdosing is difficult. The equivalent of swallowing half a vial of tablets (in a suicide attempt), for example, is not easy to achieve with rectal administration.

Disadvantages

1. Defecation decreases absorption.

   Defecation shortly after dose administration will displace the suppository and drug absorption will be terminated. The need to defecate may arise from an ordinary physiological need, or one that is induced by the placement of the suppository. Expansion of the rectal wall is an impetus for defecation. This includes the expansion caused by the presence of a suppository.

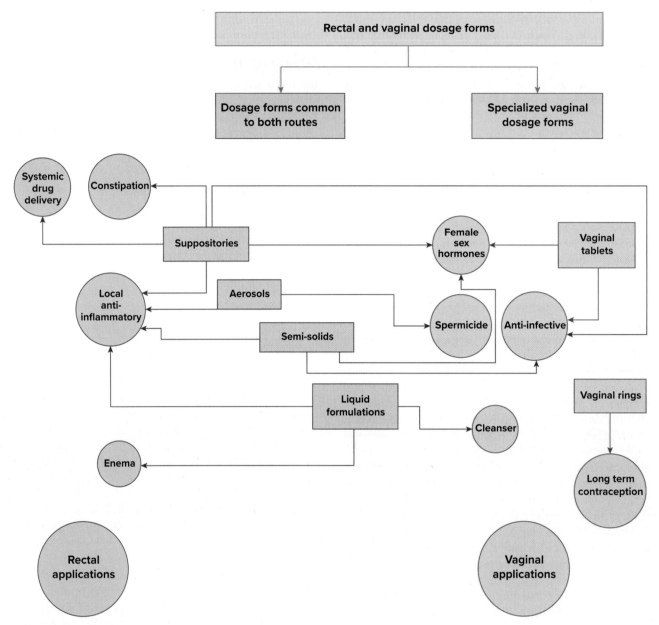

MIND MAP 24-2 Rectal and Vaginal Dosage Forms

2. Drug degradation.

   Microorganisms that normally reside in the rectum may be responsible for the degradation of certain drugs.

3. Patient acceptability.

   Patient acceptability varies by country. For example, in certain parts of Europe and South America, the use of suppositories is more acceptable than it is in the United States.

4. Higher cost.

   Suppositories are generally more expensive than the equivalent tablets or capsules. If the suppository is not commercially available, but has to be compounded, the cost may be even greater.

Future Outlook

Many new drugs are proteins and peptides. However, their oral bioavailability is poor: the extent of absorption is low and they are also degraded by proteolytic enzymes in the GIT. At the present time, these drugs are mostly administered by injection. Due to poor patient acceptance of this route of administration, alternative delivery routes are sought. Rectal administration is considered potentially viable and this area is one of intensive research. The partial avoidance of the first pass effect, is an attraction. However, the absorption of proteins and peptides, even by this route, is not very high and, for this reason, absorption enhancers are incorporated into formulations. The rest of this section, unless specifically indicated, describes research efforts.

Since metabolism of peptides can occur to a degree in the rectum, various protease inhibitors have been incorporated into rectal formulations to reduce metabolism and, thereby, improve absorption. In addition, chemical modification of the drug molecule to reduce its metabolism, has also been tried. Formulation scientists must ensure that chemical modification of the drug molecule will not introduce adverse drug reactions. While absorption of large, or complex, molecules may be improved relative to oral absorption, such absorption may not be at an ideal level. For this reason, absorption enhancers may be included in the formulation. These enhancers often modify the rectal membrane to allow a faster rate, and a greater extent, of absorption. Therefore, care must be taken to ensure that the enhancers have effects that are transitory, allowing the barrier function to return quickly to prevent the absorption of unwanted substances.

While suppositories have always been considered useful for drug administration to children, pediatric applications have recently received renewed attention. Antibiotics may be conveniently administered to children rectally; and emergency medications, such as anti-epilepsy drugs, may be administered, in this manner, to patients of all ages. This may be done when oral delivery is difficult, if not impossible, in an emergency situation. Anti-emetics are already being administered rectally because the nauseous patient may not be able to hold down the medication for long enough to allow significant absorption. Malaria medication has also received a lot of consideration with respect to rectal delivery, in recent times, especially for administration to children in Third World countries. Malaria is a scourge in tropical countries which are often poor. Artemisinin and also artesunate with mefloquine have been considered for rectal delivery by means of suppositories. For treatment of patients in rural areas, when parenteral injections are not possible, rectal administration of suppositories could work well. The melting of the suppositories at higher temperatures is a disadvantage, and mechanisms to prevent melting must be considered. In this regard, high molecular weight PEG and polyvinylpyrrolidone (PVP), with correspondingly higher melting points, may be appropriate. Drug release from such suppositories, in the rectum, occurs by a combination of dissolution and melting. Vaccines by rectal delivery are also under consideration since many infectious diseases start with a mucosal infection.

Recap Questions

1. What steps can the patient or caregiver take to ensure that hepatic first pass metabolism is largely avoided when suppositories are administered?
2. How are peptides absorbed after rectal delivery?
3. Aminophylline suppositories were used as a relatively long-acting bronchodilator. Which delivery system has largely replaced this type of suppository?
4. Name one advantage and one disadvantage of rectal drug delivery.

ANATOMY OF THE VAGINA

The vagina and related structures are shown in Figure 24-4. Apart from treating fungal and bacterial infections, to which the vagina is susceptible, other local conditions may be responsive to hormonal formulations. In addition, drugs may be applied to the vagina for absorption into the systemic system. This is possible because the vagina has extensive venous drainage which enables good drug absorption. Vaginal drainage occurs due to the presence of a venous plexus as well as other veins. These veins from the vagina drain into the external pudendal vein which drains into the pudendal vein. Blood from this vein flows into the great saphenous vein which is the major vein of the lower limb. This vein, which is the longest in the body, also receives blood from parts of the pelvic region. It drains into the femoral vein and, eventually, into the inferior vena cava. Thus, blood flows from the vaginal area to the systemic circulation, without reaching the liver and, therefore, avoids hepatic first pass metabolism.

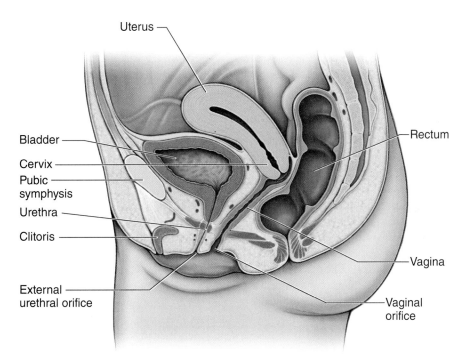

FIGURE 24-4 Structure of the vagina in relation to other organs. (Reproduced, with permission, from Morton DA, Foreman KB, Albertine KH. *The Big Picture: Gross Anatomy.* 2nd ed. New York, NY: McGraw Hill; 2019.)

VAGINAL DRUG DELIVERY SYSTEMS

Some common dosage forms have multiple applications in pharmacy. For example, creams may be applied to the hair or the skin for cosmetic, as well as drug delivery, applications. Similarly, some formulations may be used for both rectal and vaginal drug delivery and such applications have been described above in the section, Common Rectal and Vaginal Formulations. This section deals with some systems that are uniquely formulated for delivery to the vagina. Some other common dosage forms, administered vaginally, are also described in this section if used for a drug delivery application.

Vaginal Tablets

Vaginal tablets are formulated like conventional tablets but they are small in size and frequently oval, or diamond-shaped. The shape and the size facilitate easy insertion into the vagina which is done as follows. One end of the tablet is placed into an elongated insertion device. The end of the device containing the tablet is placed into the vagina. The opposite end of the device is pressed to push the tablet out of the insertion device, into the vagina.

Vaginal tablets may have an antifungal action; for example, Mycelex (which contains nystatin) or Gyne-Lotrimin (which contains clotrimazole); an antibacterial effect, for example, Terramycin-polymyxin (which contains oxytetracycline and polymyxin B sulfate). Vaginal tablets may also contain female sex hormones, for example, Vagifem (which contains estradiol).

Thin Films

Thin films similar to those described for buccal delivery (Chapter 20, Buccal and Sublingual Drug Delivery) may also be used for drug delivery to the vagina. The thin film can easily be inserted by the patient using a finger. Since the film is usually mucoadhesive, it attaches to the vaginal mucosa and remains in place over an extended time, releasing the contained drug into the vaginal tissues. This type of dosage form is in the research stage at the time of writing.

Vaginal Rings

All vaginal rings marketed at the time of writing contain female sex hormones (or their derivatives) and are used for long-term contraception. While the solid portion of the ring has a small cross-sectional area, the entire ring is much larger. It is squeezed together to form a flattened, elongated shape for insertion into the vagina (Figure 24-5). After insertion, the ring expands to touch the side walls of the vagina because it is elastic. The pressure of the ring on the vaginal wall keeps the ring in place. In the manufacturing process, the drug is loaded into the ring material. The ring substrate is latex free (to reduce allergic reactions) and usually consists of a block copolymer. A block copolymer has repeating units or blocks of, at least, two polymers. Typically, one polymer is more hydrophobic than the other. The length of each repeating polymer block controls the balance of hydrophobic and hydrophilic areas in the base and, hence, affects the drug release rate from the block copolymer. The block copolymer is

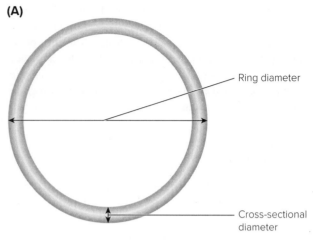

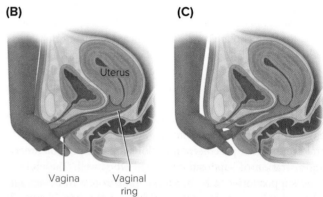

FIGURE 24-5 **A.** Vaginal ring. **B.** Insertion of vaginal ring with tip of index finger. **C.** Removal of vaginal ring by placing index finger under forward loop.

"tuned" to give the appropriate release rate, that is, the developer researches various proportions of each block to find the block copolymer with the ideal release rate.

The ring is, generally, left in place for 3 weeks (the drug release period) and is then removed. While there are marketed products, vaginal rings continue to receive much attention as an area of research. In the so-called Orange Book,[1] some of these products are listed as "rings" while others are referred to as "inserts," probably in accordance with the information supplied to the FDA by the company holding the New Drug Application. Some rings contain a single hormone, an estrogen. The Estring contains estradiol while the Femring contains estradiol acetate. Other vaginal rings contain both estrogen and progestin and are referred to as combination hormonal contraceptives. The NuvaRing is a combination hormonal contraceptive containing 2.7 mg ethinyl estradiol (an estrogen) and 11.7 mg etonogestrel (a progestin). The entire ring has an outer diameter of 54 mm (ring diameter) and a cross-sectional diameter of 4 mm (see Figure 24-5 for a description of these dimensional terms).

The copolymer used in the NuvaRing is ethylene vinyl acetate (EVA). This material consists of ethylene polymer and vinyl acetate (VA) polymer as repeating units. If the proportion of polymers is changed, the release rate would be different, as mentioned. In the case of this product, two copolymers are actually used: each contains ethylene polymer plus VA polymer. One of these copolymers has 28% VA polymer (and 72% ethylene polymer), while the other copolymer has 9% VA (and 91% ethylene). The VA polymer is more hydrophilic and displays a faster dissolution rate of the contained drug. The NuvaRing delivers etonogestrel at the rate of 0.12 mg per day and ethinyl estradiol at the rate of 0.015 mg per day. Mind Map 24-2 summarizes the more important rectal and vaginal dosage forms.

VAGINAL DRUG DELIVERY

Drugs absorbed through the vaginal mucosa avoid the hepatic first pass effect, as described above. When this occurs, a larger quantity of the absorbed drug reaches the systemic circulation. In addition, vaginal delivery avoids the acidity of the stomach and the enzymes of the GIT. For these reasons, systemically acting drugs may be effectively administered vaginally. The vaginal mucosa is similar in structure to the buccal mucosa and its absorptive properties are also similar. The vaginal surface is approximately 60 cm^2 in extent and it has a rich blood supply. The pH of vaginal fluid is in the range of 4.5 to 5.5 for women of reproductive age. When dissolved in vaginal fluid, drugs with pKa values above 5.5 will have a significant fraction in the unionized form, a form which is suitable for permeation. The acidity of vaginal fluids is maintained by lactobacilli which convert glycogen (from exfoliated and disrupted cells) into lactic acid.

Absorption may occur by the transcellular or the paracellular routes, as previously described for the oral cavity in Chapter 20, Buccal and Sublingual Drug Delivery. In addition, absorption may occur by receptor-mediated endocytosis (RME). Receptors on the surface of certain cells are primed to recognize certain drug substances, for example, hormones. When such a drug molecule attaches to the receptor, a series of biochemical events occur, resulting in the molecule being taken into the cytoplasm of the cell via endocytosis.

Vaginal administration may be used for drugs that act locally or systemically. It can also be used for the delivery of drugs to the uterus. Examples of local drug delivery include antifungal or antibacterial drugs, to treat vaginal infections, and female sex hormones, to treat atrophy of the vaginal mucosa. The latter could occur postmenopause. In recent years, new microbicides that are active against STDs, including some claimed to be effective against the human immunodeficiency virus (HIV), have been developed. Vaginal delivery would be ideal for such drugs. A novel idea is the concept of providing protection against STDs for both partners using intravaginal depot drug administration of microbicides. The latter has been referred to as "bidirectional" drug delivery. A liquid formulation of such a microbicide can also be used as a vaginal wash by HIV-positive women just prior to childbirth, to reduce perinatal transmission.

Examples of vaginal administration for systemic effect are female sex hormones and other drugs that have relevance to female physiology and disease states. The latter include bromocriptine (used, for example, to treat high prolactin levels which may be implicated in a failure to become pregnant), calcitonin (to treat osteoporosis), Luteinizing-hormone releasing-hormone (LHRH) agonists (adjuvant therapy for breast cancer), and oxytocin and prostaglandins (drugs for inducing labor). Vaginal delivery is better for all these drugs because it avoids the harsh conditions of the GIT (pH and enzymes) as well as the hepatic first pass effect. Oxytocin and calcitonin are, additionally, not well absorbed in the GIT because of their large molecular size.

Vaginal delivery may also be used to avoid certain side effects, evident when the drugs are taken orally. For example, bromocriptine displays gastrointestinal side effects, while steroids display hepatic side effects, both of which are avoided with the use of vaginal delivery. As compared to injections, pain and needle anxiety are eliminated with vaginal administration. Calcitonin and oxytocin are drugs that are conventionally administered by injection and require repeated doses.

As mentioned, a venous plexus surrounds the vagina. Drugs absorbed into this plexus and flowing with the blood, away from the vagina, pass preferentially to the uterus rather than to the general circulation. While the exact mechanism of this drug passage is not clear, the fact that such transfer exists has been demonstrated in several experiments. The passage of drugs from vagina to uterus is *functionally* similar to the passage of drugs from the small intestine to the liver. Hence, the term "first uterine pass effect" was coined, implying that it is similar to the hepatic first pass effect. Considering that this functional link between the vagina and the uterus exists, it would be an ideal mechanism to deliver drugs to the uterus.[2,3] Examples of drugs that could be usefully delivered in this manner are progesterone and danazol.

The relevance of this effect can be understood from the fact that both intramuscular and transdermal progesterone result in low systemic and low intrauterine drug levels. Vaginal progesterone delivery also results in relatively low systemic drug levels but significant intrauterine drug levels are noted, illustrating the preferential passage of the drug from the vagina to the uterus. Vaginal administration ensures sufficiently high levels of drugs, such as progesterone, within the uterus. These levels produce the required pharmacological actions, while little of the drug reaches the systemic circulation. This mechanism avoids many side effects of progesterone and is ideal since the pharmacological effects of progesterone are only needed in the uterus.

In contrast to the above positive reasons for utilizing vaginal drug delivery, there are aspects of vaginal physiology that make it less suitable for drug delivery. Fluctuating hormonal levels, especially estrogen during the menstrual cycle, lead to variations in certain physiological factors that have a significant impact on drug absorption. These factors include the thickness of the vaginal epithelial cell layer, the width of the interstitial spaces, the extent of vaginal secretions and their pH, and variations in peptidase (drug metabolizing) activity. In addition, there are also age-related changes, especially after the menopause. These relate particularly to fluid level (for dissolution of solid or semi-solid dosage forms) and the thickness of the vaginal membrane. All of these changes represent a variable, nonconsistent environment for drug absorption. This makes it difficult to predict the rate of drug absorption and the fraction of a dose that will be absorbed. Hence, it becomes more difficult to accurately estimate the dose to be administered.

Advantages

1. Avoids first pass metabolism.
2. Low enzymatic activity in the vaginal area.
3. Absorption is not affected by disturbances in the GIT.
4. One self-administered dosage form can provide continuous drug supply for weeks.
5. Painless application.
6. Use of the dosage form is discrete, although the application is done in private.
7. Because of the local effect, hormones may be administered in lower doses.

Disadvantages

1. Physiological conditions that may affect absorption can vary with the age of the patient and the stage of the menstrual cycle:
   a. Thickness of the vaginal epithelium.
   b. pH.
   c. Hormonal activity.
2. Systemic absorption, when intended, may be erratic and unpredictable.
3. The formulation may leak or slip.
4. Local irritation is possible.
5. Interference during coitus is possible.
6. Patients may have an aversion or reluctance to use this route for any indication that is not a local effect.

Recap Questions

1. Why is vaginal administration good for systemic drug delivery?
2. How is the slightly acidic pH of vaginal secretions maintained?
3. What are the differences between vaginal tablets and conventional, oral tablets?
4. Distinguish between vaginal rings and vaginal films.
5. All vaginal rings on the US market, up to the time of writing, contain drugs from only one class. Name the class of drugs that they contain.
6. Name two disadvantages of vaginal drug delivery.
7. Look up the structures of ethylene copolymer and vinyl acetate copolymer. Why is the latter more hydrophilic?

SUMMARY POINTS

- The rectum and vagina are major body cavities into which drugs may be administered and they share several similar dosage forms.
- The rectum and vagina are also different in certain respects and, for this reason, special delivery systems have been developed.
- The rectum may be used for systemic drug delivery and it is possible to attain a prolonged action of many hours from one dosage form. Depending on the placement of the dosage form, a significant fraction of the absorbed drug may avoid hepatic first pass clearance.
- Long-acting systemic drug delivery may also be attained using vaginal administration in which case the drug avoids the hepatic circulation.
- Very long-acting delivery systems, such as vaginal rings, that are unique to this route may be used for the delivery of hormones for contraception.
- The direct transmission of drugs from the vagina to the uterus is unique. Drugs delivered to the uterus in this manner largely avoid the systemic circulation. Therefore, systemic side effects are reduced.

What do you think?

1. Suppose that you are a compounding pharmacist. How would you decide whether to use a fatty, versus a hydrophilic, suppository base for a particular drug, based on the physicochemical properties of the drug?
2. Suppocire A and Suppocire AGP contain glycerides with a similar profile: triglycerides predominate and there are smaller fractions of mono- and di-glycerides. Why is the hydroxyl value different for these bases (20–30 vs 40–50, respectively)? You may refer to Table 24-1, but a full explanation is needed.
3. Two patients are given suppository formulations containing a fatty base. One of these patients is febrile (has an elevated body temperature). Explain any potential difference in drug absorption between these two patients.
4. During the development of an aerosol foam formulation, it was observed that the foam was quick breaking whereas it was intended to be a stable foam. Describe a formulation change that can be made so that the new formulation has a stable foam.
5. Large amounts of oral mannitol, which is not absorbed to a significant extent, can have a laxative effect. Explain the mechanism by which this laxative effect is brought about.
6. Name two ways in which Fleet Bisacodyl Enema is different from other Fleet enemas.
7. What is meant by the "first uterine pass effect" and why is this effect very important in obstetrics?
8. Why do you think two versions of the same copolymer, EVA, are used in one product, NuvaRing?

REFERENCES

1. Orange Book: Approved Drug Products with Therapeutic Equivalence Evaluations. https://www.accessdata.fda.gov/scripts/cder/ob/search_product.cfm. Accessed July 23, 2023.

2. De Ziegler D, Bulletti C, De Monstier B, Jääskeläinen A-S. The first uterine pass effect. *Annals of the New York Academy of Sciences.* 1997;828:291-299. doi:10.1111/j.1749-6632.1997.tb48550.x. Accessed January 26, 2018.

3. Bulletti C, de Ziegler D, Flamigni C, et al. Human targeted drug delivery in gynaecology: the first uterine pass effect. *Reproduction.* 1997;12(5):1073-1079.

BIBLIOGRAPHY

https://www.accessdata.fda.gov/drugsatfda_docs/label/2001/21252lbl.pdf. Accessed February 2, 2018.

https://www.accessdata.fda.gov/drugsatfda_docs/label/2005/021187s012lbl.pdf. Accessed January 28, 2018.

https://www.allergan.com/assets/pdf/crinone_pi. Accessed January 24, 2018.

https://www.fda.gov/drugs/drugsafety/ucm380757.htm. Accessed January 17, 2018.

Vermani K, Garg S. The scope and potential of vaginal drug delivery. *PSTT.* 2000;3:359-364.

Index

Please note that *b* denotes boxes, *f* denotes figures, *m* denotes mind maps, and *t* denotes tables.

Hydrophilic lubricant, 117, 118*t*
Hydrophilic matrix tablets, 150–151
Hydrophilic polymer, 195–196
Hydrophobic lubricant, 117, 118*t*
Hydrophobic matrix tablets, 148
Hydrophobic polymer, 195
Hydroxypropyl methyl cellulose (HPMC), 115*t*, 137, 138

I

ID injection. *See* Intradermal (ID) injection
Iluvien, 348
IM injection. *See* Intramuscular (IM) injection
Imitrex, 313
Immediate-release dosage forms, 145, 147*f*
Immediate-release products, 27
Immiscible liquids, 83
In situ soap method, 88–89
Incruse inhaler, 209, 209*f*
IND. *See* Investigational new drug application (IND)
Inderal LA, 158–159
INFeD, 198*t*
Informed consent, 260
Inhalation capsule, 139–140
Inhaled therapies, 271. *See also* Pulmonary drug delivery
Injection, 20, 165–185
    aqueous suspensions, 177–178
    dried powder formulations, 173–176
    emulsions, 172–173
    extended-release, 176–180
    freeze-dried formulations, 173–176
    general formulation considerations, 168
    microparticulate, 178–180
    oily, 176–177, 177*t*
    routes of delivery, 166–168
    solutions, 168–172
    sterilization, 180–185. *See also* Sterilization methods
    suspensions, 171–173
Innopran, 159
Inorganic nanoparticles, 191–192
Insomnia, 210–211, 296–297
Institutional review board (IRB), 259–260
Insulin, 22, 24
Intensity of action, 247
Inter-digestive migrating motor complex (MMC), 35
Intermediate testing, 221–222, 221*t*
Intermezzo, 210, 296, 297, 298*t*
International Journal of Pharmaceutical Compounding, 80
Intestinal transit time, 35–36
Intestinal villi, 29, 30*f*
Intra-arterial injection, 167
Intra-articular injection, 167
Intra-cardiac injection, 168
Intra-ocular injection, 167–168. *See also* Ophthalmic drug delivery
Intra-spinal injection, 167
Intra-vitreal inserts, 24
Intradermal (ID) injection, 167
Intradermal route of drug delivery, 14*t*
Intramuscular (IM) injection, 14*t*, 24, 167
Intraocular injections, 24
Intrathecal injection, 167
Intravenous administration, 14*t*, 23–24, 166
Intravitreal injection, 347–348
Invega, 162*t*
Invega Sustenna, 172*t*, 191, 192*t*
Investigational new drug application (IND), 258–259
Investigator's brochure, 260–261
Ionized drug, 344
Ionizing radiation techniques, 183–184
Ionotropic gelation, 195

Iontophoresis, 301, 329–330
IRB. *See* Institutional review board (IRB)
Iron oxide nanoparticle, 191
Isopropyl alcohol, 51
Isodil, 13
Isotonicity, 168, 345
Itraconazole, 46*t*
IV injections. *See* Intravenous administration
Ivabradine, 46*t*

J

Jet mill, 76
Jet nebulizer, 274
Johnson & Johnson Company, 207

K

K value, 325
Kanamycin, 34
Kaolin, 116*t*
κ carrageenan, 139
Katra, 46*t*
Kefauver-Harris Amendment, 254*t*, 255
Keflex, 55
Keratin, 23
KitchenAid, 98

L

L-dopa, 37
Lactopress Spray Dried 250, 119*t*
Lactose, 114*t*
Lake, 43
LAL. *See* Limulus amebocyte lysate (LAL)
Lamination, 122
Lanoxin, 13
Large intestine, 29, 31*f*
Large multilayer vesicle (LMV), 196, 197*f*
Large unilamellar vesicle (LUV), 196
Laser-assisted ablation, 331
Laser particle size analysis, 66
Lauriad drug delivery technology, 297
Laxative, 360
Levigation, 59
Levocetirizine dihydrochloride, 46*t*
Limulus amebocyte lysate (LAL), 185
Lining mucosa, 292
Lipid matrix nanoparticles, 194
Lipid nanocapsules, 198
Lipophilic drugs, 23
Liposome, 196–197, 200*t*, 350
Liquefied gas fill, 277–278
Liquid emulsion, 84
Liquid suppositories, 360
LMV. *See* Large multilayer vesicle (LMV)
Locking capsule, 140
Logbooks, 233
Lomudal, 140, 282
Long-term testing, 221, 221*t*
Lopinavir, 46*t*
Loramyc, 297, 298*t*
Lorsartan, 80
Lotion, 70, 320
Lubricant, 58, 96, 116–118, 118*t*
Lubritose Mannitol, 119*t*
Lucentis, 338, 347, 348
Lupron Depot, 180*t*
LUV. *See* Large unilamellar vesicle (LUV)
Lyrica, 46*t*